Math & Dosage Calculations
for Healthcare
Professionals

FOURTH EDITION

Math & Dosage Calculations
for Healthcare Professionals

Kathryn A. Booth, MS, RN, RMA (AMT), RPT, CPhT

Facilitator/Instructor, Military
to Medicine
INOVA Health System
Falls Church, Virginia

James E. Whaley, RPh, MS

Baker College
Owosso, Michigan

Susan Sienkiewicz, MA, RN

Community College of Rhode Island
Warwick, Rhode Island

Jennifer F. Palmunen, MSN, RN

Community College of Rhode Island
Warwick, Rhode Island

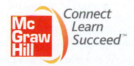

Connect
Learn
Succeed™

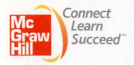

MATH & DOSAGE CALCULATIONS FOR HEALTHCARE PROFESSIONALS

Published by McGraw-Hill, a business unit of The McGraw-Hill Companies, Inc., 1221 Avenue of the Americas, New York, NY, 10020. Copyright © 2012 by The McGraw-Hill Companies, Inc. All rights reserved. Previous editions © 2002, 2007, and 2010. No part of this publication may be reproduced or distributed in any form or by any means, or stored in a database or retrieval system, without the prior written consent of The McGraw-Hill Companies, Inc., including, but not limited to, in any network or other electronic storage or transmission, or broadcast for distance learning.

Some ancillaries, including electronic and print components, may not be available to customers outside the United States.

This book is printed on acid-free paper.

1 2 3 4 5 6 7 8 9 0 RJE/RJE 1 0 9 8 7 6 5 4 3 2 1

ISBN 978-0-07-337469-7

MHID 0-07-337469-5

Vice president/Editor in chief: *Elizabeth Haefele*
Vice president/Director of marketing: *Alice Harra*
Publisher: *Kenneth S. Kasee Jr.*
Managing developmental editor: *Michelle L. Flomenhoft*
Marketing manager: *Mary B. Haran*
Lead digital product manager: *Damian Moshak*
Director, Editing/Design/Production: *Jess Ann Kosic*
Lead project manager: *Rick Hecker*
Senior buyer: *Michael R. McCormick*
Senior designer: *Srdjan Savanovic*
Senior photo research coordinator: *Lori Hancock*
Digital production coordinator: *Brent dela Cruz*
Media project manager: *Cathy L. Tepper*
Outside development house: *Melinda Bilecki*
Cover design: *Cara David Design*
Interior design: *Gino Cieslik*
Typeface: *10/12 Palatino*
Compositor: *Laserwords Private Limited*
Printer: *R. R. Donnelley*
Cover credit: © Veer
Credits: The credits section for this book begins on page Cr-1 and is considered an extension of the copyright page.

Library of Congress Cataloging-in-Publication Data

Math & dosage calculations for healthcare professionals/Kathryn A. Booth . . . [et al.].—4th ed.
   p. ; cm.
   Math and dosage calculations for healthcare professionals
   Includes index.
   Rev. ed. of: Math and dosage calculations for health care/Kathryn A. Booth, James E.
Whaley. 3rd ed. c2010.
   ISBN-13: 978-0-07-337469-7 (alk. paper)
   ISBN-10: 0-07-337469-5 (alk. paper)
   1. Pharmaceutical arithmetic—Problems, exercises, etc. I. Booth, Kathryn A., 1957-
II. Booth, Kathryn A., 1957- Math and dosage calculations for health care. III. Title: Math
and dosage calculations for healthcare professionals.
   [DNLM: 1. Drug Dosage Calculations—Problems and Exercises. 2. Pharmaceutical
Preparations—administration & dosage—Problems and Exercises. 3. Mathematics—Problems
and Exercises. QV 18.2]
RS57.H334 2012
615'.1401513—dc22

                                                                   2010046567

www.mhhe.com

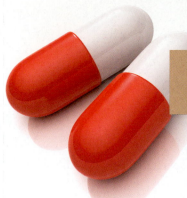

ABOUT THE AUTHORS

Kathryn A. Booth, MS, RN, RMA (AMT), RPT, CPhT, is an educator, author, and consultant and vice president and owner of Total Care Programming, a multimedia software development company. Her background includes a bachelor's degree in nursing and a master's degree in education. Her over 30 years of teaching, nursing, and healthcare experience span five states. She has authored and developed electronic media and health occupation educational textbooks and educational materials for Total Care Programming, Inc., Glencoe/McGraw-Hill, Mosby Lifeline, and McGraw-Hill Higher Education. Her most recent textbook is *Medical Assisting: Administrative and Clinical Procedures,* fourth edition, by McGraw-Hill Higher Education. Mrs. Booth has presented at numerous state and national conferences since 1994. Her current focus is to develop additional healthcare materials that will assist healthcare educators and promote the healthcare profession. To remain current, Kathy works as a nurse volunteer and teaches Medical Assisting for Military to Medicine for the Inova Health System.

James E. Whaley, RPh, MS, is currently an associate professor of health sciences and chemistry at Baker College of Owosso (Michigan) and coordinator of the Pharmacy Technician Program, which is offered at nine Baker College campuses. He routinely teaches courses in the Pharmacy Technician Program in addition to anatomy and physiology, pathophysiology, and general chemistry. Mr. Whaley has taught at Baker College of Owosso since 1995 and was the first recipient of the college's prestigious Teacher of the Year award. He has been selected as a member of Who's Who among College Teachers numerous times. Prior to coming to Baker, Mr. Whaley was twice ranked in the top 10 percent of instructors at the University of Illinois, where he was awarded a fellowship in cellular and molecular biology from the National Institutes of Health. Mr. Whaley worked as a retail pharmacist before beginning his career as an educator, and he has been a registered pharmacist since 1981.

Susan Sienkiewicz, MA, RN, is a professor of nursing and department chair of the Associate Degree Nursing Program at the Community College of Rhode Island, where she teaches nursing care of the family and dosage calculations for medication administration. She earned her bachelor's degree in nursing from Villanova University and master's degree in education from New York University.

Jennifer F. Palmunen, MSN, RN, is an assistant professor of nursing at the Community College of Rhode Island, where she teaches advanced medical-surgical nursing. She earned her associate's degree in nursing from Rockland Community College, her bachelor's degree in psychology from Sonoma State University, and her master's degree in nursing with a specialization in healthcare education from the University of Phoenix.

DEDICATION

To the future healthcare professionals using this book: may your career goals be achieved and the healthcare workforce be increased from your accomplishment.

To my first granddaughter, Kaylyn, you are truly a blessing to my life.

To my husband, Jim, for his enduring encouragement, love, friendship, and patience.

K. Booth

To my friends and colleagues at Baker College of Owosso, both past and present. Your dedication and commitment are inspirational, your support unwavering. My thanks to all of you for helping to make my days rewarding.

J. Whaley

To my students. . . . You inspire me, challenge me, motivate me!

S. Sienkiewicz

To the students who use this resource: may you have a safe and successful practice.

J. Palmunen

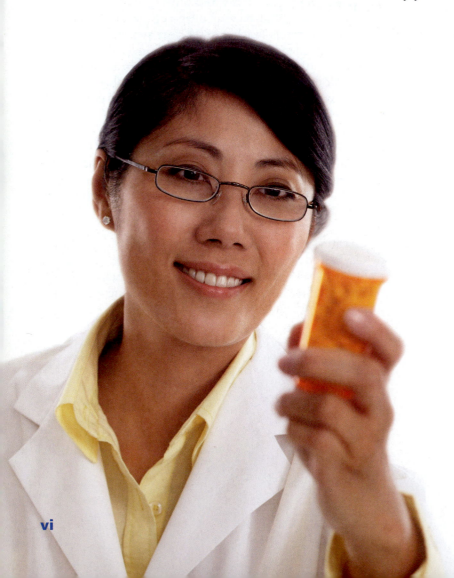

BRIEF CONTENTS

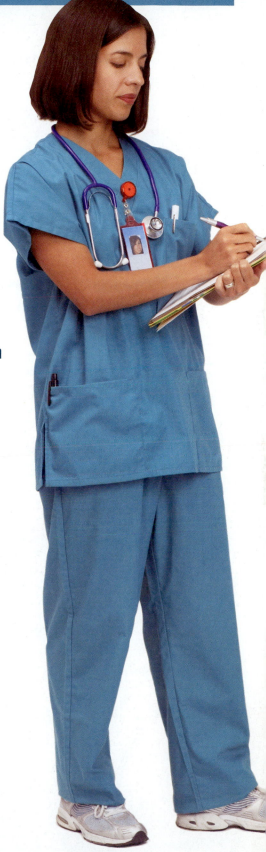

CONTENTS

Unit Two: Systems of Measurement

CHAPTER 4: METRIC SYSTEM   86

CHAPTER 5: OTHER SYSTEMS OF MEASUREMENT   98

CHAPTER 6: USING CONVERSION FACTORS   108

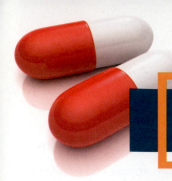

PREFACE

We've got you covered—from basic math skills to critical dosage calculations . . . from the print textbook to the digital supplements!

Welcome to the fourth edition of *Math & Dosage Calculations for Healthcare Professionals (M&DC)!* This product introduces your students to the concepts and skills they will need to move forward with their health professions or nursing curriculum. This is a critical course for many students, and the tools and resources offered with this book are meant to ensure success for all.

Here's what you and your students can expect from the new edition of *M&DC:*

- Chapters have been shortened and grouped into units to make it easier to navigate the material—this gives each chapter a clearer, better-defined purpose.
- Stronger focus on calculations that will be performed by healthcare professionals who are administering medications to patients, with less emphasis on compounding and other calculations associated with preparing medications—this allows for the incorporation of new and relevant scenarios requiring critical thinking.
- A greater emphasis on the content that is needed for a nursing curriculum through the addition of two new coauthors, Susan Sienkiewicz, MA, RN, and Jennifer Palmunen, MSN, RN, of the Community College of Rhode Island.
- Coverage of three methods of dosage calculation—proportion, formula, and dimensional analysis.
- Chapters have new learning outcomes based on the revised Bloom's Taxonomy that serve as the framework for the chapter and are emphasized throughout to tie the concepts together.
- New tabular end-of-chapter summaries are tied to the learning outcomes along with page references—these reinforce key points for review.
- Extensive examples and exercise sets, including practice with over 250 full-color, up-to-date drug label illustrations by the main drug companies and currently used by the healthcare profession—this provides an opportunity for real-world applications.
- An updated student CD-ROM with review and practice activities also tied into the learning outcomes.
- Accuracy—all of the content has gone through a rigorous, multiround accuracy check with a proven math accuracy checking vendor.
- Comprehensive digital support with ALEKS Prep for Math & Dosage and *Connect Plus*.

Here's How Your Colleagues Have Described the New Edition of *M&DC*

"This book is very comprehensive, easy-to-understand, and within our students' abilities. Key strengths include: lots of examples and practice problems, lots of example labels that look like what they will find on the shelf, and easy to understand with three different methods to do the calculations."

George Strothmann Jr., CPhT, Sanford Brown Institute

"The overall key strengths of this text are the new additions of the "Think! . . . Is It Reasonable?" sections; the variety of dosage calculation options; the way it is set up according to subject, as well the order in which the chapters are placed; and the opportunities for practice and review. The biggest key strength, I believe, is the integration of information for the administration of medications, as well as the dosage calculation."

Amy Ensign, CMA (AAMA), RMA (AMT), Baker College

"Overall it is a comprehensive review of math and dosage calculation, providing clear, easily understood explanations and practice. It provides chapters that can serve as review of basic concepts if that is needed, and it covers the daily necessary-type calculations nicely."

Margaret Gingrich, Harrisburg Area Community College

"Separating many of the chapters was a great improvement to the text, by allowing students a better opportunity to refresh some old concepts and grasp some new ones. I believe it puts the material into "bite-size" chunks that can assimilate easier. The new features (Think! . . . Is It Reasonable? and chapter summaries) are good tools for most students and help to reinforce the concepts."

Belva Matherly, CPhT, National College

"This text offers specific and concise methods of dosage calculations. The content is well-organized and the information is up-to-date."

DeLoris Larson, MSNNE, Northland College

Organization of *M&DC*, 4e

M&DC is divided into 5 units:

UNIT	COVERAGE
1: Overview of Basic Math	Chapters 1–3 focus on a review of basic math skills needed to perform dosage calculations. (Was presented as two chapters in 3e.)
2: Systems of Measurement	Chapters 4–7 focus on measurements used in dosage calculations and drug administration. (Was presented as one chapter in 3e.)
3: Principles of Medication Administration	Chapters 8–11 focus on equipment, interpreting medication orders and labels, as well as safe medication administration. (Was presented as three chapters in 3e. Chapter 11 is a brand-new chapter that focuses on principles of safe medication administration.)
4: Basic Dosage Calculations	Chapters 12–15 focus on the basic dosage calculations to include three methods: proportion method, dimensional analysis, and formula method. (Was presented as Chapters 7–10 in 3e.)
5: Calculations Used in Specialty Areas	Chapters 16–19 focus on advanced clinical calculations to include: preparation of noninjectable solutions, weight-based dosages, and critical care calculations. (Was presented as two chapters in 3e. Chapter 18 is a brand-new chapter on "high-alert" medications that includes a protocol for administration of heparin.)

New to the Fourth Edition!

One of the first things you may notice is that the design of *M&DC* has been updated and refreshed to better highlight the pedagogy and to make it easier for the reader to navigate through the material. More photos have been included, and the full-color illustrations of drug labels provided by the main drug companies have been updated to the most current labels used by the healthcare profession.

Key changes include:
- The book has been reorganized—12 chapters have been expanded to 19 by breaking the content down into smaller chunks to better fit the needs of today's courses.
- Calculations now show solving for "x" rather than solving for "?" to better reflect what is used in most math texts.

- All syringe illustrations in the book are safety syringes, have a safety needle, or have the needle cropped to better reflect what students will encounter in a real environment.
- References to *physician* have been changed to *authorized prescriber* to reflect multiple disciplines with prescriptive authority.
- The number of calculation methods has been reduced from four to three to better reflect the methods most instructors use (ratio proportion and fraction proportion have been combined into proportion; the other methods are formula and dimensional analysis).
- A new, three-step solution process has been included for the dosage calculation problems—Convert, Calculate, "Think! . . . Is It Reasonable?" and the "Think! . . . Is It Reasonable?" feature is used throughout the book to encourage critical thinking skills.
- All chapters are organized by learning outcomes, which are written using the revised version of Bloom's Taxonomy. The new tabular end-of-chapter summaries are organized by learning outcome to make it easier to review the material. And end-of-chapter exercises are also tagged to the learning outcomes.
- A Unit Assessment is now included at the end of each unit to review the material presented in that unit before moving on to the next unit.
- Additional review and practice exercises on the student CD-ROM that are now organized by learning outcome as well. CD icons are integrated throughout the text to let students know when additional practice exercises are available.
- The book is now available with ALEKS Prep for Math & Dosage and *Connect Plus*. Students can remediate on the basic math topic before class even starts with ALEKS Prep, allowing instructors to get to the dosage calculations faster. *Connect Plus* then helps students as they work through the course by providing them with additional assessment questions and interactivities, in conjunction with the integrated eBook.

Chapter-by-chapter highlights include:
- Chapters 1—7: content has been broken out into seven chapters from the three chapters presented in the previous edition.
- Chapter 8: pictures and text have been revised to demonstrate safety syringes/needles; picture of a needleless IV tubing have been added; new table on needle length, gauge, and maximum injection amount has been added; illustration of enteral feeding has been modified to clarify connection between NGT and enteral feeding pump tubing; and text has been expanded on ampules and safety maneuvers by the healthcare practitioner to prevent self-harm.
- Chapter 9: *subcut* has been added to the Abbreviation Table as the only acceptable abbreviation for subcutaneous (here and in all chapters); references to medication cards have been removed from text; some information from Chapter 9 has been moved to Chapter 11 (safe medication administration); and error-prone abbreviations have been referenced in this chapter and have been placed in Chapter 11.
- Chapter 10: updated drug labels have been added.
- Chapter 11: new chapter has been added to address multiple aspects of safe medication administration, including receiving and transcribing orders, interpreting a medication administration record, and following the *"rights"* and *"checks"* of medication administration.
- Chapter 12: ratio proportion method and fraction proportion method have been combined as "the proportion method"; proportion has been inverted to read $H/Q = D/A$, which is consistent with the common order for dosage strength (mg/mL or mg/tab *not* mL/mg or tab/mg); and the process of dosage calculation has been divided into three steps—A: Convert, B: Calculate, and C: Think! . . . Is It Reasonable. The ABCs of dosage calculation are repeated throughout the text—in step C the student is asked to estimate what the answer should be, then compare the calculated answer with the estimated answer, an important step since students are losing their sense of the value of numbers as they enter numerals into calculators and computers to generate answers.
- Chapter 13: new "Error Alert" has been added that identifies the importance of observing patients as they take their medications; and calculation of single dose and daily dose is differentiated in the end-of-chapter exercises.

- Chapter 14: parenteral equipment has been modified to have needles removed or safety needles added; maximal volume for an IM injection at the deltoid site has been corrected to 1 mL; information regarding use of MDI inhaler and transdermal patches has been expanded to include more safe administration techniques; and patient teaching box has been added.
- Chapter 15: hypotonic, hypertonic, and isotonic solutions have been differentiated; Review and Practice section regarding calculation of components of IV solutions has been added; and "Error Alert" revealing the different strengths of heparin has been added.
- Chapter 16: new chapter entitled, "Preparation of Noninjectable Solutions"; examples include: enteral feeding solutions and wound care irrigants; and Patient Education feature has been inserted that includes instructions for preparation of infant formula from dry powder.
- Chapter 17: Added Review and Practice sections on "Factors that Impact Dosing and Medication Administration," and reorganized chapter so that ideal weight calculations follow weight-based calculations.
- Chapter 18: information on insulin and heparin from Chapter 12 in the previous edition moved here with extensive revisions (ISMP lists insulin and heparin among the "high-alert medications" due to the high number of serious or lethal errors associated with these medications); new table has been inserted describing the different types of insulins, and classifying them broadly as "mealtime" or "basal;" information regarding U-500 insulin has been revised; pictures of different insulin safety syringes have been added; due to persistent over-dosage errors made from misidentifying labeled dosage strength, the heparin section has been expanded to include exercises in selecting the correct heparin dosage strength, based on the label; new labels have been added to demonstrate different dosage strengths and bottle fills; a heparin protocol has been added for weight-based IV heparin infusions, since this is common practice for IV heparin administration; and all IV dosage calculation exercises are based on use of an infusion pump, since this is now the standard of practice for administration of these medications.
- Chapter 19: separate chapter has been added for critical care IV medication calculation; information from Chapter 12 in the last edition has been extensively revised to support the rapid calculation of continuous IV infusion rates that are based on dose/weight/time; the student is taught different techniques for titrating vasoactive and antiarrhythmic medications as well as other medications commonly administered in the critical care setting; new rules and examples have been added to support this learning, and a new error alert has been added to guide calculation; critical thinking exercise has been revised to ensure the student is not led into a lethal error; and all IV dosage calculation exercises are based on use of an infusion pump, since this is now the standard of practice for administration of these medications.

For a detailed transition guide between the third and fourth editions of *M&DC*, visit www.mhhe.com/mathanddosage4e.

To the Instructor

McGraw-Hill knows how much effort it takes to prepare for a new course. Through focus groups, symposia, reviews, and conversations with instructors like you, we have gathered information about what materials you need in order to facilitate successful courses. We are committed to provide you with high-quality, accurate instructor support.

INSTRUCTOR RESOURCES

You can rely on the following materials to help you and your students work through the exercises in the book:

- Instructor Edition of the Online Learning Center at www.mhhe.com/mathanddosage4e. Your McGraw-Hill sales representative can provide you with access and show you how to "go green" with our online instructor support.

- Instructor's Manual with course overview; sample syllabi; answer keys for all exercises, which have gone through two rounds of accuracy checking; and correlations to various standards.
- A PowerPoint slide presentation for each chapter, containing teaching notes correlated to Learning Outcomes. Each presentation seeks to reinforce key concepts and provide a visual for students. The slides are excellent for in-class lectures.
- Test bank and answer key for use in classroom assessment. The comprehensive test bank includes a variety of question types, with each question linked directly to its Learning Outcome, Bloom's Taxonomy, and difficulty level. Both a Word version and a computerized version (EZ Test) of the test bank are provided.
- Executable files that were previously on Instructor CD, which allow the instructor to interact with the student CD. Using the instructor Grade Book (gradebook.exe), the instructor can open student emails and view and record the student progress on the learning activities from the student CD. Using the Test Bank editor (questioneditor.exe), the instructor can update the interactive and *Spin the Wheel* questions, adding content and additional pictures.
- Conversion Guide with a chapter-by-chapter breakdown of how the content has been revised between editions. The guide is helpful if you are currently using *M&DC* and moving to the new edition, or if you are a first-time adopter.
- Instructor Asset Map to help you find the teaching material you need with a click of the mouse. These online chapter tables are organized by Learning Outcomes and allow you to find instructor notes, PowerPoint slides, and even test bank suggestions with ease! The Asset Map is a completely integrated tool designed to help you plan and instruct your courses efficiently and comprehensively. It labels and organizes course material for use in a multitude of learning applications.
- *Connect Plus:* McGraw-Hill *Connect Plus* is a revolutionary online assignment and assessment solution, providing instructors and students with tools and resources to 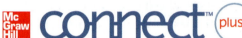 maximize their success. Through *Connect Plus*, instructors enjoy simplified course setup and assignment creation. Robust, media-rich tools and activities, all tied to the textbook Learning Outcomes ensure you'll create classes geared toward achievement. You'll have more time with your students and spend less time agonizing over course planning.
- **ALEKS Prep for Math and Dosage** is a Web-based program that focuses on content knowledge needed to be successful for the basic math topics required in a dosage calculations course. ALEKS uses **artificial intelligence** and **adaptive** questioning to precisely assess a student's preparedness and then provides personalized instruction to help students quickly attain knowledge and progress through the course. Find out more at www.aleks.com.
- **Body ANIMAT3D:** McGraw-Hill, in partnership with Nucleus Medical Media, has co-developed 3D animations on anatomy, physiology, pathophysiology, and pharmacology. These animations, presented in *Connect Plus* are offered with pre-, during-, and post-assessment assignments.
- **Medication Administration Video Series:** a strong emphasis on safe medication administration is realized in this series of 12 videos that demonstrate up-to-date practice of medication administration techniques via various routes. These videos are offered with pre-, during-, and post-assessment assignments.

McGraw-Hill Higher Education and Blackboard have teamed up. What does this mean for you?

1. **Your life, simplified.** Now you and your students can access McGraw-Hill's *Connect Plus* and Create right from within your Blackboard course—all with one single sign-on. Say goodbye to the days of logging in to multiple applications.
2. **Deep integration of content and tools.** Not only do you get single sign-on with *Connect Plus* and Create, you also get deep integration of McGraw-Hill content and content engines right in Blackboard. Whether you're choosing a book for your course or building *Connect Plus* assignments, all the tools you need are right where you want them—inside Blackboard.

3. **Seamless gradebooks.** Are you tired of keeping multiple gradebooks and manually synchronizing grades into Blackboard? We thought so. When a student completes an integrated *Connect Plus* assignment, the grade for that assignment automatically (and instantly) feeds your Blackboard grade center.

4. **A solution for everyone.** Whether your institution is already using Blackboard or you just want to try Blackboard on your own, we have a solution for you. McGraw-Hill and Blackboard can now offer you easy access to industry-leading technology and content, whether your campus hosts it, or we do. Be sure to ask your local McGraw-Hill representative for details.

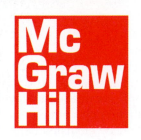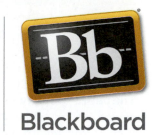

Do More

Need Help? Contact the Digital Care Support Team

Visit our Digital CARE Support website at www.mhhe.com/support. Browse the FAQs (frequently asked questions) and product documentation and/or contact a CARE support representative. The Digital CARE Support Team is available Sunday through Friday.

To the Student

Throughout the book, you will notice CD-ROM icons that indicate you should go to the CD included with the book for additional practice. This CD, organized by the learning outcomes in the book, provides exercises and games such as "Spin the Wheel," "Math Challenge," and "Key Term Concentration" to help reinforce the rules and information you have just learned in the book, along with other activities.

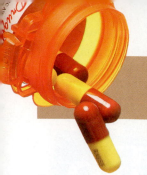

ACKNOWLEDGMENTS

Suggestions have been received from faculty and students throughout the country. This is vital feedback that is relied on with each edition. Each person who has offered comments and suggestions has our thanks.

The efforts of many people are needed to develop and improve a product. Among these people are the reviewers and consultants who point out areas of concern, cite areas of strength, and make recommendations for change. In this regard, the reviewers listed below provided feedback that was enormously helpful in preparing the fourth edition of *M&DC*.

Workshops

In 2009 and 2010, McGraw-Hill conducted 15 allied health workshops, providing an opportunity for more than 600 faculty members to gain continuing education credits as well as to provide feedback on our products.

Book Reviews

More than 75 instructors reviewed the third edition once it was published, as well as the fourth edition manuscript, providing valuable feedback that directly affected the development of the fourth edition.

Karen Amsden—RN, BSN, MSHA, Jefferson College

Michele B. Bach—MS, BA, Kansas City Kansas Community College

Ilene Borze—RN, MS, Gateway Community College

Elicia S. Collins—BSN, MSN, Atlanta Technical College

Amy Ensign—CMA, RMA, Baker College

Rhonda Evans—AND, BSN, MSN, Central Carolina Community College

Timothy Feltmeyer—MS, Erie Business Center

Thomas Fridley—CPhT, Sanford Brown Institute

Margaret Gingrich—Harrisburg Area Community College

Sheldon Guenther—BS, DC, Kansas City Kansas Community College

Betty Hassler—RMA, AS, National College

Donna J. Headrick—FNP, Barstow Community College

Elizabeth Hoffman—MA, Ed., CMA, CPT, Baker College

Pilar Perez-Jackson—CPhT, Sanford Brown Institute

Jackie H. Jones—Kennesaw State University

DeLoris P. Larson—MSNNE, Northland College

Elizabeth Laurenz—CMA, LPN, MBA, National College

Larry M. Liggan—M.Ed, PA, RMA, AHI-C, National College

Jennifer Lipke—Hibbing Community College

Ralph C. Lucki—MA, CRT, RRT, EMT-P, West Virginia Northern Community College

Sheri Lee Martin—RN, BSN, LMT, BLS, Central Georgia Technical College

Belva J. Matherly—CPhT, National College

Keith A. Monosky—PhD, MPM, EMT-P, Central Washington University

Linda W. Moore—BA, Georgia Military College

Anne F. Mullenniex—BA, MA, Ph. C, Skagit Valley College

Donna M. Olafson—MA, Kansas City Community College

Gail P. Orr—MA, RMA, National College

Peggy A. Radke—MSN, Central Community College

Ramona Gail Rice—BS, MS, Ph.D, Georgia Military College

Helen Reid—EdD, MSN, BS, BA, Trinity Valley Community College

Katherine Lippitt-Seibert—RN, Mercy College of Health Sciences

Kathleen Sheehan—AS, BS, MSN, Elms College

Kristin M. Spencer—AAS, BHS, MBA, Baker College

George W. Strothmann Jr.—CPhT, Sanford Brown Institute

Jue-Ling Tai—MS, Danville Community College

Joseph A. Tinervia—CPhT, MBA, Tulsa Job Corps Center/Tulsa Community College

Debra J. Tymcio—RT, RMA, National College

Scott David Vaillancourt—Master Certified Novell Instructor, Certified Cisco Academy Instructor, Microsoft Certified Trainer, Ultimate Medical Academy

Jane K. Walker—BBA, MSN, PhD, Walters State Community College

Olma L. Weaver—LVN, Coastal Bend College-Beeville Campus

Janet M. Westhoff—Mott Community College

Denise York—BSN, MS, Med, Columbus State Community College

Technical Editing/Accuracy Checking

Acting as consultants to our vendor, two key instructors completed a technical edit and review of all content in the final manuscript and again in the book page proofs.

Elizabeth Hoffman, MA, Ed., CMA, CPT, Baker College

Keith Monosky, PhD, MPM, EMT-P, Central Washington University

Acknowledgments from the Authors

To the students and instructors who use this book, your feedback and suggestions have made *M&DC* a better learning tool for all.

We especially want to thank the editorial team at McGraw-Hill—Liz Haefele, Ken Kasee, and Michelle Flomenhoft—for their enthusiastic support and their willingness to go the extra mile to get this book revised. We would also like to thank freelance editor Melinda Bilecki for her excellent contributions.

The EDP staff was also outstanding; senior designer Srdj Savanovic created an impressive new design, which was implemented through the production process by Rick Hecker, lead project manager; Michael McCormick, senior buyer; Lori Hancock, photo research coordinator; and Cathy Tepper, media project manager.

We also appreciate the many efforts of Mary Haran, marketing manager, who helps people stay aware of the latest information on *M&DC*.

We would also like to give special thanks to Linda Moore and Ramona Rice at Georgia Military College for preparing the Instructor's Manual.

And to our families.

The Authors

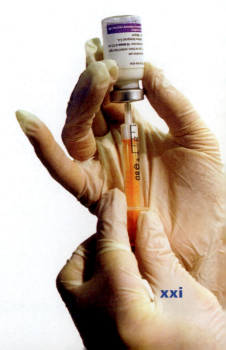

GUIDED TOUR

Chapter Opener

The **chapter opener** sets the stage for what will be learned in the chapter.

    Learning Outcomes are written to reflect the revised version of Bloom's Taxonomy and to establish the key points the student should focus on in the chapter. In addition, major chapter heads are structured to reflect the Learning Outcomes and are numbered accordingly.

    Key terms are first introduced in the chapter opener so the student can see them all in one place.

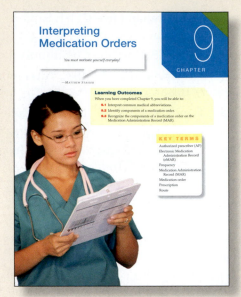

Rules and Examples

Rules state important formulas and facts for completing calculations. The **Examples** that follow illustrate these rules.

RULE 2-2	Always write a zero to the left of the decimal point when the decimal number has no whole-number part. Using the zero makes the decimal point more noticeable. Never place a trailing zero after the decimal point when working with medication dosages. Using zeros correctly helps to prevent medication errors.

Example	Write the following fractions in decimal form.
	 a. $\frac{4}{10}$
	     $\frac{4}{10} = 0.4$ Do *not* write .4.
	 b. $\frac{25}{1000}$
	     $\frac{25}{1000} = 0.025$ Do *not* write .025.
	 c. 100/25
	     $\frac{100}{25} = 4$ Do *not* write 4.0.

RULE 13-1	Always question and/or verify when your calculation indicates to give a portion of a tablet when the tablet is not scored.
Example 1	Do not administer $\frac{1}{2}$ of an unscored tablet.
Example 2	Do not administer $\frac{1}{3}$ or $\frac{1}{4}$ of a tablet scored for division in two.

Methods of Dosage Calculations

Three methods of dosage calculation are included in this edition, as compared to the previous edition. The methods are color-coded so you can easily find the method of problem solving that best fits your learning style or has been specified by your instructor. These methods are reinforced on the card inserted at the back of the book.

PROPORTION METHOD

EXAMPLE 1   The order is to give the patient 15 mg codeine PO now. You have 30 mg scored tablets available.

STEP A: CONVERT
The desired dose (D) is 15 mg. The dose on hand H is 30 mg, and the dosage unit Q is 1 tablet. Because the desired dose and the dose on hand have the same units, no conversion needed.

STEP B: CALCULATE
Follow Procedure Checklist 12-1.

  1. Fill in the proportion.

$$\frac{H}{Q} = \frac{D}{A} \quad \text{or} \quad \frac{\text{Dose on hand}}{\text{Dosage unit}} = \frac{\text{Desired dose}}{\text{Amount to administer}}$$

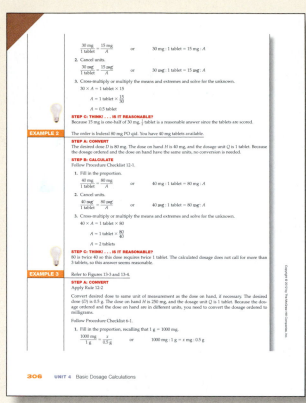

$$\frac{30 \text{ mg}}{1 \text{ tablet}} = \frac{15 \text{ mg}}{A} \qquad \text{or} \qquad 30 \text{ mg} : 1 \text{ tablet} = 15 \text{ mg} : A$$

2. Cancel units.

$$\frac{30 \text{ mg}}{1 \text{ tablet}} = \frac{15 \text{ mg}}{A} \qquad \text{or} \qquad 30 \text{ mg} : 1 \text{ tablet} = 15 \text{ mg} : A$$

3. Cross-multiply or multiply the means and extremes and solve for the unknown.

$$30 \times A = 1 \text{ tablet} \times 15$$

$$A = 1 \text{ tablet} \times \frac{15}{30}$$

$$A = 0.5 \text{ tablet}$$

STEP C: THINK! . . . IS IT REASONABLE?
Because 15 mg is one-half of 30 mg, $\frac{1}{2}$ tablet is a reasonable answer since the tablets are scored.

EXAMPLE 2 The order is Inderal 80 mg PO qid. You have 40 mg tablets available.

STEP A: CONVERT
The desired dose D is 80 mg. The dose on hand H is 40 mg, and the dosage unit Q is 1 tablet. Because the dosage ordered and the dose on hand have the same units, no conversion is needed.

STEP B: CALCULATE
Follow Procedure Checklist 12-1.

1. Fill in the proportion.

$$\frac{40 \text{ mg}}{1 \text{ tablet}} = \frac{80 \text{ mg}}{A} \qquad \text{or} \qquad 40 \text{ mg} : 1 \text{ tablet} = 80 \text{ mg} : A$$

2. Cancel units.

$$\frac{40 \text{ mg}}{1 \text{ tablet}} = \frac{80 \text{ mg}}{A} \qquad \text{or} \qquad 40 \text{ mg} : 1 \text{ tablet} = 80 \text{ mg} : A$$

3. Cross-multiply or multiply the means and extremes and solve for the unknown.

$$40 \times A = 1 \text{ tablet} \times 80$$

$$A = 1 \text{ tablet} \times \frac{80}{40}$$

$$A = 2 \text{ tablets}$$

STEP C: THINK! . . . IS IT REASONABLE?
80 is twice 40 so this dose requires twice 1 tablet. The calculated dosage does not call for more than 3 tablets, so this answer seems reasonable.

EXAMPLE 3 Refer to Figures 13-3 and 13-4.

STEP A: CONVERT
Apply Rule 12-2

Convert desired dose to same unit of measurement as the dose on hand, if necessary. The desired dose (D) is 0.5 g. The dose on hand H is 250 mg, and the dosage unit Q is 1 tablet. Because the dosage ordered and the dose on hand are in different units, you need to convert the dosage ordered to milligrams.

Follow Procedure Checklist 6-1.

1. Fill in the proportion, recalling that 1 g = 1000 mg.

$$\frac{1000 \text{ mg}}{1 \text{ g}} = \frac{x}{0.5 \text{ g}} \qquad \text{or} \qquad 1000 \text{ mg} : 1 \text{ g} = x \text{ mg} : 0.5 \text{ g}$$

Copyright © 2012 by The McGraw-Hill Companies, Inc.

M&DC, 3e	M&DC, 4e
Ratio Proportion	
	Proportion
Fraction Proportion	
Formula	Formula
Dimensional Analysis	Dimensional Analysis

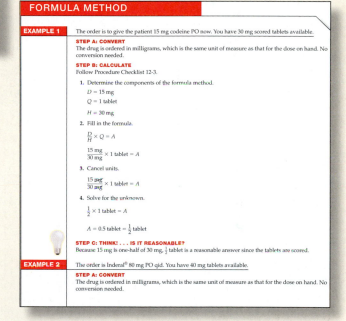

DIMENSIONAL ANALYSIS

EXAMPLE 1 The order is to give the patient 15 mg codeine PO now. You have 30 mg scored tablets available.

STEP A: CONVERT
The unit of measurement for the desired dose and the dose on hand are both milligrams. No conversion factor needed.

STEP B: CALCULATE
Follow Procedure Checklist 12-2.

1. The unit of measure for the amount to administer will be tablets.

$$A \text{ tablets} =$$

2. No conversion factor needed.

3. The dosage unit is 1 tablet. The dosage on hand is 30 mg.

$$A \text{ tablets} = \frac{1 \text{ tablet}}{30 \text{ mg}}$$

4. The dosage ordered is 15 mg.

$$A \text{ tablets} = \frac{1 \text{ tablet}}{30 \text{ mg}} \times \frac{15 \text{ mg}}{1}$$

5. Cancel units.

$$A \text{ tablets} = \frac{1 \text{ tablet}}{30 \text{ mg}} \times \frac{15 \text{ mg}}{1}$$

6. Solve the equation.

$$A \text{ tablets} = \frac{1 \text{ tablet}}{30} \times \frac{15}{1}$$

$$A = 0.5 \text{ tablet} = \frac{1}{2} \text{ tablet}$$

STEP C: THINK! . . . IS IT REASONABLE?
Because 15 mg is one-half of 30 mg, $\frac{1}{2}$ tablet is an appropriate answer since the tablets are scored.

EXAMPLE 2 The order is Inderal® 80 mg PO qid. You have 40 mg tablets available.

STEP A: CONVERT
The unit of measurement for the desired dose and the dose on hand are both milligrams. No conversion factor needed.

FORMULA METHOD

EXAMPLE 1 The order is to give the patient 15 mg codeine PO now. You have 30 mg scored tablets available.

STEP A: CONVERT
The drug is ordered in milligrams, which is the same unit of measure as that for the dose on hand. No conversion needed.

STEP B: CALCULATE
Follow Procedure Checklist 12-3.

1. Determine the components of the formula method.

$$D = 15 \text{ mg}$$

$$Q = 1 \text{ tablet}$$

$$H = 30 \text{ mg}$$

2. Fill in the formula.

$$\frac{D}{H} \times Q = A$$

$$\frac{15 \text{ mg}}{30 \text{ mg}} \times 1 \text{ tablet} = A$$

3. Cancel units.

$$\frac{15 \text{ mg}}{30 \text{ mg}} \times 1 \text{ tablet} = A$$

4. Solve for the unknown.

$$\frac{1}{2} \times 1 \text{ tablet} = A$$

$$A = 0.5 \text{ tablet} = \frac{1}{2} \text{ tablet}$$

STEP C: THINK! . . . IS IT REASONABLE?
Because 15 mg is one-half of 30 mg, $\frac{1}{2}$ tablet is a reasonable answer since the tablets are scored.

EXAMPLE 2 The order is Inderal® 80 mg PO qid. You have 40 mg tablets available.

STEP A: CONVERT
The drug is ordered in milligrams, which is the same unit of measure as that for the dose on hand. No conversion needed.

LEARNING LINK Recall the components of a medication order addressed in Chapter 9: name of patient, patient's date of birth, date and time the order is written, drug name, drug dose, route, time and/or frequency of medication administration, and signature of authorized prescriber (AP). (See Table 9-3.)

Learning Aids

Learning Links refer students to an earlier chapter for a quick review when concepts are repeated.

Patient Education boxes teach students about clear and accurate communication with their patients.

PATIENT EDUCATION

Patient education, although not one of the six basic rights of medication administration, is critical to the patient's right to know. Patients should always be provided with basic information regarding their medications.

1. Explain the purpose of a medication and its side effects.
2. Review the dose, route, frequency, and time that the physician has prescribed.
3. When appropriate, be certain that the patient understands how to self-administer the medication.
4. If the patient is taking liquid oral medications at home, emphasize the importance of using calibrated spoons and measuring cups.

Error Alert! boxes point out common errors to students so they can focus on avoiding them and doing correct calculations instead.

Critical Thinking on the Job boxes contain real-world scenarios that help students apply math and dosage calculations to the healthcare profession. Students must read the scenarios and then answer critical thinking questions to determine what they would do to solve the scenario presented.

A **three-step solution process** has been included for the dosage calculation problems—Convert, Calculate, "Think! . . . Is It Reasonable?," and the "Think! . . . Is It Reasonable?" feature is used throughout the book to encourage critical thinking skills.

CD-ROM references are included throughout the book to direct students to related exercises for review, reinforcement, and evaluation.

ERROR ALERT!

Always Be Certain That You Are Dispensing the Correct Medication

Many drugs have names that are very similar. Read the order carefully and, when in doubt, contact the authorized prescriber. The following list gives just a few examples of how similar the names of different drugs can look and sound. It is especially easy to confuse them when they are written rather than printed.

Acular®—Ocular
Benadryl®—Bentyl®
Cafergot®—Carafate®
Darvon®—Diovan®
Digitoxin—digoxin
Eurax—Urex®

Iodine—Lodine®
Nicobid—Nitrobid®
Pavabid—Pavased
Phenaphen—Phenergan®
Quinidine—Quinine
Uracel—Uracil

CRITICAL THINKING ON THE JOB

The Importance of the Right Drug

A patient is brought to the hospital with a severe thumb laceration. The attending physician verbally orders lidocaine 1% solution 2 mL as a local anesthetic. The healthcare professional picks up a vial labeled lidocaine 1% with epinephrine and draws up 2 mL. He then says, "This is lidocaine 1% solution 2 mL," but neither mentions the epinephrine nor shows the physician the label.

A while later, the patient expresses concern about continuing numbness in his thumb. After locating the vial, the staff member realized that the patient received epinephrine, a vasoconstricting drug, in addition to the lidocaine. The patient is reassured that feeling will return to his thumb, although not quite as quickly as was first anticipated.

 Think! . . . Is It Reasonable? What could have been done to prevent the patient from losing feeling in his thumb?

GO TO . . . Open the CD-ROM that accompanies your textbook, and select Chapter 11, Parts of a Prescription (LO 11.1). Review the animation and example problems, then complete the practice problems. Continue to the next section of the book once you have mastered the information presented.

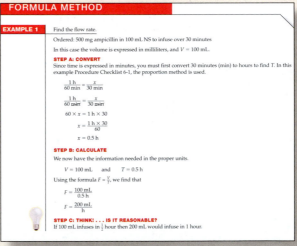

FORMULA METHOD

EXAMPLE 1   Find the flow rate.

Ordered: 500 mg ampicillin in 100 mL NS to infuse over 30 minutes

In this case the volume is expressed in milliliters, and $V = 100$ mL.

STEP A: CONVERT

Since time is expressed in minutes, you must first convert 30 minutes (min) to hours to find T. In this example Procedure Checklist 6-1, the proportion method is used.

$$\frac{1\,h}{60\,min} = \frac{x}{30\,min}$$

$$\frac{1\,h}{60\,\cancel{min}} = \frac{x}{30\,\cancel{min}}$$

$$60 \times x = 1\,h \times 30$$

$$x = \frac{1\,h \times 30}{60}$$

$$x = 0.5\,h$$

STEP B: CALCULATE

We now have the information needed in the proper units.

$$V = 100\,mL \quad and \quad T = 0.5\,h$$

Using the formula $F = \frac{V}{T}$, we find that

$$F = \frac{100\,mL}{0.5\,h}$$

$$F = \frac{200\,mL}{h}$$

STEP C: THINK! . . . IS IT REASONABLE?

If 100 mL infuses in $\frac{1}{2}$ hour then 200 mL would infuse in 1 hour.

Review and Practice

Review and Practice exercises follow every section in each chapter, giving students an immediate opportunity to apply new concepts.

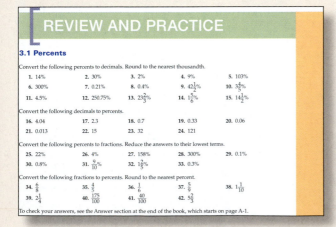

REVIEW AND PRACTICE

3.1 Percents

Convert the following percents to decimals. Round to the nearest thousandth.

1. 14%	2. 30%	3. 2%	4. 9%	5. 103%
6. 300%	7. 0.21%	8. 0.4%	9. $42\frac{1}{2}$%	10. $3\frac{4}{5}$%
11. 4.5%	12. 250.75%	13. $23\frac{2}{3}$%	14. $1\frac{5}{6}$%	15. $14\frac{1}{2}$%

Convert the following decimals to percents.

16. 4.04	17. 2.3	18. 0.7	19. 0.33	20. 0.06
21. 0.013	22. 15	23. 32	24. 121	

Convert the following percents to fractions. Reduce the answers to their lowest terms.

25. 22%	26. 4%	27. 158%	28. 300%	29. 0.1%
30. 0.8%	31. $\frac{9}{10}$%	32. $1\frac{2}{5}$%	33. 0.3%	

Convert the following fractions to percents. Round to the nearest percent.

34. $\frac{6}{8}$	35. $\frac{4}{5}$	36. $\frac{1}{6}$	37. $\frac{5}{9}$	38. $1\frac{1}{10}$
39. $2\frac{1}{4}$	40. $\frac{175}{100}$	41. $\frac{40}{100}$	42. $5\frac{2}{3}$	

To check your answers, see the Answer section at the end of the book, which starts on page A-1.

End-of-Chapter Resources

Tabular **end-of-chapter summaries** are tied to the learning outcomes along with page references—these reinforce key points for the students to review.

    Homework Assignments provide at least one of every type of problem introduced in the chapter. Answers are NOT provided in the back of the book so that instructors can assign these as an introduction, a review, or even a chapter quiz.

    The **Chapter Review** section offers additional exercises for reinforcement of the chapter content. It falls into these categories: Check Up, Critical Thinking Applications, Case Study, and Internet Activities.

    Unit Assessments are presented at the end of each of the five units. In each chapter, all of the calculations have been grouped together to allow students the opportunity to practice a specific skill. In the "real world," however, students will be faced with a variety of situations in which they will need to use each of these skills at various times throughout the day. This assessment requires students to use skills practiced in each of the chapters in the unit. If they have trouble with some of these calculations, it will help them to identify areas where more practice is needed. If they do well, they can move forward with the confidence that they are prepared for the next unit.

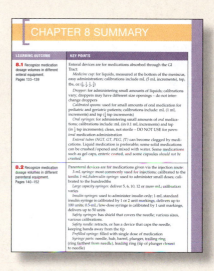

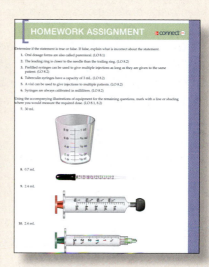

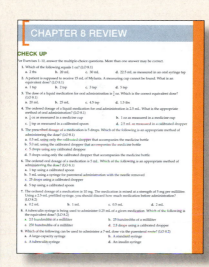

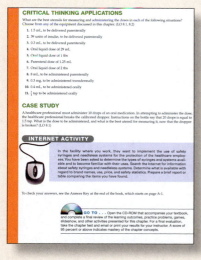

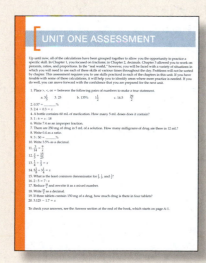

A COMMITMENT TO ACCURACY

You have a right to expect an accurate textbook, and McGraw-Hill invests considerable time and effort to make sure that we deliver one. Listed below are the many steps we take to make sure this happens.

OUR ACCURACY VERIFICATION PROCESS

First Round — *Development Reviews*

STEP 1: Numerous **health professions instructors** review the current edition and the draft manuscript and report on any errors that they may find. The authors make these corrections in their final manuscript. The manuscript is then fully accuracy-checked by a trusted **math vendor.**

Second Round—*Page Proofs*

STEP 2: Once the manuscript has been typeset, the **authors** check their manuscript against the page proofs to ensure that all illustrations, graphs, examples, and exercises have been correctly laid out on the pages. The same **math vendor** rechecks the pages to make sure corrections have been made and does a spot check to rework exercises.

STEP 3: An outside panel of **peer instructors** consults with the math vendor to further ensure accuracy. The authors add these corrections to their review of the page proofs.

STEP 4: A **proofreader** adds a triple layer of accuracy assurance in pages by looking for errors; then a confirming, corrected round of page proofs is produced.

Third Round—*Confirming Page Proofs*

STEP 5: The **author team** reviews the confirming round of page proofs to make certain that any previous corrections were properly made and to look for any errors they might have missed on the first round.

STEP 6: The **project manager,** who has overseen the book from the beginning, performs another proofread to make sure that no new errors have been introduced during the production process.

Final Round—*Printer's Proofs*

STEP 7: The **project manager,** performs a final proofread of the textbook during the printing process, providing a final accuracy review.

In addition, all supplements undergo a proofreading and technical editing stage to ensure their accuracy, in concert with the main text.

RESULTS

What results is a textbook that is as accurate and error-free as is humanly possible, and our authors and publishing staff are confident that our many layers of quality assurance have produced textbooks that are the leaders of the industry for their integrity and correctness. Please view the Acknowledgments section for more details on the many people involved in this process.

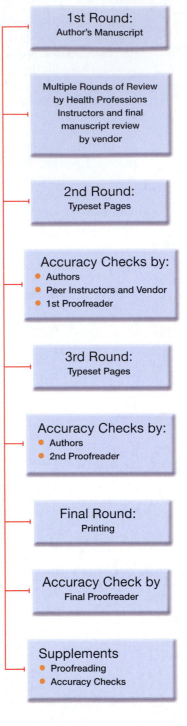

The following test covers basic mathematical concepts that you will need to understand and calculate dosages. This test will help you determine which concepts you need to review before continuing. You should already be able to perform basic operations—addition, subtraction, multiplication, and division—with whole numbers. The test covers fractions, decimals, percents, ratios, and proportions.

Take two hours to answer the following 72 questions. Then check your answers on page A-1. Review the questions you answered incorrectly to learn more about any basic math weaknesses. Then, as needed, review that content in Chapters 1 through 3. Each question (or group of questions) has an "LO" listed to indicate the learning outcome addressed by the question. If you need to review, these LO indicators will help you find the appropriate material in the text.

1. Convert $\frac{14}{3}$ to a mixed number. (LO 1.1)

2. Convert $3\frac{7}{8}$ to a fraction. (LO 1.1)

3. Convert $\frac{8}{5}$ to a mixed number. (LO 1.1)

4. Convert $2\frac{3}{4}$ to a fraction. (LO 1.1)

Find the missing numerator in the following equations. (LO 1.2, 3.4)

5. $\frac{2}{7} = \frac{x}{21}$

6. $1\frac{1}{8} = \frac{x}{16}$

7. Reduce $\frac{40}{100}$ to lowest terms. (LO 1.3)

8. Which fraction has the greater value, $\frac{3}{8}$ or $\frac{2}{6}$? (LO 1.5)

9. Reduce $\frac{48}{10}$ and rewrite the answer as a mixed number. (LO 1.1, 1.3)

10. Which number has a greater value, $3\frac{1}{3}$ or $3\frac{1}{4}$? (LO 1.5)

Calculate the following. Reduce fractions to lowest terms and rewrite any fractions as mixed numbers. (LO 1.1, 1.2, 1.3, 1.4, 1.6, 1.7, 1.8, 1.9)

11. $\frac{4}{5} + \frac{3}{8}$

12. $1\frac{1}{3} + \frac{5}{7}$

13. $\frac{7}{10} - \frac{1}{4}$

14. $8\frac{1}{4} - 2\frac{1}{3}$

15. $\frac{3}{5} \times \frac{1}{9}$

16. $3\frac{1}{5} \times 4\frac{3}{8}$

17. $\frac{2}{3} \div \frac{4}{5}$

18. $5\frac{1}{4} \div 2\frac{5}{8}$

19. $\frac{1}{4} + \frac{1}{3}$

20. $2\frac{3}{8} - \frac{3}{4}$

21. $7\frac{1}{2} \times \frac{3}{4}$

22. $3\frac{1}{3} \div 2$

23. Which number has the lesser value, 1.01 or 1.009? (LO 2.1)

24. Round 14.42 to the nearest whole number. (LO 2.2)

25. Round 6.05 to the nearest tenth. (LO 2.2)

26. Round 19.197 to the nearest hundredth. (LO 2.2)

27. Convert $3\frac{4}{5}$ to a decimal number. If necessary, round to the nearest tenth. (LO 2.3)

28. Convert 0.045 to a fraction or a mixed number. Reduce to lowest terms. (LO 2.4)

29. Which number has a greater value, 1.015 or 1.0105?

30. Convert $7\frac{1}{8}$ to a decimal number.

31. Round 3.08 to the nearest whole number.

32. Convert 3.6 to a fraction or mixed number. Reduce to lowest terms.

Calculate the following. (LO 2.5, 2.6, 2.7)

33. $7.289 + 8.011$	34. $0.012 + 0.9 + 4.2$
35. $19.1 - 4.4$	36. $100.03 - 0.6$
37. 0.07×3.2	38. $0.4 \div 0.02$
39. $6 - 1.025$	40. 1.4×1.5

41. $1.05 \div 2$

42. Convert 0.8 percent to a decimal number. (LO 3.1)

43. Convert 0.99 to a percent. (LO 3.1)

44. Convert 260 percent to a fraction or mixed number. (LO 3.1)

45. Convert $1\frac{1}{8}$ to a percent. (LO 2.3, 3.1)

46. Convert 7 : 12 to a fraction. (LO 3.2)

47. Convert $\frac{10}{50}$ to a ratio. Reduce to lowest terms. (LO 3.2)

48. Convert 1 : 12 to a decimal. Round to the nearest hundredth, if necessary. (LO 3.2)

49. Convert 0.4 to a ratio. Reduce to lowest terms. (LO 3.2)

50. Convert 3 : 8 to a percent. Round to the nearest percent, if necessary. (LO 3.1)

51. Convert 0.5 percent to a ratio. Reduce to lowest terms. (LO 3.2)

52. Convert 8:3 to a mixed number. (LO 3.2)

53. Convert 0.15 to a ratio. Reduce to lowest terms. (LO 3.2)

54. Convert 1.05 to a percent. (LO 3.1)

55. Convert 1.5% to a fraction. Reduce to lowest terms. (LO 3.1)

Find the missing value in the following proportions. (LO 3.4)

56. $8 : 16 = x : 8$

57. $\frac{5}{9} = \frac{x}{27}$

58. $8 : 12 = x : 9$

59. $\frac{2}{7} = \frac{x}{28}$

60. $\frac{x}{4} = \frac{8}{32}$

61. A healthcare professional is instructed to give a patient $1\frac{1}{2}$ teaspoons of cough syrup 4 times a day. How many teaspoons of cough syrup will be given each day? (LO 3.4)

62. A healthcare professional tries to keep the equivalent of 12 bottles of a medication on hand. The hospital's first floor has $1\frac{1}{2}$ bottles, the second floor has $1\frac{3}{4}$ bottles, the third floor has $3\frac{1}{4}$ bottles, and the supply closet has 3 bottles. Is there enough medication on hand? If not, how much should be ordered? (LO 1.6)

63. A bottle contains 75 milliliters (mL) of a liquid medication. Since the bottle was opened, one patient has received 3 doses of 2.5 mL. A second patient has received 4 doses of 2.2 mL. How much medication remains in the bottle? (LO 2.5, 2.6)

64. A tablet contains 0.125 milligram (mg) of medication. A patient receives 3 tablets a day for 5 days. How many milligrams of medication does the patient receive over the 5 days? (LO 2.6)

65. An IV bag contained 1000 mL of a liquid. The liquid was administered to a patient, and now there is 400 mL left in the bag after 3 hours. How much IV fluid did the patient receive each hour? (LO 3.4)

66. The patient is taking 0.5 mg of medication 4 times a day. How many milligrams would the patient receive after $1\frac{1}{2}$ days? (LO 2.6, 3.4)

67. The patient took 0.88 microgram (mcg) every morning and 1.2 mcg each evening for 4 days. What was the total amount of medication taken? (LO 2.5, 2.6)

68. Write a ratio that represents that 500 mL of solution contains 5 mg of drug. (LO 3.3)

69. Write a ratio that represents that every tablet in a bottle contains 25 mg of drug. (LO 3.3)

70. Write a ratio that represents that 3 mL of solution contains 125 mg of drug. (LO 3.4)

71. A patient takes 5 mL of a medication twice a day. How long will 120 mL last? (LO 3.4)

72. Write a ratio that represents 2 mg of drug in 1 mL of a liquid. (LO 3.2)

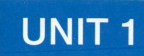

UNIT 1

Overview of Basic Math

1 Fractions

He who is ashamed of asking is ashamed of learning.

—Danish proverb

Learning Outcomes

When you have completed Chapter 1, you will be able to:

1.1 Produce fractions and mixed numbers in the proper form.

1.2 Produce and identify equivalent fractions.

1.3 Determine the simplest form of a fraction.

1.4 Find the least common denominator.

1.5 Compare the values of fractions.

1.6 Add fractions.

1.7 Subtract fractions.

1.8 Multiply fractions.

1.9 Divide fractions.

KEY TERMS

Complex fraction

Denominator

Equivalent fractions

Least common denominator

Mixed number

Numerator

Prime number

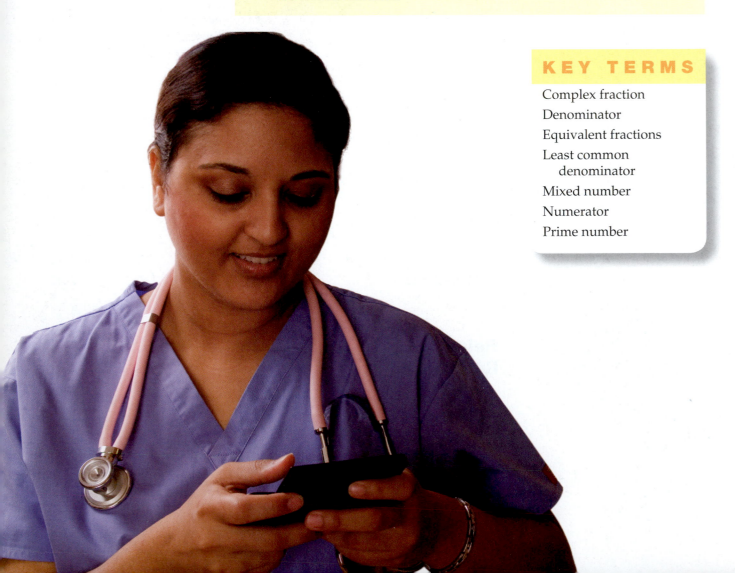

INTRODUCTION

Basic math skills, such as working with fractions, are the building blocks for accurate dosage calculations. To prepare yourself mathematically, you must be confident in your math skills; so do not be afraid to ask for help while you are learning these important concepts. Remember that a minor mistake in basic math can mean major errors in the patient's medication.

1.1 Fractions and Mixed Numbers

Fractions measure a portion or part of a whole amount. They are written in two ways: as common fractions or as decimals. In medical settings, it is sometimes necessary to convert from one type of fraction to another.

Common Fractions

A common fraction represents parts of a whole. It consists of two numbers and a fraction bar, and it is written in the form:

$$\frac{\text{Numerator}}{\text{Denominator}}$$

The **denominator**—the bottom part of the fraction—represents the whole. It can *never* equal zero. Suppose the whole is 1 yard (yd). You could express the denominator in many ways: as 1 (the yard as a whole), 3 (the yard as 3 feet), or 36 (the yard as 36 inches).

The **numerator**—the top part of the fraction—represents parts of the whole. If you buy 2 feet (ft) of fabric out of a yard, you can express the numerator as 2 feet (ft) with the denominator as 3 feet (ft). The fraction $\frac{2}{3}$ represents how much of a yard of fabric you buy, or 2 of 3 ft. If you buy less fabric, say, 9 inches (in.), you can express the numerator as 9 with the denominator as 36 inches (in.). The fraction $\frac{9}{36}$ represents how much of a yard of fabric you buy, or 9 of 36 inches (in.).

Suppose you are working with a medicine tablet that is scored (marked) for division in two parts, and you must administer one part of that tablet each day. The denominator represents the whole tablet. The numerator represents one part, the amount that you administer each day. The fraction, or part, of the tablet that you must administer each day is written as:

$$\frac{\text{Numerator}}{\text{Denominator}} = \frac{1 \text{ part}}{2 \text{ parts}} = \frac{1}{2}$$

This number is read *one-half*. The denominator is 2, since two parts make up the whole. If you administer 1 part each day, you administer $\frac{1}{2}$ of the tablet.

If you have trouble remembering which number is the numerator and which is the denominator, note that the words *denominator* and *down* begin with the letter d. The <u>d</u>enominator is <u>d</u>own, under the fraction bar.

The fraction $\frac{2}{3}$, read as *two-thirds*, means two parts out of the three parts that make up the whole. The fraction bar also means *divided by*. Thus, $\frac{2}{3}$ can be read as "two divided by three," or $2 \div 3$. This definition is important when you change fractions to decimals.

Sometimes fractions show the relationship between part of a group and the whole group. For example, in a group of 15 patients with hyperthyroidism, 9 patients respond well to a medication. The other 6 patients show no change. The number of patients in the full group, 15, is the whole, or the denominator. You write the fraction of patients who respond well to the medication as:

$$\frac{\text{Part}}{\text{Whole}} = \frac{\text{respond well}}{\text{whole group}} = \frac{9}{15}$$

Similarly, the fraction of patients who show no change is:

$$\frac{\text{Part}}{\text{Whole}} = \frac{\text{show no change}}{\text{whole group}} = \frac{6}{15}$$

RULE 1-1	When the denominator is 1, the fraction equals the number in the numerator.
Example	$\frac{4}{1} = 4$ $\frac{100}{1} = 100$ Check these equations by treating each fraction as a division problem. $4 \div 1 = 4$ $100 \div 1 = 100$

GO TO . . . Open the CD-ROM that accompanies your textbook, and select Chapter 1, Fractions (LO 1.1). Review the animation and example problems; then complete the practice problems. Continue to the next section of the book once you have mastered the information presented.

Mixed Numbers

Fractions with a value greater than 1 are more properly written as mixed numbers. A **mixed number** combines a whole number with a fraction. Examples include $2\frac{2}{3}$ (two and two-thirds), $1\frac{7}{8}$ (one and seven-eighths) and $12\frac{31}{32}$ (twelve and thirty-one thirty-seconds).

RULE 1-2	**1.** If the numerator of the fraction is less than the denominator, the fraction has a value less than (<) 1.
	2. If the numerator of the fraction is equal to the denominator, the fraction has a value equal to (=) 1.
	3. If the numerator of the fraction is greater than the denominator, the fraction has a value greater than (>) 1. Fractions with a value greater than one may be written as a mixed number.

GO TO . . . Open the CD-ROM that accompanies your textbook, and select Chapter 1, Mixed Numbers (LO 1.1). Review the animation and example problems; then complete the practice problems. Continue to the next section of the book once you have mastered the information presented.

Example 1	**a.** The fraction $\frac{8}{9}$ is less than 1 because the numerator (8) is less than the denominator (9). This can be written $\frac{8}{9} < 1$.
	b. The fraction $\frac{3}{4}$ is less than 1 because the numerator (3) is less than the denominator (4). This can be written $\frac{3}{4} < 1$.

Example 2	**a.** $\frac{12}{12}$ is equal to 1 because the numerator (12) is equal to the denominator (12). This can be written $\frac{12}{12} = 1$.
	b. $\frac{32}{32}$ is equal to 1 because the numerator (32) is equal to the denominator (32). This can be written $\frac{32}{32} = 1$.
Example 3	**a.** $\frac{8}{5}$ is greater than 1 because the numerator (8) is greater than the denominator (5). This can be written $\frac{8}{5} > 1$.
	b. $\frac{11}{4}$ is greater than 1 because the numerator (11) is greater than the denominator (4). This can be written $\frac{11}{4} > 1$.

RULE 1-3	To convert a fraction to a mixed number:
	1. Divide the numerator by the denominator. The result will be a whole number plus a remainder.
	2. Write the remainder as the numerator over the original denominator.
	3. Combine the whole number and the fractional remainder. This mixed number equals the original fraction.
	Reminder: This rule is only applied when the numerator is greater than the denominator.
Example 1	Convert $\frac{11}{4}$ to a mixed number.
	1. Divide the numerator by the denominator:
	$11 \div 4 = 2 \text{ R3}$ (R3 means a *remainder* of 3.)
	The result is the whole number 2 with a remainder of 3.
	2. Write the remainder as the numerator over the original denominator of 4.
	$\dfrac{\text{Remainder}}{\text{Denominator}} = \dfrac{3}{4}$
	3. Combine the whole number and the fractional remainder:
	$2 + \dfrac{3}{4} = 2\dfrac{3}{4}$
	The mixed number $2\frac{3}{4}$ equals the original fraction $\frac{11}{4}$.
Example 2	Convert $\frac{23}{7}$ to a mixed number.
	1. $23 + 7 = 3 \text{ R2}$
	The result is the whole number 3 with a remainder of 2
	2. $\dfrac{\text{Remainder}}{\text{Denominator}} = \dfrac{2}{7}$
	3. $3 + \dfrac{2}{7} = 3\dfrac{2}{7}$
	The fraction $\frac{23}{7}$ equals the mixed number $3\frac{2}{7}$.

GO TO . . . Open the CD-ROM that accompanies your textbook, and select Chapter 1, Converting Fractions (LO 1.1). Review the animation and example problems; then complete the practice problems. Continue to the next section of the book once you have mastered the information presented.

You can also convert mixed numbers to fractions. This is often necessary before you use the number in a calculation.

RULE 1-4	To convert a mixed number to a fraction: **1.** Multiply the whole number by the denominator of the fraction. **2.** Add the product from step 1 to the numerator of the fraction. **3.** Write the sum from step 2 over the original denominator. The result is a fraction equal to the original mixed number. You can also use this equation for converting a mixed number to a fraction: $$\text{Whole number} \left(\frac{\text{numerator}}{\text{denominator}} \right) = \frac{(\text{whole number} \times \text{denominator}) + \text{numerator}}{\text{denominator}}$$
Example 1	Convert $5\frac{1}{3}$ to a fraction. The whole number is 5. The denominator of the fraction is 3. The numerator of the fraction is 1 **1.** Multiply the whole number by the denominator of the fraction. $5 \times 3 = 15$ **2.** Add the product from step 1 to the numerator of the fraction. $15 + 1 = 16$ **3.** Write the sum from step 2 over the original denominator. $\dfrac{16}{3}$ Thus, $5\frac{1}{3} = \frac{16}{3}$.
Example 2	Convert $10\frac{7}{8}$ to a fraction. The whole number is 10. The denominator is 8. The numerator is 7. **1.** $10 \times 8 = 80$ **2.** $80 + 7 = 87$ **3.** $\dfrac{87}{8}$ Thus, $10\frac{7}{8} = \frac{87}{8}$.

GO TO . . . Open the CD-ROM that accompanies your textbook, and select Chapter 1, Converting Mixed Numbers (LO 1.1). Review the animation and example problems; then complete the practice problems. Continue to the next section of the book once you have mastered the information presented.

While performing a calculation, a healthcare professional adds the following numbers: $21\frac{3}{4}$, $12\frac{1}{2}$, and $1\frac{1}{2}$. He calculates an answer of $49\frac{1}{4}$. Before he accepts this answer as correct, however, he asks himself "Is this reasonable?" In order to answer this question, he does a quick estimation. First, he adds the whole numbers from each of the mixed numbers in the problem: $21 + 12 + 1 = 34$. Then he rounds each mixed number up to a whole number and adds them: $22 + 13 + 2 = 37$. He recognizes that the correct answer to the problem must be between 34 and 37, so his original answer is incorrect. He likely entered one of the numbers into his calculator incorrectly. When he repeats the original calculation, he now comes up with an answer of $35\frac{3}{4}$. This is between the values that he expected based on his estimate, so it is a reasonable answer to the problem.

Think! . . . Is It Reasonable? When performing calculations, there are many steps where an error might be made. In this case, a number had been entered incorrectly into a calculator. While errors like this can happen to anyone, they can usually be detected by performing a quick check to see if the answer is reasonable. Throughout this text you will be asked to "Think! . . . Is It Reasonable?" on a number of examples in each chapter. This question is included as a reminder, but you should develop the habit of asking yourself the same question *every time you perform a calculation.* When performing a calculation, analyze the problem and try to estimate a reasonable range for the answer. This critical thinking skill can help you to detect errors and should become a part of every calculation you perform.

REVIEW AND PRACTICE

1.1 Fractions and Mixed Numbers

1. What is the numerator in $\frac{17}{100}$?

2. What is the numerator in $\frac{8}{3}$?

3. What is the denominator in $\frac{4}{100}$?

4. What is the denominator in $\frac{60}{1}$?

5. Twelve patients are in a hospital ward. Four have type A blood.
   a. What fraction of the patients have type A blood?
   b. What fraction of the patients do not have type A blood?

6. Twenty patients are in a hospital ward. Six have diabetes.
   a. What fraction of the patients have diabetes?
   b. What fraction of the patients do not have diabetes?

7. Write this expression as a fraction: $16 \div 3$

8. Write this expression as a fraction: $4 \div 15$

9. Write this expression as a fraction: $3 \div 4$

10. Insert <, >, or = to make a true statement, where < means less than, > means greater than, and = means equal to.

   a. $\frac{14}{14}$ 1

   b. $\frac{24}{32}$ 1

   c. $\frac{125}{100}$ 1

11. Insert <, >, or = to make a true statement, where < means less than, > means greater than, and = means equal to.

   a. $\frac{24}{3}$ 1

   b. $\frac{75}{100}$ 1

   c. $\frac{18}{18}$ 1

Convert the following fractions to mixed or whole numbers.

12. $\frac{43}{6}$

13. $\frac{17}{3}$

14. $\frac{100}{20}$

15. $\frac{50}{50}$

16. $\frac{8}{5}$

17. $\frac{167}{25}$

18. $\frac{16}{12}$

Convert the following mixed numbers to fractions.

19. $2\frac{16}{17}$

20. $8\frac{8}{9}$

21. $1\frac{1}{10}$

22. $4\frac{1}{8}$

23. $103\frac{2}{3}$

24. $6\frac{7}{8}$

25. $8\frac{1}{5}$

To check your answers, see the Answer section at the end of the book, which starts on page A-1.

1.2 Equivalent Fractions

Two fractions may have the same value even when they are written differently. These are known as **equivalent fractions.** Suppose you and a friend are sharing a pizza equally, dividing it in half. If you cut the pizza into eight slices, you will each get four pieces, or $\frac{4}{8}$ of the whole pizza. If you cut the pizza into six slices, you will each get three pieces, or $\frac{3}{6}$. And if you cut the pizza into four slices, you will each get two slices, or $\frac{2}{4}$. Whether you get $\frac{4}{8}$, $\frac{3}{6}$, or $\frac{2}{4}$ of the pizza, you still have the same amount: one-half or $\frac{1}{2}$ of the pizza (see Figure 1-1). Thus, $\frac{4}{8} = \frac{3}{6} = \frac{2}{4} = \frac{1}{2}$. These four fractions are equivalent fractions.

CONVERTING FRACTIONS Equivalent fractions help you compare measurements more easily. They also help you add and subtract fractions that have different denominators.

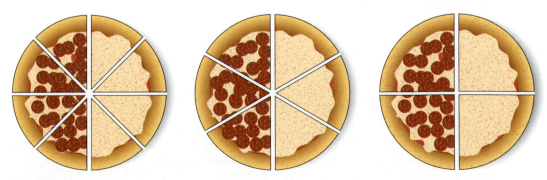

Figure 1-1 Equivalent fractions.

RULE 1-5	To find an equivalent fraction, multiply or divide both the numerator and denominator by the same number. *Exception:* The numerator and denominator cannot be multiplied or divided by zero.
Example 1	Find equivalent fractions for $\frac{2}{4}$. $$\frac{2 \times 2}{4 \times 2} = \frac{4}{8} \qquad \frac{2 \times 3}{4 \times 3} = \frac{6}{12} \qquad \frac{2 \div 2}{4 \div 2} = \frac{1}{2} \qquad \frac{2 \times 10}{4 \times 10} = \frac{20}{40}$$ Thus, $\frac{2}{4} = \frac{4}{8} = \frac{6}{12} = \frac{1}{2} = \frac{20}{40}$ These are equivalent fractions.
Example 2	Find equivalent fractions for $\frac{4}{7}$. $$\frac{4 \times 3}{7 \times 3} = \frac{12}{21} \qquad \frac{4 \times 5}{7 \times 5} = \frac{20}{35} \qquad \frac{4 \times 10}{7 \times 10} = \frac{40}{70} \qquad \frac{4 \times 100}{7 \times 100} = \frac{400}{700}$$ Thus, $\frac{4}{7} = \frac{12}{21} = \frac{20}{35} = \frac{40}{70} = \frac{400}{700}$. These are equivalent fractions. **Think! . . . Is It Reasonable?** In this case, the original numerator was greater than $\frac{1}{2}$ of the denominator. Since this was true for the original fraction, it should also be true for all of the equivalent fractions.
Example 3	Find some equivalent fractions for 4 To find equivalent fractions for a whole number, first write the whole number as a fraction. Then proceed as before. $$4 = \frac{4}{1}$$ $$\frac{4 \times 2}{1 \times 2} = \frac{8}{2} \qquad \frac{4 \times 3}{1 \times 3} = \frac{12}{3} \qquad \frac{4 \times 4}{1 \times 4} = \frac{16}{4} \qquad \frac{4 \times 5}{1 \times 5} = \frac{20}{5}$$ Thus, $4 = \frac{4}{1} = \frac{8}{2} = \frac{12}{3} = \frac{16}{4} = \frac{20}{5}$. These are some equivalent fractions.
Example 4	Find some equivalent fractions for $1\frac{4}{6}$. To find equivalent fractions for a mixed number, first convert the mixed number to a fraction. **1.** $1 \times 6 = 6$ **2.** $6 + 4 = 10$ **3.** $1\frac{4}{6} = \frac{10}{6}$ Now follow the same steps used in Examples 1 through 3. $$\frac{10 \times 2}{6 \times 2} = \frac{20}{12} \qquad \frac{10 \times 3}{6 \times 3} = \frac{30}{18} \qquad \frac{10 \div 2}{6 \div 2} = \frac{5}{3} \qquad \frac{10 \times 10}{6 \times 10} = \frac{100}{60}$$ Thus, $1\frac{4}{6} = \frac{10}{6} = \frac{20}{12} = \frac{30}{18} = \frac{5}{3} = \frac{100}{60}$.

GO TO . . . Open the CD-ROM that accompanies your textbook, and select Chapter 1, Equivalent Fractions (LO 1.2). Review the animation and example problems; then complete the practice problems. Continue to the next section of the book once you have mastered the information presented.

FINDING MISSING NUMERATORS Suppose you want to convert a fraction into an equivalent one with a specific denominator. To convert $\frac{1}{5}$ to tenths, find the missing value in $\frac{1}{5} = \frac{x}{10}$. The x stands for the number you want to find.

In this case multiply the numerator in the original fraction by the denominator in the new fraction. Then divide the result by the original denominator. The original numerator is 1 and the denominator is 10.

$$1 \times 10 = 10$$

The original denominator is 5.

$$10 \div 5 = 2$$

$$x = 2 \quad \text{The numerator for the new fraction.}$$

RULE 1-6	To find the missing numerator in an equivalent fraction:
	a. Multiply the original numerator by the denominator of the new fraction.
	b. Divide the product from step a by the original denominator.

Example 1	$\frac{2}{3} = \frac{x}{12}$
	a. Multiply the original numerator by the denominator of the new fraction.
	$2 \times 12 = 24$
	b. Divide the product from step a by the original denominator.
	$24 \div 3 = 8$
	Thus, $x = 8$ and $\frac{2}{3} = \frac{8}{12}$

Example 2	$\frac{28}{60} = \frac{x}{15}$
	a. Multiply the original numerator by the denominator of the new fraction.
	$28 \times 15 = 420$
	b. Divide the product from step a by the original denominator.
	$420 \div 60 = 7$
	Thus, $x = 7$ and $\frac{28}{60} = \frac{7}{15}$
	Thus, $\frac{28}{60} = \frac{28 \div 4}{60 \div 4} = \frac{7}{15}$ and $x = 7$
	Think! . . . Is It Reasonable? In the original fraction, the numerator (28) was slightly less than $\frac{1}{2}$ the value of the denominator (60). Based on this observation, is 7 a reasonable answer?

Example 3	$2\frac{1}{2} = \frac{x}{6}$
	First convert the mixed number into a fraction.
	$2\frac{1}{2} = \frac{(2 \times 2) + 1}{2} = \frac{5}{2}$
	The equation is now $\frac{5}{2} = \frac{x}{6}$.
	a. Multiply the original numerator by the denominator of the new fraction.
	$5 \times 6 = 30$
	b. Divide the product from step a by the original denominator.
	$30 \div 2 = 15$
	Thus, $x = 15$ and $2\frac{1}{2} = \frac{15}{6}$

GO TO . . . Open the CD-ROM that accompanies your textbook, and select Chapter 1, Equivalent Fractions–Finding the Numerator (LO 1.2). Review the animation and example problems; then complete the practice problems. Continue to the next section of the book once you have mastered the information presented.

REVIEW AND PRACTICE

1.2 Equivalent Fractions

Find three equivalent fractions for each of the following.

1. $\frac{4}{5}$
2. $\frac{1}{10}$
3. $\frac{4}{2}$
4. $\frac{15}{9}$
5. 9

6. 24
7. $2\frac{1}{3}$
8. $3\frac{6}{9}$
9. $\frac{7}{12}$
10. $4\frac{1}{4}$

Find the missing numerator in the following equations:

11. $\frac{3}{8} = \frac{x}{16}$
12. $\frac{1}{3} = \frac{x}{27}$
13. $\frac{16}{24} = \frac{x}{6}$
14. $\frac{18}{15} = \frac{x}{5}$
15. $3 = \frac{x}{4}$

16. $5 = \frac{x}{12}$
17. $1\frac{5}{16} = \frac{x}{160}$
18. $4\frac{2}{8} = \frac{x}{4}$
19. $\frac{8}{12} = \frac{x}{24}$
20. $\frac{32}{16} = \frac{x}{4}$

To check your answers, see the Answer section at the end of the book, which starts on page A-1.

1.3 Simplifying Fractions

The last section showed how to find equivalent fractions by multiplying or dividing the numerator and denominator by the same number. When you divide, you simplify (or reduce) a fraction. Reduced or simplified equivalent fractions may be easier to use when you are performing a calculation. It is considered proper form to express your final answer in a fraction that is reduced to its lowest terms.

RULE 1-7	To reduce a fraction to its lowest terms, find the largest whole number that divides evenly into both the numerator and the denominator. When no whole number except 1 divides evenly into them, the fraction is reduced to its lowest terms.
Example 1	Reduce $\frac{10}{15}$ to its lowest terms. Both 10 and 15 are divisible by 5. $$\frac{10 \div 5}{15 \div 5} = \frac{2}{3}$$ No whole number other than 1 divides evenly into *both* 2 and 3. Thus, $\frac{10}{15}$ has been reduced to its lowest terms, $\frac{2}{3}$.

Example 2	Reduce $\frac{24}{30}$ to its lowest terms.
	Both 24 and 30 are divisible by 6.
	$$\frac{24 \div 6}{30 \div 6} = \frac{4}{5}$$
	No whole number other than 1 divides evenly into *both* 4 and 5. Thus, $\frac{24}{30}$ has been reduced to its lowest terms, $\frac{4}{5}$.

GO TO . . . Open the CD-ROM that accompanies your textbook, and select Chapter 1, Reducing Fractions (LO 1.3). Review the animation and example problems; then complete the practice problems. Continue to the next section of the book once you have mastered the information presented.

ERROR ALERT!

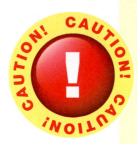

Reducing a Fraction Does Not Automatically Mean You Have Simplified It to Its Lowest Terms

More than one number may divide evenly into both the numerator and the denominator. For example, both 18 and 42 are even numbers. To reduce $\frac{18}{42}$, you can divide by 2, so that:

$$\frac{18 \div 2}{42 \div 2} = \frac{9}{21}$$

You are not done, though. Both 9 and 21 are divisible by 3, so that:

$$\frac{18}{42} = \frac{9}{21} = \frac{9 \div 3}{21 \div 3} = \frac{3}{7}$$

Some fractions are easy to reduce. Looking at $\frac{2}{4}$, you can guess that 2 divides evenly into both the numerator and the denominator, so that $\frac{2 \div 2}{4 \div 2} = \frac{1}{2}$. In other cases, you may have to use several steps. See Table 1-1 for numbers divisible by 2, 3, 4, 5, 6, 8, 9, or 10.

Prime numbers are whole numbers other than 1 that can be evenly divided only by themselves and 1. The first 10 prime numbers are 2, 3, 5, 7, 11, 13, 17, 19, 23, and 29. If either the numerator or the denominator of a fraction is a prime number, and if the other term is not divisible by that prime number, then the fraction is in lowest terms. For example, $\frac{17}{24}$ is in lowest terms. However, you can simplify $\frac{17}{34}$ to $\frac{1}{2}$, dividing both the numerator and denominator by 17.

TABLE 1-1 Is a Number Divisible by 2, 3, 4, 5, 6, 8, 9, or 10?

NUMBER	HINT	EXAMPLE
2	Even numbers (numbers ending with 2, 4, 6, 8, or 0) are divisible by 2.	112; 734; 2936; 10,118; 356, 920
3	If the sum of the digits of a number is divisible by 3, then the number is divisible by 3.	37,887 The sum of the digits is 3 + 7 + 8 + 8 + 7 = 33; 33 is divisible by 3.
4	If the last two digits of a number are divisible by 4, the entire number is divisible by 4.	126,936 The last two digits form a number, 36, that is divisible by 4.
5	Any number that ends with 5 or 0 is divisible by 5.	735 12,290
6	Combine the rules for 2 and 3 If a number is even *and* the sum of its digits is divisible by 3 then the number is divisible by 6.	582 The number is even. The sum of its digits, 5 + 8 + 2 = 15, is divisible by 3.
8	If the last three digits are divisible by 8, then the entire number is divisible by 8.	42,376 Here, 376 is divisible by 8.
9	If the sum of the digits is a multiple of 9, the number is divisible by 9.	42,705 4 + 2 + 7 + 0 + 5 = 18, which is divisible by 9.
10	If a number ends with 0, then the number is divisible by 10.	640

[REVIEW AND PRACTICE

1.3 Simplifying Fractions

Reduce the following fractions to their lowest terms.

1. $\frac{10}{12}$ 2. $\frac{3}{6}$ 3. $\frac{27}{81}$ 4. $\frac{11}{22}$ 5. $\frac{10}{100}$

6. $\frac{55}{100}$ 7. $\frac{4}{5}$ 8. $\frac{6}{17}$ 9. $\frac{21}{27}$ 10. $\frac{35}{50}$

11. $\frac{48}{90}$ 12. $\frac{49}{84}$ 13. $\frac{10}{28}$ 14. $\frac{5}{8}$ 15. $\frac{33}{99}$

16. $\frac{25}{35}$ 17. $\frac{18}{48}$ 18. $\frac{49}{77}$ 19. $\frac{8}{32}$ 20. $\frac{24}{44}$

To check your answers, see the Answer section at the end of the book, which starts on page A-1.

1.4 Finding Common Denominators

A *common denominator* is any number that is a common multiple of all the denominators in a group of fractions. The **least common denominator** (LCD) is the smallest of these numbers. Before you can add and subtract fractions with different denominators, you must first convert them to equivalent fractions with a common denominator. To compare fractions with different denominators, you must also convert them to equivalent fractions with a common denominator.

RULE 1-8	To find the least common denominator (LCD) of a group of fractions:
	1. List the multiples of each denominator.
	2. Compare the lists. Any numbers that appear on all lists are common denominators.
	3. The smallest number that appears on all the lists is the LCD.
	Once you have found the LCD, you can convert each fraction to an equivalent fraction with the LCD as the denominator.

Example 1

Find the least common denominator of $\frac{1}{3}$ and $\frac{1}{2}$. Then convert each to an equivalent fraction with the LCD.

1. The number 3 divides evenly into 3, <u>6</u>, 9, <u>12</u>, 15, 18, and 21. The number 2 divides evenly into 2, 4, <u>6</u>, 8, 10, <u>12</u>, 14, 16, and <u>18</u>.

2. The numbers 6, 12, and 18 are common denominators.

3. The smallest number that appears on both lists is 6. It is the least common denominator and is divisible by both 3 and 2.

    Now convert $\frac{1}{3}$ and $\frac{1}{2}$ so that $\frac{1}{3} = \frac{x}{6}$, and $\frac{1}{2} = \frac{x}{6}$.

4. To convert $\frac{1}{3}$ to the equivalent fraction $\frac{x}{6}$.

    a. $6 \div 3 = 2$

    b. $\frac{1}{3} = \frac{1 \times 2}{3 \times 2} = \frac{2}{6}$

5. To convert $\frac{1}{2}$ to the equivalent fraction $\frac{x}{6}$.

    $6 \div 2 = 3$

    $\frac{1}{2} = \frac{1 \times 3}{2 \times 3} = \frac{3}{6}$

The least common denominator is 6 Using this denominator the equivalent fractions are $\frac{1}{3} = \frac{2}{6}$ and $\frac{1}{2} = \frac{3}{6}$.

Example 2

Find the least common denominator of $\frac{1}{4}$, $\frac{1}{6}$, and $\frac{1}{8}$. Then convert each to an equivalent fraction with the LCD.

1. The number 4 divides evenly into 4, 8, 12, 16, 20, and <u>24</u>

    The number 6 divides evenly into 6, 12, 18, and <u>24</u>

    The number 8 divides evenly into 8, 16, and <u>24</u>

2. The number 24 is a common denominator.

3. In this case, 24 is the LCD.

4. $\frac{1}{4} = \frac{x}{24}$

    $24 \div 4 = 6$

    $\frac{1}{4} = \frac{1 \times 6}{4 \times 6} = \frac{6}{24}$

5. $\frac{1}{6} = \frac{x}{24}$

    $24 \div 6 = 4$

$$\frac{1}{6} = \frac{1 \times 4}{6 \times 4} = \frac{4}{24}$$

6. $\frac{1}{8} = \frac{x}{24}$

$$24 \div 8 = 3$$

$$\frac{1}{8} = \frac{1 \times 3}{8 \times 3} = \frac{3}{24}$$

The least common denominator is 24. Using this denominator, we see the equivalent fractions are:

$$\frac{1}{4} = \frac{6}{24}$$

$$\frac{1}{6} = \frac{4}{24}$$

$$\frac{1}{8} = \frac{3}{24}$$

GO TO . . . Open the CD-ROM that accompanies your textbook, and select Chapter 1, Finding the LCD (LO 1.4). Review the animation and example problems; then complete the practice problems. Continue to the next section of the book once you have mastered the information presented.

You may find it difficult to find common denominators of fractions with large denominators. However, you can simply multiply the individual denominators to find a common denominator.

RULE 1-9	To convert fractions with large denominators to equivalent fractions with a common denominator:
	1. List the denominators of all the fractions.
	2. Multiply the denominators. The product is a common denominator. Convert each fraction to an equivalent one with the common denominator.
Example 1	Convert $\frac{1}{7}$ and $\frac{1}{19}$ to equivalent fractions with a common denominator.
	1. The denominators are 7 and 19.
	2. Multiply 7×19. The common denominator is 133.
	$\dfrac{1}{7} = \dfrac{1 \times 19}{7 \times 19} = \dfrac{19}{133}$ and $\dfrac{1}{19} = \dfrac{1 \times 7}{19 \times 7} = \dfrac{7}{133}$
	The equivalent fractions are $\frac{19}{133}$ and $\frac{7}{133}$.
Example 2	Convert $\frac{2}{37}$ and $\frac{7}{90}$ to equivalent fractions with a common denominator.
	1. The denominators are 37 and 90.
	2. $37 \times 90 = 3330$
	$\dfrac{2 \times 90}{37 \times 90} = \dfrac{180}{3330}$ and $\dfrac{7 \times 37}{90 \times 37} = \dfrac{259}{3330}$
	The equivalent fractions are $\frac{180}{3330}$ and $\frac{259}{3330}$.

GO TO . . . Open the CD-ROM that accompanies your textbook, and select Chapter 1, Converting Fractions–Large Denominators (LO 1.4). Review the animation and example problems; then complete the practice problems. Continue to the next section of the book once you have mastered the information presented.

REVIEW AND PRACTICE

1.4 Common Denominators

For each set of fractions, find the least common denominator. Then convert each fraction to an equivalent fraction with the LCD.

1. $\frac{1}{3}$ and $\frac{1}{7}$

2. $\frac{1}{5}$ and $\frac{1}{8}$

3. $\frac{1}{25}$ and $\frac{1}{40}$

4. $\frac{1}{24}$ and $\frac{1}{36}$

5. $\frac{1}{2}$ and $\frac{1}{12}$

6. $\frac{1}{6}$ and $\frac{1}{18}$

7. $\frac{5}{6}$ and $\frac{4}{7}$

8. $\frac{3}{4}$ and $\frac{5}{8}$

9. $\frac{1}{9}$ and $\frac{1}{36}$

10. $\frac{5}{24}$ and $\frac{9}{96}$

11. $\frac{4}{5}$ and $\frac{9}{11}$

12. $\frac{5}{6}$ and $\frac{7}{12}$

13. $\frac{11}{30}$ and $\frac{21}{80}$

14. $\frac{5}{48}$ and $\frac{7}{72}$

15. $\frac{1}{2}, \frac{1}{3},$ and $\frac{1}{4}$

16. $\frac{1}{6}, \frac{4}{9},$ and $\frac{13}{24}$

17. $\frac{2}{3}, \frac{4}{9},$ and $\frac{7}{15}$

18. $\frac{1}{4}, \frac{5}{6},$ and $\frac{7}{16}$

19. $\frac{1}{5}, \frac{3}{10},$ and $\frac{7}{20}$

20. $\frac{1}{6}, \frac{5}{24},$ and $\frac{9}{40}$

To check your answers, see the Answer section at the end of the book, which starts on page A-1.

1.5 Comparing Fractions

Suppose a home patient is to take $\frac{3}{4}$ tablespoon (tbs) of medication with lunch. You learn that the patient took $\frac{2}{3}$ tbs. Did the patient take too little, too much, or just the right amount?

To determine this answer, you must be able to compare fractions by comparing the numerators of the equivalent fractions. For this example the equivalent fractions are:

$$\frac{3}{4} = \frac{9}{12} \qquad \frac{2}{3} = \frac{8}{12}$$

$\frac{9}{12}$ is more than $\frac{8}{12}$, so the patient did not take enough.

RULE 1-10

To compare fractions:

1. Write all fractions as equivalent fractions with a common denominator.

2. Write the fractions in order by the size of the numerator. The fraction with the largest numerator is the largest in the group.

3. Restate the comparisons with the original fractions.

Example 1

Order from smallest to largest: $\frac{1}{5}$, $\frac{4}{5}$, and $\frac{3}{10}$.

1. Write the fractions as equivalent fractions with a common denominator. The least common denominator of $\frac{1}{5}$, $\frac{4}{5}$, and $\frac{3}{10}$ is 10.

$$\frac{1}{5} = \frac{x}{10} = \frac{1 \times 2}{5 \times 2} = \frac{2}{10}$$

$$\frac{4}{5} = \frac{x}{10} = \frac{4 \times 2}{5 \times 2} = \frac{8}{10}$$

$$\frac{3}{10} = \frac{3}{10}$$

If you have difficulty with this step, review "Equivalent Fractions" and "Finding Common Denominators" in this chapter.

2. Order the fractions by the size of their numerators, in this case, from smallest to largest.

$$\frac{2}{10} \quad \frac{3}{10} \quad \frac{8}{10}$$

Insert the proper comparison signs.

$$\frac{2}{10} < \frac{3}{10} < \frac{8}{10}$$

3. Restate with the original equivalent fractions.

$$\frac{1}{5} < \frac{3}{10} < \frac{4}{5}$$

Example 2

Order from largest to smallest: $1\frac{7}{8}$, $\frac{6}{3}$, 2, $\frac{2}{8}$.

First, convert all whole and mixed numbers to fractions:

$$1\frac{7}{8} = \frac{15}{8}$$

$$2 = \frac{2}{1}$$

If you have difficulty with this step, review "Producing Fractions and Mixed Numbers in the Proper Form" in this chapter.

1. Write all fractions as equivalent fractions with a common denominator. The LCD for this set of fractions is 24

$$1\frac{7}{8} = \frac{15}{8} = \frac{x}{24} = \frac{15 \times 3}{8 \times 3} = \frac{45}{24}$$

$$\frac{6}{3} = \frac{x}{24} = \frac{6 \times 8}{3 \times 8} = \frac{48}{24}$$

$$2 = \frac{2}{1} = \frac{x}{24} = \frac{2 \times 24}{1 \times 24} = \frac{48}{24}$$

$$\frac{2}{8} = \frac{x}{24} = \frac{2 \times 3}{8 \times 3} = \frac{6}{24}$$

2. Write the fractions in order by the size of their numerator.

$$\frac{48}{24} \quad \frac{48}{24} \quad \frac{45}{24} \quad \frac{6}{24}$$

Insert the proper comparison signs.

$$\frac{48}{24} = \frac{48}{24} > \frac{45}{24} > \frac{6}{24}$$

3. Restate with the original equivalent fractions.

$$2 = \frac{6}{3} > 1\frac{7}{8} > \frac{2}{8}$$

GO TO . . . Open the CD-ROM that accompanies your textbook, and select Chapter 1, Comparing Fractions (LO 1.5). Review the animation and example problems; then complete the practice problems. Continue to the next section of the book once you have mastered the information presented.

REVIEW AND PRACTICE

1.5 Comparing Fractions

Insert >, <, or = to make a true statement.

1. $\dfrac{1}{5}$ $\dfrac{3}{5}$

2. $\dfrac{7}{9}$ $\dfrac{4}{9}$

3. $\dfrac{2}{8}$ $\dfrac{1}{4}$

4. $\dfrac{7}{10}$ $\dfrac{7}{20}$

5. $\dfrac{3}{24}$ $\dfrac{1}{8}$

6. $\dfrac{11}{3}$ $\dfrac{13}{9}$

7. 1 $\dfrac{2}{3}$

8. $\dfrac{9}{4}$ 2

9. $\dfrac{3}{12}$ $\dfrac{13}{36}$

10. $1\dfrac{1}{12}$ $1\dfrac{5}{12}$

11. $3\dfrac{3}{5}$ $3\dfrac{2}{5}$

12. $1\dfrac{3}{4}$ $1\dfrac{7}{8}$

13. $2\dfrac{1}{10}$ $2\dfrac{1}{8}$

14. $3\dfrac{1}{5}$ $2\dfrac{5}{8}$

15. $\dfrac{9}{5}$ $1\dfrac{8}{10}$

Place in order from largest to smallest.

16. $\dfrac{3}{4}, \dfrac{2}{5}, \dfrac{5}{6}, \dfrac{4}{7}$

17. $\dfrac{1}{3}, \dfrac{4}{7}, \dfrac{5}{9}, \dfrac{1}{2}$

18. $1\dfrac{3}{16}, \dfrac{9}{8}, \dfrac{5}{2}, 2\dfrac{1}{10}$

19. $2\dfrac{1}{2}, \dfrac{5}{3}, \dfrac{12}{9}, 1\dfrac{5}{6}$

20. $\dfrac{1}{2}, \dfrac{3}{5}, \dfrac{6}{7}, \dfrac{5}{8}$

21. A home patient is supposed to take $\dfrac{2}{3}$ tbs of medication with lunch. You learn that the patient took $\dfrac{1}{2}$ tbs. Did the patient take too little, too much, or just the right amount?

22. You want to prepare 150 units of a solution that consists of 25 units of medication mixed with 125 units of water. You find an already prepared solution that has 1 unit of medication for every 5 units of water. Can you use 150 units of the already prepared solution? Explain your answer.

23. Of 12 patients in the north wing, 8 have high blood pressure. Of 15 patients in the east wing, 9 have high blood pressure. Which wing has a larger portion of patients with high blood pressure?

24. You give George his medication once every 8 hours (h). You give Martha the same medication 4 times a day. Who receives medication more often? (In this problem, a day means 24 h.)

25. You have $1\dfrac{3}{4}$ h until your shift starts. Your friend has $1\dfrac{7}{12}$ h. Who has more time before his or her shift starts?

To check your answers, see the Answer section at the end of the book, which starts on page A-1.

1.6 Adding Fractions

Suppose you gave a patient $\dfrac{1}{2}$ tbs of medication with breakfast, $\dfrac{3}{8}$ tbs with lunch, $\dfrac{3}{4}$ tbs with dinner, and another $\dfrac{3}{8}$ tbs at bedtime. To determine the total amount of medication you have given the patient, you must add the fractions. Review Rule 1-11 and then solve this problem in the Review and Practice 1.6, question 24.

RULE 1-11	To add fractions: **1.** Rewrite any mixed numbers as fractions. **2.** Write equivalent fractions with common denominators. The LCD will be the denominator of your answer. **3.** Add the numerators. The sum will be the numerator of your answer. *Reminder:* Answers should be reported in the proper form. If the answer has a value greater than 1, convert it to a mixed number. If the fraction in the answer can be reduced to lower terms, do so.
Example 1	Add $\frac{2}{6} + \frac{3}{6}$. **1.** There are no mixed numbers. **2.** The fractions already have a common denominator. The denominator of the answer is 6. **3.** Add the numerators: $2 + 3 = 5$. The numerator of the answer is 5. The answer is $\frac{5}{6}$. It is already in the proper form.
Example 2	Add $3\frac{1}{4} + 2\frac{1}{2}$. **1.** Rewrite any mixed numbers as fractions. $3\frac{1}{4} = \frac{13}{4}$ $2\frac{1}{2} = \frac{5}{2}$ **2.** Write equivalent fractions with common denominators. The LCD of the fractions is 4. The denominator of the answer is 4. You don't need to change $\frac{13}{4}$. An equivalent fraction for $\frac{5}{2}$ is $\frac{10}{4}$. **3.** Add the numerators. $13 + 10 = 23$ The numerator of the answer is 23. The answer is $\frac{23}{4}$. The proper form for this answer is $5\frac{3}{4}$. **Think! . . . Is It Reasonable?** The mixed numbers being added in this example were a little greater than 3 and 2. The answer is between 5 and 6.
Example 3	Add $1\frac{7}{8} + \frac{2}{3}$. **1.** Rewrite any mixed numbers as fractions. $1\frac{7}{8} = \frac{15}{8}$. $\frac{2}{3}$ is not a mixed number. **2.** Write equivalent fractions with common denominators. The LCD of the fractions is 24. The denominator of the answer is 24. An equivalent fraction for $\frac{15}{8}$ is $\frac{45}{24}$. An equivalent fraction for $\frac{2}{3}$ is $\frac{16}{24}$.

3. Add the numerators.

$$45 + 16 = 61$$

The numerator of the answer is 61.

The answer is $\frac{61}{24}$. The proper form for this answer is $2\frac{13}{24}$.

Example 4	Add $1\frac{2}{5} + \frac{1}{2}$.

1. Rewrite any mixed numbers as fractions:

$1\frac{2}{5} = \frac{7}{5}$. $\frac{1}{2}$ is not a mixed number.

2. Write equivalent fractions with common denominators.

The LCD of the fractions is 10.

The denominator of the answer is 10.

An equivalent fraction for $\frac{7}{5}$ is $\frac{14}{10}$.

An equivalent fraction for $\frac{1}{2}$ is $\frac{5}{10}$.

3. Add the numerators.

$$14 + 5 = 19$$

The numerator of the answer is 19.

The answer is $\frac{19}{10}$. The proper form for this answer is $1\frac{9}{10}$.

GO TO . . . Open the CD-ROM that accompanies your textbook, and select Chapter 1, Adding Fractions (LO 1.6). Review the animation and example problems; then complete the practice problems. Continue to the next section of the book once you have mastered the information presented.

REVIEW AND PRACTICE

1.6 Adding Fractions

Find the following sums. (Rewrite answers in the proper form.)

1. $\frac{1}{8} + \frac{3}{8}$ 2. $\frac{1}{7} + \frac{3}{7}$ 3. $\frac{1}{7} + \frac{2}{14}$ 4. $\frac{2}{5} + \frac{4}{15}$ 5. $\frac{1}{6} + \frac{3}{8}$

6. $\frac{4}{10} + \frac{2}{25}$ 7. $\frac{5}{8} + \frac{7}{12}$ 8. $\frac{5}{6} + \frac{7}{9}$ 9. $2 + \frac{4}{5}$ 10. $\frac{8}{11} + 3$

11. $1\frac{1}{2} + \frac{1}{3}$ 12. $2\frac{3}{8} + \frac{1}{5}$ 13. $\frac{7}{9} + \frac{9}{12}$ 14. $1\frac{2}{5} + 4\frac{3}{7}$ 15. $2\frac{1}{8} + 1\frac{1}{2}$

16. $\frac{1}{2} + \frac{1}{5} + \frac{1}{8}$ 17. $\frac{1}{3} + \frac{1}{4} + \frac{1}{5}$ 18. $\frac{3}{4} + \frac{3}{8} + \frac{7}{12}$ 19. $\frac{1}{2} + \frac{2}{3} + \frac{3}{5}$ 20. $\frac{1}{4} + \frac{2}{5} + \frac{3}{10}$

21. The patient's chart indicates that he weighed 158 pounds (lb) at the end of April. He then gained $\frac{3}{4}$ lb in May and $1\frac{1}{2}$ lb in June. What did he weigh at the end of June?

22. $2\frac{1}{2}$ ounces (oz), $3\frac{3}{4}$ oz, and 5 oz were used from a bottle of solution in the office laboratory. What is the total amount of solution used?

23. Since breakfast, Kelly drank $1\frac{1}{4}$ cups of water, $\frac{2}{3}$ cup of juice, and $\frac{3}{4}$ cup of milk. How much liquid has Kelly had since breakfast?

24. During the day, you gave one of your patients $\frac{1}{2}$ tbs of medication with breakfast, $\frac{3}{8}$ tbs with lunch, $\frac{3}{4}$ tbs with dinner, and $\frac{3}{8}$ tbs at bedtime. What is the total amount of medication you gave your patient?

25. You are observing your patient's sleep pattern over the past 24 h. She slept $7\frac{1}{2}$ h at night, $1\frac{3}{4}$ h after breakfast, and $2\frac{1}{4}$ h after lunch. She also had a $\frac{1}{4}$ h nap before lunch and a $\frac{1}{4}$ h nap after dinner. How many hours did she sleep?

To check your answers, see the Answer section at the end of the book, which starts on page A-1.

1.7 Subtracting Fractions

Subtracting fractions is similar to adding fractions.

RULE 1-12	To subtract fractions: 1. Rewrite any mixed numbers as fractions. 2. Write equivalent fractions with common denominators. The LCD will be the denominator of your answer. 3. Subtract the numerators. The difference will be the numerator of your answer. *Reminder:* Answers should be reported in the proper form. If the answer has a value greater than 1, convert it to a mixed number. If the fraction in the answer can be reduced to lower terms, do so.

Example 1	Subtract $\frac{2}{6} - \frac{3}{12}$.
	
	1. There are no mixed numbers.
	
	2. Write equivalent fractions with common denominators.
	
	   The LCD of the fractions is 12.
	
	   The denominator of the answer is 12.
	
	   An equivalent fraction for $\frac{2}{6}$ is $\frac{4}{12}$.
	
	   You don't need to change $\frac{3}{12}$.
	
	3. Subtract the numerators.
	
	   $4 - 3 = 1$
	
	   The numerator of the answer is 1.
	
	   The answer is $\frac{1}{12}$. It is already in the proper form.

Example 2	Subtract $3\frac{1}{4} - 2\frac{1}{2}$.
	1. Rewrite any mixed numbers as fractions.
	$3\frac{1}{4} = \frac{13}{4}$ $\qquad$ $2\frac{1}{2} = \frac{5}{2}$
	2. Write equivalent fractions with common denominators.
	The LCD of the fractions is 4.
	The denominator of the answer is 4.
	You don't need to change $\frac{13}{4}$.
	An equivalent fraction for $\frac{5}{2}$ is $\frac{10}{4}$.
	3. Subtract the numerators.
	$13 - 10 = 3$
	The numerator of the answer is 3.
	The answer is $\frac{3}{4}$. It is already in the proper form.
Example 3	Subtract $9\frac{3}{4} - 2\frac{3}{8}$.
	1. Rewrite any mixed numbers as fractions.
	$9\frac{3}{4} = \frac{39}{4}$ $\qquad$ $2\frac{3}{8} = \frac{19}{8}$
	2. Write equivalent fractions with common denominators.
	The LCD of the fractions is 8.
	The denominator of the answer is 8.
	An equivalent fraction for $\frac{39}{4}$ is $\frac{78}{8}$.
	You don't need to change $\frac{19}{8}$.
	3. Subtract the numerators.
	$78 - 19 = 59$
	The numerator of the answer is 59.
	The answer is $\frac{59}{8}$. Written as a mixed number, this is $7\frac{3}{8}$.

Think! . . . Is It Reasonable? The mixed numbers being subtracted in this example were a little less than 10 and a little greater than 2. The answer is a little greater than 7.

Example 4	Subtract $6 - 1\frac{1}{2}$.
	1. Rewrite any mixed numbers as fractions.
	6 is not a mixed number.
	$1\frac{1}{2} = \frac{3}{2}$
	2. Write equivalent fractions with common denominators.
	The LCD of the fractions is 2.
	The denominator of the answer is 2.
	An equivalent fraction for 6 is $\frac{12}{2}$.
	You don't need to change $\frac{3}{2}$.
	3. Subtract the numerators.
	$12 - 3 = 9$
	The numerator of the answer is 9.
	The answer is $\frac{9}{2}$. The proper form for the answer is $4\frac{1}{2}$.

GO TO . . . Open the CD-ROM that accompanies your textbook, and select Chapter 1, Subtracting Fractions (LO 1.7). Review the animation and example problems; then complete the practice problems. Continue to the next section of the book once you have mastered the information presented.

REVIEW AND PRACTICE

1.7 Subtracting Fractions

Find the following differences.

1. $7\frac{7}{15} - 4\frac{4}{15}$

2. $\frac{7}{25} - \frac{2}{25}$

3. $\frac{11}{3} - \frac{2}{6}$

4. $\frac{4}{7} - \frac{3}{21}$

5. $\frac{5}{6} - \frac{4}{9}$

6. $\frac{3}{4} - \frac{1}{6}$

7. $1\frac{7}{8} - \frac{1}{4}$

8. $2\frac{5}{8} - \frac{1}{2}$

9. $6\frac{1}{3} - \frac{5}{6}$

10. $4\frac{1}{2} - \frac{3}{4}$

11. $14\frac{9}{10} - 3\frac{1}{3}$

12. $6\frac{6}{7} - 2\frac{3}{5}$

13. $24\frac{1}{8} - 3\frac{3}{16}$

14. $8\frac{7}{10} - 3\frac{3}{4}$

15. $6 - \frac{2}{3}$

16. $7 - \frac{3}{7}$

17. $5 - \frac{3}{5}$

18. $\frac{2}{3} - \frac{1}{2}$

19. $10\frac{1}{5} - \frac{7}{15}$

20. $7\frac{2}{3} - \frac{7}{12}$

21. You give a patient $\frac{3}{4}$ cup (c) of juice, but he only drinks $\frac{3}{8}$ c. How much juice remains?

22. You give a patient $1\frac{1}{4}$ c of water to drink before supper. When you bring in the meal, you see that $\frac{5}{8}$ c remains in the glass. How much water did the patient drink?

23. At the beginning of the day, you have $6\frac{1}{2}$ bottles of a medication on hand. At the end of the day, $2\frac{3}{4}$ bottles remain. How much of the medication was used during the day?

24. Brenda weighed $153\frac{1}{2}$ lb when she began a diet. The first month she lost $2\frac{3}{4}$ lb. The second month she lost $4\frac{1}{2}$ lb. The third month she lost $2\frac{1}{2}$ lb. What does she weigh now? (*Hint:* You can subtract each month separately, or you can calculate her total weight loss first.)

25. The patient's temperature is $101\frac{1}{2}$ degrees. The patient's normal temperature is $98\frac{3}{4}$ degrees. How many degrees above normal is this patient's temperature?

To check your answers, see the Answer section at the end of the book, which starts on page A-1.

1.8 Multiplying Fractions

Unlike adding and subtracting fractions, multiplying fractions does not need a common denominator. Think about what $\frac{2}{3} \times \frac{1}{2}$ means. This problem could be read as "two-thirds times one-half" or "two-thirds of one-half." In Figure 1-2a, a pizza is divided into six slices. Half of the pizza (three slices) has pepperoni. When you look for $\frac{2}{3}$ of $\frac{1}{2}$ of the pizza, you are looking for two-thirds of the pepperoni half.

In Figure 1-2b, two-thirds of the pepperoni half also has mushrooms. The mushroom slices represent $\frac{2}{3}$ of $\frac{1}{2}$ of the pizza, or $\frac{2}{3} \times \frac{1}{2}$. They also represent $\frac{2}{6}$ of the entire pizza. Thus, $\frac{2}{3} \times \frac{1}{2} = \frac{2}{6} = \frac{1}{3}$.

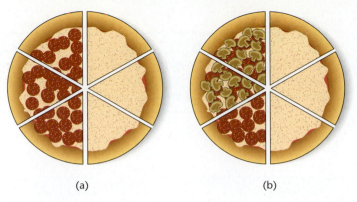

Figure 1-2 Multiplying fractions.

RULE 1-13	To multiply fractions: **1.** Convert any mixed or whole numbers to improper fractions. **2.** Multiply the numerators. Then multiply the denominators. **3.** Reduce the product to its lowest terms.
Example 1	Multiply $\frac{1}{6} \times \frac{3}{4}$. **1.** There are no mixed or whole numbers. **2.** The product of the numerators is $1 \times 3 = 3$. The product of the denominators is $6 \times 4 = 24$. Thus, $\frac{1}{6} \times \frac{3}{4} = \frac{3}{24}$. **3.** $\frac{3}{24}$ reduces to $\frac{1}{8}$.
Example 2	Multiply $\frac{1}{2} \times \frac{7}{3} \times \frac{4}{9}$. The only difference from Example 1 is that now you are multiplying three numerators and three denominators. $$\frac{1}{2} \times \frac{7}{3} \times \frac{4}{9} = \frac{1 \times 7 \times 4}{2 \times 3 \times 9} = \frac{28}{54}$$ $\frac{28}{54}$ reduces to $\frac{14}{27}$.
Example 3	Multiply $1\frac{4}{7} \times 2\frac{3}{5}$. **1.** First convert the mixed numbers to improper fractions. $$1\frac{4}{7} = \frac{11}{7} \quad \text{and} \quad 2\frac{3}{5} = \frac{13}{5}$$ **2.** Now multiply the numerators and denominators. $$1\frac{4}{7} \times 2\frac{3}{5} = \frac{11}{7} \times \frac{13}{5} = \frac{11 \times 13}{7 \times 5} = \frac{143}{35}$$ **3.** $\frac{143}{35}$ converts to $4\frac{3}{35}$.

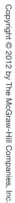

Example 4	Multiply $3 \times \frac{2}{3}$

First convert 3 to the improper fraction $\frac{3}{1}$. Now solve.

$$3 \times \frac{2}{3} = \frac{3}{1} \times \frac{2}{3} = \frac{3 \times 2}{1 \times 3} = \frac{6}{3}$$

$\frac{6}{3}$ reduces to 2.

GO TO . . . Open the CD-ROM that accompanies your textbook, and select Chapter 1, Multiplying Fractions (LO 1.8). Review the animation and example problems; then complete the practice problems. Continue to the next section of the book once you have mastered the information presented.

Reducing terms provides a shortcut that makes multiplying fractions easier. It lets you work with smaller numbers, decreasing the potential for arithmetic errors. If you divide both the numerator and the denominator of a fraction by the same number, you have not changed the fraction's value. You already use this rule to reduce a fraction. This rule also applies to two or more fractions that are being multiplied.

To multiply $\frac{8}{21} \times \frac{7}{16}$, you could multiply the numerators and multiply the denominators.

$$\frac{8}{21} \times \frac{7}{16} = \frac{8 \times 7}{21 \times 16} = \frac{56}{336}$$

$\frac{56}{336}$ reduces to $\frac{1}{6}$, although that may not be immediately clear to you. By reducing terms before multiplying, however, you work with smaller numbers.

RULE 1-14	To reduce terms when you are multiplying fractions, divide both a numerator and a denominator by the same number. You may reduce terms only if a numerator and denominator can both be divided evenly.
Example 1	Reduce terms to solve $\frac{8}{21} \times \frac{7}{16}$.

Both the numerator 8 and the denominator 16 can be divided evenly by 8. You can now write the problem as:

$$\frac{\overset{1}{\cancel{8}}}{21} \times \frac{7}{\underset{2}{\cancel{16}}} \qquad \text{which is equivalent to} \qquad \frac{1}{21} \times \frac{7}{2}$$

The slash marks indicate that 8 and 16 were reduced. In this case, they were divided by 8, reducing 8 and 16 to 1 and 2, respectively. Both the numerator 7 and the denominator 21 are divisible by 7. After you reduce again, you can rewrite the problem as:

$$\frac{\overset{1}{\cancel{8}}}{\underset{3}{\cancel{21}}} \times \frac{\overset{1}{\cancel{7}}}{\underset{2}{\cancel{16}}} \qquad \text{which is equivalent to} \qquad \frac{1}{3} \times \frac{1}{2}$$

Now when you solve, the answer will already be in lowest terms.

$$\frac{8}{21} \times \frac{7}{16} = \frac{\overset{1}{\cancel{8}}}{\underset{3}{\cancel{21}}} \times \frac{\overset{1}{\cancel{7}}}{\underset{2}{\cancel{16}}} = \frac{1}{3} \times \frac{1}{2} = \frac{1}{6}$$

Example 2

$$\frac{27}{36} \times \frac{4}{5}$$

In this problem, one of the fractions has not been reduced to lowest terms. Both 27 and 36 are divisible by 9.

$$\frac{\overset{3}{\cancel{27}}}{\underset{4}{\cancel{36}}} \times \frac{4}{5} \qquad \text{becomes} \qquad \frac{3}{4} \times \frac{4}{5}$$

You can also reduce the numerator 4 and what had begun as the denominator 36. The problem now becomes:

$$\frac{\overset{3}{\cancel{27}}}{\underset{\underset{1}{\cancel{4}}}{\cancel{36}}} \times \frac{\overset{1}{\cancel{4}}}{5} = \frac{3}{\cancel{4}} \times \frac{\overset{1}{\cancel{4}}}{5} = \frac{3}{1} \times \frac{1}{5} = \frac{3}{5}$$

The answer $\frac{3}{5}$ is already reduced to lowest terms.

Example 3

$$2\frac{1}{2} \times \frac{8}{15} \times \frac{45}{4}$$

First convert the mixed number $2\frac{1}{2}$ to the improper fraction $\frac{5}{2}$. Now the problem becomes:

$$\frac{5}{2} \times \frac{8}{15} \times \frac{45}{4}$$

Both the numerator 45 and the denominator 15 are divisible by 15. Both the numerator 8 and the denominator 2 are divisible by 2.

$$\frac{5}{\underset{1}{\cancel{2}}} \times \frac{\overset{4}{\cancel{8}}}{\underset{1}{\cancel{15}}} \times \frac{\overset{3}{\cancel{45}}}{4} = \frac{5}{1} \times \frac{4}{1} \times \frac{3}{4}$$

You have another opportunity to reduce both a numerator and a denominator by 4. The problem now becomes:

$$\frac{5}{\underset{1}{\cancel{2}}} \times \frac{\overset{4}{\cancel{8}}}{\underset{1}{\cancel{15}}} \times \frac{\overset{3}{\cancel{45}}}{4} = \frac{5}{1} \times \frac{\overset{1}{\cancel{4}}}{1} \times \frac{3}{\underset{1}{\cancel{4}}} = \frac{5}{1} \times \frac{1}{1} \times \frac{3}{1} = \frac{15}{1} = 15$$

If you are not sure what numbers will divide evenly into both the numerator and the denominator, review Table 1-1.

GO TO . . . Open the CD-ROM that accompanies your textbook, and select Chapter 1, Reducing Terms–Reducing Fractions (LO 1.8) . Review the animation and example problems; then complete the practice problems. Continue to the next section of the book once you have mastered the information presented.

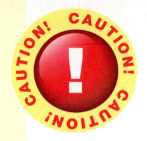

Avoid Reducing Too Many Terms

A term that you plan to reduce may be a factor in more than one numerator or more than one denominator. Each time you reduce a term, you must reduce it from *one numerator* **and** *one denominator*.

Suppose you are multiplying $\frac{7}{12} \times \frac{8}{20}$. You can reduce 4 from the numerator 8. You can also reduce either of the denominators (12 or 20) by 4, but not both. Either of the following is correct.

$$\frac{7}{\underset{3}{\cancel{12}}} \times \frac{\overset{2}{\cancel{8}}}{20} \quad \text{or} \quad \frac{7}{12} \times \frac{\overset{2}{\cancel{8}}}{\underset{5}{\cancel{20}}}$$

However, *you cannot reduce by 4 as follows* in this problem:

$$\frac{7}{\underset{3}{\cancel{12}}} \times \frac{\overset{2}{\cancel{8}}}{\underset{5}{\cancel{20}}}$$

If the problem were $\frac{5}{12} \times \frac{9}{24}$, where the numerator can be reduced by 3 twice, then you could reduce 3 twice in the denominators. Thus,

$$\frac{5}{12} \times \frac{9}{24} = \frac{5}{\underset{4}{\cancel{12}}} \times \frac{\overset{\overset{1}{\cancel{3}}}{\cancel{9}}}{\underset{8}{\cancel{24}}} = \frac{5}{4} \times \frac{1}{8} = \frac{5}{32}$$

REVIEW AND PRACTICE

1.8 Multiplying Fractions

Find the following products. (Rewrite answers in the proper form.)

1. $\frac{1}{6} \times \frac{1}{8}$ 2. $\frac{2}{7} \times \frac{3}{5}$ 3. $\frac{1}{2} \times \frac{6}{8}$ 4. $\frac{6}{9} \times \frac{1}{6}$ 5. $\frac{3}{8} \times \frac{4}{9}$

6. $\frac{5}{12} \times \frac{6}{15}$ 7. $\frac{10}{14} \times \frac{7}{5}$ 8. $\frac{5}{3} \times \frac{9}{10}$ 9. $\frac{9}{8} \times \frac{8}{2}$ 10. $\frac{4}{3} \times \frac{15}{8}$

11. $1\frac{7}{8} \times \frac{4}{5}$ 12. $3\frac{1}{3} \times \frac{9}{15}$ 13. $3\frac{6}{8} \times 5\frac{2}{9}$ 14. $1\frac{5}{6} \times 7\frac{4}{5}$ 15. $\frac{7}{16} \times \frac{4}{3} \times \frac{1}{2}$

16. $\frac{5}{7} \times \frac{3}{10} \times \frac{3}{4}$ 17. $\frac{11}{32} \times \frac{4}{22} \times 12$ 18. $5 \times \frac{7}{15} \times \frac{3}{14}$ 19. $\frac{12}{25} \times \frac{8}{9} \times \frac{15}{16}$ 20. $\frac{49}{20} \times \frac{12}{7} \times \frac{5}{21}$

21. A bottle of liquid medication contains 24 doses. If the hospital has a supply of $9\frac{3}{4}$ bottles of the medication, how many doses are available?

22. A tablet contains $\frac{1}{4}$ grain (gr) of a medication. If you give a patient $1\frac{1}{2}$ tablets 3 times per day, how many grains of the medication are you giving to the patient each day?

23. A patient is supposed to take $\frac{1}{3}$ teaspoon (tsp) of medicine 4 times per day. However, the patient misunderstood the directions and took $\frac{1}{4}$ tsp of medicine 3 times per day.

    a. How much medicine should the patient have taken per day?

    b. How much medicine did the patient take per day?

    c. What is the difference per day between the two amounts?

24. For 4 days, you give a patient $1\frac{1}{2}$ oz of a medication 5 times per day. How much medication did you give the patient over the 4 days?

25. One tablet contains 500 milligrams (mg) of medication. How many milligrams are in $3\frac{1}{2}$ tablets?

To check your answers, see the Answer section at the end of the book, which starts on page A-1.

1.9 Dividing Fractions

You have now learned most of the steps needed to divide fractions. Suppose you have $\frac{3}{4}$ bottle of liquid medication available. The regular dose you would give a patient is $\frac{1}{16}$ bottle, and you want to know how many doses remain in the bottle. You solve this problem by dividing fractions.

You want to solve $\frac{3}{4} \div \frac{1}{16}$, where $\frac{3}{4}$ is the dividend, $\frac{1}{16}$ is the divisor, and your answer is the quotient. The problem is read, "three-quarters divided by one-sixteenth," where you are finding out how many times $\frac{1}{16}$ goes into $\frac{3}{4}$.

To solve this problem, multiply the dividend $\frac{3}{4}$ by the reciprocal of the divisor $\frac{1}{16}$. You find the *reciprocal* of a fraction by inverting it—flipping it so that the numerator becomes the denominator and the denominator becomes the numerator. The reciprocal of $\frac{1}{16}$ is $\frac{16}{1}$. Thus,

$$\frac{3}{4} \div \frac{1}{16} = \frac{3}{4} \times \frac{16}{1}$$

You now solve this as a multiplication problem.

$$\frac{3}{\underset{1}{\cancel{4}}} \times \frac{\overset{4}{\cancel{16}}}{1} = \frac{3}{1} \times \frac{4}{1} = \frac{12}{1} = 12$$

The bottle has 12 doses remaining.

RULE 1-15	To divide fractions:
	1. Convert any mixed or whole numbers to improper fractions.
	2. Invert (flip) the divisor to find its reciprocal.
	3. Multiply the dividend by the reciprocal of the divisor and reduce.
Example 1	Divide $\frac{1}{2} \div \frac{1}{4}$.
	1. The problem has no mixed or whole numbers.
	2. Invert (flip) the divisor $\frac{1}{4}$ to find its reciprocal $\frac{4}{1}$.

3. Multiply the dividend by the reciprocal of the divisor.

$$\frac{1}{2} \div \frac{1}{4} = \frac{1}{2} \times \frac{4}{1} = \frac{1}{\cancel{2}} \times \frac{\cancel{4}^{2}}{1} = \frac{2}{1} = 2$$

Example 2

Divide $1\frac{1}{2} \div \frac{1}{4}$.

1. Convert the mixed number to a fraction.

$$1\frac{1}{2} = \frac{3}{2}$$

2. Invert (flip) the divisor $\frac{1}{4}$ to find its reciprocal $\frac{4}{1}$.

3. Multiply the dividend by the reciprocal of the divisor.

$$1\frac{1}{2} \div \frac{1}{4} = \frac{3}{2} \div \frac{1}{4} = \frac{3}{2} \times \frac{\cancel{4}^{2}}{1} = \frac{3}{1} \times \frac{2}{1} = \frac{6}{1} = 6$$

Example 3

You may have to simplify a **complex fraction,** in which the numerator and the denominator are themselves fractions. The main fraction bar will often be wider and darker than the fraction bars within the numerator and the denominator. You can simply rewrite a complex fraction as an ordinary division problem and proceed.

Simplify $\frac{\frac{7}{10}}{\frac{3}{5}}$.

Here $\frac{7}{10}$ is the numerator and $\frac{3}{5}$ is the denominator. Rewrite the complex fraction as a regular division problem, then solve.

$$\frac{\frac{7}{10}}{\frac{3}{5}} = \frac{7}{10} \div \frac{3}{5} = \frac{7}{10} \times \frac{5}{3} = \frac{7}{\cancel{10}_{2}} \times \frac{\cancel{5}^{1}}{3} = \frac{7}{2} \times \frac{1}{3} = \frac{7}{6} = 1\frac{1}{6}$$

Example 4

Divide $20\frac{1}{6} \div 4$

1. Convert $20\frac{1}{6}$ to $\frac{121}{6}$. Change the whole number 4 to $\frac{4}{1}$.

2. $\frac{121}{6} \div \frac{4}{1}$

Flip (invert) the divisor $\frac{4}{1}$ to find its reciprocal $\frac{1}{4}$.

3. Multiply $\frac{121}{6} \times \frac{1}{4} = \frac{121}{24}$. Reduce answer to proper form $5\frac{1}{24}$.

GO TO . . . Open the CD-ROM that accompanies your textbook, and select Chapter 1, Dividing Fractions (LO 1.9). Review the animation and example problems; then complete the practice problems. Continue to the next section of the book once you have mastered the information presented.

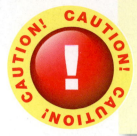

ERROR ALERT!

Write Division Problems Carefully to Avoid Mistakes

Be sure to find the reciprocal of the correct fraction. You want the reciprocal of the divisor when you convert the problem from division to multiplication.

$$\frac{2}{3} \div \frac{4}{5} = \frac{2}{3} \times \frac{5}{4} \qquad \text{not} \qquad \frac{3}{2} \times \frac{4}{5}$$

REVIEW AND PRACTICE

1.9 Dividing Fractions

Find the following quotients. (Rewrite the answers in proper form.)

1. $\frac{4}{9} \div \frac{5}{7}$

2. $\frac{3}{11} \div \frac{4}{5}$

3. $\frac{3}{8} \div \frac{1}{2}$

4. $\frac{1}{6} \div \frac{3}{4}$

5. $\frac{3}{5} \div \frac{2}{8}$

6. $\frac{6}{9} \div \frac{5}{11}$

7. $\frac{9}{10} \div \frac{3}{5}$

8. $\frac{7}{12} \div \frac{21}{36}$

9. $1\frac{3}{4} \div \frac{2}{3}$

10. $\frac{7}{8} \div 1\frac{3}{4}$

11. $4\frac{2}{9} \div 2\frac{3}{8}$

12. $3\frac{1}{2} \div 1\frac{1}{4}$

13. $1\frac{7}{8} \div 9$

14. $6 \div \frac{5}{8}$

15. $\dfrac{\frac{9}{12}}{\frac{4}{6}}$

16. $\dfrac{\frac{2}{9}}{\frac{1}{8}}$

17. $\frac{2}{7} \div \frac{1}{4}$

18. $\frac{7}{10} \div \frac{3}{5}$

19. $5 \div \frac{4}{5}$

20. $\dfrac{\frac{4}{5}}{\frac{3}{8}}$

21. A bottle of pills has 40 tablets scored so that each tablet can be divided into four pieces. If a typical dose is $\frac{1}{4}$ tablet, how many doses does the bottle contain?

22. A healthcare professional administered doses of $2\frac{1}{2}$ milliliters (mL) of medication from a bottle that contained 150 mL. How many $2\frac{1}{2}$ mL doses was the healthcare professional able to give from the bottle?

23. A patient is told to drink the equivalent of 8 glasses of water each day. How many times must the patient drink $\frac{1}{2}$ glass of water to reach the daily goal?

24. A healthcare professional opens a case that has a total of 84 oz of medication. If each vial in the case holds $1\frac{3}{4}$ oz, how many vials are in the case?

25. How many $\frac{2}{3}$ h periods of time are in $8\frac{1}{2}$ h?

To check your answers, see the Answer section at the end of the book, which starts on page A-1.

LEARNING OUTCOME	KEY POINTS

1.1 Produce fractions and mixed numbers in the proper form. Pages 3–8	▶ The numerator of a proper fraction is always smaller than the denominator.
	  • Examples of proper fractions are $\frac{1}{2}, \frac{2}{3}, \frac{4}{15}$.
	▶ A mixed number is made up of a number and a fraction.
	  • Examples of mixed numbers are $3\frac{1}{2}, 2\frac{5}{8}, 12\frac{3}{4}$.
	▶ A fraction with a numerator greater than the denominator is called an improper fraction.
	  • Examples of improper fractions are $\frac{12}{5}, \frac{7}{3}, \frac{5}{2}$.
	▶ It is sometimes necessary to use an improper fraction while performing calculations, but the answer should always be reported as a proper fraction or a mixed number.
	  • For example, an answer of $\frac{5}{2}$ should be rewritten as $2\frac{1}{2}$.

1.2 Produce and identify equivalent fractions. Pages 8–11	▶ In order to perform calculations with fractions, it is sometimes necessary to convert a fraction to an equivalent fraction. ▶ Equivalent fractions are fractions that have the same value but that are written indifferent ways. • The fractions $\frac{1}{3}, \frac{2}{6}, \frac{3}{9}$, and $\frac{4}{12}$ are all equivalent. ▶ Changing a fraction to an equivalent may be necessary before adding or subtracting fractions.
1.3 Determine the simplest form of a fraction. Pages 11–13	▶ The simplest form of a fraction is the equivalent fraction with the lowest numerator and denominator. ▶ After performing calculations involving fractions, the answer should always be reduced to its simplest form. • For example, if you perform a calculation and come up with an answer of $\frac{4}{8}$, the proper answer would be this fraction reduced to its simplest form, which is $\frac{1}{2}$.
1.4 Find the least common denominator. Pages 13–16	▶ Fractions must be converted into equivalent fractions with the same denominator before they can be added or subtracted. • Before subtracting $\frac{1}{3}$ from $\frac{5}{6}$ you will need to find a common denominator. ▶ The least common denominator is the lowest multiple of all denominators in the problem.

1.5 Compare the values of fractions. Pages 16–18	▶ Changing a fraction to an equivalent fraction can make it easier to compare the values of fractions. • It is easier to compare $\frac{5}{8}$ and $\frac{6}{8}$ than it is $\frac{5}{8}$ and $\frac{3}{4}$.
1.6 Add fractions Pages 18–21	▶ Change mixed numbers to improper fractions before adding them. • For example, before adding $3\frac{2}{5} + 1\frac{4}{5}$, rewrite the problem as $\frac{17}{5} + \frac{9}{5}$. ▶ Convert fractions to equivalent fractions with a common denominator before adding them. • For example, before adding $\frac{2}{3} + \frac{1}{4}$, rewrite the problem as $\frac{8}{12} + \frac{3}{12}$.
1.7 Subtract fractions Pages 21–23	▶ Change mixed numbers to improper fractions before subtracting them. • For example, before subtracting $3\frac{2}{5} - 1\frac{4}{5}$, rewrite the problem as $\frac{17}{5} - \frac{9}{5}$. ▶ Convert fractions to equivalent fractions with a common denominator before subtracting them. • For example, before subtracting $\frac{2}{3} - \frac{1}{4}$, rewrite the problem as $\frac{8}{12} - \frac{3}{12}$.
1.8 Multiply fractions Pages 23–27	▶ Fractions do NOT need common denominators when they are multiplied. ▶ Change mixed numbers to improper fractions before multiplying. • Before multiplying $1\frac{2}{3} \times \frac{3}{8}$, rewrite the problem as $\frac{5}{3} \times \frac{3}{8}$. ▶ To multiply fractions, you multiply the numerators and then the denominators. • $\frac{5}{6} \times \frac{7}{8}$ is equal to 5×7 (the numerators) over 6×8 (the denominators).
1.9 Divide fractions Pages 28–30	▶ Fractions do NOT need common denominators when they are divided. ▶ Change mixed numbers to improper fractions before dividing. • Before dividing $1\frac{2}{3} \div \frac{3}{8}$, rewrite the problem as $\frac{5}{3} \div \frac{3}{8}$. ▶ To divide fractions, you multiply the fraction you are dividing into (the dividend) by the *reciprocal* of the fraction that you are dividing by (the divisor). • $\frac{5}{6} \div \frac{7}{8}$ is equal to $\frac{5}{6} \div \frac{8}{7}$

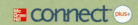
Convert the following mixed numbers to fractions. (LO 1.1)

1. $3\frac{1}{5}$

2. $5\frac{2}{3}$

3. $8\frac{5}{8}$

Reduce the following fractions to their lowest terms. Convert improper fractions to mixed numbers when necessary. (LO 1.3)

4. $\frac{14}{42}$

5. $\frac{12}{45}$

6. $\frac{42}{8}$

Find the least common denominator for each set of fractions, and then write equivalent fractions that use the common denominator. (LO 1.2, 1.4)

7. $\frac{3}{4}$ and $\frac{5}{6}$

8. $\frac{3}{5}$, $\frac{2}{3}$, and $\frac{3}{4}$

Place >, <, or = between the following pairs of fractions to make a true statement. (LO 1.5)

9. $\frac{4}{9}$ $\frac{2}{5}$

10. $\frac{14}{25}$ $\frac{3}{5}$

Perform the following calculations. Give the answer in the proper form. (LO 1.6 to 1.9)

11. $\frac{3}{2} + \frac{1}{3}$

12. $\frac{5}{8} \times \frac{4}{9}$

13. $3\frac{2}{5} - 1\frac{1}{5}$

14. $\frac{5}{7} + \frac{11}{14} + \frac{16}{21}$

15. $\frac{3}{8} \div \frac{2}{3}$

16. $\frac{5}{9} \times \frac{3}{10}$

17. $\frac{4}{9} - \frac{1}{3}$

18. $\frac{7}{15} \div 1\frac{5}{9}$

CHAPTER 1 REVIEW

CHECK UP

Convert the following mixed numbers to fractions. (LO 1.1)

1. $2\frac{3}{8}$ **2.** $1\frac{2}{7}$ **3.** $9\frac{9}{10}$ **4.** $12\frac{11}{12}$

Reduce the following fractions to their lowest terms. Convert improper fractions to mixed numbers when necessary. (LO 1.1, 1.3)

5. $\frac{12}{36}$ **6.** $\frac{39}{48}$ **7.** $\frac{45}{9}$ **8.** $\frac{58}{8}$

Find the least common denominator. Then write an equivalent fraction for each. (LO 1.2, 1.4)

9. $\frac{3}{10}$ and $\frac{4}{5}$ **10.** $\frac{5}{6}$ and $\frac{4}{9}$ **11.** $\frac{3}{8}, \frac{3}{4}$, and $\frac{1}{6}$ **12.** $\frac{7}{10}, \frac{1}{4}$, and $\frac{2}{3}$

Place >, <, or = between the following pairs of fractions to make a true statement. (LO 1.5)

13. $\frac{3}{10}$ ___ $\frac{3}{16}$ **14.** $\frac{3}{2}$ ___ $\frac{8}{5}$ **15.** $1\frac{2}{3}$ ___ $1\frac{16}{24}$ **16.** $\frac{4}{25}$ ___ $\frac{16}{75}$

Perform the following calculations. Give the answer in the proper form. (LO 1.1, 1.6, to 1.9)

17. $\frac{9}{4} + \frac{2}{3}$ **18.** $\frac{3}{5} + \frac{12}{5}$ **19.** $\frac{2}{10} + \frac{1}{100} + \frac{4}{50}$ **20.** $6 + \frac{5}{8} + \frac{1}{3} + \frac{5}{12}$

21. $\frac{11}{9} - \frac{1}{3}$ **22.** $\frac{4}{5} - \frac{3}{4}$ **23.** $3\frac{1}{4} - 1\frac{7}{8}$ **24.** $3 - \frac{2}{7}$

25. $\frac{5}{6} \times \frac{2}{3}$ **26.** $\frac{7}{9} \times \frac{3}{14}$ **27.** $2\frac{2}{5} \times \frac{10}{3}$ **28.** $\frac{3}{8} \times 11$

29. $\frac{1}{7} \div \frac{3}{4}$ **30.** $\frac{12}{13} \div \frac{3}{52}$ **31.** $2\frac{5}{8} \div \frac{1}{6}$ **32.** $\frac{1}{3} \div 1\frac{1}{4}$

33. A medical unit has 18 patients. Eight have type O blood. Five have type A blood. Two have type AB blood. Three have type B blood. Write the fractions that describe the portions of the medical unit patients that have each blood type. (LO 1.1)

34. A patient is supposed to receive $\frac{1}{2}$ cup (c) of medication 3 times per day. Instead, the patient receives $\frac{1}{3}$ c twice per day. During the day, how much medicine does the patient receive? How does that amount compare with the amount ordered? (LO 1.2, 1.4, 1.5, 1.6)

35. During the day, Brian drank $\frac{3}{4}$ c of water 7 times, 1 c of milk 2 times, and $\frac{1}{2}$ c of juice 3 times. How much liquid did Brian consume? (LO 1.2, 1.4, 1.6)

36. A bottle contains 48 mL of liquid medication. If the average dose is $\frac{3}{4}$ mL, how many doses does the bottle contain? (LO 1.9)

CRITICAL THINKING APPLICATIONS

A healthcare professional is asked to arrange a set of instruments on a tray in order from smallest to largest on the basis of the instruments' diameters. The diameters are marked $\frac{1}{4}, \frac{7}{16}, \frac{1}{2}, \frac{1}{8}, \frac{1}{16}, \frac{3}{16}$, and $\frac{5}{16}$. How should the healthcare professional arrange the instruments? Look at the pattern of increase in these measurements. Are any instruments missing in the sequence? If so, which ones? (LO 1.2, 1.4, 1.5)

CASE STUDY

A healthcare professional is tracking the weight of a patient who is retaining fluids because of congestive heart failure. On day 3, the patient is given a diuretic. Here is a summary of the weight changes that occurred. In the column marked "change," write the amount of weight change since the previous measurement. Use a plus (+) sign to indicate weight gained and a minus sign (−) to indicate weight lost. Day 2 has been completed as an example. (LO 1.2, 1.4, 1.6, 1.7)

time	weight in lb	change
Day 1, 8:00 a.m.	$142\frac{1}{2}$	n/a
Day 2, 8:00 a.m.	144	$+1\frac{1}{2}$
Day 3, 8:00 a.m.	$145\frac{3}{4}$	
Day 3, 8:00 a.m.	Patient receives diuretic Lasix (furosemide) 40 mg	
Day 3, 2:00 p.m.	$144\frac{3}{4}$	
Day 3, 4:00 p.m.	Lasix 40 mg	
Day 4, 8:00 a.m.	$142\frac{3}{4}$	
Day 4, 8:00 a.m.	Lasix 20 mg	
Day 4, 4:00 p.m.	$140\frac{1}{2}$	

To check your answers, see the Answer section at the end of the book, which starts on page A-1.

INTERNET ACTIVITY

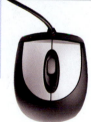

Search the Web for more practice problems with fractions. You might search for "help with fractions," "working with fractions," or "games with fractions."

GO TO . . . Open the CD-ROM that accompanies your textbook, and review the learning outcomes, practice problems, games, slideshow, and other activities presented for this chapter. For a final evaluation, take the chapter test and email or print your results for your instructor. A score of 95 percent or above indicates mastery of the chapter concepts.

2 CHAPTER

Decimals

Learning is not attained by chance, it must be sought for with ardor and attended to with diligence.

—ABIGAIL ADAMS

Learning Outcomes

When you have completed Chapter 2, you will be able to:

2.1 Write decimals and compare their value.

2.2 Apply the rules for rounding decimals.

2.3 Convert fractions into decimals.

2.4 Convert decimals into fractions.

2.5 Add and subtract decimals.

2.6 Multiply decimals.

2.7 Divide decimals.

KEY TERMS

Divisor
Dividend
Quotient

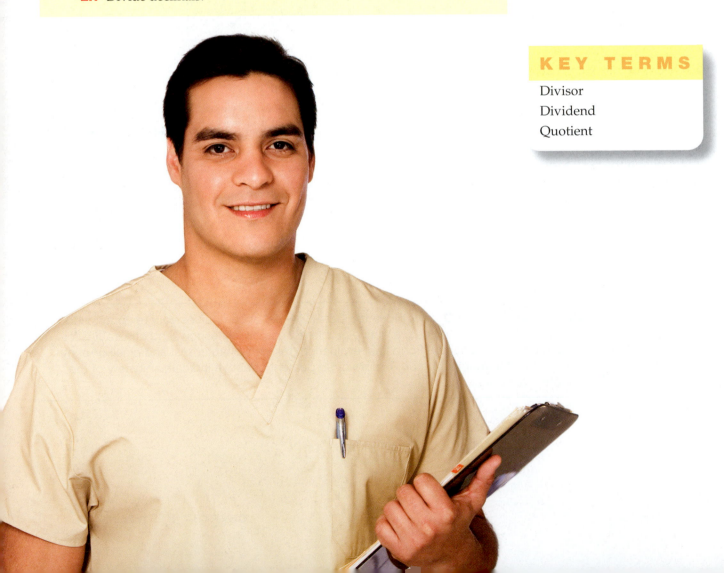

INTRODUCTION

In Chapter 1 you were asked to review your mathematical skills for writing and using fractions. In this chapter you will be practicing many of the same skills for numbers containing decimals. As was true with fractions, it is important that you are comfortable working with decimals before learning how to perform dosage calculations.

2.1 Decimals

The decimal system provides another way to represent whole numbers and their fractional parts. Healthcare professionals use decimals in their daily work. The metric system, which is decimal-based, is used in dosage calculations, instrument calibrations, and general charting work. You must be able to work with decimals and convert fractions and mixed numbers to decimals.

In the decimal system, the location of a digit relative to the decimal point determines its value. The decimal point separates the whole number from the decimal fraction.

Writing and Comparing Decimals

Each position in a decimal number has a place value. You already know values to the left of a decimal point. The places to the right of a decimal point represent fractions.

The number 1542.567 is read "one thousand five hundred forty-two *and* five hundred sixty-seven thousandths." Note that when you are writing decimal numbers using words or speaking decimal numbers, the word *and* replaces the decimal point. All numbers to the right of the decimal point are read and written as whole numbers with the place value of the decimal number written last. See Table 2-1.

TABLE 2-1 Decimal Place Values

The number 1542.567 can be represented as follows:

WHOLE NUMBER				DECIMAL POINT	DECIMAL FRACTION		
Thousands	Hundreds	Tens	Ones	.	Tenths	Hundredths	Thousandths
1	5	4	2	.	5	6	7

RULE 2-1

To write a decimal number:

1. Write the whole-number part to the left of the decimal point.

2. Write the decimal fraction part to the right of the decimal point. Decimal fractions are equivalent to fractions that have denominators of 10, 100, 1000, and so forth.

3. Use zero as a placeholder to the right of the decimal point just as you use zero for whole numbers. The decimal number 1.203 represents 1 ones, 2 tenths, 0 hundredths, and 3 thousandths.

Example 1

Decimal	Description	Mixed Number
12.5	Twelve and five tenths	$12\frac{5}{10}$
206.34	Two hundred six and thirty-four hundredths	$206\frac{34}{100}$

0.33	Thirty-three hundredths	$\frac{33}{100}$
1.125	One and one hundred twenty-five thousandths	$1\frac{125}{1000}$

Example 2

Write $3\frac{4}{10}$ in decimal form.

$3\frac{4}{10}$ is 3 ones and 4 tenths. In decimal form, $3\frac{4}{10} = 3.4$.

Example 3

Write $20\frac{7}{100}$ in decimal form.

$20\frac{7}{100}$ is 2 tens, 0 ones, 0 tenths, and 7 hundredths. In decimal form, $20\frac{7}{100} = 20.07$.

GO TO . . . Open the CD-ROM that accompanies your textbook and select Chapter 2, Writing Decimals (LO 2.1). Review the animation and example problems; then complete the practice problems. Continue to the next section of the book once you have mastered the information presented.

RULE 2-2

Always write a zero to the left of the decimal point when the decimal number has no whole-number part. Using the zero makes the decimal point more noticeable. Never place a trailing zero after the decimal point when working with medication dosages. Using zeros correctly helps to prevent medication errors.

Example

Write the following fractions in decimal form.

a. $\frac{4}{10}$

$\frac{4}{10} = 0.4$ Do *not* write .4.

b. $\frac{25}{1000}$

$\frac{25}{1000} = 0.025$ Do *not* write .025.

c. 100/25

$\frac{100}{25} = 4$ Do *not* write 4.0.

GO TO . . . Open the CD-ROM that accompanies your textbook, and select Chapter 2, Using Zeros (LO 2.1). Review the animation and example problems; then complete the practice problems. Continue to the next section of the book once you have mastered the information presented.

COMPARING DECIMALS   The more places a number is to the right of the decimal point, the smaller its value. For example, 0.3 is $\frac{3}{10}$, or three-tenths; 0.03 is $\frac{3}{100}$, or three-hundredths; and 0.003 is $\frac{3}{1000}$, or three-thousandths. Think of it like this: $\frac{3}{10}$ is similar to three dimes and $\frac{3}{100}$ is similar to three cents. If a dollar is divided further into 1000 parts, $\frac{3}{1000}$ (three thousandths) is very small.

RULE 2-3	To compare the values of a group of decimal numbers:
	1. Look first at the whole-number part. The decimal number with the greatest whole number is the greatest decimal number.
	2. If the whole numbers of two decimals are equal, compare the digits in the tenths place. The tenths place is the first place to the right of the decimal point.
	3. If the tenths places are equal, move to the right and compare the hundredths place digits.
	4. Continue moving to the right, comparing digits until one is greater than the other. This will be the larger number. Zeros added to the right of the last nonzero digit after the decimal point do not change the value of the number.
Example 1	Which is larger, 2.1 or 2.3? The whole number 2 is the same in both numbers. Move one space to the right of the decimal. Compare the tenths digits. Because 3 > 1, $2.3 > 2.1$
Example 2	Which is larger, 0.3 or 0.05? There is no whole number. Move one space to the right of the decimal. Compare the tenths digits. Because 3 > 0, $0.3 > 0.05$
Example 3	Which is larger, 0.121 or 0.13? There is no whole number. Move one space to the right of the decimal. Compare the tenths digits. These digits are equal. Move one space to the right and compare the hundredths digits. Because 3 > 2, $0.13 > 0.121$

GO TO . . . Open the CD-ROM that accompanies your textbook, and select Chapter 2, Comparing Decimal Numbers (LO 2.1). Review the animation and example problems; then complete the practice problems. Continue to the next section of the book once you have mastered the information presented.

REVIEW AND PRACTICE

2.1 Writing and Comparing Decimals

Write the following fractions in decimal form.

1. $\dfrac{2}{10}$ 2. $\dfrac{17}{100}$ 3. $6\dfrac{5}{10}$ 4. $7\dfrac{19}{100}$

5. $\dfrac{3}{1000}$ 6. $\dfrac{23}{1000}$ 7. $5\dfrac{67}{1000}$ 8. $7\dfrac{151}{1000}$

Place > or < between each pair of decimals to make a true statement.

9. 4.27   4.02   **10.** 12.25   12.18   **11.** 0.4   0.6   **12.** 2.22   2.20

13. 0.0170   0.0172   **14.** 0.3001   0.2998   **15.** 5.41   5.34   **16.** 34.58   34.85

17. 0.7 0.9   **18.** 0.67   0.53   **19.** 0.0542   0.0524   **20.** 0.6891   0.8619

To check your answers, see the Answer section at the end of the book, which starts on page A-1.

2.2 Rounding Decimals

In healthcare settings, you will usually round decimals to the nearest tenth or hundredth, especially if you use a calculator. The answer you get may contain many more decimal places than you need, and you must round the answer. For example, $10 \div 6 = 1.66666666666. \ldots$ In some circumstances you will be asked to round to the nearest tenth, which is 1.7. In other situations your may need to round to the nearest hundredth, which is 1.67. For example, standard syringes are calibrated in tenths of a milliliter, while tuberculin syringes are calibrated in hundredths.

RULE 2-4	To round decimals: **1.** Underline the place value to which you want to round. **2.** Look at the digit to the right of this target place value. If this digit is 4 or less, do not change the digit in the target place value. If this digit is 5 or more, round the digit in the target place value up one unit. **3.** Drop all digits to the right of the target place value.
Example 1	Round 2.42 to the nearest tenth. **1.** Underline the tenths place (the target place value): 2.4̲2. **2.** The digit to the right of the tenths place is 2. Do not change the digit in the tenths place. **3.** Drop the digits to the right of the tenths place. The number 2.42 rounded to the nearest tenth equals 2.4.
Example 2	Round 0.035 to the nearest hundredth. **1.** 0.03̲5 **2.** The digit to the right of the hundredths place is 5. Round the digit in the hundredths place up one unit: 0.04. **3.** The number 0.035 rounded to the nearest hundredth equals 0.04.
Example 3	Round 3.99 to the nearest tenth. **1.** 3.9̲9 **2.** The digit to the right of the tenths place is 9. Round the digit in the tenths place up one unit. When 9 is rounded up, it becomes 10. Place the 0 in the tenths place, and carry the 1 to the ones place. When 1 is added to the ones place, 3 becomes 4 the rounded number becomes 4.0̲0. **3.** The number 3.99 rounded to the nearest tenth equals 4.

GO TO . . . Open the CD-ROM that accompanies your textbook, and select Chapter 2, Rounding Decimals (LO 2.2). Review the animation and example problems; then complete the practice problems. Continue to the next section of the book once you have mastered the information presented.

REVIEW AND PRACTICE

2.2 Rounding Decimals

Round to the nearest tenth.

1. 14.34   **2.** 3.45   **3.** 0.86   **4.** 0.19

5. 1.007   **6.** 0.2083   **7.** 152.68

Round to the nearest hundredth.

8. 9.293   **9.** 55.168   **10.** 4.0060   **11.** 2.2081

12. 5.5195   **13.** 11.999   **14.** 767.4562

Round to the nearest whole number.

15. 11.493   **16.** 19.98   **17.** 2.099   **18.** 50.505

19. You are preparing a syringe to administer 3.75 mL of medication. The syringe is calibrated in tenths. How much medication should you draw into the syringe?

20. A healthcare professional is preparing a syringe for an injection. The calculations indicate that 0.38 mL should be given to the patient. The syringe is calibrated in hundredths. How much medication should the healthcare professional draw into the syringe?

To check your answers, see the Answer section at the end of the book, which starts on page A-1.

2.3 Converting Fractions into Decimals

Conversions between fractions and decimals is important in healthcare settings. When you convert fractions, the equivalent decimals are greater than 1. When you convert fractions to decimals, think of the fractions as division problems. You can write $\frac{1}{4}$ as $1 \div 4$. Reducing fractions first (if possible) often makes the division easier.

RULE 2-5	To convert a fraction to a decimal, divide the numerator by the denominator.
Example 1	Convert $\frac{3}{4}$ to a decimal. Divide the numerator by the denominator. $\begin{array}{r} 0.75 \\ 4\overline{)3.00} \\ \underline{2\,8} \\ 20 \\ \underline{20} \end{array}$ $\qquad \frac{3}{4} = 0.75$
Example 2	Convert $\frac{2}{3}$ to a decimal. $\begin{array}{r} 0.666 \\ 3\overline{)2.000} \\ \underline{1\,8} \\ 20 \\ \underline{18} \\ 20 \\ \underline{18} \\ 2\ldots \end{array}$ Sometimes the decimal repeats rather than terminates, as with $\frac{2}{3}$. In such cases, you round, for example, to the nearest hundredth. $\frac{2}{3} \approx 0.67$
Example 3	Convert $\frac{8}{5}$ to a decimal. $\begin{array}{r} 1.6 \\ 5\overline{)8.0} \\ \underline{5} \\ 3.0 \\ \underline{3.0} \end{array}$ $\qquad \frac{8}{5} = 1.6$
Example 4	Convert $1\frac{7}{8}$ to a decimal. $\begin{array}{r} 0.875 \\ 8\overline{)7.000} \\ \underline{6\,4} \\ 60 \\ \underline{56} \\ 40 \\ \underline{40} \end{array}$ $\qquad 1\frac{7}{8} = 1 + \frac{7}{8} = 1 + 0.875 = 1.875$

GO TO . . . Open the CD-ROM that accompanies your textbook, and select Chapter 2, Converting Fractions to Decimals (LO 2.3). Review the animation and example problems; then complete the practice problems. Continue to the next section of the book once you have mastered the information presented.

REVIEW AND PRACTICE

2.3 Converting Fractions into Decimals

Convert the following numbers into decimals. Where necessary, round to the nearest thousandth.

1. $\frac{2}{5}$ 2. $\frac{7}{20}$ 3. $\frac{9}{12}$ 4. $\frac{12}{24}$ 5. $\frac{1}{3}$

6. $\frac{4}{9}$ 7. $\frac{15}{27}$ 8. $\frac{21}{36}$ 9. $\frac{12}{8}$ 10. $\frac{11}{5}$

11. $\frac{7}{3}$ 12. $\frac{9}{8}$ 13. $1\frac{4}{5}$ 14. $2\frac{1}{10}$ 15. $6\frac{3}{4}$

16. $3\frac{1}{2}$ 17. $\frac{7}{8}$ 18. $\frac{9}{45}$ 19. $\frac{20}{7}$ 20. $7\frac{2}{3}$

To check your answers, see the Answer section at the end of the book, which starts on page A-1.

2.4 Converting Decimals into Fractions

Sometimes you need to convert a decimal to a fraction, especially when you use a calculator that provides decimals, but you need a fraction. When you work with decimals, treat the number to the left of the decimal point as a whole number and the number to the right of the decimal point as a fraction. For example, 12.5 is twelve and five tenths, or $12\frac{5}{10}$. The place value of the digit farthest to the right of the decimal point is the denominator. For 12.5, this place value is the tenths place. The denominator is 10. The numerator is 5, the number to the right of the decimal point.

RULE 2-6

To convert a decimal to a fraction or mixed number:

1. Write the number to the left of the decimal point as the whole number.

2. Write the number to the right of the decimal point as the numerator of the fraction.

3. Use the place value of the digit farthest to the right of the decimal point as the denominator.

4. Reduce the fraction part to its lowest terms.

Example 1	Convert 3.75 to a mixed number.
	1. Write the number to the left of the decimal point, 3, as the whole number.
	2. Write the number to the right of the decimal point, 75, as the numerator of the fraction.
	3. The digit farthest to the right of the decimal point, 5, is in the hundredths place. Thus, the denominator is 100. The mixed number is $3\frac{75}{100}$.
	4. Reduce to lowest terms: $3\frac{75}{100} = 3\frac{3}{4}$.
Example 2	Convert 0.015 to a fraction.
	1. The number to the left of the decimal point is 0, so 0.015 has no whole number.
	2. The number 015 is to the right of the decimal point. Because 015 = 15, write 15 as the numerator of the fraction.
	3. The digit farthest to the right of the decimal point is 5, in the thousandths place. The denominator is 1000. The fraction is $\frac{15}{1000}$.
	4. $\frac{15}{1000} = \frac{3}{200}$

ERROR ALERT!

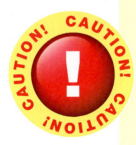

Always Write a Zero to the Left of the Decimal When Writing a Number That Is Less Than Zero

When converting a fraction such as 1/5 to a decimal, you might be tempted to write the answer as .2 instead of 0.2. After all, the zero does not change the value of the number. By doing this, however, you will run the risk of missing the decimal point when referring to the number at a later time and reading the number as a 2. While including a zero does not change the value, it does serve a purpose. It brings attention to the decimal, which could otherwise be mistaken for a stray mark. This can lead to avoidable errors.

GO TO . . . Open the CD-ROM that accompanies your textbook, and select Chapter 2, Converting Decimals to Fractions (LO 2.4). Review the animation and example problems; then complete the practice problems. Continue to the next section of the book once you have mastered the information presented.

2.4 Converting Decimals into Fractions

Convert the following decimals to fractions or mixed numbers. Reduce the answer to its lowest terms.

1. 1.2	**2.** 98.6	**3.** 0.3	**4.** 0.442	**5.** 5.03
6. 0.301	**7.** 100.04	**8.** 206.070	**9.** 10.68	**10.** 7.44

To check your answers, see the Answer section at the end of the book, which starts on page A-1.

2.5 Adding and Subtracting Decimals

When you add or subtract decimals, you align them by their place value, just as you do to add or subtract whole numbers.

RULE 2-7	To add or subtract decimals: **1.** Write the problem vertically, as you would with whole numbers. Align the decimal points. **2.** Add or subtract, starting from the right. Include the decimal point in your answer.
Example 1	Add 2.47 + 0.39. **1.** Write the problem vertically. Align the decimal points. $$\begin{array}{r} 2.47 \\ +\ 0.39 \\ \hline \end{array}$$ **2.** Add. $$\begin{array}{r} 2.47 \\ +\ 0.39 \\ \hline 2.86 \end{array}$$
Example 2	Subtract 52.04 − 14.31. Align the decimal points. $$\begin{array}{r} 52.04 \\ -14.31 \\ \hline 37.73 \end{array}$$ When the decimals have an unequal number of places, add zeros to the end of the decimal fraction so that all numbers are the same length past the decimal point. Writing zeros after the last digit to the right of the decimal point does not change the number's value. Including these zeros helps prevent errors in calculations.

Example 3	Add 14.3 + 1.56 + 9 + 0.352. Align the numbers. (Rewrite 9 as 9.0 to help you align it properly.) Fill in zeros so that all decimal fractions are of equal length. Then add.

$$
\begin{array}{r}
14.3 \\
1.56 \\
9.0 \\
+\ 0.352 \\
\end{array}
\qquad
\begin{array}{r}
14.300 \\
1.560 \\
9.000 \\
+\ 0.352 \\
\hline
25.212 \\
\end{array}
$$

Think! . . . Is It Reasonable? Estimate the range that the answer should fall into. To do this, round all numbers down to whole numbers and add. 14 + 1 + 9 + 0 = 24. Then round both numbers up and add. 15 + 2 + 9 + 1 = 27. The answer must be between 24 and 27, and the answer is 25.212.

Example 4	Subtract 7.3 − 1.005. Align the numbers. Fill in zeros so that all decimal fractions are of equal length. Then subtract.

$$
\begin{array}{r}
7.3 \\
-\ 1.005 \\
\end{array}
\qquad
\begin{array}{r}
7.300 \\
-\ 1.005 \\
\hline
6.295 \\
\end{array}
$$

Example 5	Subtract 10 − 0.75.

$$
\begin{array}{r}
10.00 \\
-\ 0.75 \\
\hline
9.25 \\
\end{array}
$$

GO TO . . . Open the CD-ROM that accompanies your textbook, and select Chapter 2, Adding and Subtracting Decimals (LO 2.5). Review the animation and example problems; then complete the practice problems. Continue to the next section of the book once you have mastered the information presented.

REVIEW AND PRACTICE

2.5 Adding and Subtracting Decimals

Add or subtract the following pairs of numbers.

1. 7.58 + 3.24
2. 143.05 + 22.07
3. 13.561 + 0.099
4. 24.102 + 2.410
5. 2.01 + 0.5

6. 2.30 + 0.005
7. 0.075 + 0.73
8. 4 + 0.025
9. 31.64 − 17.39
10. 16.250 − 1.625

11. 5.66 − 0.09
12. 14.7 − 0.9
13. 1.22 − 0.4
14. 12.2 − 0.972
15. 8 − 0.076

16 12 − 0.02
17. 8.67 + 0.93
18. 121.04 + 56.75
19. 70.22 − 4.23
20. 526.10 − 7.41

21. Steve's temperature on Wednesday morning was 101.4 degrees Fahrenheit (101.4°F). By Thursday afternoon, it was 99.5°F. By how many degrees had his temperature changed?

22. While waiting to see her father, Helene ate at the hospital cafeteria, where she spent $1.30 for a soda, $2.65 for a bowl of soup, and $3.50 for a garden salad. How much did Helene spend?

23. You are supposed to administer 9 grams (g) of a medication. You give the patient one tablet with 4.5 grams (g) and a second tablet with 2.25 grams (g). How much more medication should you administer?

24. A bottle of liquid medication contains 50 mL. The following amounts are given to patients from the bottle: 2.5 mL, 3.1 mL, 1.75 mL, 3 mL, and 2.25 mL. How much medication remains in the bottle?

25. Your patient weighed 70.57 kilograms (kg) 2 months ago. His weight then increased by 2.3 kg one month and 1.75 kg the next month. What is this patient's current weight in kilograms?

To check your answers, see the Answer section at the end of the book, which starts on page A-1.

2.6 Multiplying Decimals

Multiplying decimals is similar to multiplying whole numbers, except you must determine where to place the decimal point.

RULE 2-8	To multiply decimals:
	1. First multiply without considering the decimal points, as if the numbers were whole numbers.
	2. Count the total number of places to the right of the decimal points in *both* numbers.
	3. To place the decimal point in the answer, start at its right end. Move the decimal point to the left the same number of places as the answer from step 2.

Example 1

Multiply 3.42×2.5.

When you are multiplying, the decimal points *do not* need to line up as they do for adding and subtracting.

1. First multiply without considering the decimal points.

$$
\begin{array}{r}
3.42 \\
\times\ 2.5 \\
\hline
1710 \\
684 \\
\hline
8550
\end{array}
$$

2. Count the total number of decimal places (to the right of the decimal point) in the numbers. The number 3.42 has two decimal places; 2.5 has one decimal place. The numbers have a total of three decimal places.

3. Place the decimal point in the answer. Start at the right of the answer 8550. Move the decimal point three places to the left: 8.550. *After* placing the decimal point, you can drop the final zero so that the answer is 8.55.

 Think! . . . Is It Reasonable? Estimate the range that the answer should fall into. To do this, multiply the whole numbers. $3 \times 2 = 6$. Then round both numbers up and multiply. $4 \times 3 = 12$. The answer must be between 6 and 12, and the answer is 8.55.

Example 2

Multiply 0.001 × 0.02

1. Multiply.
$$\begin{array}{r} 0.001 \\ \times\ 0.02 \\ \hline 2 \end{array}$$

2. The number 0.001 has three decimal places, and 0.02 has two decimal places. The numbers have a total of five decimal places.

3. Start to the right of the answer 2. Move the decimal point five places to the left. Insert zeros to the left of 2 in order to correctly place the decimal point. The correct answer is 0.00002.

GO TO . . . Open the CD-ROM that accompanies your textbook, and select Chapter 2, Multiplying Decimals (LO 2.6). Review the animation and example problems; then complete the practice problems. Continue to the next section of the book once you have mastered the information presented.

REVIEW AND PRACTICE

2.6 Multiplying Decimals

Multiply the following numbers.

1. 7.4×8.2
2. 8.21×1.1
3. 4.2×0.3
4. 3.04×0.04
5. 0.55×0.5
6. 0.027×0.4
7. 0.003×0.02
8. 0.25×0.75
9. 1.03×14
10. 12×0.09
11. 0.004×15.5
12. 0.004×40.01
13. 5.2×3.1

14. A patient is given 7.5 mL of liquid medication 5 times per day. How many milliliters does she receive per day?

15. A small syringe is used to give a patient 0.28 mL of medication 4 times per day for 4 days. How much medication does he receive over the 4 days?

16. A tablet has a strength of 0.25 milligram (mg) of medication. You give the patient $1\frac{1}{2}$ tablets 3 times per day. How many milligrams of medication do you give the patient each day? (Hint: Convert $1\frac{1}{2}$ to decimal form first.)

17. A tablet has a strength of 0.4 mg of medication. If you give the patient $\frac{1}{4}$ tablet twice a day, how many milligrams of medication does the patient receive per day?

18. A case of isopropyl alcohol contains 12 bottles. Each bottle contains 15.95 oz. How many ounces of alcohol are in each case?

To check your answers, see the Answer section at the end of the book, which starts on page A-1.

2.7 Dividing Decimals

The key to dividing decimals correctly is to place the decimal point properly. Recall that the dividend is the number that will be divided. If the divisor is a decimal, you want to convert the problem to one in which the divisor is a whole number.

RULE 2-9	To divide decimals:
	1. Move the decimal point to the right the same number of places in both the divisor (the number you are dividing by) and the dividend (the number you are dividing into) until the divisor is a whole number. Insert zeros as necessary.
	3. Complete the division as you would with whole numbers. Align the decimal point of the quotient with the decimal point of the dividend if needed.

Example 1

Divide 0.8 ÷ 0.02.

(dividend) (divisor)

1. Move the decimal point two places to the right in both the divisor and the dividend. The divisor is now a whole number.

$$0.02\overline{).80}$$

2. Complete the division.

$$\begin{array}{r} 40 \\ 2\overline{)80} \\ 80 \end{array}$$ so 0.8 ÷ 0.02 = 40

Think! . . . Is It Reasonable? When performing division, a quick check for "reasonable" is to compare the values of the numbers.

- If the divisor is greater than the dividend your answer should be less than 1.

- If the dividend is greater than the divisor, your answer should be greater than 1.

The dividend is greater than the divisor, so the answer should be greater than 1 and the answer is 40.

Example 2

Divide 0.066 ÷ 0.11.

1. $0.11.\overline{)0.06.6}$

Move the decimal point two places to the right so that the divisor is a whole number.

2. $\begin{array}{r} 0.6 \\ 11\overline{)6.6} \\ 6.6 \end{array}$

Align the decimal point of the quotient with the decimal point of the dividend. Here, 0.066 ÷ 0.11 = 0.6

GO TO . . . Open the CD-ROM that accompanies your textbook, and select Chapter 2, Dividing Decimals (LO 2.7). Review the animation and example problems; then complete the practice problems. Continue to the next section of the book once you have mastered the information presented.

Placing Decimals Correctly

A practitioner was instructed to give 0.25 gram (g) of medication for every 1.0 kilogram (kg) of body weight. A baby she was treating weighed 6.25 kg. She set up this calculation:

$$
\begin{array}{r}
6.25 \\
\times\ 0.25 \\
\hline
3125 \\
1250 \\
\hline
156.25
\end{array}
$$

Think! . . . Is It Reasonable? What mistake did the healthcare professional make? What could have happened if the mistake was not corrected?

REVIEW AND PRACTICE

2.7 Dividing Decimals

Divide the following numbers. When necessary, round to the nearest thousandth.

1. $3.2 \div 1.6$ **2.** $48.6 \div 1.8$ **3.** $24.5 \div 0.2$ **4.** $0.004 \div 0.002$

5. $1.25 \div 0.5$ **6.** $0.32 \div 0.8$ **7.** $0.05 \div 4$ **8.** $12.6 \div 4$

9. $40 \div 0.8$ **10.** $0.44 \div 4.4$ **11.** $29.05 \div 100$ **12.** $3.48 \div 1000$

13. $39.666 \div 0.03$ **14.** $54.54 \div 0.009$ **15.** $59.48 \div 66.93$ **16.** $84.3 \div 68.48$

17. A bottle holds 60 mL of medication. If the average dose is 0.75 mL, how many doses does the bottle hold?

18. A bottle contains 32 oz of medication. If the average dose is 0.4 oz, how many doses does the bottle contain?

19. A patient received a total of 2.25 g of a medication. If the patient received the total over a 3-day period and was given 3 doses per day, what was the strength of each dose?

20. A patient weighs 197.5 lb. The patient's goal is to weigh 152.5 lb a year from now. How much weight should the patient lose per month to be successful?

To check your answers, see the Answer section at the end of the book, which starts on page A-1.

CHAPTER 2 SUMMARY

LEARNING OUTCOME	KEY POINTS

2.1 Write decimals and compare their value. Pages 37–40.	▶ The places to the right of a decimal represent fractions, and each position has a place value.
	
	   • For example, numbers in the first position after the decimal represent a fraction with a denominator of 10. If there are two places after the decimal, they represent a fraction with a denominator of 100.
	
	▶ When comparing numbers that contain decimals, you first compare the value of the numbers to the left of the decimal.
	
	   • For example, when comparing the value of 3.15 and 5.65 it is not necessary to look at the numbers to the right of the decimal. 5 is greater than 3, so 5.65 is greater than 3.15.
	
	▶ When the numbers to the left of the decimal are the same, you compare values to the right of the decimal moving one place at a time until you find one value greater than another.
	
	   • For example, when comparing 25.025 and 25.04, you would compare values starting at the first place after the decimal. The first place of the two numbers contains the same value, so you proceed to the second, where 4 is greater than 2. Therefore, 25.04 is greater than 25.025.

2.2 Apply the rules for rounding decimals. Pages 40–42.	▶ When rounding, you must look at the first digit to the right of the place value that you are rounding to. If this digit is 5 or more, round up. If it is less than 5, round down. • For example, to round 2.7384 to the hundredths place, you look at the digit to the right of the 3. This digit, 8, is greater than 5, so you round the number up to 2.74.
2.3 Convert fractions into decimals. Pages 42–43.	▶ To convert a fraction to a decimal, divide the numerator by the denominator. • For example, to convert 1/5 to a decimal you would divide 1 by 5. $1 \div 5 = 0.2$.
2.4 Convert decimals into fractions. Pages 43–45.	▶ To convert a decimal to a fraction, write the numbers to the right of the decimal as the numerator and the place value of the number furthest to the right as the denominator. • For example, to convert 0.12 to a fraction, the numerator is 12 (the numbers to the right of the decimal) and the denominator is 100 (the place value of the 2). The equivalent fraction for 0.12 is $\frac{12}{100}$.

2.5 Add and subtract decimals. Pages 45–47.	▶ To add and subtract decimals, it is first necessary to align the decimals vertically before adding or subtracting. • For example, to add 10.3 + 3.05: $$\begin{array}{r} 10.3 \\ +\ 3.05 \\ \hline 13.35 \end{array}$$
2.6 Multiply decimals. Pages 47–48.	▶ To multiply decimals, first multiply the numbers, then determine the position of the decimal. The decimal in your answer should be placed so that the number of digits to the right of the decimal is equal to the total number of decimal places in the numbers that were multiplied. • For example, to multiply 1.05×3.1 you first multiply $105 \times 31 = 3255$. You then determine the position of the decimal. Since the numbers that were multiplied contained a total of 3 decimal places, the decimal should be placed 3 places from the right in your answer. The answer is 3.255.
2.7 Divide decimals. Pages 49–50.	▶ To divide decimals, first move the decimal to the right the same number of places in both the divisor and dividend until the divisor is a whole number. • Example: $3.2 \div 0.4 = 32 \div 4 = 8$

Copyright © 2012 by The McGraw-Hill Companies, Inc.

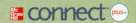
Place >, <, or = between the following pairs of fractions to make a true statement. (LO 2.1)

1. 0.017   0.09

2. 3.092   3.27

Round to the nearest hundredth. (LO 2.2)

3. 1.1834

4. 17.526

Round to the nearest tenth. (LO 2.2)

5. 6.158

6. 0.135

Round to the nearest whole number. (LO 2.2)

7. 12.185

8. 1.518

Convert the following fractions to decimals. (LO 2.3)

9. $2\frac{1}{8}$

10. $\frac{12}{5}$

Convert the following decimals to fractions. Reduce the answers to lowest terms. (LO 2.4)

11. 1.35

12. 0.025

Perform the following calculations. (LO 2.5 to 2.7)

13. 4.25×1.2

14. $1.86 \div 0.3$

15. $3.26 + 0.015$

16. 0.325×2.8

17. $12.05 - 7.6$

18. $10.5 \div 1.5$

19. $0.321 + 0.0075$

20. $3.65 - 0.125$

21. During the day, a patient drank the following quantities of fluid: $1\frac{1}{2}$ cups, 2.4 cups, $1\frac{3}{4}$ cups, and 1.2 cups.

    a. Convert each of the measurements into fractions. Add the fractions to find the total volume of fluid.

    b. Convert each of the measurements into decimals. Add the decimals to find the total volume of fluid.

CHECK UP

Place >, <, or = between the following pairs of decimals to make a true statement. (LO 2.1)

1. 5.7   5.09
2. 0.04   0.004
3. 6.3 6   300
4. 9.033   9.303

Round to the nearest hundredth. (LO 2.2)

5. 0.229
6. 7.091
7. 46.001
8. 9.885

Round to the nearest tenth. (LO 2.2)

9. 4.34
10. 3.65
11. 6.991
12. 0.073

Round to the nearest whole number. (LO 2.2)

13. 8.96
14. 20.6
15. 0.931
16. 12.449

Convert the following fractions to decimals. (LO 2.3)

17. $\frac{7}{14}$
18. $\frac{5}{8}$
19. $2\frac{3}{5}$
20. $\frac{32}{4}$

Convert the following decimals to fractions. Reduce the answers to lowest terms. (LO 2.4)

21. 0.82
22. 0.65
23. 3.5
24. 1.001

Perform the following calculations. (LO 2.4 to 2.7)

25. 7.23 + 12.38
26. 4.59 + 0.2
27. 0.031 + 0.99
28. 12 + 0.004 + 1.7

29. 7.49 − 0.38
30. 4.28 − 3.39
31. 0.852 − 0.61
32. 14.01 − 0.788

33. 2.3 × 4.9
34. 0.33 × 0.002
35. 5 × 0.999
36. 12.01 × 1.005

37. 38.85 ÷ 2.1
38. 4.875 ÷ 3.25
39. 2.2 ÷ 0.11
40. 1.4 ÷ 0.07

41. A bottle contains 48 mL of liquid medication. If the average dose is 1.2 mL, how many doses does the bottle contain?

CRITICAL THINKING APPLICATIONS

A healthcare professional is asked to arrange a set of instruments in order from smallest to largest on the basis of each instrument's diameter. The diameters are marked 0.875, 0.25, 0.625, 1.0, 0.75, 0.125, and 0.375. How should the healthcare professional arrange the instruments? Look at the pattern of increase in these measurements. Are any missing in the sequence? If so, which ones? (LO 2.1)

CASE STUDY

A healthcare professional is tracking the weight of a patient who is retaining fluids because of congestive heart failure. On day 3, the patient is given a diuretic. Here is a summary of the weight changes that occurred. In the column marked "Change," write the amount of weight change since the previous measurement. Use a plus (+) sign to indicate weight gained and a minus sign (−) to indicate weight lost. Day 2 has been completed as an example. (LO 2.3, 2.4)

time	weight in lbs	change
Day 1, 8:00 a.m.	142.5	n/a
Day 2, 8:00 a.m.	144	+1.5
Day 3, 8:00 a.m.	145.75	
Day 3, 8:00 a.m.	Patient receives diuretic Lasix (furosemide) 40 mg	
Day 3, 2:00 p.m.	144.75	
Day 3, 4:00 p.m.	lasix 40 mg	
Day 4, 8:00 a.m.	142.75	
Day 4, 8:00 a.m.	Lasix 20 mg	
Day 4, 4:00 p.m.	140.5	

To check your answers, see the Answer section at the end of the book, which starts on page A-1.

INTERNET ACTIVITY

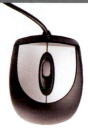

Search the Web for more practice problems with decimals. You might search for "working with decimals," "decimal practice," or "decimal games."

GO TO . . . Open the CD-ROM that accompanies your textbook and review the learning outcomes practice problems, games, slideshow, and other activities presented for this chapter. For a final evaluation, take the chapter test and email or print your results for your instructor. A score of 95 percent or above indicates mastery of the chapter concepts.

3 CHAPTER

Relationships of Quantities: Percents, Ratios, and Proportions

If what you're working for really matters, you'll give it all you've got.

—NIDO QUBEIN

Learning Outcomes

When you have completed Chapter 3, you will be able to:

3.1 Convert values to and from a percent.

3.2 Convert values to and from a ratio.

3.3 Write proportions

3.4 Use proportions to solve for an unknown quantity.

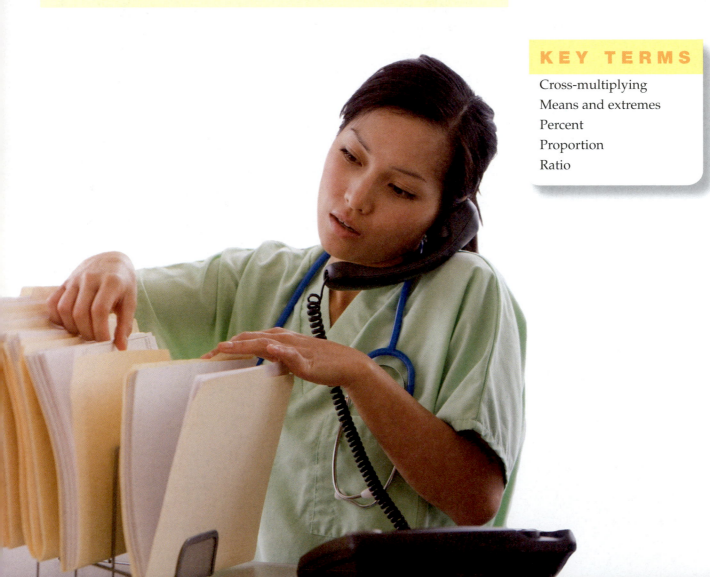

INTRODUCTION

As a healthcare professional, you will need to know how to determine the amount of drug contained in a quantity of a product such as a tablet or a solution. For example, you may need to calculate how much drug is in $2\frac{1}{2}$ tablets, or in 300 mL of an IV solution. To do this, you must have a keen understanding of percents, ratios, and proportions. Additionally the process of finding the missing value in a proportion problem (included in this chapter) is the necessary first step in many dosage calculations. So in preparation for your health career, give Chapter 3 all you've got!

3.1 Percents

Percents, like decimals and fractions, provide a way to express the relationship of parts to a whole. Indicated by the symbol %, **percent** literally means "per 100" or "divided by 100" The whole is always 100 units, just as a test is worth 100 points. A grade of 75% means that 75 per 100 points are answered correctly. Table 3-1 shows the same number expressed as a decimal, a fraction, and a percent. A number less than 1 is expressed as less than 100 percent. A number greater than 1 is expressed as greater than 100 percent. Any expression of 1 (for instance, 1.0 or $\frac{5}{5}$) equals 100 percent.

TABLE 3-1 Comparing Decimals, Fractions, and Percents

WORDS	DECIMAL	FRACTION	PERCENT
Eight hundredths	0.08	$\frac{8}{100}$	8%
Twenty-three hundredths	0.23	$\frac{23}{100}$	23%
Seven-tenths	0.7	$\frac{7}{10}$	70%
One		$\frac{1}{1}$	100%
One and five-tenths or one and one-half	1.5	$1\frac{5}{10}$ or $1\frac{1}{2}$	150%

Converting Values to and from a Percent

Converting between percents and decimals requires dividing and multiplying by 100. Converting a percent to a decimal is similar to dividing a number by 100—you move the decimal point two places to the left. If the percent is a fraction or a mixed number, first convert it to a decimal (see Chapter 2 for review). Then divide by 100, moving the decimal point two places to the left.

RULE 3-1	To convert a percent to a decimal, remove the percent symbol. Then divide the remaining number by 100 by moving the decimal point two places to the left.
Example 1	Convert 42 percent to a decimal. $42\% = 42.\% = .42. = 0.42$ Insert the zero before the decimal point for clarity.

Example 2	Convert 175 percent to a decimal. $175\% = 175.\% = 1.\underset{\smile}{75}. = 1.75$
Example 3	When you move the decimal point to the left, you may need to insert zeros. Convert 0.3 percent to a decimal. $0.3\% = 000.3\% = 0.\underset{\smile}{00}3 = 0.003$
Example 4	Convert $25\frac{1}{2}$ percent to a decimal. $25\frac{1}{2}\% = 25\frac{5}{10}\% = 25.5\% = .\underset{\smile}{25}5 = 0.255$ Add a zero in front of the decimal point for clarity.
Example 5	Convert $\frac{3}{4}$ percent to a decimal. First convert $\frac{3}{4}$ to a decimal. $\frac{3}{4} = 4\overline{)3.00}^{\,0.75} = 0.75$ $\frac{3}{4}\% = 0.75\% = 000.75\% = 0.\underset{\smile}{00}75 = 0.0075$ **Think! . . . Is It Reasonable?** When dividing a number by 100, you move the decimal point two places to the left and insert zeros when necessary. In this case, $0.75\% = 0.0075$.

GO TO . . . Open the CD-ROM that accompanies your textbook, and select Chapter 3, Convert Percent to Decimal (LO 3.1). Review the animation and example problems; then complete the practice problems. Continue to the next section of the book, once you have mastered the information presented.

Converting a decimal to a percent is similar to multiplying a number by 100—you move the decimal point two places to the right. Because $100\% = 1.00$, multiplying a number by 100 percent does not change its value.

RULE 3-2	To convert a decimal into a percent, multiply the decimal by 100. Then add the percent symbol.
Example 1	Convert 1.42 to a percent. $1.42 \times 100\% = 142\%$ You can write this as $1.42 = 1.\underset{\smile}{42}.\% = 142\%$.
Example 2	Convert 0.02 to a percent. $0.02 \times 100\% = 2\%$ You can write this as $0.02 = 0.\underset{\smile}{02}.\% = 2\%$.

Example 3	When you move the decimal point to the right, you may need to insert zeros. Convert 0.8 to a percent.
	$0.8 \times 100\% = 80\%$

You can write this as $0.8 = 0.80 = 0.80.\% = 80\%$.

Think! . . . Is It Reasonable? Percents are based on hundredths. Therefore, numbers must be written to *at least* two decimal places (hundredths) before you move the decimal and express them as a percent.

Think! . . . Is It Reasonable? When you multiply a number by 100, you move the decimal point two places to the right. Since percents are based on hundredths, numbers must be written with at least two decimal places (hundredths) before you can move the decimal and express them as a percent. In this example, 0.8 is first rewritten with an extra zero (0.80) and then as 80%.

GO TO . . . Open the CD-ROM that accompanies your textbook, and select Chapter 3, Convert Decimal to Percent (LO 3.1). Review the animation and example problems; then complete the practice problems. Continue to the next section of the book, once you have mastered the information presented.

Because percent means "per 100" or "divided by 100," you can easily convert percents to equivalent fractions.

RULE 3-3	To convert a percent to an equivalent fraction, write the value of the percent as the numerator and 100 as the denominator. Then reduce the fraction to its lowest terms.
Example 1	Convert 8 percent to an equivalent fraction. $$8\% = \frac{8}{100} = \frac{\overset{2}{\cancel{8}}}{\underset{25}{\cancel{100}}} = \frac{2}{25}$$
Example 2	Convert 130 percent to an equivalent mixed number. $$130\% = \frac{130}{100} = \frac{\overset{13}{\cancel{130}}}{\underset{10}{\cancel{100}}} = \frac{13}{10} = 1\frac{3}{10}$$
Example 3	Change 0.6 percent to an equivalent fraction. $$0.6\% = \frac{0.6}{100}$$ To reduce a fraction, it must not include a decimal point. To eliminate the decimal point, multiply it by $\frac{10}{10}$. (Remember that a fraction with the same number in the numerator and denominator is equal to 1.) $$\frac{0.6}{100} \times \frac{10}{10} = \frac{6}{1000} = \frac{3}{500}$$

Example 4	Change $\frac{3}{4}$ percent to an equivalent fraction. $$\frac{3}{4}\% = \frac{3}{4} \div 100 = \frac{3}{4} \times \frac{1}{100} = \frac{3}{400}$$ For a review of division with fractions, see Chapter 1.

GO TO . . . Open the CD-ROM that accompanies your textbook, and select Chapter 3, Convert Percent to Fraction (LO 3.1). Review the animation and example problems; then complete the practice problems. Continue to the next section of the book, once you have mastered the information presented.

RULE 3-4	To convert a fraction to a percent, first convert the fraction to a decimal. Round the decimal to the nearest hundredth. Then follow the rule for converting a decimal to a percent.
Example 1	Convert $\frac{1}{2}$ to a percent. First convert $\frac{1}{2}$ to a decimal. $$\frac{1}{2} = 1 \div 2 = 0.5$$ Now convert the decimal to a percent. $$\frac{1}{2} = 0.5 = 0.5 \times 100\% = 50\%$$ You can write this as $0.5 = 0.50 = 0.50.\% = 50\%$.
Example 2	Convert $\frac{2}{3}$ to a percent. Convert $\frac{2}{3}$ to a decimal. Round to the nearest hundredth. $$\frac{2}{3} = 2 \div 3 = 0.666 = 0.67$$ Now convert to a percent. $$\frac{2}{3} = 0.67 = 0.67 \times 100\% = 67\%$$ You can write this as $0.67 = 0.67.\% = 67\%$.
Example 3	Convert $1\frac{3}{4}$ to a percent. $$1\frac{3}{4} = \frac{7}{4} = 1.75 = 1.75 \times 100\% = 175\%$$ You can write this as $1\frac{3}{4} = 1.75.\% = 175\%$. An alternative method for converting a fraction to a percent is to multiply the fraction by 100 percent.
Example 4	Convert $\frac{1}{2}$ to a percent. $$\frac{1}{2} \times 100\%$$ $$\frac{1}{2} \times \frac{100\%}{1} = \frac{100\%}{2} = 50\%$$

Example 5	Convert $\frac{2}{3}$ to a percent.
	$$\frac{2}{3} \times \frac{100\%}{1} = \frac{200\%}{3} = 66.66\% \text{ rounded to } 67\%.$$
Example 6	Convert $1\frac{3}{4}$ to a percent.
	Change $1\frac{3}{4}$ to the fraction $\frac{7}{4}$.
	$$\frac{7}{4} \times \frac{100\%}{1} = \frac{700\%}{4} = 175\%$$

GO TO . . . Open the CD-ROM that accompanies your textbook, and select Chapter 3, Convert Fraction to Percent (LO 3.1). Review the animation and example problems; then complete the practice problems. Continue to the next section of the book, once you have mastered the information presented.

REVIEW AND PRACTICE

3.1 Percents

Convert the following percents to decimals. Round to the nearest thousandth.

1. 14%	**2.** 30%	**3.** 2%	**4.** 9%	**5.** 103%
6. 300%	**7.** 0.21%	**8.** 0.4%	**9.** $42\frac{1}{2}\%$	**10.** $3\frac{4}{5}\%$
11. 4.5%	**12.** 250.75%	**13.** $23\frac{2}{3}\%$	**14.** $1\frac{5}{6}\%$	**15.** $14\frac{1}{2}\%$

Convert the following decimals to percents.

16. 4.04	**17.** 2.3	**18.** 0.7	**19.** 0.33	**20.** 0.06
21. 0.013	**22.** 15	**23.** 32	**24.** 121	

Convert the following percents to fractions. Reduce the answers to their lowest terms.

25. 22%	**26.** 4%	**27.** 158%	**28.** 300%	**29.** 0.1%
30. 0.8%	**31.** $\frac{9}{10}\%$	**32.** $1\frac{2}{5}\%$	**33.** 0.3%	

Convert the following fractions to percents. Round to the nearest percent.

34. $\frac{6}{8}$	**35.** $\frac{4}{5}$	**36.** $\frac{1}{6}$	**37.** $\frac{5}{9}$	**38.** $1\frac{1}{10}$
39. $2\frac{1}{4}$	**40.** $\frac{175}{100}$	**41.** $\frac{40}{100}$	**42.** $5\frac{2}{3}$	

To check your answers, see the Answer section at the end of the book, which starts on page A-1.

3.2 Ratios

Ratios, like fractions, express the relationship of a part to the whole. They may relate a quantity of liquid drug to a quantity of a solution, such as an injection or an IV. Ratios can also be used to express how much drug is in a tablet or a capsule.

Like a fraction, a ratio has two parts. The first part of the ratio is like the numerator of a fraction, and represents parts of the whole. The second part of the ratio is like the denominator of a fraction, and represents the whole. The two parts are separated by a colon. For example, if a tablet contains 250 mg of drug, the ratio 250 mg:1 tablet could be used to represent the tablet. This same tablet could also be expressed as a fraction: 250 mg of drug would be the numerator, 1 tablet would be the denominator. For example, $\frac{250 \text{ mg}}{1 \text{ tablet}}$.

Converting Values to and from a Ratio

You use only whole numbers when you write a ratio. Correct ratios include 8 : 1, 2 : 5, and 1 : 100 Incorrect ratios include 2.5 : 10, 1 : 4.5, and $3\frac{1}{2}$: 100

Ratios are sometimes expressed in lowest terms. Just as $\frac{4}{100}$ reduces to $\frac{1}{25}$, the ratio 4 : 100 can be written 1 : 25. Similarly, you reduce 2 : 10 to 1 : 5 and 10 : 12 to 5 : 6.

RULE 3-5	Reduce a ratio as you would a fraction. Find the largest whole number that divides evenly into both values *A* and *B*.
Example 1	Reduce 2 : 12 to its lowest terms. Both values 2 and 12 are divisible by 2. $2 \div 2 = 1 \qquad 12 \div 2 = 6$ Thus, 2 : 12 is written 1 : 6.
Example 2	Reduce 10 : 15 to its lowest terms. Both values 10 and 15 are divisible by 5. $10 \div 5 = 2 \qquad 15 \div 5 = 3$ $10 : 15 = 2 : 3$

GO TO . . . Open the CD-ROM that accompanies your textbook, and select Chapter 3, Reducing Ratios (LO 3.2). Review the animation and example problems; then complete the practice problems. Continue to the next section of the book, once you have mastered the information presented.

Because a ratio relates two quantities, value *A* and value *B*, ratios can be written as fractions. Within this textbook for simplicity when two numbers are expressed as *A* : *B*, this is a ratio. When two numbers are expressed as $\frac{A}{B}$ or *A/B*, this is a fraction.

RULE 3-6	To convert a ratio to a fraction, write value *A* (the first number) as the numerator and value *B* (the second number) as the denominator, so that $A : B = \frac{A}{B}$.

Example	Convert the following ratios to fractions. **a.** $1:2 = \frac{1}{2}$ **d.** $7:3 = \frac{7}{3}$ **b.** $4:5 = \frac{4}{5}$ **e.** $8:5 = \frac{8}{5}$ **c.** $1:100 = \frac{1}{100}$

GO TO . . . Open the CD-ROM that accompanies your textbook, and select Chapter 3, Convert Ratio to Fraction (LO 3.2). Review the animation and example problems; then complete the practice problems. Continue to the next section of the book, once you have mastered the information presented.

RULE 3-7	To convert a fraction to a ratio, write the numerator as the first value *A* and the denominator as the second value *B*. $$\frac{A}{B} = A:B$$ Convert a mixed number to a ratio by first writing the mixed number as a fraction.
Example	Convert the following to ratios. **a.** $\frac{7}{12} = 7:12$ **d.** $\frac{47}{12} = 47:12$ **b.** $\frac{3}{10} = 3:10$ **e.** $3\frac{1}{3} = \frac{10}{3} = 10:3$ **c.** $\frac{3}{2} = 3:2$ **f.** $2\frac{1}{2} = \frac{5}{2} = 5:2$

GO TO . . . Open the CD-ROM that accompanies your textbook, and select Chapter 3, Convert Fraction to Ratio (LO 3.2). Review the animation and example problems; then complete the practice problems. Continue to the next section of the book, once you have mastered the information presented.

RULE 3-8	To convert a ratio to a decimal: **1.** Write the ratio as a fraction. **2.** Convert the fraction to a decimal. (See Chapter 2.)

Example 1	Convert 1 : 10 to a decimal.
	1. Write the ratio as a fraction.
	$1 : 10 = \dfrac{1}{10}$
	2. Convert the fraction to a decimal.
	$\dfrac{1}{10} = 1 \div 10 = 0.1$
	Thus, $1 : 10 = \frac{1}{10} = 0.1$.
Example 2	Convert 3 : 2 to a decimal.
	1. $3 : 2 = \dfrac{3}{2}$
	2. $\dfrac{3}{2} = 3 \div 2 = 1.5$
	Thus, $3 : 2 = \frac{3}{2} = 1.5$.

GO TO . . . Open the CD-ROM that accompanies your textbook, and select Chapter 3, Convert Ratio to Decimal (LO 3.2). Review the animation and example problems; then complete the practice problems. Continue to the next section of the book, once you have mastered the information presented.

RULE 3-9	To convert a decimal to a ratio:
	1. Write the decimal as a fraction. (See Chapter 2.)
	2. Reduce the fraction to lowest terms.
	3. Restate the fraction as a ratio by writing the numerator as value *A* and the denominator as value *B*; in the form *A* : *B*.
Example 1	Convert 0.8 to a ratio.
	1. Write the decimal as a fraction.
	$0.8 = \dfrac{8}{10}$
	2. Reduce the fraction to lowest terms.
	$\dfrac{8}{10} = \dfrac{\overset{4}{\cancel{8}}}{\underset{5}{\cancel{10}}} = \dfrac{4}{5}$
	3. Restate the number as a ratio.
	$\dfrac{4}{5} = 4 : 5$
	Thus, $0.8 = \frac{8}{10} = \frac{4}{5} = 4 : 5$.

Example 2	Convert 0.05 to a ratio.
	1. $0.05 = \dfrac{5}{100}$
	2. $\dfrac{5}{100} = \dfrac{\overset{1}{\cancel{5}}}{\underset{20}{\cancel{100}}} = \dfrac{1}{20}$
	3. $\dfrac{1}{20} = 1:20$
	Thus, $0.05 = \dfrac{1}{20} = 1:20$.
Example 3	Convert 2.5 to a ratio.
	1. $2.5 = 2\dfrac{5}{10} = \dfrac{25}{10}$
	2. $\dfrac{25}{10} = \dfrac{\overset{5}{\cancel{25}}}{\underset{2}{\cancel{10}}} = \dfrac{5}{2}$
	3. $\dfrac{5}{2} = 5:2$
	Thus, $2.5 = \dfrac{5}{2} = 5:2$.

 GO TO . . . Open the CD-ROM that accompanies your textbook, and select Chapter 3, Convert Decimal to Ratio (LO 3.2). Review the animation and example problems; then complete the practice problems. Continue to the next section of the book, once you have mastered the information presented.

LEARNING LINK   Recall from Rule 3.3 on page 59 that you can write a percent as a fraction with the denominator of 100. This step helps you to convert a ratio to a percent and a percent to a ratio.

RULE 3-10	To convert a ratio to a percent:
	1. Convert the ratio to a decimal.
	2. Write the decimal as a percent by multiplying the decimal by 100 and adding the percent symbol.
Example 1	Convert $1:50$ to a percent.
	1. Convert the ratio to a decimal.
	$1:50 = \dfrac{1}{50} = 0.02$
	2. Multiply 0.02 by 100 and add the percent symbol.
	$0.02 = 100\% = 2\%$
	$1:50 = \dfrac{1}{50} = 0.02 = 2\%$

Example 2	Convert 2 : 3 to a percent.
	1. $2 : 3 = \frac{2}{3} = 0.67$
	2. $0.67 \times 100\% = 67\%$
	$2 : 3 = \frac{2}{3} = 0.67 = 67\%$

Example 3	Convert 5 : 2 to a percent.
	1. $5 : 2 = \frac{5}{2} = 2.5 = 2.50$
	2. $2.50 \times 100\% = 250\%$
	$5 : 2 = \frac{5}{2} = 2.50 = 250\%$

Think! . . . Is It Reasonable? When a fraction or ratio with a value of less than 1 is converted to a percent, it will be less than 100 percent. If the fraction or ratio is greater than 1, it will equal over 100 percent.

GO TO . . . Open the CD-ROM that accompanies your textbook, and select Chapter 3, Convert Ratio to Percent (LO 3.2). Review the animation and example problems; then complete the practice problems. Continue to the next section of the book, once you have mastered the information presented.

RULE 3-11	To convert a percent to a ratio:
	1. Write the percent as a fraction.
	2. Reduce the fraction to lowest terms.
	3. Write the fraction as a ratio by writing the numerator as value *A* and the denominator as value *B*, in the form *A : B*.

Example 1	Convert 25 percent to a ratio.
	1. Write the percent as a fraction.
	$25\% = \frac{25}{100}$
	2. Reduce the fraction.
	$\frac{25}{100} = \frac{1}{4}$
	3. Restate the fraction as a ratio. Write the numerator as value *A* and the denominator as value *B*.
	$\frac{1}{4} = 1 : 4$
	Thus, $25\% = \frac{1}{4} = 1 : 4$.

Example 2	Convert 450 percent to a ratio.

1. $450\% = \dfrac{450}{100}$

2. $\dfrac{450}{100} = \dfrac{45}{10} = \dfrac{9}{2}$

3. $\dfrac{9}{2} = 9 : 2$

Thus, $450\% = \dfrac{9}{2} = 9 : 2$.

Example 3	Convert 0.3 percent to a ratio.

1. Write the percent as a fraction. In this case, rewrite the fraction without decimal points.

$0.3\% = \dfrac{0.3}{100} = \dfrac{3}{1000}$

2. $\dfrac{3}{1000}$ is reduced to lowest terms.

3. $\dfrac{3}{1000} = 3 : 1000$

Thus, $0.3\% = \dfrac{3}{1000} = 3 : 1000$.

GO TO . . . Open the CD-ROM that accompanies your textbook, and select Chapter 3, Convert Percent to Ratio (LO 3.2). Review the animation and example problems; then complete the practice problems. Continue to the next section of the book, once you have mastered the information presented.

REVIEW AND PRACTICE

3.2 Ratios

Convert the following ratios to fractions or mixed numbers.

1. $3 : 4$ **2.** $4 : 9$ **3.** $5 : 3$ **4.** $10 : 1$ **5.** $1 : 20$

6. $1 : 250$ **7.** $4 : 12$

Convert the following fractions to ratios.

8. $\dfrac{2}{3}$ **9.** $\dfrac{6}{7}$ **10.** $\dfrac{5}{4}$ **11.** $\dfrac{7}{3}$ **12.** $1\dfrac{7}{8}$

13. $3\dfrac{1}{3}$ **14.** $\dfrac{6}{10}$ **15.** $\dfrac{18}{27}$ **16.** $\dfrac{1}{50}$ **17.** $\dfrac{1}{75}$

18. $5\dfrac{4}{5}$

Convert the following ratios to decimals. Round to the nearest hundredth, if necessary.

19. $1 : 4$ **20.** $1 : 8$ **21.** $3 : 4$ **22.** $2 : 5$ **23.** $50 : 1$

24. $25 : 2$ **25.** $8 : 3$ **26.** $5 : 6$ **27.** $5 : 75$

Convert the following decimals to ratios.

28. 0.9   **29.** 0.3   **30.** 0.01   **31.** 0.45   **32.** 6

33. 2.4   **34.** 8   **35.** 9.8

Convert the following ratios to percents. If necessary, round to the nearest percent.

36. $1 : 4$ **37.** $1 : 25$ **38.** $2 : 9$ **39.** $7 : 17$ **40.** $20 : 1$

41. $15 : 2$ **42.** $3 : 8$

Convert the following percents to ratios.

43. 14 %   **44.** 65 %   **45.** 400 %   **46.** 175 %   **47.** 0.6 %

48. 0.18 %   **49.** 84 %   **50.** 0.57 %

To check your answers, see the Answer section at the end of the book, which starts on page A-1.

ERROR ALERT!

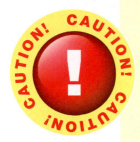

Do Not Forget the Units of Measurement

Including units in the dosage strength will help you to avoid some common errors. Consider the case in which we have two solutions of a drug. One of the solutions contains 1 g of drug in 50 mL; the other contains 1 mg of drug in 50 mL. While both of these solutions have ratio strengths of 1 : 50, they are obviously different from each other. To distinguish between them, the first solution could be written as 1 g : 50 mL while the second is written 1 mg : 50 mL.

3.3 Proportions

A **proportion** is a mathematical statement that two ratios are equal. Because ratios are often written as fractions, a proportion is also a statement that two fractions are equal.

Writing Proportions

You have learned that 2 : 3 is read "two to three." The proportion 2 : 3 = 4 : 6 reads "two is to three as four is to six." A double colon in a proportion means as and can be used in place of the equals sign. For example, the proportion 2:3 :: 4:6 would also read, "two is to three as four is to six." In this text we will use the = sign when writing proportions. This **proportion** states that the relationship of 2 to 3 is the same as the relationship of 4 to 6. By now, you know that 2 divided by 3 is the same as 4 divided by 6 *When you write proportions, do not reduce the ratios to their lowest terms.*

You can write proportions by using either ratios or fractions. Thus, 2 : 3 = 4 : 6 is the same as $\frac{2}{3} = \frac{4}{6}$

RULE 3-12	To change a proportion from ratios to fractions convert both ratios to fractions.
Example 1	Write 3 : 4 = 9 : 12 as a proportion using fractions. Convert both ratios to fractions. Here 3 : 4 becomes $\frac{3}{4}$ and 9 : 12 becomes $\frac{9}{12}$, so that: $$3 : 4 = 9 : 12 \rightarrow \frac{3}{4} = \frac{9}{12}$$

Copyright © 2012 by The McGraw-Hill Companies, Inc.

Example 2	Write $5 : 10 = 50 : 100$ as a proportion using fractions.
	$5 : 10 = 50 : 100 \rightarrow \dfrac{5}{10} = \dfrac{50}{100}$
Example 3	Write $8 : 6 = 4 : 3$ as a proportion using fractions.
	$8 : 6 = 4 : 3 \rightarrow \dfrac{8}{6} = \dfrac{4}{3}$

GO TO . . . Open the CD-ROM that accompanies your textbook, and select Chapter 3, Convert Proportions from Ratios to Fractions (LO 3.3). Review the animation and example problems; then complete the practice problems. Continue to the next section of the book, once you have mastered the information presented.

RULE 3-13	To change a proportion from fractions to ratios, convert each fraction to a ratio.
Example 1	Write $\dfrac{5}{6} = \dfrac{10}{12}$ using ratios.
	Convert each fraction to a ratio.
	$\dfrac{5}{6} = 5 : 6$ and $\dfrac{10}{12} = 10 : 12$ so $5 : 6 = 10 : 12$
Example 2	Write $\dfrac{3}{8} = \dfrac{9}{24}$ using ratios.
	$\dfrac{3}{8} = 3 : 8$ and $\dfrac{9}{24} = 9 : 24$, so that $3 : 8 = 9 : 24$
Example 3	Write $\dfrac{10}{2} = \dfrac{5}{1}$ using ratios.
	$\dfrac{10}{2} = 10 : 2$ and $\dfrac{5}{1} = 5 : 1$ so that $10 : 2 = 5 : 1$

GO TO . . . Open the CD-ROM that accompanies your textbook, and select Chapter 3, Convert Proportions from Fractions to Ratios (LO 3.3). Review the animation and example problems; then complete the practice problems. Continue to the next section of the book, once you have mastered the information presented.

REVIEW AND PRACTICE

3.3 Proportions

Write the following proportions using fractions.

1. $4 : 5 = 8 : 10$	**2.** $5 : 12 = 10 : 24$	**3.** $1 : 10 = 100 : 1000$	**4.** $2 : 3 = 20 : 30$
5. $50 : 25 = 10 : 5$	**6.** $6 : 4 = 18 : 12$	**7.** $5 : 24 = 10 : 48$	**8.** $75 : 100 = 150 : 200$
9. $4 : 16 = 16 : 64$	**10.** $125 : 100 = 375 : 300$		

Write the following proportions using ratios.

11. $\dfrac{3}{4} = \dfrac{75}{100}$ **12.** $\dfrac{1}{5} = \dfrac{3}{15}$ **13.** $\dfrac{8}{4} = \dfrac{2}{1}$ **14.** $\dfrac{8}{7} = \dfrac{24}{21}$ **15.** $\dfrac{18}{16} = \dfrac{9}{8}$

16. $\dfrac{10}{1} = \dfrac{40}{4}$ **17.** $\dfrac{5}{7} = \dfrac{15}{21}$ **18.** $\dfrac{45}{5} = \dfrac{9}{1}$ **19.** $\dfrac{1}{100} = \dfrac{100}{10,000}$ **20.** $\dfrac{36}{12} = \dfrac{72}{24}$

To check your answers, see the Answer section at the end of the book, which starts on page A-1.

3.4 Using Proportions to Solve for an Unknown Quantity

You often work with proportions to calculate dosages. When you know three of four values of a proportion, you can solve the proportion to determine the unknown quantity. The proportion can be set up using either ratios or fractions—both methods lead to the same answer. Which method you select is a matter of personal preference.

It is not enough to learn to find the unknown quantity. You must also learn to set up the proportion correctly. If you set up the proportion incorrectly, you could give the wrong amount of medication, with serious consequences for the patient. Use critical thinking skills to select the appropriate information and set up the proportion. In later chapters, you will learn to read physician's orders and drug labels, the sources for the information that goes into the proportion. The remainder of this chapter focuses on finding unknown quantities.

Means and Extremes

When you set up a proportion in the form $A : B = C : D$, the values A and D are the **extremes.** The values B and C are the **means.** If you have trouble remembering which is which, think, "Extremes are on the ends. Means are in the middle."

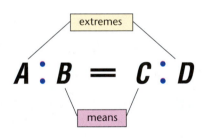

In any true proportion, the product of the means always equals the product of the extremes.

RULE 3-14

To determine if a proportion is true:

1. Multiply the means.

2. Multiply the extremes.

3. Compare the product of the means with the product of the extremes. If the products are equal, the proportion is true.

Example 1	Determine if 1 : 2 = 3 : 6 is a true proportion. **1.** Multiply the means: 2 × 3 = 6 **2.** Multiply the extremes: 1 × 6 = 6 **3.** Compare the products of the means and the extremes. 6 = 6 The statement 1 : 2 = 3 : 6 is a true proportion.
Example 2	Determine if 100 : 40 = 50 : 20 is a true proportion. **1.** 40 × 50 = 2000 **2.** 100 × 20 = 2000 **3.** 2000 = 2000 The proportion 100 : 40 = 50 : 20 is true.
Example 3	Determine if 100 : 20 = 5 : 4 is a true proportion. **1.** 20 × 5 = 100 **2.** 100 × 4 = 400 **3.** 400 ≠ 100 The proportion 10 : 20 = 5 : 4 is not a true proportion.

GO TO . . . Open the CD-ROM that accompanies your textbook, and select Chapter 3, Determine if a Proportion is True (LO 3.4). Review the animation and example problems; then complete the practice problems. Continue to the next section of the book, once you have mastered the information presented.

By definition, both sides of an equation are equal. If you perform the same calculation on both sides of an equation, the two sides will still be equal. For instance, consider the equation:

$$4 \times 2 = 8$$

You can add 3 to both sides or subtract 5 from both sides of the equation, and the resulting equations are still true.

$$(4 \times 2) + 3 = 8 + 3 \qquad (4 \times 2) - 5 = 8 - 5$$
$$11 = 11 \qquad\qquad 3 = 3$$

You can also multiply or divide both sides by the same nonzero number and the sides remain equal.

$$(4 \times 2) \times 6 = 8 \times 6 \qquad (4 \times 2) \div 4 = 8 \div 4$$
$$48 = 48 \qquad\qquad 2 = 2$$

Now you can use the means and extremes to help you find an unknown quantity in a proportion. Suppose you have the proportion

$$2 : 4 = x : 12$$

where x represents the unknown quantity. The product of the means equals the product of the extremes.

$$4 \times x = 2 \times 12$$
$$4 \times x = 24$$

To find the value of x, you must write the equation so that x stands alone on one side of the equal sign. Here you simply divide both sides by the number before x, or 4

$$4 \times x = 24$$
$$\frac{4 \times x}{4} = \frac{24}{4}$$
$$x = 6$$

Check that the proportion is now true:

$$2 : 4 = 6 : 12$$
$$4 \times 6 = 24 \qquad \text{and} \qquad 2 = 12 = 24$$

Because $4 \times 6 = 2 \times 12$, the proportion is true. *Remember,* taking the time to check your work will help you avoid errors.

RULE 3-15	To find the unknown quantity in a proportion: **1.** Write an equation setting the product of the means equal to the product of the extremes. **2.** Solve the equation for the unknown quantity. **3.** Restate the proportion, inserting the unknown quantity. **4.** Check your work. Determine if the proportion is true.
Example	Find the unknown quantity in $25 : 5 = 50 : x$ **1.** Write an equation setting the product of the means equal to the product of the extremes. $5 \times 50 = 25 \times x$ $250 = 25 \times x$ **2.** Solve the equation. Here, divide both sides by 25. $\dfrac{250}{25} = \dfrac{25 \times x}{25}$ $10 = x$ **3.** Restate the proportion, inserting the unknown quantity. $25 : 5 = 50 : 10$ **4.** Check your work. $5 \times 50 = 25 \times 10$ $250 = 250$ The unknown quantity is 10.

GO TO . . . Open the CD-ROM that accompanies your textbook, and select Chapter 3, Find Missing Values (Unknown Quantities) in Proportions using Ratios (LO 3.4). Review the animation and example problems; then complete the practice problems. Continue to the next section of the book, once you have mastered the information presented.

CANCELING UNITS IN PROPORTIONS   It is important to include units when you are writing ratios and proportions. Including units, and learning how to cancel like units, will help you to determine the correct units for the answer when you solve problems using proportions. For example, you have a solution containing 200 mg of drug in 5 mL, and you are asked to determine how many milliliters of a solution contain 500 mg of drug. You can solve the problem by using the following two ratios.

200 mg : 5 mL

500 mg : x

If the units of the first parts of the two ratios are the same, they can be dropped or canceled. Likewise, if the units from the second part of the two ratios are the same, they can be canceled. In this case, the units for the first part of each ratio are milligrams. Canceling the units leaves us with the following proportion.

200 : 5 mL = 500 : x

The product of the means equals the product of the extremes.

5 mL × 500 = 200 × x

We then divide both sides of the equation by 200 so that x stands alone.

$$\frac{5 \text{ mL} \times 500}{200} = \frac{200 \times x}{200}$$

12.5 mL = x

There are 500 mg of the drug in 12.5 mL of the solution.

Think! . . . Is It Reasonable? There is 200 mg for every 5 mL, and we need 500 mg of medication, which is $2\frac{1}{2}$ times the 200 mg. Our solution of 12.5 mL is $2\frac{1}{2}$ times the 5 mL of solution.

RULE 3-16	If the units in the first part of the ratios in a proportion are the same, the units can be canceled. If the units in the second part of the ratios in a proportion are the same, the units can be canceled.
Example 1	If 100 mL of solution contains 20 mg of drug, how many milligrams of the drug will be in 500 mL of the solution?

Start by setting up the ratios.

20 mg : 100 mL   and x : 500 mL

Compare the units used in the two ratios to see if any can be canceled. In this case, the units for the second part of both ratios are milliliters. These can be canceled when we set up the proportion.

20 mg : 100 = x : 500

Now solve for x, the unknown quantity.

1. $100 \times x = 20 \text{ mg} \times 500$

2. $\dfrac{100 \times x}{100} = \dfrac{20 \text{ mg} \times 500}{100}$

3. $x = 100 \text{ mg}$

The second solution will contain 100 mg of drug in 500 mL of solution.

Example 2

15 g of drug is dissolved in 300 mL of solution. If you need 45 g of the drug, how many milliliters of the solution are needed?

Set up the ratios.

$\qquad$ 15 g : 300 mL $\quad$ and $\quad$ 45 g : x

Cancel units and set up the proportion.

$\qquad$ 15 : 300 mL = 45 : x

Solve for the unknown quantity.

1. 300 mL $\times$ 45 = 15 $\times$ x

2. $\dfrac{300 \text{ mL} \times 45}{15} = \dfrac{15 \times x}{15}$

3. 900 mL = x

You will need 900 mL of the solution to have 45 g of drug.

GO TO . . . Open the CD-ROM that accompanies your textbook, and select Chapter 3, Canceling Units in a Proportion Using Ratios (LO 3.4). Review the animation and example problems; then complete the practice problems. Continue to the next section of the book, once you have mastered the information presented.

CRITICAL THINKING ON THE JOB

Setting Up the Correct Proportion

A physician's order calls for a patient to receive 250 mg of amoxicillin oral suspension 3 times a day. Amoxicillin oral suspension is a dry medication that is mixed with water before being given to the patient. Each 5 mL of suspension contains 125 mg of drug. The healthcare professional needs to calculate how many milliliters he will need to give the patient for each dose. He sets up the proportion as 5 mL/125 mg = 250 mg/x.

Think! . . . Is It Reasonable? What mistake did the healthcare professional make? How should it be corrected? What dose should the patient receive?

Cross-Multiplying

When a proportion is written with fractions, you can use a method, known as **cross-multiplying** to determine if it is true. Cross-multiplying is multiplying the numerator from each fraction by the denominator of the other. If the proportion is true, the products must be equal.

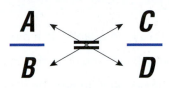

Cross-multiplying

RULE 3-17	To determine if a proportion written with fractions is true: **1.** Cross-multiply. Multiply the numerator of the first fraction with the denominator of the second fraction. Then multiply the denominator of the first fraction with the numerator of the second fraction. **2.** Compare the products. The products must be equal.
Example 1	Determine if $\frac{2}{5} = \frac{10}{25}$ is a true proportion. **1.** Cross-multiply. $\frac{2}{5} \diagup\!\!\!\!\!\diagdown \frac{10}{25} \rightarrow 2 \times 25 = 5 \times 10$ **2.** Compare the products on both sides of the equal sign. $50 = 50$ $\frac{2}{5} = \frac{10}{25}$ is a true proportion.
Example 2	Determine if $\frac{100}{1000} = \frac{500}{5000}$ is a true proportion. **1.** $\frac{100}{1000} \diagup\!\!\!\!\!\diagdown \frac{500}{5000} \rightarrow 100 \times 5000 = 1000 \times 500$ **2.** $500{,}000 = 500{,}000$ $\frac{100}{1000} = \frac{500}{5000}$ is a true proportion.
Example 3	Determine if $\frac{5}{8} = \frac{40}{72}$ is a true proportion. **1.** $\frac{5}{8} \diagup\!\!\!\!\!\diagdown \frac{40}{72} \rightarrow 5 \times 72 = 8 \times 40$ **2.** $360 \neq 320$ The proportion $\frac{5}{8} = \frac{40}{72}$ is not true.

GO TO . . . Open the CD-ROM that accompanies your textbook, and select Chapter 3, Determine if Proportion Using Fractions is True (LO 3.4). Review the animation and example problems; then complete the practice problems. Continue to the next section of the book, once you have mastered the information presented.

In the previous section, you learned to use means and extremes to find an unknown quantity in a proportion that was written using ratios. As you might expect, you can cross-multiply to find the unknown quantity in a proportion expressed with fractions.

RULE 3-18	To find the unknown quantity in a proportion written with fractions:
	1. Cross-multiply. Write an equation setting the products equal to each other.
	2. Solve the equation to find the unknown quantity.
	3. Restate the proportion, inserting the unknown quantity.
	4. Check your work. Determine if the proportion is true.

Example 1

Find the unknown quantity in $\frac{3}{5} = \frac{6}{x}$

1. Cross-multiply.

$$\frac{3}{5} \diagtimes \frac{6}{x} \rightarrow 3 \times x = 5 \times 6$$

$$3 \times x = 30$$

2. Solve the equation. Here, divide both sides by 3.

$$\frac{3 \times x}{3} = \frac{30}{3}$$

$$x = 10$$

3. Restate the proportion, inserting the unknown quantity.

$$\frac{3}{5} = \frac{6}{10}$$

4. Check your work by cross-multiplying.

$$3 \times 10 = 5 \times 6$$

$$30 = 30$$

The unknown quantity is 10.

Example 2

Find the unknown quantity in $\frac{25}{5} = \frac{50}{x}$

1. $\frac{25}{5} \diagtimes \frac{50}{x} \rightarrow 25 \times x = 5 \times 50$

$$25 \times x = 250$$

2. $\frac{25 \times x}{25} = \frac{250}{25}$

$$x = 10$$

3. $\frac{25}{5} = \frac{50}{10}$

4. $25 \times 10 = 5 \times 50$

$$250 = 250$$

The unknown quantity is 10.

GO TO . . . Open the CD-ROM that accompanies your textbook, and select Chapter 3, Find Missing Value (Unknown Quantity) in Proportions Using Fractions (LO 3.4). Review the animation and example problems; then complete the practice problems. Continue to the next section of the book, once you have mastered the information presented.

CANCELING UNITS IN PROPORTIONS WRITTEN WITH FRACTIONS Just as we were able to cancel units in proportions written as ratios, we can cancel them in proportions written as fractions. Now, however, we need to compare the units used in the top and bottom of the two fractions in the proportion. For example, you have a solution containing 200 mg of drug in 5 mL, and you are asked to determine how many milliliters of a solution contain 500 mg of drug. You can solve the problem by using the following two fractions. Must make sure that the labels are in like positions. In this case, mg is placed in the numerator in both fractions.

$$\frac{200 \text{ mg}}{5 \text{ mL}} \qquad \frac{500 \text{ mg}}{x}$$

Because the units for both numerators of the fraction are milligrams, they can be canceled. Canceling the units leaves us with the following proportion.

$$\frac{200}{5 \text{ mL}} = \frac{500}{x}$$

The unknown quantity can now be found by cross-multiplying and solving the equation as before.

RULE 3-19	If the units of the numerator of the two fractions are the same, they can be dropped or canceled before you set up a proportion. Likewise, if the units from the denominator of the two fractions are the same, they can be canceled.
Example 1	If 100 mL of solution contains 20 mg of drug, how many milligrams of the drug will be in 500 mL of the solution?

Start by setting up the fractions.

$$\frac{20 \text{ mg}}{100 \text{ mL}} \quad \text{and} \quad \frac{x}{500 \text{ mL}}$$

Compare the units used in the two fractions to see if any can be canceled. In this case, the units for the denominators of both fractions are milliliters. These can be canceled when you set up the proportion.

$$\frac{20 \text{ mg}}{100} = \frac{x}{500}$$

Now solve for x, the unknown quantity.

1. $100 \times x = 20 \text{ mg} \times 500$

2. $\dfrac{100 \times x}{100} = \dfrac{20 \text{ mg} \times 500}{100}$

3. $x = 100$ mg

The second solution will contain 100 mg of drug in 500 mL of solution.

Example 2

15 grams of drug is dissolved in 300 mL of solution. If you need 45 g of the drug, how many milliliters of the solution are needed?

Set up the fractions.

$$\frac{15 \text{ g}}{300 \text{ mL}} \quad \text{and} \quad \frac{45 \text{ g}}{x}$$

Cancel units and set up the proportion.

$$\frac{15}{300 \text{ mL}} = \frac{45}{x}$$

Solve for the missing value.

1. $300 \text{ mL} \times 45 = 15 \times x$

2. $\dfrac{300 \text{ mL} \times 45}{15} = \dfrac{15 \times x}{15}$

3. $900 \text{ mL} = x$

You will need 900 mL of the solution to have 45 g of drug.

 GO TO . . . Open the CD-ROM that accompanies your textbook, and select Chapter 3, Canceling Units in a Proportion using Fractions (LO 3.4). Review the animation and example problems; then complete the practice problems. Continue to the next section of the book, once you have mastered the information presented.

CRITICAL THINKING ON THE JOB

Confusing Multiplying Fractions with Cross-Multiplying

A healthcare professional is preparing a 5% solution of dextrose in batches of 500 cubic centimeters or milliliters (mL). She sets up the calculation as follows: $\frac{5 \text{ g}}{100 \text{ mL}} = \frac{x}{500 \text{ mL}}$. Distracted by a call, she returns to the calculation and computes:

$$5 \times x = 100 \times 500 = 50{,}000$$

This calculation leads to:

$$x = 10{,}000$$

Think! . . . Is It Reasonable? What mistake did the healthcare professional make? How could she have avoided this mistake?

3.4 Using Proportions to Solve for an Unknown Quantity

Determine if the following proportions are true.

1. $6 : 12 = 12 : 24$

2. $3 : 8 = 9 : 32$

3. $5 : 75 = 15 : 250$

4. $8 : 100 = 20 : 250$

5. $6 : 18 = 18 : 54$

6. $\dfrac{7}{16} = \dfrac{28}{48}$

7. $\dfrac{6}{9} = \dfrac{24}{36}$

8. $\dfrac{100}{250} = \dfrac{150}{375}$

9. $\dfrac{50}{125} = \dfrac{125}{300}$

10. $\dfrac{60}{96} = \dfrac{80}{108}$

Find the missing value.

11. $10 : x = 5 : 8$

12. $10 : 4 = 20 : x$

13. $4 : 25 = 16 : x$

14. $x : 15 = 100 : 75$

15. $21 : 27 = x : 45$

16. $100 : x = 50 : 2$

17. $3 : 12 = x : 36$

18. $33 : 39 = 55 : x$

19. $x : 24 : = 5 : 30$

20. $18 : x = 27 : 6$

21. $\dfrac{3}{15} = \dfrac{x}{5}$

22. $\dfrac{2}{x} = \dfrac{8}{100}$

23. $\dfrac{x}{20} = \dfrac{120}{100}$

24. $\dfrac{50}{75} = \dfrac{100}{x}$

25. $\dfrac{10}{3} = \dfrac{x}{60}$

26. $\dfrac{x}{4} = \dfrac{4}{16}$

27. $\dfrac{25}{x} = \dfrac{75}{3}$

28. $\dfrac{2}{3} = \dfrac{6}{x}$

29. $\dfrac{x}{9} = \dfrac{18}{27}$

30. $\dfrac{25}{125} = \dfrac{x}{150}$

31. A patient must take 3 tablets per day for 14 days. How many tablets should the pharmacy supply to fill this order?

32. If 15 mL of solution contains 75 mg of drug, how many milligrams of drug are in 60 mL of solution?

33. A healthcare professional is instructed to administer 600 mL of a solution every 8 h. How many hours will be needed to administer 1800 mL of the solution?

34. Two tablets contain a total of 50 mg of drug. How many milligrams of drug are in 10 tablets?

35. If 250 mL of solution contains 90 mg of drug, there is 450 mg of drug in how many milliliters of solution?

To check your answers, see the Answer section at the end of the book, which starts on page A-1.

CHAPTER 3 SUMMARY

LEARNING OUTCOME	KEY POINTS

3.1 Convert values to and from a percent. Pages 57–61	▶ A value expressed as a percent represents the value divided by 100.
	  • Example: 15% is equal to 0.15 or 15 hundredths.
	▶ Fractions can be converted to percents by dividing the numerator by the denominator, multiplying by 100, and then adding the percent sign.
	  • Example: To convert $\frac{3}{4}$ to a percent, divide 3 by 4 and then multiply by 100%. $(3 \div 4) \times 100\% = 75\%$.
	▶ Decimals can be converted into a percent by multiplying them by 100 and then adding the percent sign.
	  • Example: To convert 0.125 to a percent, multiply by 100%. $0.125 \times 100\% = 12.5\%$.

3.2 Convert values to and from a ratio. Pages 62–68	▶ A ratio is another way to write a fraction. ▶ A ratio contains 2 numbers separated by a colon. The number before the colon is the numerator of the fraction, the number after the colon is the denominator. • Example: The fraction $\frac{5}{8}$ is equal to the ratio $5 : 8$.
3.3 Write proportions. Pages 68–70	▶ Proportions state that two fractions or two ratios are equal to each other. ▶ Proportions can be written using either ratios or fractions. • Example: $2 : 3 = 6 : 9$ and $\frac{2}{3} = \frac{6}{9}$ are the same proportion written in two different ways.

3.4 Use proportions to solve for an unknown quantity. Pages 70–79	▶ When 3 of the 4 values in a proportion are known, the unknown value can be calculated.
	▶ Proportions using ratios can be are solved by multiplying means and extremes.
	  • Example: To solve for the unknown in $2 : 4 = 3 : x$, multiply the means $(4 \times 3 = 12)$ then the extremes $(2 \times x = 2x)$. Write an equation using the products $(2x = 12)$ and then solve for the unknown $(x = 6)$
	▶ Proportions using fractions are solved by cross-multiplying.
	  • Example: To solve for the unknown in $\frac{2}{3} = \frac{x}{12}$, cross-multiply $(3 \times x = 2 \times 12)$ and then solve for the unknown $(x = 8)$.

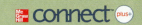
In each row of the table below, use the information to calculate the equivalent values. When necessary, round decimals to the nearest hundredth. Round percents to the nearest tenth of a percent. Do not reduce ratios or fractions. (LO 3.1, 3.2)

	fraction	decimal	reatio	percent
1		0.625		
2	$\frac{5}{2}$			
3			3 : 5	
4				35%
5	$\frac{1}{6}$			
6		11.4		
7				18.5%
8			6 : 20	

Find the missing value: (LO 3.3, 3.4)

9. $2 : x = 6 : 15$

10. $x : 8 = 3 : 12$

11. $5 : 8 = x : 40$

12. $\frac{1}{6} = \frac{x}{18}$

13. $\frac{4}{12} = \frac{2}{x}$

14. $\frac{15}{x} = \frac{6}{8}$

15. If 1 tablet contains 30 mg of drug, how many milligrams of drug do 5 tablets contain?

16. If 10 g of drug is in 250 mL of solution, how many grams of drug are in 1000 mL of solution?

17. If 3 tablets contain 45 mg of drug, how many milligrams of drug are in 1 tablet?

18. If 60 mg of drug is in 500 mL of solution, how many milliliters of solution contain 36 mg of drug?

19. If 80 mg of drug is in 480 mL of solution, how many milliliters of solution contain 60 mg of drug?

20. If 3 capsules contain 60 mg of drug, how many capsules contain 100 mg of drug?

CHECK UP

In each row of the table below, use the information to calculate the equivalent values. For instance, in row 1, convert the ratio 2 : 3 to a fraction, a decimal, and a percent. Where necessary, round decimals to the nearest hundredth. Round percents to the nearest percent. Do not reduce ratios and fractions. (LO 3.1, 3.2)

	fraction	decimal	reatio	percent
1			2 : 3	
2	$\frac{5}{4}$			
3				28%
4		0.03		
5	$\frac{40}{8}$			
6			4 : 12	
7	$\frac{9}{27}$			
8		1.4		
9				0.5%
10			3 : 50	
11				25%
12		6		
13	$\frac{1}{9}$			
14				150%
15			6 : 97	
16		12.8		

Find the missing value. (LO 3.4)

17. $1 : 10 = 4 : x$ **18.** $3 : 27 = x : 9$ **19.** $x : 6 = 8 : 12$ **20.** $5 : x = 10 : 50$

21. $\frac{4}{8} = \frac{24}{x}$ **22.** $\frac{x}{14} = \frac{5}{70}$ **23.** $\frac{3}{x} = \frac{30}{20}$ **24.** $\frac{1}{25} = \frac{x}{125}$

25. If 1 tablet contains 25 mg of drug, how many milligrams of drug are in 3 tablets? (LO 3-3, 3-4)

26. If 100 mL of drug is in 600 mL of solution, how many milliliters of drug are in 1800 mL of solution? (LO 3.3, 3.4)

27. A solution contains 5 grams of dextrose in 100 cc of solution. How many grams (g) of dextrose are in 500 cc of solution? (LO 3.3, 3.4)

28. A solution contains 1 g of drug for every 50 mL of solution. How much solution would you need to give a patient to administer 3 g of drug? (LO 3.3, 3.4)

29. 10 mL of a liquid medication contains 250 mg of drug. How many milliliters contain 50 mg of drug? (LO 3.3, 3.4)

30. If 30 g of drug is in 100 mL of solution, how many grams of drug is in 350 mL of solution? (LO 3.3, 3.4)

CRITICAL THINKING APPLICATIONS

A healthcare professional has just finished preparing 250 mL of a solution containing 6 grams of drug in every 100 mL when he learns that the physician wants a solution containing 8 grams of drug in 100 mL of solution. How many additional grams of drug should the healthcare professional add to the first solution he prepared? (LO 3.3, 3.4)

CASE STUDY

A physician's order calls for Ceclor® oral suspension 750 mg to be given daily for 14 days. The daily dosage is to be divided into 3 equal doses per day. Ceclor® oral suspension is a drug that is mixed with solvent before it is administered. (LO 3.3, 3.4)

1. How many milligrams of drug should be given in each dose?

2. If 5 mL of solution contains 125 mg of drug, how many milliliters should be given in each dose?

INTERNET ACTIVITY

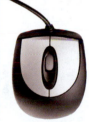

To obtain a better understanding of solutions, lotions, creams, suspensions, and ointments, search for these terms on the Internet. Find their definitions and at least three example medications of each type. You can start with an online dictionary such as found on www.refdesk.com and then search websites such as www.fda.gov or www.rxlist.com for example medications.

To check your answers, see the Answer section at the end of the book, which starts on page A-1.

GO TO . . . Open the CD-ROM that accompanies your textbook, and complete a final review of the learning outcomes, practice problems, games, slideshow, and other activities presented for this chapter. For a final evaluation, take the chapter test and email or print your results for your instructor. A score of 95 percent or above indicates mastery of the chapter concepts.

UNIT ONE ASSESSMENT

Up until now, all of the calculations have been grouped together to allow you the opportunity to practice a specific skill. In Chapter 1, you focused on fractions; in Chapter 2, decimals. Chapter 3 allowed you to work on percents, ratios, and proportions. In the "real world," however, you will be faced with a variety of situations in which you will need to use each of these skills at various times throughout the day. Problems will not be sorted by chapter. This assessment requires you to use skills practiced in each of the chapters in this unit. If you have trouble with some of these calculations, it will help you to identify areas where more practice is needed. If you do well, you can move forward with the confidence that you are prepared for the next unit.

1. Place >, <, or = between the following pairs of numbers to make a true statement.

   a. $3\frac{1}{5}$ 3. 25   b. 135% $1\frac{1}{2}$ c. 14.5 $\frac{29}{2}$

2. $0.57 = $ _____%

3. $2.4 \div 0.3 = x$

4. A bottle contains 60 mL of medication. How many 5 mL doses does it contain?

5. $1 : 6 = x : 18$

6. Write 7.4 as an improper fraction.

7. There are 250 mg of drug in 5 mL of a solution. How many milligrams of drug are there in 12 mL?

8. Write 0.4 as a ratio.

9. $3 : 50 = $ _____%

10. Write 3.5% as a decimal.

11. $\frac{3}{14} = \frac{9}{x}$

12. $\frac{x}{5} = \frac{15}{25}$

13. $\frac{1}{4} \div \frac{1}{3} = x$

14. $5\frac{1}{8} + 3\frac{1}{4} = x$

15. What is the least common denominator for $\frac{2}{5}$, $\frac{1}{3}$, and $\frac{1}{2}$?

16. $2 : 5 = 7 : x$

17. Reduce $\frac{18}{4}$ and rewrite it as a mixed number.

18. Write $\frac{23}{4}$ as a decimal.

19. If three tablets contain 150 mg of a drug, how much drug is there in four tablets?

20. $3.125 - 1.7 = x$

To check your answers, see the Answer section at the end of the book, which starts on page A-1.

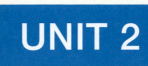

UNIT 2

Systems of Measurement

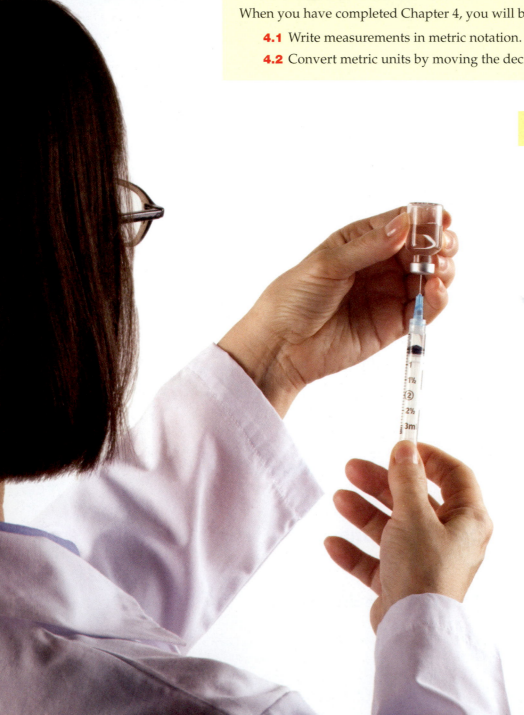

Metric System

Practice is the best instruction of them all.

—Publilius Syrus

Learning Outcomes

When you have completed Chapter 4, you will be able to:

4.1 Write measurements in metric notation.

4.2 Convert metric units by moving the decimal.

KEY TERMS

Centi (c)
Gram (g)
Kilo (k)
Liter (L)
Meter (m)
Micro (mc)
Milli (m)

INTRODUCTION

The metric system is the most commonly used system of measurement in the healthcare system. Drugs are most often labeled and ordered in milligrams, although there are some that will be measured in micrograms or **grams**. Injections are usually measured in milliliters. Intravenous solutions may be measured in liters. Knowing how to accurately convert units within the metric system is an essential skill for anyone performing dosage calculations. Practice these concepts until you are certain you understand.

4.1 Metric System

The metric system is the most widely used system of measurement in the world today. The system, which was defined in 1792, gets its name from the **meter,** the basic unit of length. A meter is approximately 3 inches (8.56 cm) longer than a yard. It may be helpful to visualize the relationship of the metric system to measurements you already know. (See Figure 4-1.)

Units of measurement in the metric system are sometimes referred to as SI units, an abbreviation for International System of Units. This system was established in 1960 to make units of measurement for the metric system standard throughout the world. Table 4-1 lists the basic metric units for length, weight, and volume.

Notice that meter and gram are abbreviated with lowercase letters, but **liter** is abbreviated with an uppercase L. Using the uppercase L minimizes the chance of confusing the lowercase letter L (l) with the digit 1. You will use length mostly when expressing measurements such as patient height, infant head circumference, and lesion or wound size. However, you will use weight and volume frequently when you calculate dosages. Most dosages and drug strengths are expressed using the metric system.

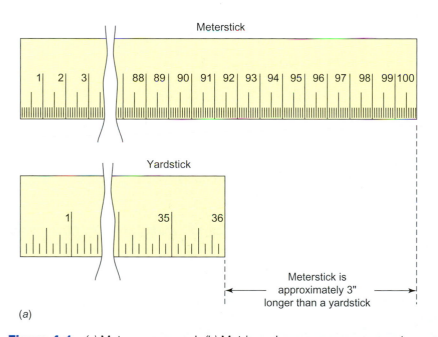

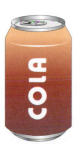

Height: 4¾ inches or 12 centimeters

Diameter: 2½ inches or 6.35 centimeters

Weight (full): ¾ pound or 0.36 kilograms

Weight (empty): ½ ounce or 15 grams

Volume: 12 ounces or 355 milliliters

(a) (b)

Figure 4-1 *(a)* Meter versus yard. *(b)* Metric and common measurements comparison.

TABLE 4-1 Basic Units of Metric Measurement		
TYPE OF MEASURE	**BASIC UNIT**	**ABBREVIATION**
Length	meter	m
Weight (or mass)	gram	g (or gm)
Volume	liter	L

Metric Notation

Like the decimal system, the metric system is based on multiples of 10. The greater confidence you have working with decimals, the more comfortable you will be working with metric units. (To review decimals, see Chapter 2.)

A prefix before the basic unit indicates relative size. For example, **kilo-** indicates that you multiply the basic unit by 1000. A kilometer is 1000 meters, a kilogram is 1000 grams, and a kiloliter is 1000 liters. When you divide 1 meter into 1000 equal lengths, each length is 1 millimeter. The prefix **milli-** means one-thousandth. A millimeter is one-thousandth of a meter, a milliliter is one-thousandth of a liter, and a milligram is one-thousandth of a gram.

As a healthcare provider, you will most often use the metric prefixes **kilo-**, **centi-**, **milli-**, and **micro-**. Table 4-2 shows how these prefixes are combined with the base units and their value relative to the base unit.

TABLE 4-2 Common Metric Prefixes

Prefix	kilo-	base unit	centi-	milli-	micro-
Value	× 1000	—	÷ 100	÷ 1000	÷ 1,000,000
Length	kilometer km 1000 m	meter m 1 m	centimeter cm 0.01 m	millimeter mm 0.001 m	micrometer mcm 0.000001 m
Weight (Mass)	kilogram kg 1000 g	gram g 1 g	centigram cg 0.01 g	milligram mg 0.001 g	microgram mcg 0.000001 g
Volume	kiloliter kL 1000 L	liter L 1 L	centiliter cL 0.01 L	milliliter mL 0.001 L	microliter mcm 0.000001 L

RULE 4-1	Use Arabic numerals, with decimals to represent any fractions.
Example	Write 1.25 g to represent $1\frac{1}{4}$ g.

RULE 4-2	If the quantity is less than 1, include a 0 before the decimal point. Delete any other zeros that are not necessary.
Example	Do not write .750; instead, write 0.75, adding a zero before the decimal point and deleting the unnecessary zero at the end.

RULE 4-3	Write the unit after the quantity with a space between them.
Example	Write 30 mg, not mg 30 or 30mg.

RULE 4-4	Use lowercase letters for metric abbreviations. However, use uppercase L to represent liter.
Example	Write mg, not MG. Write mL, not ml. While ml is technically correct, you will avoid errors if you use an uppercase L.

Considering Rules 4-1 to 4-4, we will determine the correct metric notation for six and two-eighths milliliters. First, $6\frac{2}{8}$ must be converted to decimals.

$$6\frac{2}{8} = 6.25$$

 LEARNING LINK   Recall from Chapter 1 (Rule 1-5) and Chapter 2 (Rule 2-5) that $\frac{2}{8}$ can be reduced to $\frac{1}{4}$ and $\frac{1}{4} = 0.25$.

Next, write the unit after the quantity, leaving a space between them and using the abbreviation mL for milliliters. So:

6.25 mL is correct metric notation for six and two-eighths milliliters.

Now consider how you would write one-half milligram.

$$\frac{1}{2} = 0.50$$

Place a zero in front of the decimal point, and delete any unnecessary zeros.

0.5

Place the unit after the quantity with a space between them.

0.5 mg is correct metric notation for one-half milligram.

GO TO . . . Open the CD-ROM that accompanies your textbook, and select Chapter 4, Representing Fractions (LO 4.1). Using a Zero before the Decimal Point (LO 4.1), Writing the Unit (LO 4.1), and Metric Abbreviations (LO 4.1). Review the animation and example problems, then complete the practice problems. Continue to the next section of the book once you have mastered the information presented.

REVIEW AND PRACTICE

4.1 Metric Notation

In Exercises 1–10, select the correct metric notation.

1. Two and one-half kilograms
   a. 2.5 Kg   **b.** 2.05 kg   **c.** $2\frac{1}{2}$ kg   **d.** 2.5 kg

2. Seven-tenths of a milliliter
   a. $\frac{7}{10}$ mL   **b.** .7mL   **c.** ml 0.7   **d.** 0.7 mL

3. Four-hundredths of a gram

    a. 400 G   **b.** 0.4g   **c.** 0.04 g   **d.** .04 g

4. Thirty-one millimeters

    a. 31mm   **b.** 0.031 mm   **c.** 31.0 mlm   **d.** 31 mm

5. Eight liters

    a. 8.0 l   **b.** 8 L   **c.** 8.0L   **d.** 0.8 l

6. One hundred twenty-five micrograms

    a. 125 mg   **b.** 0.125 mcg   **c.** 125 mcg   **d.** 125mg

7. Seventy-eight centimeters

    a. 78 ctm   **b.** 78.0 Cm   **c.** 0.78 cm   **d.** 78 cm

8. Two hundred fifty microliters

    a. mcL 250   **b.** 250 mcL   **c.** 25.0 mcL   **d.** 250 mL

9. Nine and one-quarter milligrams

    a. $9\frac{1}{4}$ mg   **b.** 9.25mg   **c.** 9.25 mg   **d.** 9.25 mgm

10. Four-tenths of a liter

    a. 0.4 L   **b.** $\frac{4}{10}$ L   **c.** 0.40 L   **d.** 0.40 l

In Exercises 11–20, write the indicated amounts with correct metric notation.

11. Four and one-half milliliters _____   **12.** Sixty-two hundredths of a gram _____

13. Three-quarters of a milliliter _____   **14.** Seven-tenths of a meter _____

15. Twelve liters _____   **16.** Nine-twelfths of a kilogram _____

17. One hundred fifty-seven kilometers _____   **18.** Seven and three-quarters centimeters _____

19. Ninety-three micrograms _____   **20.** Eight-hundredths of a milligram _____

To check your answers, see the Answer section at the end of the book, which starts on page A-1.

4.2   Converting Within the Metric System

Recall from Chapter 2 that when you multiply a decimal number by 100, you move the decimal point two places to the right and get a larger number. When you divide a decimal number by 100, you move the decimal point two places to the left and get a smaller number.

Converting one metric unit of measurement to another is similar to multiplying and dividing decimal numbers. For example, if you travel 1 kilometer, you travel 1000 meters. When you convert from the larger unit of measurement (kilometer) to the smaller unit (meter), the quantity of units increases. Therefore, you multiply, moving the decimal point to the right.

If you convert from meters to kilometers, the quantity of units decreases. If you travel 1000 meters, you travel 1 kilometer. When you convert from a smaller unit (meter) to a larger unit (kilometer), the quantity of units decreases. Therefore, you divide, moving the decimal point to the left.

When you calculate dosages, you will work most often with four metric units of weight and three metric units of volume. The four units of weight are kilogram (kg), gram (g), milligram (mg), and microgram (mcg). Two of the units of volume are liter (L) and milliliter (mL). The third is cubic centimeter (cc), which is equivalent to milliliter (mL). Although the abbreviation cc for cubic centimeter may be seen in practice, it should not be used. Instead use the abbreviation mL for milliliter.

When you convert a quantity from one unit of metric measurement to another:

1. Move the decimal point to the right if you convert from a larger to a smaller unit.

2. Move the decimal point to the left if you convert from a smaller to a larger unit.

Table 4-3 and Figure 4-2 will help you determine both the direction and the number of places to move the decimal point when you convert between units of metric measurement. For example, milliliter is three places to the right of liter, the basic unit. To convert a quantity from liters (larger) to milliliters (smaller), move the decimal point three places to the right. Similarly, to convert a quantity from grams (smaller) to kilograms (larger), move the decimal point three places to the left.

TABLE 4-3 Metric System Place Values and Units

	KILO-	BASE UNIT	CENTI-	MILLI-	MICRO-
Meaning	1000	1	$\frac{1}{100}$ 0.01	$\frac{1}{1000}$ 0.001	$\frac{1}{1,000,000}$ 0.000001
Commonly used units and abbreviations	kilograms (kg)	grams (g) meters (m) liters (L)	centimeters (cm)	milligrams (mg) millimeters (mm) milliliters (mL)	micrograms (mcg)

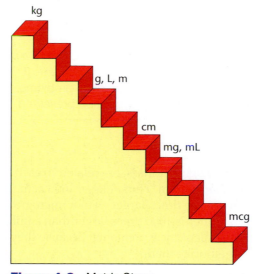

Figure 4-2 Metric Steps.

Example 1

Convert 4 L to milliliters (mL).

Move the decimal point for 4 (or 4.0) three places to the right to find the number of milliliters. Add zeros as necessary to help you with your calculation.

    4 L = 4.000 L = 4000 mL

Think! . . . Is It Reasonable? A milliliter (mL) is smaller than a liter (L); a quantity will have more milliliters than liters. Using Figure 4-2, you can see that milliliter is three steps to the right of liter.

Example 2	How many meters (m) are in 75 mm? A meter (m) is larger than a millimeter (mm); a quantity will have fewer meters than millimeters. Using Figure 4-2, you can see that meter is three steps to the left of millimeter. Write 75 as 75.0, and move the decimal point in 75 three places to the left. Add zeros as necessary. 75 mm = 75.0 mm = 0.075 m
Example 3	Convert 4.5 mcg to milligrams (mg). You are converting from a smaller unit to a larger one. Use Figure 4-2 or divide 4.5 by 1000, moving the decimal point three places to the left. 4.5 mcg ÷ 1000 = 0004.5 mcg ÷ 1000 = 0.0045 mg
Example 4	Convert 62 kg to grams (g). You are converting from a larger unit to a smaller one. Use Figure 4-2 or multiply 62 by 1000, moving the decimal point three places to the right. 62 kg × 1000 = 62.000 kg × 1000 = 62,000 g
Example 5	Convert 300 mg to grams (g). You are converting from a smaller unit to a larger one. Use Figure 4-2 or divide 300 by 1000, moving the decimal point three places to the left. 300 mg ÷ 1000 = 0300.0 mg ÷ 1000 = 0.3 g

GO TO . . . Open the CD-ROM that accompanies your textbook, and select Chapter 4, Converting Between Metric Measurements (LO 4.2). Review the animation and example problems, then complete the practice problems. Continue to the next section of the book once you have mastered the information presented.

The four units of weight, or mass, are related to each other by a factor of 1000. A kilogram is 1000 times larger than a gram. Thus, 1 kg = 1000 g. In turn, a gram is 1000 times larger than a milligram, which is 1000 times larger than a microgram. The same relationship is true for liters and milliliters; a liter is 1000 times larger than a milliliter. Table 4-4 lists four of the most commonly used equivalent measurements. Because they are so important to dosage calculations, you should memorize them.

TABLE 4-4 Equivalent Metric Measurements	
1 kg = 1000 g	1 mg = 1000 mcg
1 g = 1000 mg	1 L = 1000 mL

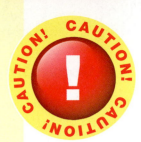

Remember: The Larger the Unit, the Smaller the Quantity; the Smaller the Unit, the Larger the Quantity

You may be tempted to multiply when you convert from a smaller unit to a larger unit, thinking that you are increasing in size. If you find yourself confused, think about conversions you have made all your life.

For example, a dollar bill is a larger unit of money than a quarter, which is a larger unit of money than a penny. When you write their relationship, look at how the quantity changes:

1 dollar bill = 4 quarters = 100 pennies

When you convert from the larger unit to the smaller one, the quantity increases. Writing the money relationship as:

100 pennies = 4 quarters = 1 dollar bill

shows you that as the unit increases in size, the quantity decreases. You see the same relationship with units of time and in the metric system:

1 hour = 60 minutes = 3600 seconds

1 g = 1000 mg = 1,000,000 mcg

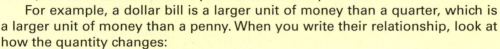

CRITICAL THINKING ON THE JOB

Placing the Decimal Point Correctly

A child suffering from congestive heart failure is rushed into an emergency room. The physician orders 0.05 mg of Lanoxin® for the child. The healthcare professional quickly calculates that 0.05 mg = 500 mcg. Lanoxin® is available for injection in quantities of 500 mcg. The nurse hands the syringe to the doctor.

Fortunately, the doctor catches the error before the Lanoxin® is administered. The child should be given 50 mcg, not 500 mcg of Lanoxin®. As it turns out, Lanoxin® is available as an elixir in doses of 50 mcg. This quantity should be administered. The larger dose of 500 mcg could be fatal to the child.

Think! . . . Is It Reasonable? How can the attending healthcare professional ensure that she converted the quantity correctly. How should the problem have been solved? Why is it important in this situation?

ERROR ALERT!

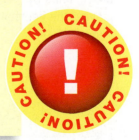

Converting Quantities for Medications

When you convert quantities from one unit of measure to another within the metric system, pay close attention to the decimal point. For example, when going from milligrams (mg) to micrograms (mcg), the quantity should be multiplied by 1000; the decimal should move three places to the right. If you move the decimal the wrong direction a dangerous error can occur.

REVIEW AND PRACTICE

4.2 Converting Within the Metric System

In Exercises 1–20. complete the conversions.

1. 7 g = _____ mg
2. 1200 mg = _____ g
3. 23 g = _____ kg
4. 8 kg = _____ g
5. 8.01 L = _____ mL
6. 100 mL = _____ L
7. 3.6 m = _____ mm
8. 5233 mm = _____ m
9. 500 m = _____ km
10. 3.25 km = _____ m
11. 0.25 mg = _____ mcg
12. 462 mg = _____ mcg
13. 250 mcg = _____ mg
14. 75 mcg = _____ mg
15. 0.06 g = _____ mcg
16. 0.5 g = _____ mcg
17. 8000 mcg = _____ g
18. 20,000 mcg = _____ g
19. 562 mm = _____ cm
20. 4.32 cm = _____ m

To check your answers, see the Answer section at the end of the book, which starts on page A-1.

CHAPTER 4 SUMMARY

LEARNING OUTCOME	KEY POINTS
4.1 Write measurements in metric notation. Pages 87–90	▶ The base units of the metric system are the gram (for weight) liter (for volume) and meter (for length). ▶ Grams, liters, and meters are abbreviated using a single letter—g, L, or m. • The L is capitalized to avoid confusing it with the number 1. ▶ Metric prefixes can be combined with the base unit. • For example, milligram is written mg. This combines the prefix for milli- with the abbreviation for the base unit gram. ▶ The metric prefixes used in dosage calculations are kilo, centi, milli, and micro.
4.2 Convert metric units by moving the decimal. Pages 90–94	▶ When converting to a larger unit the decimal is moved to the left, giving you a smaller number. • When converting 250 mg to grams you are converting to a larger unit, so you move the decimal to the left. 250 mg = 0.25 g. ▶ When converting to a smaller unit the decimal is moved to right, giving you a larger number. • When converting liters to milliliters you are converting to a smaller unit, so you move the decimal to the right. 1.8 L = 1800 mL.

HOMEWORK ASSIGNMENT

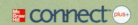

Write the indicated amounts using the proper abbreviations. (LO 4.1)

1. Twenty-five micrograms _____

2. Seven and one-half milliliters _____

3. Eighty-two centimeters _____

4. Three-hundredths of a gram _____

5. Two and three-quarters liters _____

Perform the following conversions. (LO 4.2)

6. 3.5 g = _____ mg

7. 30 mg = _____ g

8. 1.2 kg = _____ g

9. 0.25 mg = _____ mcg

10. 350 g = _____ kg

11. 0.5 L = _____ mL

12. 180 mL = _____ L

13. 1.2 mm = _____ cm

14. 5 mcg = _____ mg

15. 36 cm = _____ m

CHECK UP

In Exercises 1–8, write the indicated amounts, using numerals and abbreviations. (LO 4.1)

1. Twenty-five and one-half kilograms

2. Forty-five hundredths of a centimeter

3. Forty micrograms

4. Three-quarters of a liter

5. Nine-tenths of a milligram

6. One and one-half millimeters

7. Three hundred seventy-five thousandths of a gram

8. Twelve milliliters

In Exercises 9–20, calculate the conversions. (LO 4.2)

9. 0.06 g = _____ mg

10. 125 mcg = _____ mg

11. 0.004 km = _____ m

12. 0.75 cm = _____ mm

13. 965 mL = _____ L

14. 0.008 L = _____ mL

15. 0.32 kg = _____ g

16. 0.05 mg = _____ mcg

17. 988 m = _____ km

18. 1725 cm = _____ km

19. 368 mg = _____ g

20. 247 g = _____ kg

CRITICAL THINKING APPLICATIONS

A patient is given a prescription for 0.5 g of a medication. The medication is available in both 250 mg and 400 mg tablets. Which product should be use? How many tablets would the patient take for each dose? (LO 4.2)

CASE STUDY

A patient suffering from a cold is given a prescription for 15 mL of cough suppressant every 8 h for 10 days. The patient will be using a household measuring device to measure the dose of medication. (LO 4.2)

1. How many milliliters of medication will the patient take in one day?

2. If the medication is supplied in 0.5 L bottles, how many bottles will the patient need to complete the 10 days of treatment?

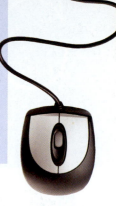

There are many other metric prefixes that were not covered in this chapter. Use the Internet to look up the meaning of the following metric prefixes.

1. mega
2. pico
3. zetta
4. nano
5. hecto

To check your answers, see the Answer section at the end of the book, which starts on page A-1.

GO TO . . . Open the CD-ROM that accompanies your textbook, and complete a final review of the learning outcomes, practice problems, games, slideshow, and other activities presented for this chapter. For a final evaluation, take the chapter test and email or print your results for your instructor. A score of 95 percent or above indicates mastery of the chapter concepts.

5 CHAPTER

Other Systems of Measurement

The purpose of learning is growth, and our minds, unlike our bodies, can continue growing as we continue to live.

—MORTIMER ADLER

Learning Outcomes

When you have completed Chapter 5, you will be able to:

5.1 Write measurements and equivalent measures using the apothecary system.

5.2 Write measurements and equivalent measures using the household system.

5.3 Recognize equivalent measurements used in dosage calculations.

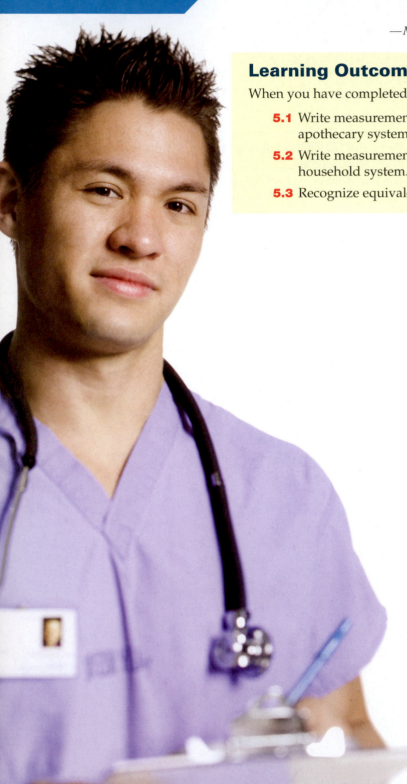

KEY TERMS

Dram

Grain

International unit (IU)

Milliequivalents (mEq)

Minim

Ounce

Unit

INTRODUCTION

While the metric system is the most commonly used system, there are other systems of measurement that you will need to be familiar with when performing dosage calculations. Each of these systems is less common than they once were, but are still used in some circumstances. In this chapter you will be introduced to the commonly used units for the apothecary and household systems of measurement. You will also learn how and when quantities are expressed using milliequivalents (mEq) and units. An understanding of each of these systems is essential to anyone dispensing or administering medications.

5.1 Apothecary System

The apothecary system is an old system of measurement. Used first by apothecaries (early pharmacists), it traveled across Europe from Greece and Rome to France and England. Eventually, it crossed the Atlantic to colonial America. The common measures of gallon, quart, pint and fluid ounce are derived from the apothecary system. Certain medications, especially older ones such as aspirin and morphine, are sometimes labeled and ordered using apothecary units. Apothecary units are less familiar and can be confused with metric units, thus causing them to be infrequently used. Metric units are preferred for dosage calculations in most cases.

Units of Measure

The basic unit of weight in the apothecary system is the grain (gr). Originally, the grain was defined as the weight of a single grain of wheat, hence its name. Other units of weight used in the apothecary system include the ounce and pound, which are still commonly used. Table 5-1 shows the relationship between these units.

TABLE 5-1 Equivalent Apothecary Measurements	
WEIGHTS	VOLUMES
1 ounce = 480 grains	60 minims = 1 dram
16 ounces = 1 pound	8 drams = 1 fluid ounce

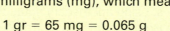

ERROR ALERT!

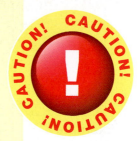

Do Not Confuse Grains and Grams

Because they have names and abbreviations that are similar, **grains** (gr) and grams (g) are easily confused. A grain is a measure in the apothecary system; a gram is a measure in the metric system. If you are not sure whether an order refers to grains or grams, check with the physician or pharmacist. For most conversions, 1 grain equals either 60 or 65 milligrams (mg), which means:

$$1 \text{ gr} = 60 \text{ mg} = 0.06 \text{ g} \qquad \text{or} \qquad 1 \text{ gr} = 65 \text{ mg} = 0.065 \text{ g}$$

In either case, 1 grain is significantly smaller than 1 gram. Medications that are measured in grains do not all use the same conversion. However, typically their labels list the metric units as well.

Three units of volume in the apothecary system are the **minim,** the **dram,** and the **ounce.** The symbols to represent these three units (shown in parenthesis) are error prone and should not be used. The minim was originally defined as the volume of a drop of wine. The apothecary ounce has become part of the common system of measures used in the United States. There are 8 ounces (oz) to 1 cup (c) in our commonly used household system of measures. Minims are seldom used these days, although many syringes continue to have marks that indicate minims.

Do Not Confuse Symbols of the Apothecary System

Note that the symbols for (ʒ) dram and (ʒ) ounce are very similar to one another. These similarities are the reason the two symbols should NOT be used in practice and are considered error prone. If seen on any order or document, check with physician or other authorized prescriber before proceeding.

Apothecary Notation

The system of apothecary notation has special rules that combine fractions, Roman and Arabic numerals, symbols, and abbreviations. Even the order in which information is written differs from the order most familiar to you. Recall that Roman numerals may be written with a bar above them.

Converting from grains in the apothecary system to milligrams in the metric system is much like converting from minutes to seconds (see Figure 5-1).

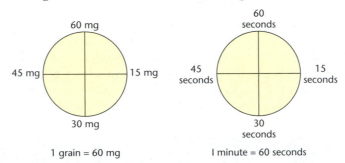

1 grain = 60 mg   1 minute = 60 seconds

Figure 5-1 Converting from grains to milligrams is much like converting from minutes to second. One-quarter of a minute is 15 seconds, and one-quarter of a grain is 15 milligrams!

RULE 5-1	When you are writing a value in the apothecary system: **1.** Write values with lowercase Roman numerals such as i or ii. Roman numerals are discussed in more detail in Chapter 9. **2.** For values that are not whole numbers, use fractions or mixed numbers, not Roman numerals or decimals. **3.** Use the abbreviation "gr" to represent grain. For ounces write either the term "ounce" or the abbreviation "oz.". The units dram and minim should be written out and are not abbreviated. **4.** When using the abbreviation for grain along with Roman numerals, the unit is written before the quantity.
Example 1	Write *four grains,* using apothecary notation. Use lowercase Roman numerals to represent four as iv. Abbreviate grains as gr, and place it before the quantity: gr iv or gr iv.
Example 2	Write *two and one-half grains,* using apothecary notation. Use a mixed number to represent the value because it is not a whole number: gr $2\frac{1}{2}$.

GO TO . . . Open the CD-ROM that accompanies your textbook, and select Chapter 5, Writing Values in the Apothecary System (LO 5.1). Review the animation and example problems, then complete the practice problems. Continue to the next section of the book once you have mastered the information presented.

5.1 Apothecary System

In Exercises 1-6, write the amounts using the units or abbreviations of the apothecary system.

1. Seven grains
2. Eight ounces
3. Five drams

4. Fourteen grains
5. One-half grain
6. Five and one-half ounces

In Exercises 7-10, write the equivalent apothecary measurement.

7. One ounce 5 _____ grains
8. Sixty minims 5 _____ drams

9. Eight drams 5 _____ fluid ounces
10. One pound 5 _____ ounces

To check your answers, see the Answer section at the end of the book, which starts on page A-1.

5.2 Household System

Patients who take medication at home are more likely to use everyday household measures than metric ones. Many over-the-counter medications provide instructions for patients relying on household measures. For instance, a patient will be told to take two teaspoons of a cough syrup.

While the household system may be the most familiar one to patients, in practice it is the least accurate. For instance, patients who take a teaspoon of a syrup will often use everyday spoons that vary in size, rather than baking or other calibrated spoons. Instructions for over-the-counter medications can even invite inaccuracies. A patient may be told to mix a rounded teaspoon of powder with a quantity of water. The interpretation of *rounded* will vary from patient to patient.

Units of Measure

Basic units of volume in the household system, in increasing size, include the drop, teaspoon, tablespoon, ounce, cup, pint, quart, and gallon. Of these, the four smallest measures are most commonly used for medications. Table 5-2 summarizes the equivalent measures of the household measurements most likely to be encountered in a medical setting.

When one is specifically discussing medications, the word *ounce* generally implies volume; it represents fluid ounce. In other contexts, *ounce* may represent a unit of weight, as does *pound*.

Household Notation

As with the metric system, household notation places the quantity in Arabic numerals before the abbreviation for the unit. Table 5-3 summarizes the standard abbreviations.

TABLE 5-2 Equivalent Household Measurements	
WEIGHTS	**VOLUMES**
1 pound = 16 ounces	1 cup = 8 fluid ounces
	1 pint = 16 fluid ounces
	1 ounce = 2 tablespoons
	1 tablespoon = 3 teaspoons

TABLE 5-3 Abbreviations for Household Measures

UNIT OF MEASUREMENT	ABBREVIATION
Drop(s)	gt, gtt
Teaspoon	tsp or t
Tablespoon	tbsp, tbs or T
Ounce	oz
Cup	cup or c
Pint	pt
Quart	qt
Gallon	gal
Pound	lb

Example 1	Write *six drops,* using household notation. Write the quantity with Arabic numerals before the abbreviation for the unit: 6 gtt.
Example 2	Write *twelve ounces,* using household notation. Write the quantity with Arabic numerals before the abbreviation for the unit: 12 oz.

GO TO . . . Open the CD-ROM that accompanies your textbook, and select Chapter 5, Writing Values in the Household System (LO 5.2). Review the animation and example problems, then complete the practice problems. Continue to the next section of the book once you have mastered the information presented.

REVIEW AND PRACTICE

5.2 Household System

In Exercises 1-6, write the quantity with the appropriate abbreviations.

1. Two teaspoons

2. Three and one-half tablespoons

3. Seventy-five pounds

4. Four fluid ounces

5. Two drops

6. One gallon

In Exercises 7-10, write the equivalent household measurement.

7. Two pints = _____ mL

8. Four tablespoons = _____ oz

9. Two tablespoons = _____ teaspoons

10. Thirty-two ounces = _____ pounds

To check your answers, see the Answer section at the end of the book, which starts on page A-1.

5.3 Equivalent Measurements

Units of measurement found in both the apothecary and the household systems are equal: an apothecary ounce equals a household ounce. Unlike the metric system, neither the apothecary system nor the household system is based on multiples of 10. When performing dosage calculations, sometimes it will be necessary to convert units from one system to another. In order to do this, you must become familiar with their equivalent measures. Keep in mind these equivalent measures are approximations (see Table 5-4).

TABLE 5-4 Approximate Equivalent Measures for the Metric, Apothecary, and Household Systems		
1 teaspoon = 5 mL*	1 tablespoon = 15 mL*	1 fl oz = 30 mL*
1 pint = 480 mL	1 pound = 454 g	1 gr = 60 mg*
1 kg = 2.2 lb	1 oz = 30 g*	
1 cup = 8 fl oz	1 fl oz = 2 tablespoons	15 gr = 1 g*

*Indicates approximation. See Error Alert for more information.

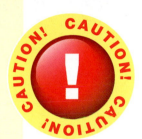

ERROR ALERT!

Equivalent Measure Approximations

The equivalent measures shown in Table 5-4 are approximations. The exact value of apothecary units are usually rounded when performing dosage calculations. Note the following:

- Household teaspoons and tablespoons are not uniform in size, although measuring spoons will have the volume indicated.
- A pint is actually equal to 473 mL, but 480 mL is used for most calculations.
- The ounce (weight) is slightly greater than 30 g; the ounce (volume) is slightly less than 30 mL.
- One grain is actually equal to 64.8 mg. The conversion 1 grain = 60 mg is the one most often used when performing dosage calculations. For some medications (aspirin, acetaminophen, iron) the conversion that is typically used is 1 grain = 65 mg.

Example 1	How many teaspoons of solution are contained in 1 ounce (oz) of solution? From Table 5-4, you can see that 1 ounce contains 2 tablespoons. In turn, each tablespoon contains 3 teaspoons. Therefore, $1 \text{ oz} = 2 \times 1 \text{ tbsp} = 2 \times 3 \text{ tsp} = 6 \text{ tsp}$ One ounce of solution contains six teaspoons of solution.
Example 2	How many tablespoons are in $\frac{1}{2}$ cup of solution? Convert 1 cup to ounces, then ounces to tablespoons. From Table 5-4, you know that 1 cup = 8 oz and 1 oz = 2 tbsp: $\frac{1}{2} \text{ cup} = \frac{1}{2} \times 1 \text{ cup} = \frac{1}{2} \times 8 \text{ oz} = 4 \text{ oz}$ $= 4 \times 1 \text{ oz} = 4 \times 2 \text{ tbsp} = 8 \text{ tbsp}$ One-half cup of solution contains eight tablespoons of solution.

Milliequivalents and Units

Some drugs are measured in **milliequivalents** (mEq). A unit of measure based on the chemical combining power of the substance, one milliequivalent is defined as $\frac{1}{1000}$ of an equivalent weight of a chemical. Electrolytes, such as sodium and potassium, are often measured in milliequivalents. Sodium bicarbonate and potassium chloride are examples of drugs that are prescribed in milliequivalents. You do not need to learn to convert from milliequivalent to another system of measurement.

Medications such as insulin, heparin, and penicillin are measured in *USP units*. A **unit** is the amount of a medication required to produce a certain effect. *The size of a unit varies for each drug.* Some medications, such as vitamins, are measured in standardized units called **international units** (IU). These IUs represent the amount of medication needed to produce a certain effect, but they are standardized by international agreement. As with milliequivalent, you do not need to convert from units to other measures. Medications that are ordered in units will also be labeled in units.

GO TO . . . Open the CD-ROM that accompanies your textbook, and select Chapter 5, Recognizing Equivalent Measurements (LO 5.3). Review the animation and example problems, then complete the practice problems. Continue to the next section of the book once you have mastered the information presented.

REVIEW AND PRACTICE

5.3 Equivalent Measurements

1. 3 kg = _____ lb

2. 30 mL = _____ tablespoons

3. 30 gr = _____ g

4. 180 mg = _____ gr

5. 3 pt = _____ mL

6. 2 teaspoons = _____ mL

7. 120 mL = _____ fl oz

8. 3 tablespoons = _____ mL

9. 1 lb = _____ g

10. 2 oz = _____ g

To check your answers, see the Answer section at the end of the book, which starts on page A-1.

ERROR ALERT!

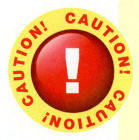

Milliequivalents (mEq) Conversions

Some minerals, especially potassium, are available as over-the-counter medications. Certain patients may elect to take the over-the-counter version to save money. Prescription potassium is ordered in mEq and the over-the- counter version is available in mcg or mgs. Converting between mEq and mcg or mg is tricky and can lead to errors. There are several forms of potassium (potassium gluconate, potassium citrate, etc.) and each convert differently. Always check with the physician or pharmacist to ensure the proper conversion is made based on the form of the medication.

CHAPTER 5 SUMMARY

LEARNING OUTCOME	KEY POINTS
5.1 Write measurements and equivalent measures using the apothecary system. Pages 99–101	▶ Units of volume for the apothecary system include the minim, dram, and fluid ounce. ▶ Units of weight for the apothecary system include grains, ounces, and pounds. For example write gr iv NOT iv gr.
5.2 Write measurements and equivalent measures using the household system. Pages 101–103	▶ Units of volume for the household system include the drop, teaspoon, tablespoon, fluid ounce, cups, pints, and quarts. ▶ Units of weight for the household system include the ounce and pound, which are the same as those used in the apothecary system.
5.3 Recognize equivalent measurements for the metric, apothecary, and household systems. Pages 103–105	▶ While metric units are the most commonly used units in dosage calculations, there are times when other systems are used. ▶ In order to perform dosage calculations, it is essential to know the equivalent measures needed for converting between the systems of measurement.

HOMEWORK ASSIGNMENT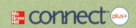

Write the equivalent measurement. (LO 5.1, 5.2, 5.3)

1. 1 oz = _____ gr
2. 1 lb = _____ g
3. 1 tsp = _____ mL
4. 1 c = _____ oz
5. 1 g = _____ gr
6. 1 gr = _____ mg
7. 1 kg = _____ lb
8. 1 oz = _____ tbsp
9. 1 lb = _____ oz
10. 1 T = _____ mL

CHAPTER 5 REVIEW

CHECK UP

In Exercises 1–8, write the indicated amounts, using numerals and abbreviations. (LO 5.1, 5.2)

1. Fourteen and one-quarter ounces

2. Two tablespoons

3. Fifteen grains

4. Three and one-half gallons

5. Two drops

6. Seventy five pounds

7. One and one-half teaspoons

8. Two pints

In Exercises 9-20, write the equivalent measurement. (LO 5.1, 5.2, 5.3)

9. 1 oz = _____ gr

10. 1 tbs = _____ mL

11. 1 oz = _____ mL

12. 1 oz = _____ tbsp

13. 1 pt = _____ mL

14. 1 gr = _____ mg

15. 1 cup = _____ oz

16. 1 kg = _____ lb

17. 1 lb = _____ oz

18. 1 T = _____ t

19. 1 pt = _____ oz

20. 1 tsp = _____ mL

CRITICAL THINKING APPLICATIONS

A patient suffering from a cold is given a prescription for 2 teaspoons of cough suppressant every 6 h for 8 days. The patient will be using a teaspoon to measure the dose of medication. (LO 5.3)

1. How many teaspoons of cough suppressant should the patient take each day?

2. How many eight ounce bottles of medication will the patient need to complete the order?

3. If the medication is supplied in pint bottles, how many bottles will the patient need during the 10 days?

CASE STUDY

The package insert for a medication states that the patient should be given 5 mL of medication for every 50 kg that they weigh. If the patient weighs 66 lb, how many mL of medication should they be given? (LO 5.3)

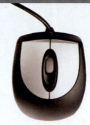

Find a reliable metric conversion chart on the Internet, and use it to convert the following.

1. Your weight in pounds to your weight in kilograms.
2. A 2-tbsp dose of medication to ounces.

To check your answers, see the Answer section at the end of the book, which starts on page A-1.

GO TO . . . Open the CD-ROM that accompanies your textbook, and complete a final review of the learning outcomes, practice problems, games, slideshow, and other activities presented for this chapter. For a final evaluation, take the chapter test and email or print your results for your instructor. A score of 95 percent or above indicates mastery of the chapter concepts.

6 CHAPTER

Using Conversion Factors

Knowing is not enough; we must apply. Willing is not enough; we must do.

—GOETHE

KEY TERMS

Conversion factor
Proportions
Dimensional analysis

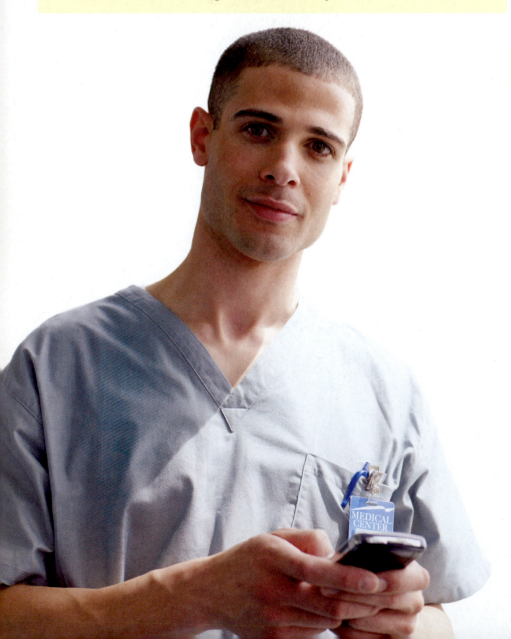

INTRODUCTION

One of the most crucial skills needed for calculating dosages is the ability to perform conversions. To do this, you will apply the material that has been presented in earlier chapters. Two methods for performing conversions will be presented in this chapter—the proportion method and dimensional analysis. You will notice that the methods are different only in the initial setup of the problem. While practicing these methods, you should decide which works best for you. In later chapters you will learn how to use these same methods for dosage calculations.

6.1 Writing Conversion Factors from Equivalent Measurements

In Chapters 4 and 5 you learned the systems of measurement that are most commonly used in dosage calculations—the metric, apothecary, and household systems.

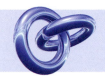 **LEARNING LINK** Recall the equivalent measures presented in Table 5-4 in Chapter 5. You will use these equivalent measurements when writing conversion factors, so it is important that you learn them.

A **conversion factor** is a fraction or ratio made of two quantities that are equal to each other but expressed in different units. For example, if you wished to convert between days and weeks, you would start by recalling that 1 week is equal to 7 days. You can write 4 conversion factors from this relationship:

1 week/7 days
7 days/1 week
1 week:7 days
7 days: 1 week

The conversion factor that you would write depends on two factors—the method that you are using (fractions or ratios) and whether you are converting from days to weeks or from weeks to days.

RULE 6-1	Writing Conversion Factors
	When you are writing conversion factors:
	1. The two quantities in the conversion factor must be equal to each other.
	2. When writing conversion factors using fractions, the quantity containing the units that you wish to convert *to* goes in the numerator of the conversion factor and the quantity containing the units that you are converting *from* goes in the denominator of the conversion factor.
	3. When writing conversion factors using ratios, write the conversion factor with the units that you are converting to *before* the colon in the conversion factor. The quantity that you are converting *from* goes after the colon in the conversion factor.
Example	Write a conversion factor for converting from milliliters to ounces.
	According to Table 5-4 on page 103, 30 mL is equivalent to 1 oz. Since we wish to convert to ounces, the quantity with ounces must be the numerator of the conversion factor when using fractions. When using ratios the ounces must be before the colon.
	1 oz/30 mL
	1 oz: 30 mL

GO TO . . . Open the CD-ROM that accompanies your textbook, and select Chapter 6, Writing Conversion Factors (LO 6.1). Review the animation and example problems, then complete the practice problems. Continue to the next section of the book once you have mastered the information presented.

REVIEW AND PRACTICE

6.1 Writing Conversion Factors from Equivalent Measurements

Write the conversion factor that would be used to convert from:

1. grains to milligrams
2. pounds to grams
3. milliliters to teaspoons
4. grams to milligrams
5. ounces to tablespoons
6. kilograms to pounds
7. milliliters to liters
8. cups to milliliters
9. milligrams to micrograms
10. tablespoons to milliliters

To check your answers, see the Answer section at the end of the book, which starts on page A-1.

6.2 Converting Units Using the Proportion Method

Cross-multiplying when using fractions, and multiplying the means and extremes when using ratios, can be used to convert from one unit to another if you know a conversion factor. One of the fractions in your proportion is the conversion factor itself. The other fraction contains the unknown value in the numerator (before the colon) and the value that you wish to convert in the denominator (after the colon).

 LEARNING LINK Recall from Chapter 3 (Rules 3-15 and 3-18) you can solve proportions for an unknown value by cross-multiplying or multiplying the means and extremes.

PROPORTION METHOD

Procedure Checklist 6-1
Converting by the Proportion Method

1. Write a conversion factor with the units needed in the answer in the numerator (before the colon) and the units you are converting from in the denominator (after the colon).
2. Write a fraction or ratio with the unknown, x, in the numerator (before the colon) and the number that you need to convert in the denominator (after the colon).
3. Set the two factors up as a proportion.
4. Cancel units.
5. Cross-multiply when using fractions or multiply the means and extremes when using ratios, then solve for the unknown value.

EXAMPLE 1	Convert 66 lb to kilograms.

Follow Procedure Checklist 6-1.

1. Table 5-4 in Chapter 5 tells us that 1 kg is equal to 2.2 lb. Since we are converting to kilograms, kilograms must appear in the numerator (before the colon) of our conversion factor. Our conversion factor is 1 kg/2.2 lb using fractions or 1 kg : 2.2 lb using ratios.

2. The other fraction or ratio for our proportion has the unknown x for a numerator (before the colon) and 66 lb as the denominator (after the colon): $\frac{x}{66 \text{ lb}}$ or x: 66 lb.

3. Setting the two fractions or ratios into a proportion gives us the following equation:

   Using Fractions: **Using Ratios:**

   $$\frac{x}{66 \text{ lb}} = \frac{1 \text{ kg}}{2.2 \text{ lb}} \qquad\qquad x: 66 \text{ lb} = 1 \text{ kg}: 2.2 \text{ lb}$$

4. Cancel units.

   $$\frac{x}{66} = \frac{1 \text{ kg}}{2.2} \qquad\qquad x: 66 = 1 \text{ kg}: 2.2$$

5. Solve for the unknown by cross-multiplying or multiplying the means and extremes.

   $$2.2 \times x = 1 \text{ kg} \times 66$$

   $$\frac{2.2 \times x}{2.2} = \frac{1 \text{ kg} \times 66}{2.2}$$

   $$x = 30 \text{ kg}$$

EXAMPLE 2	A patient needs to take 10 mL of a medication, but is going to be measuring the medication with a teaspoon. How many teaspoons should he use?

Follow Procedure Checklist 6-1.

1. Table 5-4 in Chapter 5 tells us that 5 mL is equal to 1 tsp. Since we are converting to teaspoons, our conversion factor is $\frac{1 \text{ tsp}}{5 \text{ mL}}$ or 1 tsp: 5 mL.

2. The other fraction or ratio for our proportion is $\frac{x}{10 \text{ mL}}$ or x: 10 mL

3. Setting the two fractions or ratios into a proportion gives us either of the following equations:

   Using Fractions: **Using Ratios:**

   $$\frac{x}{10 \text{ mL}} = \frac{1 \text{ tsp}}{5 \text{ mL}} \qquad\qquad x: 10 \text{ mL} = 1 \text{ tsp}: 5 \text{ mL}$$

4. Cancel units.

   $$\frac{x}{10} = \frac{1 \text{ tsp}}{5} \qquad\qquad x: 10 = 1 \text{ tsp}: 5$$

5. Solve for the unknown.

   $$5 \times x = 1 \text{ tsp} \times 10$$

   $$\frac{5 \times x}{5} = \frac{1 \text{ tsp} \times 10}{5}$$

   $$x = 2 \text{ tsp}$$

EXAMPLE 3	A medication order calls for 0.2 milligrams of a drug. The product is labeled in micrograms, so it will be necessary to convert the 0.2 milligrams into micrograms before performing the dosage calculation.

Follow Procedure Checklist 6-1.

1. As we learned in Chapter 3, 1000 micrograms equals 1 milligram. The conversion factor is $\frac{1000 \text{ mcg}}{1 \text{ mg}}$ or 1000 mcg : 1 mg.

2. The other factor for our proportion is $\frac{x}{0.2 \text{ mg}}$ or x: 0.2 mg.

3. Setting the two fractions or ratios into a proportion gives us the following equations:

Using Fractions:

$$\frac{x}{0.2 \text{ mg}} = \frac{1000 \text{ mcg}}{1 \text{ mg}}$$

Using Ratios:

$$x : 0.2 \text{ mg} = 1000 \text{ mcg} : 1 \text{ mg}$$

4. Cancel units.

$$\frac{x}{0.2} \times \frac{1000 \text{ mcg}}{1}$$

$$x : 0.2 = 1000 \text{ mcg} : 1$$

5. Solve for the unknown.

$$1 \times x = 0.2 \times 1000 \text{ mcg}$$

$$x = 200 \text{ mcg}$$

GO TO . . . Open the CD-ROM that accompanies your textbook, and select Chapter 6, Converting by the Proportion Method (LO 6.2). Review the animation and example problems, then complete the practice problems. Continue to the next section of the book once you have mastered the information presented.

ERROR ALERT!

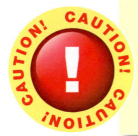

Always Include Units When Using Conversion Factors

It is important to always include units when you use conversion factors. Errors can be made by using the wrong form of the conversion factor. If you include units and follow the rules for canceling them, you will be able to recognize when the wrong form of the conversion factor was used. Never take shortcuts by leaving off units!

REVIEW AND PRACTICE

6.2 Converting Units Using the Proportion Method

In Exercises 1-11, convert the measures from one unit of measurement to another.

1. 30 mL = _____ tbsp
2. 125 mL = _____ tsp
3. 120 mL = _____ tsp
4. 240 mL = _____ L
5. 15 mg = gr _____
6. gr 15 = _____ mg
7. 10 mg = _____ g
8. 2.5 g = gr _____
9. 42 kg = _____ lb
10. 44 lb = _____ kg
11. 6 oz = _____ mL

12. During the total course of his treatment, a patient will receive 720 mL of medication. How many pints will he receive?

13. If an order calls for the patient to receive 2 tsp of cough syrup, how many milliliters of syrup should the patient receive?

14. A patient weighs 65 kg. How many pounds does she weigh?

15. A patient weighs 187 lb. How many kilograms does he weigh?

16. A physician orders 2 ounces of liquid medication. How many tablespoons should the patient take?

17. A patient drinks 4 c of liquid during the morning. How many milliliters did the patient drink?

18. An order is for gr iii of medication. How many milligrams should the patient be given?

19. A physician orders that a patient be given 10 mg of medication 3 times per day. How many grains of medication should the patient be given per day?

20. An order calls for 1.5 tbsp of medicated mouthwash. How many milliliters of medicated mouthwash should the patient receive?

To check your answers, see the Answer section at the end of the book, which starts on page A-1.

6.3 Converting Units Using Dimensional Analysis

The **dimensional analysis** (DA) method for using conversion factors is a modification of the proportion method. Sometimes the DA method is also known as the *factor method* or *factor analysis*. When you are using DA, the unknown value *x* stands alone on one side of the equation. The conversion factor multiplied by the number being converted is placed on the other side of the equation.

DIMENSIONAL ANALYSIS

Procedure Checklist 6-2
Converting by Dimensional Analysis

1. Determine the unit of measure for the answer, and place it as the unknown on one side of the equation.

2. On the other side of the equation, write a conversion factor with the units of measure for the answer on top and the units you are converting from on the bottom.

3. Multiply the numerator of the conversion factor by the number that is being converted divided by 1.

4. Cancel the units on the right side of the equation. The remaining unit of measure on the right side of the equation should match the unknown unit of measure on the left side of the equation.

5. Solve the equation.

EXAMPLE 1

Convert 66 lb to kilograms.

Follow Procedure Checklist 6-2.

1. The unit of measure for the answer is kilograms.

$x \text{ kg} =$

2. Our conversion factor is $\frac{1 \text{ kg}}{2.2 \text{ lb}}$. Place it on the other side of an equal sign.

$x \text{ kg} = \frac{1 \text{ kg}}{2.2 \text{ lb}}$

Copyright © 2012 by The McGraw-Hill Companies, Inc.

3. Multiplying the numerator of the conversion factor by 66 lb gives us the following equation.

$$x \text{ kg} = \frac{1 \text{ kg}}{2.2 \text{ lb}} \times \frac{66 \text{ lb}}{1}$$

4. Cancel units. The remaining unit on both sides is kilograms.

$$x \text{ kg} = \frac{1 \text{ kg}}{2.2 \text{ lb}} \times \frac{66 \text{ lb}}{1}$$

5. Solve for the unknown.

$$x = 30 \text{ kg}$$

EXAMPLE 2

A patient needs to take 10 mL of a medication, but is going to be measuring the medication with a teaspoon. How many teaspoons should he use?

Follow Procedure Checklist 6-2.

1. The unit of measure for the answer is teaspoons.

$$x \text{ tsp}$$

2. Our conversion factor is $\frac{1 \text{ tsp}}{5 \text{ mL}}$. Place it on the other side of an equal sign.

$$x \text{ tsp} = \frac{1 \text{ tsp}}{5 \text{ mL}}$$

3. Multiplying the numerator of the conversion factor by 10 mL gives us the following equation.

$$x \text{ tsp} = \frac{1 \text{ tsp}}{5 \text{ mL}} \times \frac{10 \text{ mL}}{1}$$

4. Cancel units. The remaining units indicate we are solving for teaspoons.

$$x \text{ tsp} = \frac{1 \text{ tsp}}{5 \text{ mL}} \times \frac{10 \text{ mL}}{1}$$

5. Solve for the unknown.

$$x = 2 \text{ tsp}$$

EXAMPLE 3

A medication order calls for 0.2 milligrams of a drug. The product is labeled in micrograms, so it will be necessary to convert the 0.2 milligrams into micrograms before performing the dosage calculation.

Follow Procedure Checklist 6-2.

1. The unit of measure for the answer is tablespoons.

$$x \text{ mcg}$$

2. Our conversion factor is $\frac{1000 \text{ mcg}}{1 \text{ mg}}$. Place it on the other side of an equal sign.

$$x \text{ mcg} = \frac{1000 \text{ mcg}}{1 \text{ mg}}$$

3. Multiplying the numerator of the conversion factor by 60 mL gives us the following equation.

$$x \text{ mcg} = \frac{1000 \text{ mcg}}{1 \text{ mg}} \times \frac{0.2 \text{ mg}}{1}$$

4. Cancel units. The remaining units indicate we are solving for tablespoons.

$$x \text{ mcg} = \frac{1000 \text{ mcg}}{1 \text{ mg}} \times \frac{0.2 \text{ mg}}{1}$$

5. Solve for the unknown.

$$x = 200 \text{ mcg}$$

GO TO . . . Open the CD-ROM that accompanies your textbook, and select Chapter 6, Converting Using the Dimensional Analysis Method (LO 6.3). Review the animation and example problems, then complete the practice problems. Continue to the next section of the book once you have mastered the information presented.

CRITICAL THINKING ON THE JOB

Selecting the Correct Conversion Factor

Greg is teaching a patient how much liquid medication to take. The physician has ordered 30 mL of Milk of Magnesia, but the patient will be using teaspoons to measure her medication. Using a conversion chart, Greg confuses 1 tbsp with 1 tsp, and he reads 1 tsp = 15 mL. Using the incorrect information, he calculates the dose as follows:

$$\frac{x}{30 \text{ mL}} = \frac{1 \text{ tsp}}{15 \text{ mL}}$$

$$x \times 15 = 1 \text{ tsp} \times 30$$

$$x = 2 \text{ tsp}$$

Greg tells the patient to take 2 tsp of Milk of Magnesia. This amount is only one-third of the amount that the physician ordered; the patient does not get the relief desired.

Think! . . . Is It Reasonable? What mistake did Greg make? How could the error have been avoided? What is the correct dose the patient should receive?

REVIEW AND PRACTICE

6.3 Converting Units Using Dimensional Analysis

In Exercises 1–11, convert the measures from one unit of measurement to another. When necessary, round to the nearest tenth.

1. 30 mL = _____ tbsp
2. 125 mL = _____ tsp
3. 120 mL = _____ tsp
4. 240 mL = _____ L
5. 15 mg = gr _____
6. gr 15 = _____ mg
7. 10 mg = _____ g
8. 2.5 g = gr _____
9. 42 kg = _____ lb
10. 44 lb = _____ kg
11. 6 oz = _____ mL

12. During the total course of his treatment, a patient will receive 720 mL of medication. How many pints will he receive?

13. If an order calls for the patient to receive 2 tsp of cough syrup, how many milliliters of syrup should the patient receive?

14. A patient weighs 65 kg. How many pounds does she weigh?

15. A patient weighs 187 lb. How many kilograms does he weigh?

16. A physician orders 2 ounces of liquid medication. How many tablespoons should the patient take?

17. A patient drinks 4 c of liquid during the morning. How many milliliters did the patient drink?

18. An order is for gr iii of medication. How many milligrams should the patient be given?

19. A physician orders that a patient be given 10 mg of medication 3 times per day. How many grains of medication should the patient be given per day?

20. An order calls for 1.5 tbsp of medicated mouthwash. How many milliliters of medicated mouthwash should the patient receive?

To check your answers, see the Answer section at the end of the book, which starts on page A-1.

CHAPTER 6 SUMMARY

LEARNING OUTCOME	KEY POINTS

6.1 Write conversion factors from equivalent measurements. Pages 109–110	▶ Conversion factors can be written as either fractions or ratios.
	  • 1 tsp/5 mL and 1 tsp:5 mL are the same conversion factor written in different ways
	▶ The two measurements in a conversion factor are equal to one another but written with different units.
	  • The measurements in the conversion factors $\frac{1\ \text{tsp}}{5\ \text{mL}}$ and 1 tsp : 5 mL are equal to one another: 1 tsp = 5 mL.

6.2 Convert units using the proportion method. Pages 110–113	▶ Units can be converted using proportions expressed as either ratios or fractions.
	  • When using fractions, you cross-multiply.
	  • When using ratios, you use means and extremes.
	▶ When using fractions, the conversion factor should have the unit being converted to in the numerator and the unit being converted from in the denominator.
	  • To use fractions for converting to pounds from kilograms, use the conversion factor 2.2 lb/1 kg.

LEARNING OUTCOME	KEY POINTS
	▶ When using ratios, the conversion factor should have the unit being converted to before the colon and the unit being converted from after the colon.
	• To use ratios for converting to pounds from kilograms, use the conversion factor 2.2 lb : 1 kg.
	▶ In order to avoid errors, it is important to always include units when setting up proportions for converting units.
	• 1 g/1000 mg is a conversion factor. 1/1000 is a fraction but not a conversion factor.
6.3 Convert units using dimensional analysis. Pages 113–116	▶ In dimensional analysis, the measurement to be converted is multiplied by a conversion factor that is expressed as a fraction.
	▶ The conversion factor will have the unit being converted to in the numerator and the unit converted from in the denominator.
	• To convert 3 teaspoons to milliliters with dimensional analysis, multiply 3 tsp $\times$ 5 mL/1 tsp.
	▶ In order to avoid errors, it is important to always include units when setting up multiplication problems for converting units.

HOMEWORK ASSIGNMENT

Perform the following conversions using either the proportion method or dimensional analysis. (LO 6.1, 6.2, 6.3)

1. 3.5 g = _____ mg

2. 30 mg = _____ gr

3. 3 tbsp = _____ mL

4. 0.25 mg = _____ mcg

5. 110 lb = _____ kg

6. 3 tsp = _____ mL

7. 180 mL = _____ oz

8. 1.2 mm = _____ cm

9. 5 gr = _____ mg

10. 600 mL = _____ L

CHAPTER 6 REVIEW

CHECK UP

In Exercises 1–8, write conversion factors for each pair of units. (LO 6.1)

1. kilograms and pounds

2. ounces and milliliters

3. micrograms and milligrams

4. grains and milligrams

5. teaspoons and milliliters

6. milliliters and liters

7. tablespoons and ounces

8. tablespoons and milliliters

In Exercises 9–18, calculate the conversions (LO 6.2, 6.3).

9. $8 \text{ g} = \text{gr} \underline{\hspace{1cm}}$

10. $2\frac{1}{2} \text{ gr} = \underline{\hspace{1cm}} \text{ mg}$

11. $90 \text{ mL} = \underline{\hspace{1cm}} \text{ tbsp}$

12. $5 \text{ tsp} = \underline{\hspace{1cm}} \text{ mL}$

13. $8 \text{ oz} = \underline{\hspace{1cm}} \text{ mL}$

14. $1200 \text{ mL} = \underline{\hspace{1cm}} \text{ oz}$

15. $540 \text{ mg} = \text{gr} \underline{\hspace{1cm}}$

16. $\text{gr} \frac{3}{4} = \underline{\hspace{1cm}} \text{ mg}$

17. $178.2 \text{ lb} = \underline{\hspace{1cm}} \text{ kg}$

18. $47 \text{ kg} \underline{\hspace{1cm}} \text{ lb}$

19. An order is placed for gr v of medication. If the medication is supplied in milligrams, how many milligrams should be given? (For this example, use gr i = 65 mg.) (LO 6.1, 6.2, 6.3)

20. If a patient weighs 44 lb, how many kilograms does she weigh? (LO 6.1, 6.2, 6.3)

21. A physician orders $\frac{1}{2}$ oz of medication for a patient. How many milliliters of medication should the patient be given? (LO 6.1, 6.2, 6.3)

22. The maximum dose of a medication is 3 tbsp. What is the maximum number of milliliters that the patient should be given? (LO 6.1, 6.2, 6.3)

23. A physician tells a patient to drink 2400 mL of fluid per day. How many quarts of liquid should this patient drink? (LO 6.1, 6.2, 6.3)

24. Several months ago, a patient weighed 95 kg. When he comes in for his next appointment, he tells you he has lost 11 lb. If he is correct, how many kilograms should he weigh? (LO 6.1, 6.2, 6.3)

CRITICAL THINKING APPLICATIONS

A patient is given a prescription for 7.5 mL of cough suppressant every 4 h for 10 days. The patient will be using a device that is calibrated in teaspoons. (LO 6.1, 6.2, 6.3)

1. How much medication should the patient take for each dose?

2. If the medication is supplied in 200 mL bottles, how many bottles will the patient need during the 10 days?

CASE STUDY

You are doing an inventory of medications on hand. For one product you have open bottles containing 350 mL, 85 mL, 220 mL, and 175 mL on hand. You also have a full pint bottle of the medication. (LO 6.1, 6.2, 6.3)

1. How many milliliters total do you have available?

2. You need to order enough of the medication so that you have at least two liters on hand. How many pint bottles do you need to order?

INTERNET ACTIVITY

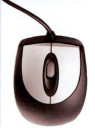

Find a reliable metric conversion chart on the Internet, and use it to convert the following.

1. A two liter bottle to quarts.
2. A 250 mL bottle to ounces.
3. A 2.4 ounce bottle to mL.

To check your answers, see the Answer section at the end of the book, which starts on page A-1.

GO TO . . . Open the CD-ROM that accompanies your textbook, and complete a final review of the learning outcomes, practice problems, games, slideshow, and other activities presented for this chapter. For a final evaluation, take the chapter test and email or print your results for your instructor. A score of 95 percent or above indicates mastery of the chapter concepts.

7 CHAPTER

Temperature and Time

Learning is not a spectator sport.

—ANONYMOUS

Learning Outcomes

When you have completed Chapter 7, you will be able to:

7.1 Convert temperatures between the Celsius and Fahrenheit systems.

7.2 Convert times between conventional and 24-hour systems.

KEY TERMS

Conventional time
24-hour time
Celsius
Fahrenheit

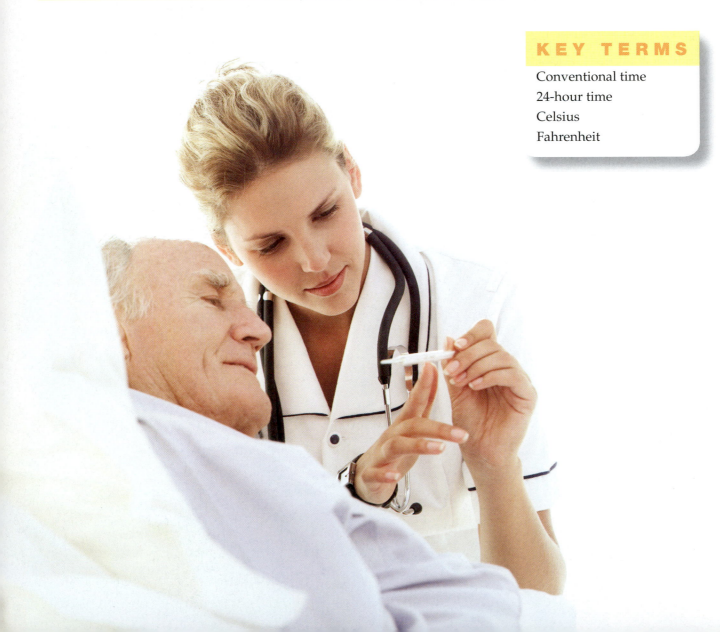

INTRODUCTION

Temperature and time are both commonly expressed in two different ways. Temperature can be expressed using either the Fahrenheit scale or the Celsius scale. Time is usually given using the conventional system of AM and PM, but in certain settings (such as the military and when charting drug administration) the 24-hour clock is used. As a healthcare professional you must be able to convert accurately between these systems.

7.1 Converting Temperature

Both the **Fahrenheit** (F) and **Celsius** (C) temperature scales are used in healthcare settings. If you examine the two thermometers in Figure 7-1, you will notice that the Fahrenheit scale sets the temperature at which water freezes at 32 degrees, or 32°F. It also measures the temperature at which water boils as 212°F. On the Celsius scale, water freezes at 0°C and boils at 100°C. In Fahrenheit, average body temperature is 98.6°F. In Celsius, average body temperature is 37°C.

As a healthcare worker, you may need to convert between these two temperature scales. The following formula can be used for converting between the two systems:

$$5F - 160 = 9C$$

In this formula, F represents the temperature in degrees Fahrenheit and C represents the temperature in degrees Celsius.

You may also use these formulas to convert between temperature scales.

From Fahrenheit to Celsius use:

$$\frac{°F - 32}{1.8} = °C$$

From Celsius to Fahrenheit use:

$$(1.8 \times °C) + 32 = °F$$

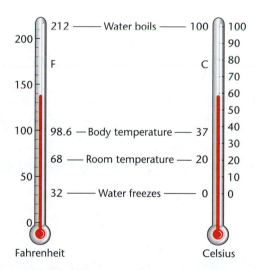

Figure 7-1 Fahrenheit and Celsius scales.

RULE 7-1

Converting between Temperature Systems

Use any of the following formulas to convert a temperature from Fahrenheit to Celsius or Celsius to Fahrenheit.

$5F - 160 = 9C$ (to convert between systems)

$\frac{°F - 32}{1.8} = °C$ (to convert from °F to °C) $(1.8 \times °C) + 32 = °F$ (to convert from °C to °F)

Example 1

Convert 98.6°F to degrees Celsius.

Substituting 98.6 for *F* in the first formula gives us:

$(5 \times 98.6) - 160 = 9C$ (Multiply before subtracting.)

$493 - 160 = 9C$

$333 = 9C$ (Since $\frac{9}{9}$ equals 1, divide both sides by 9 to solve for *C*.)

$\dfrac{333}{9} = \dfrac{9C}{9}$

$37 = C$

Thus 98.6°F = 37°C; both measures represent normal body temperature.

Example 2

Convert 100°C to degrees Fahrenheit.

Substituting 100 for *C* in the first formula gives us:

$5F - 160 = 9 \times 100$

$5F - 160 = 900$ (Add 160 to both sides.)

$5F = 900 + 160$

$\dfrac{5F}{5} = \dfrac{1060}{5}$ (Since $\frac{5}{5}$ equals 1, divide both sides by 5 to solve for *F*.)

$F = 212$

So 100°C = 212°F; both measures represent the boiling point of water.

Example 3

Convert 98.6°F to degrees Celsius.

Substituting 98.6 for °F in the second formula gives:

$\dfrac{98.6 - 32}{1.8} = \dfrac{66.6}{1.8} = 37$

So 98.6°F = 37°C; both measures represent normal body temperature.

Example 4

Convert 37°C to degrees Fahrenheit.

Substituting 37 for °C in the third formula gives:

$(1.8 \times 37) + 32 = 66.6 + 32 = 98.6$

Thus 37°C = 98.6°F.

GO TO . . . Open the CD-ROM that accompanies your textbook, and select Chapter 7, Converting Between Temperature Systems (LO 7.1). Review the animation and example problems, then complete the practice problems. Continue to the next section of the book once you have mastered the information presented.

7.1 Converting Temperature

In Exercises 1–10, convert the temperatures. Round to the nearest tenth, when necessary.

1. 34°C = _____°F   **2.** 41°C = _____°F   **3.** 95°F = _____°C

4. 102°F = _____°C   **5.** 45.3°F = _____°C   **6.** 212°F = _____°C

7. 25°C = _____°F   **8.** 100°C = _____°F   **9.** 59°F = _____°C

10. 67°C = _____°F

To check your answers, see the Answer section at the end of the book, which starts on page A-1.

7.2 Converting Time

Many healthcare facilities use the clock with 24-hours (h), known as military, international, or **24-hour** (24 h) time. A **conventional** 12 h clock is a source of errors in administering medication. On the 12 h clock, each time occurs twice a day. For instance, the hour 10:00 is recorded as both 10:00 a.m. and 10:00 p.m. The abbreviation "a.m." means *ante meridian* or before noon; "p.m." means *post meridian* or after noon. If these abbreviations are not clearly marked, the patient could receive medication at the wrong time.

The 24 h clock (military time) bypasses this opportunity for error. Each time occurs only once per day. In military time, 10:00 a.m. is written as 1000, whereas 10:00 p.m. is written as 2200. (See Figure 7-2.)

When you write the time using a 12 h clock, you separate the hour from the minutes by a colon. You write a single digit for hours 1 through 9. You then add a.m. or p.m. to indicate before or after noon. When you write the time using a 24 h clock, you use a four-digit number with no colon. The first two digits represent the hour; the last two digits, the minutes.

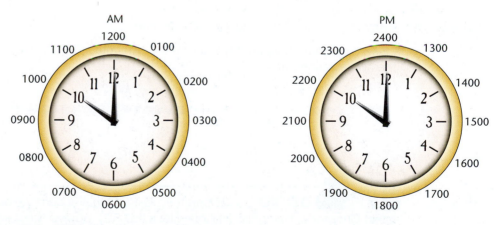

Figure 7-2 Military time is based on a 24-hour clock.

RULE 7-2	When you are using a 24-hour clock for time: **1.** Write 00 as the first two digits to represent the first hour after midnight. **2.** Write 01, 02, 03, . . . , 09 as the first two digits to represent the hours 1:00 a.m. through 9:00 a.m. **3.** Add 12 to the first two digits to represent the hours 1:00 p.m. through 11:00 p.m., so that 13, 14, 15, . . . , 23 represent these hours. **4.** Write midnight as either 2400 or 0000.
Example 1	Convert 9:00 a.m. to 24-hour time. Remove the colon and the abbreviation a.m. Write the hour 9 with two digits, starting with zero. 9:00 a.m. = 0900
Example 2	Convert 12:19 a.m. to 24-hour time. Remove the colon and the abbreviation a.m. Because this time occurs in the first hour after midnight, use 00 for the hour. 12:19 a.m. = 0019
Example 3	Convert 4:28 p.m. to 24-hour time. Remove the colon and the abbreviation p.m. Because this time is after noon, add 12 to the hour. 4:28 p.m. = 1628
Example 4	Convert 1139 to 12-hour (conventional) time. Insert a colon to separate the hour from the minutes. Because this time occurs before noon, add a.m. following the time. 1139 = 11:39 a.m.
Example 5	Convert 1515 to 12-hour (conventional) time. Insert a colon to separate the hour from the minutes. Subtract 12 from the hour, and add the abbreviation p.m. 1515 = 3:15 p.m.

GO TO . . . Open the CD-ROM that accompanies your textbook, and select Chapter 7, Using the 24-hour Clock (LO 7.2). Review the animation and example problems, then complete the practice problems. Continue to the next section of the book once you have mastered the information presented.

RULE 7-3	To state the time using 24-hour time: **1.** Say *zero* if the first digit is a zero. **2.** Say *zero zero* if the first two digits are both zero. **3.** If the minutes are represented by 00, then say *hundred* after you say the hour.
Example 1	State the time 0900. Say *zero nine* for the hours and *hundred* for the minutes. Thus, 0900 is stated as *zero nine hundred.*
Example 2	State the time 1139. Say *eleven* for the hours and *thirty-nine* for the minutes. Thus, 1139 is stated as *eleven thirty-nine.*
Example 3	State the time 0023. Say *zero zero* for the hours and *twenty-three* for the minutes. Thus, 0023 is stated *zero zero twenty-three.*

GO TO . . . Open the CD-ROM that accompanies your textbook, and select Chapter 7, Stating 24-hour Time (LO 7.2). Review the animation and example problems, then complete the practice problems. Continue to the next section of the book once you have mastered the information presented.

REVIEW AND PRACTICE

7.2 Converting Time

In Exercises 1–10, convert the times to 24-hour time.

1. 2:35 a.m.	**2.** 7:57 a.m.	**3.** 12:08 a.m.	**4.** 12:55 a.m.	**5.** 1:49 p.m.
6. 3:14 p.m.	**7.** 11:54 p.m.	**8.** 10:19 p.m.	**9.** 6:59 p.m.	**10.** 4:26 a.m.

In Exercises 11–20, convert the times to 12-hour (conventional) time.

11. 0011	**12.** 0036	**13.** 0325	**14.** 0849	**15.** 1313
16. 1527	**17.** 2145	**18.** 2359	**19.** 2037	**20.** 1818

To check your answers, see the Answer section at the end of the book, which starts on page A-1.

LEARNING OUTCOME	KEY POINTS
7.1 Convert temperatures between the Celsius and Fahrenheit systems. Pages 121–123	▶ Storage requirements for medications are usually indicated in Celsius; thermostats are often calibrated in Fahrenheit. It is therefore necessary to be able to convert temperatures accurately. ▶ There are many formulas for converting temperature. Learn the one that works best for you. • $5F - 160 = 9C$ • $\dfrac{(°F - 32)}{1.8} = °C$ • $(1.8 \times °C) + 32 = °F$
7.2 Convert times between conventional and 24-hour systems. Pages 123–125	▶ Conventional time uses a.m. and p.m. to indicate before noon or after noon. • 7:00 a.m. is in the morning, or before noon; 7:00 p.m. is in the evening, or after noon. ▶ When using the 24 h clock, time is indicated with four digits and without the use of a.m. or p.m. • 7:00 in the morning is written 0700; 7:00 in the evening is 1900. ▶ The first two digits in 24-hour time indicate hours since midnight. The last two digits are for minutes. • 0415 is 4 hours and 15 minutes past midnight.

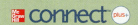
Perform the following conversions. (LO 7.1)

1. 41°F = _____ °C

2. 36°C = _____ °F

3. 70°F = _____ °C

4. 10°C = _____ °F

Convert the following times to 24-hour time. (LO 7.2)

5. 5:30 p.m.

6. 11:15 a.m.

Convert the following times to conventional time. (LO 7.2)

7. 0730

8. 1234

CHECK UP

Convert the following temperatures to Celsius. Round to the nearest tenth, when necessary. (LO 7.1)

1. 97.6°F   **2.** 72°F   **3.** 57.4°F   **4.** 82.8°F

Convert the following temperatures to Fahrenheit. Round to the nearest tenth, when necessary. (LO 7.1)

5. 24°C   **6.** 43.8°C   **7.** 15.6°C   **8.** 8.8°C

Convert the following times to 24-hour time. (LO 7.2)

9. 3:21 a.m.   **10.** 4:42 p.m.   **11.** 10:47 p.m.   **12.** 11:20 a.m.

Convert the following times to conventinal time. (LO 7.2)

13. 0029   **14.** 1417   **15.** 2053   **16.** 0912

CRITICAL THINKING APPLICATIONS

A medication order calls for a drug to be given every 8 hours. The patient takes the first dose at 7:30 a.m. (LO 7.2)

1. At what times will the patient take the next two doses? (Use conventional time)

2. At what times will the patient take the next two doses? (Use 24-hour time)

CASE STUDY

The state health department requires that certain medications be stored between 36°F and 41°F. The refrigerator in the medication room has a Celsius thermometer. What temperature range is appropriate, using the Celsius thermometer? (LO 7.1)

INTERNET ACTIVITY

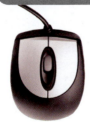

Many medications are labeled to be stored at "Controlled Room Temperature". The guidelines for this temperature are established by the United States Pharmacopeia (USP). Search the USP web site (usp.org) for the meaning of Controlled Room Temperature in Celsius and Fahrenheit.

To check your answers, see the Answer section at the end of the book, which starts on page A-1.

GO TO . . . Open the CD-ROM that accompanies your textbook, and complete a final review of the learning outcomes, practice problems, games, slideshow, and other activities presented for this chapter. For a final evaluation, take the chapter test and email or print your results for your instructor. A score of 95 percent or above indicates mastery of the chapter concepts.

UNIT TWO ASSESSMENT

1. 150 mcg = _____ mg

2. 44 lb = _____ kg

3. 15°C = _____ °F

4. 4 fl oz = _____ mL

5. $2\frac{1}{2}$ tsp = _____ mL

6. 2400 mL = _____ L

7. 8 grains = _____ mg

8. 1530 = _____ (in conventional time)

9. 3.4 m = _____ cm

10. 2 oz = _____ tbsp

11. 8 kg = _____ g

12. 0.6 L = _____ oz

13. 55°F = _____ °C

14. 2:15 p.m. = _____ (in military time)

15. 2 cups = _____ mL

16. When Bill had a physical a year ago, he weighed 185 pounds. The clinic now weighs patients in kilograms, and Bill weighs 82.5 kg now. Did his weight change? If yes, how much has he lost or gained in the past year?

17. A patient receives a four-ounce bottle of cough syrup. The instructions are to take $1\frac{1}{2}$ teaspoons four times a day. How many days will the bottle of cough syrup last?

18. The label on a bottle of extra-strength aspirin states that there are 7.5 grains of aspirin in one tablet. Approximately how many milligrams of aspirin will a patient receive if he takes two tablets?

19. The following orders been filled from a 1 pt bottle of medication: 2 fl oz, 45 mL, 3 fl oz, and 180 mL. You receive an order for 4 ounces of the medication. Is there enough remaining in the bottle to fill the order?

20. A coworker shares a recipe with you for making lasagna. The recipe comes from a relative in Italy and says to bake the lasagna at 220°C for 90 minutes.
    a. What temperature (in °F) would you cook the lasagna at?
    b. If you start the lasagna at 5:45 p.m., what time will it be done (in military time)?

To check your answers, see the Answer section at the end of the book, which starts on page A-1.

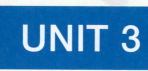

UNIT 3

Principles of Medication Administration

8

CHAPTER

Equipment for Dosage Measurement

Nothing will work unless you do.

—*Maya Angelou*

Learning Outcomes

When you have completed Chapter 8 you will be able to:

8.1 Recognize medication dosage volumes in different enteral equipment.

8.2 Recognize medication dosage volumes in different parenteral equipment.

KEY TERMS

Ampule
Calibrated spoons
Calibrations
Cartridges
Eccentric
Enteral
Hypodermic syringes
Jejunostomy tube
Leading ring
Meniscus
Nasogastric
Parenteral
Percutaneous endoscopic (PEG) tube
Trailing ring
Transdermal
Vial

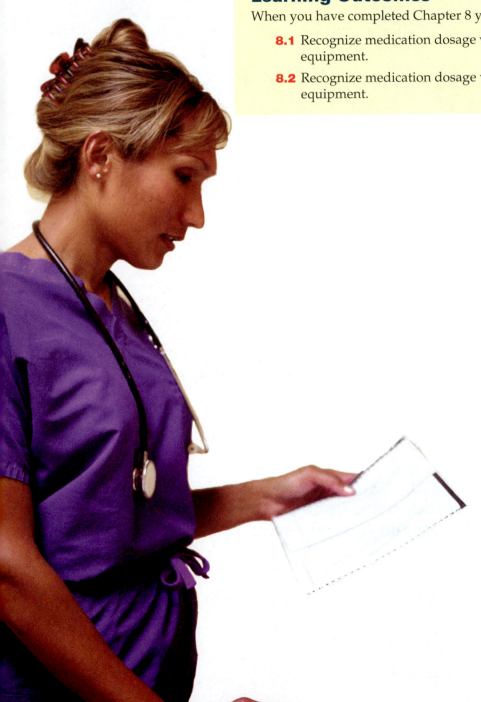

INTRODUCTION

To prepare the correct dosage of medications, you must know the equipment you will be using. You will be required to accurately select and read this equipment. This chapter will introduce you to common equipment used to prepare dosages and administer medications.

8.1 Enteral Medication Administration Devices

Many medications are available in liquid form and can be administered via the **enteral** route. Enteral medications are absorbed in the gastrointestinal tract. This includes medications that are administered orally or through a tube into the stomach or intestines. Several types of equipment are used to measure and administer enteral liquid medications. These include medicine cups, droppers, calibrated spoons, and oral syringes.

Each measuring device has a series of **calibrations,** or marks numbered at varying intervals. Calibrations enable you to measure the amount of liquid in the device. When you choose a measuring device, compare its calibrations with the desired dose of medication. They may represent different units of measurement. If your equipment does not match the order, then you will have to convert the order to the unit of measurement you will use to administer the medication. For example, a patient is required to take 10 mL of a medication. You have available a container that is marked in teaspoons only. In this case you will have to obtain a different container that is marked in milliliters or convert the amount of medication (10 mL) to teaspoons.

Medicine Cups

Medicine cups are used to measure oral liquid medications and administer them to patients. Cups provide a measured dose that is easy for most patients to swallow. Usually, medicine cups are plastic and measure up to 1 fluid ounce, or its equivalent. To make dose calculation easier, most cups are typically marked with metric, household, and apothecary systems of measurement. Thus, cups include units such as tablespoons (tbsp), teaspoons (tsp), milliliters (mL), drams (dr), and ounces (oz). Although sometimes marked on medication cups, the dram is an outdated unit of measurement and is rarely, if ever, used in medication administration.

Use the two views of a cup shown in Figure 8-1 to compare the different calibrations. In Figure 8-1A, milliliters are displayed in units of 5. Teaspoons and tablespoons are marked in units of 1 or $\frac{1}{2}$. On the other side of the cup in Figure 8-1B, ounces are displayed in units of $\frac{1}{8}$ or $\frac{1}{4}$, and drams are marked in units of 1 or 2. You can see that 5 mL is equivalent to 1 tsp. The slight curve in the surface of a liquid is the **meniscus.** The quantity of liquid is measured at the bottom of the meniscus, not by the higher levels at the edges. (Refer to Figure 8-2.)

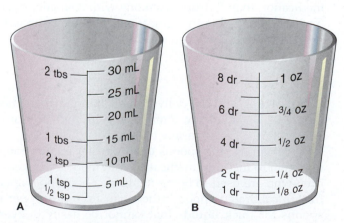

Figure 8-1 Two views of a medicine cup.

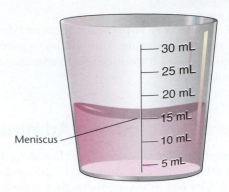

Meniscus

Figure 8-2 Fluid in a medicine cup should be measured at the bottom of the meniscus. This medicine cup contains 15 mL of liquid.

RULE 8-1

Do not use medicine cups for doses less than 5 mL, even if the cup has calibrations smaller than 5 mL. Instead, use a dropper, calibrated spoon, or oral syringe to ensure accuracy.

GO TO . . . Open the CD-ROM that accompanies your textbook, and, select Chapter 8, Using Proper Equipment (LO 8.1). Review the animation and example problems, then complete the practice problems. Continue to the next section of the book once you have mastered the information presented.

Droppers

Droppers help you measure and administer small amounts of oral liquid medication. You may also use them to deliver certain liquid medications to the eyes, ears, and nose. Droppers are especially helpful with oral pediatric doses. A product that requires a dropper is often packaged with a special dropper calibrated for the specified dose. The indicated units of measurement (calibrations) are usually milliliters (mL), cubic centimeters, drops, or even teaspoons. (Recall that 1 mL = 1 cc.) See Figure 8-3 for various types of droppers.

Droppers have different-size openings. The diameter of the opening affects the size of the individual drops. For example, 3 drops from a dropper with a large opening provides more medication than 3 drops from one with a smaller opening. So do not interchange droppers that are packaged with medications. However, separate calibrated droppers can be reused if properly cleaned between uses.

Calibrated Spoons

In some cases, you can deliver small amounts of medication by using **calibrated spoons** (see Figure 8-4). Spoons are often used with pediatric or elderly patients. They come in many sizes, calibrated to a variety of doses.

You can use the spoons to administer medication directly into the mouth. You can also use them to measure medication into food or a beverage for a child or elderly patient. Children who are used to being fed from a household spoon may accept medication if it comes from a calibrated spoon rather than from a dropper or a medicine cup. You can also use spoons for thick liquids that cannot be easily delivered through the small openings of a dropper.

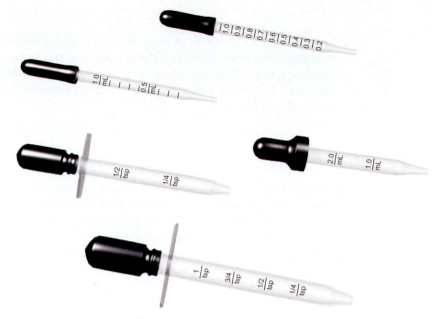

Figure 8-3 Droppers come in various sizes with different calibrations.

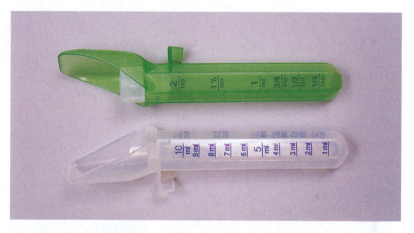

Figure 8-4 Calibrated spoons.

PATIENT EDUCATION

Patients who take oral medications at home need instruction in the proper use of medicine cups, droppers, and calibrated spoons.

1. To measure the correct dose by using a medicine cup, locate the appropriate calibration on the cup. While being careful not to tilt the cup, pour the liquid medication. The cup should be on a flat surface, such as a table, while you pour. If the flat surface is not already at eye level, then bend down to check the measurement at eye level for accuracy. The measurement should be read at the lowest level of the meniscus. Also check the expiration date of the medication and the medication itself for changes in clarity, color, or consistency.

2. Measure the proper amount in the calibrated dropper before delivery. Hold the dropper in a vertical position when delivering liquid. Count slowly, allowing drops to form fully.

(Continued)

3. Use calibrated spoons for medications that are measured by teaspoons, tablespoons, or milliliters. Do not measure medication with household spoons used for eating. They vary in size and are not reliable measures. Measuring spoons used for baking are acceptable, but not as accurate as calibrated spoons.

Oral Syringes

For small quantities of liquid, especially less than 5 mL, oral syringes provide accurate readings. Generic oral syringes are often calibrated for milliliters and teaspoons, with additional calibrations between these numbers (see Figure 8-5). Oral syringes are designed with safety features to keep them from being confused with hypodermic syringes. Oral syringes often have **eccentric,** or off-center, tips that have a different shape and size than the tips of hypodermic syringes. Oral syringes may be tinted, whereas hypodermic syringes are clear.

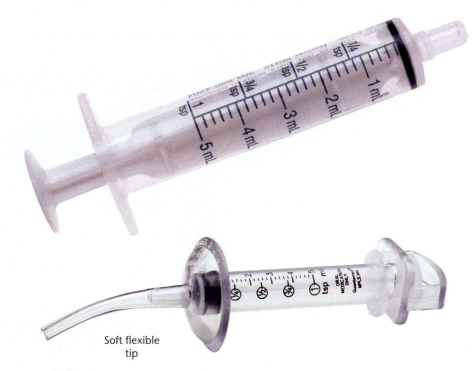

Soft flexible tip

Figure 8-5 Oral syringes.

Oral syringes are not to be confused with hypodermic syringes. Oral syringes are not sterile. Some oral syringes include a small cap that must be removed before administering medication orally to prevent choking. To administer sterile medications, you must use a sterile syringe.

RULE 8-2

1. Never attach a needle to an oral syringe.

2. Never inject an oral dose.

3. In emergencies, you may use a hypodermic syringe without a needle to measure and administer liquid oral doses, but never while its needle is attached.

GO TO . . . Open the CD-ROM that accompanies your textbook and select Chapter 8, Hypodermic VS Oral Syringe (LO 8.1). Review the animation and example problems, then complete the practice problems. Continue to the next section of the book once you have mastered the information presented.

Other Equipment for Enteral Medications

Sometimes oral medications, intended for absorption in the stomach or intestines, cannot be delivered orally. The patient may have difficulty swallowing or some condition or trauma that prevents taking the medication orally.

Liquid medications are preferred for **nasogastric** tubes, which delivers medication into the stomach (see Figure 8-6). Sometimes, you can crush a solid medication, adding water to transport it through the tube. Consult your facility for the appropriate procedure. Many solid oral medications, such as gelcaps and extended-release medications, may *not* be crushed. See Chapter 13 for further discussion about these medications.

There are other tubes used to deliver medications directly to the stomach or intestines. A **percutaneous** (through the skin) **endoscopic gastrostomy (PEG) tube** delivers medication and nutrients directly to the stomach. A **jejunostomy tube** delivers medication and nutrients directly to the small intestine.

No matter what equipment is used to administer medication, it must be measured accurately using the equipment's calibrations.

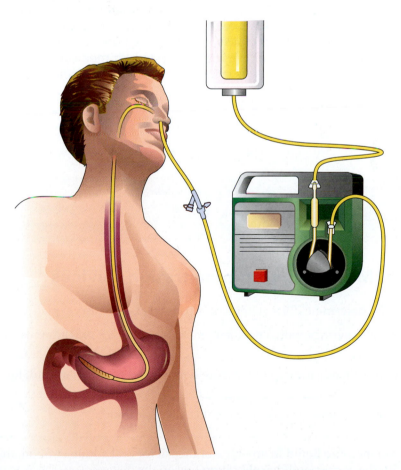

Figure 8-6   A nasogastric tube delivers medication into the stomach.

The Utensil You Use Must Provide the Calibration You Need to Accurately Measure the Dose

Suppose the volume of the dose is less than 0.5 mL. The calibrations on the utensil must measure increments of less than 0.5 mL. Otherwise, you cannot accurately measure the medication. Using a utensil that is marked in 1-mL increments and estimating the halfway point is not accurate.

CRITICAL THINKING ON THE JOB

Use the Correct Dropper

A baby with a fever is prescribed acetaminophen for home administration. The healthcare professional tells the baby's father that he will be given a bottle of liquid acetaminophen and a medicine dropper for measuring the prescribed number of drops. The father is told to give the baby 8 drops of medicine at regular intervals.

At home, the father accidentally drops and breaks the dropper. He remembers, though, that he has a dropper from another medication. He uses it instead to measure the acetaminophen. The second dropper is much smaller than the one that came with the acetaminophen. The baby receives a smaller dose than prescribed, even though the father administers the prescribed 8 drops.

Two nights later, the baby's symptoms are not relieved. The father calls the physician, who asks if he has been delivering the number of prescribed drops. The physician prescribes a stronger medication. The baby has suffered needlessly and now is exposed to a stronger medication for no reason.

Think! . . . Is It Reasonable? How could this error have been avoided?

REVIEW AND PRACTICE

8.1 Enteral Medication Administration Devices

For Exercises 1–14, determine if the statement is true or false. If false, explain why it is incorrect.

1. You may use a syringe with a needle to measure liquid for oral administration.

   _____

2. You may use a medicine cup to measure liquid doses of less than 1 mL for oral administration.

   _____

3. Oral and hypodermic syringes are identical in appearance.

   _____

4. When you measure liquid in any type of utensil for oral administration, the dose volume must be level with the corresponding calibration line on the device.

   _____

5. If the dropper supplied by a drug manufacturer for a specific medication is not available, you may substitute a dropper supplied for another medication, as long as the replacement dropper has never been used.

_____

6. If a patient does not have a calibrated spoon, then any household spoon may be substituted.

_____

7. Measuring utensils are often calibrated with more than one system of measurement.

_____

8. A prescribed dose of liquid oral medication cannot be dispensed reliably without calibrated cups, spoons, oral syringes, or droppers.

_____

9. When you calculate volume and dosage, it is helpful to remember that 1 mL is equal to 1.5 cubic centimeters.

_____

10. If a prescribed dose and the calibrated device used for administering that dose use different systems of measurement, then the device cannot be used.

_____

11. Measure the quantity of liquid in a measuring cup by the higher levels at the edge.

_____

12. Droppers may be used to deliver certain liquid medications to the eyes and ears but not the nose.

_____

13. Measuring spoons used for baking are acceptable for measuring liquid medication.

_____

14. Gelcaps and extended-release medications may be delivered through a nasogastric tube as long as they are crushed and flushed with water.

_____

For Exercises 15–20, convert the dosage ordered to the same units as those marked on calibrated utensils. You may wish to refer to the conversion factors in Chapter 5. There may be more than one correct answer for each conversion.

15. The prescribed dose is 2 tbs. Which of the following is *not* equivalent, as marked on the medicine cup?
    a. 30 mL   b. 1 oz   c. 6 tsp   d. 15 mL

16. An oral medication comes in a bottle labeled 10 units per cubic centimeter. The dose to be administered is 50 units. Which of the following is a correct dose?
    a. 50 mL   b. 500 mL   c. 5 mL   d. 0.5 mL

17. Which of the following statements about calibrated droppers is true?
    a. 0.25 mL equals 25 drops.   c. 1 mL equals 10 drops.
    b. 0.25 mL equals 5 drops.   d. The number of drops in each milliliter varies per dropper.

18. The dose to be given is 5 mL. The medicine cup is labeled in tablespoons, teaspoons, and ounces. Which of the following is a correct dose?
    a. 1 tsp   b. $\frac{1}{3}$ tsp   c. $\frac{1}{3}$ tsp   d. $\frac{1}{3}$ oz

19. An oral medication comes in a bottle labeled 200 mg per 5 mL. The dose to be administered is 600 mg. Which of the following is a correct dose?
    a. 1 tsp   b. 2 tsp   c. 1 tbs   d. 2 tbs

20. The dose to be given is 15 mL. The dose cup is labeled in tablespoons, teaspoons, and ounces. Which of the following is a correct dose?
    a. 3 tsp   b. 1 tbs   c. $\frac{1}{2}$ oz   d. All the above

To check your answers, see the Answer Key at the end of the book, which starts on page A-1.

Many medications must be administered **parenterally,** bypassing the digestive tract. (*Parenterally* means "outside the intestines.") While parenteral dosage forms include topical and **transdermal** (through the skin) medications, inhalers, and sublingual tablets, the term most often refers to injections. The most common injection routes are *intravenous* (IV), *intramuscular* (IM), *intradermal* (ID), and *subcutaneous* (SC). See Chapters 14 and 15 for more information about these methods of injection. Different **hypodermic syringes** are used to administer injections. These syringes are calibrated with different measurements. The type of syringe you use depends on the type and amount of medication to be administered. Remember 1 milliliter (mL) equals 1 cubic centimeter (cc). Although cc is an "error prone" abbreviation (see Chapter 11) you may see the abbreviation cc printed on a syringe.

Standard Syringes

The 3-mL syringe is one of the most common standard syringes used for parenteral administration. Standard syringes have scales calibrated in milliliters. Syringes with smaller capacities may have divisions of tenths, two-tenths, or even hundredths of a milliliter, allowing for measurement of small doses. The 3-mL syringe in Figure 8-7 is calibrated in tenths; it has 10 calibrations for each milliliter. Calibrations for half and whole milliliters are numbered. Standard syringes may also be marked with a minim scale from the apothecary system. However, the metric system is almost always used.

Any healthcare worker who uses a syringe must be familiar with its calibrations so that the correct dose is administered. On all syringes, the zero calibration is the edge of the barrel closest to the needle. The barrel is filled with liquid up to the point of the wide ring, known as the **leading ring,** on the tip of the plunger closest to the needle. Liquid in the barrel does not go past this ring. While the leading ring might have a raised middle, measure from the ring itself. Do *not* measure from the **trailing ring,** which is the ring farther from the needle.

Safety Syringes

Safety syringes have the same components as their standard counterparts: a needle, a hub, a barrel, and a plunger. See Figures 8-8 and 8-9. However, their needles are protected by plastic shields. These shields help prevent needlestick injury. Although safety syringes do not guarantee that healthcare workers will not receive accidental needlesticks, the syringes reduce the chances of such accidents. Some safety syringes have needles that retract into the syringe at the end of the injection. Safety syringes come in all sizes with various calibrations. They are calibrated in milliliters or units. Smaller-capacity safety syringes are divided into tenths, two-tenths, and hundredths of a milliliter.

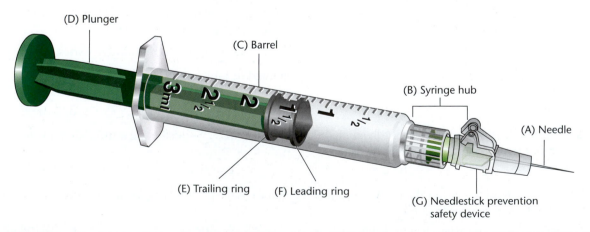

Figure 8-7 The parts of a standard syringe include (A) the needle, (B) the syringe hub, (C) the barrel that contains the liquid, (D) the plunger, (E) the trailing ring, (F) the plunger tip, also called the leading ring, and (G) needlestick prevention safety device.

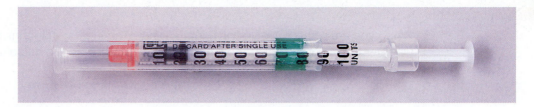

Figure 8-8 This 100-unit insulin safety syringe has a shield that covers the needle, minimizing needlestick injuries.

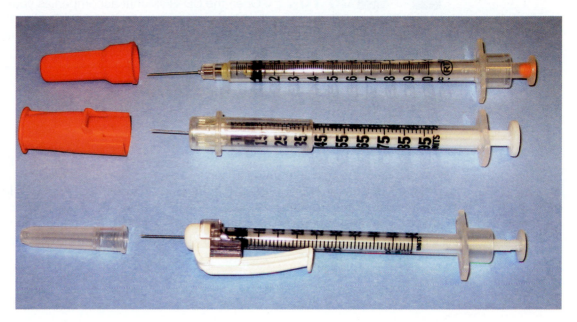

Figure 8-9 All syringes should have a safe-needle device. Shown here are three insulin syringes before activation. From top to bottom; VanishPoint, Monoject, and SafetyGlide.

Prefilled Syringes

Prefilled syringes are shipped from the manufacturer filled with a single dose of medication. If the patient is given only a portion of the dose, the remainder must be discarded before the medication is administered. Prefilled syringes have the same parts as a standard syringe: a needle, a syringe hub, a barrel, and a plunger (see Figure 8-8). Shown in Figure 8-10 is a syringe prefilled with normal saline. This syringe would most likely be used to flush an IV. Always check any prefilled syringe you use carefully. They may be marked in units other than milliliters (mL) and they may contain more medication than the markings indicate. You may need to perform a calculation and discard any excess before administration.

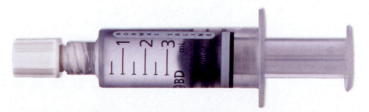

Figure 8-10 Prefilled syringe. Notice the calibration marks indicate milliliters and the syringe is filled beyond the 3 mL mark.

GO TO . . . Open the CD-ROM that accompanies your textbook and select Chapter 8, Examining the Markings on Syringes (LO 8.2). Review the animation and example problems, then complete the practice problems. Continue to the next section of the book once you have mastered the information presented.

Insulin Syringes

Insulin syringes are used only to measure and administer insulin. Insulin is measured in units. Insulin syringes are unique. They are calibrated in the amount of medication in units rather than calibrated by volume (milliliters). Whether for adults or children, insulin doses are smaller than many other doses. In turn, insulin syringes are calibrated in smaller increments. The most common strength of insulin is U-100; it contains 100 units of insulin per 1 mL. Insulin syringes are marked with "U-100", indicating that they are calibrated for use with U-100 insulin only.

Figure 8-11 shows a standard U-100 insulin syringe. It contains up to 100 units (1 mL) of U-100 insulin. The larger numbers mark increments of 10 units. The smaller calibrations indicate every 2 units. Many 100-unit syringes have two scales–one on the right showing the even number unit line and one on the left showing the odd number unit lines. Not all insulin syringes are marked with these increments. Figure 8-12 shows a syringe that holds up to 50 units of U-100 insulin. The larger numbers show increments of 5 units, and the smaller calibrations show increments of 1 unit. This syringe is often used to measure and administer pediatric or adult doses of insulin that are less than 50 units. (See Figure 8-13 for a comparison.)

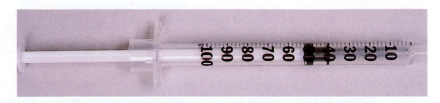

Figure 8-11   A standard insulin syringe can hold up to 100 units of insulin.

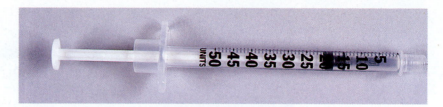

Figure 8-12 This insulin syringe can hold up to 50 units of insulin.

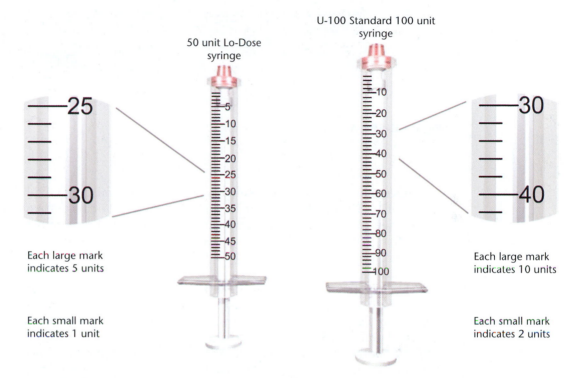

Figure 8-13 When comparing a 50 unit 0.5 mL versus standard 100 unit (1 mL) insulin syringe, always check the calibrations carefully.

GO TO . . . Open the CD-ROM that accompanies your textbook and select Chapter 8, Use Insulin Syringe Only (LO 8.2). Review the animation and example problems, then complete the practice problems. Continue to the next section of the book once you have mastered the information presented.

Tuberculin Syringes

Tuberculin syringes are used to administer subcutaneous injections as well as the intradermal purified protein derivative (PPD) skin test that determines if a person has been exposed to tuberculosis. More than that, they are simply small syringes used when small doses of medication—less than 1 mL—are administered. Vaccines, heparin, pediatric medicines, and allergen extracts are typically administered with a tuberculin syringe.

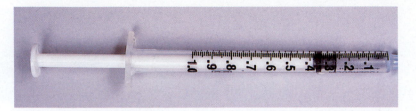

Figure 8-14 A 1-mL tuberculin syringe.

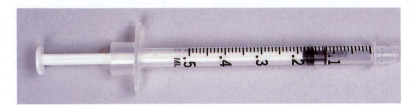

Figure 8-15 A 0.5-mL tuberculin syringe.

Tuberculin syringes usually hold a total volume of 1 mL and are calibrated in hundredths of a milliliter. The numbering is slightly different from that of the other syringes. In Figure 8-14, the marked numbers represent tenths of a milliliter. The first number, located on the tenth calibration, is 0.1 mL. Each smaller calibration represents one-hundredth (0.01) of a milliliter. Some syringes are even smaller. The tuberculin syringe in Figure 8-15 holds a total volume of 0.5 mL.

Measuring the correct dose with a tuberculin syringe requires extreme care. The calibrations are close together and marked with a number only at every one-tenth or two-tenths calibration. Be sure the leading ring is aligned with the proper calibration. See Figure 8-16 to become familiar with these calibrations. Sometimes tuberculin syringes are also calibrated with the apothecary scale in minims although these calibrations are not used very often. You must always take great care when reading any syringe to ensure you are reading the correct scale.

Syringes for Established Intravenous Lines

Some syringes are used to administer medication through already established intravenous lines that deliver medication and fluids directly into a patient's veins. Figure 8-17 shows an example of such a syringe.

Adding medication through existing lines has several advantages. Using the injection ports, IV medications can be administered quickly without the patient being punctured repeatedly. Because the syringes do not have needles, accidental needlesticks to patients and healthcare workers are avoided. An intravenous system with needleless syringes allows more than one drug to be administered at a time, provided that the drugs are compatible. Needleless syringes also enable you to deliver drugs on a periodic basis and to dilute the medication. Although these syringes are needleless, they still have calibrations that must be read carefully.

Large-Capacity Syringes

Although the maximal volume of an IM injection is 3 mL in any one site, not all medications can be delivered in doses of 3 mL or less. Larger volumes of medications may

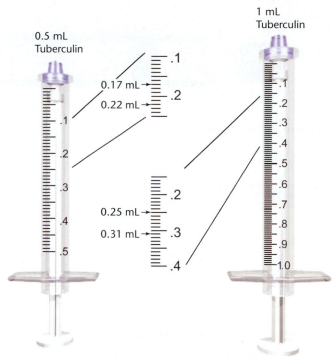

0.5 mL
Tuberculin

1 mL
Tuberculin

0.17 mL →

0.22 mL →

0.25 mL →

0.31 mL →

0.5 mL Tuberculin vs 1 mL Tuberculin syringe

Figure 8-16   Both syringes are calibrated to 0.01 mL. Each number indicates 0.1 mL.

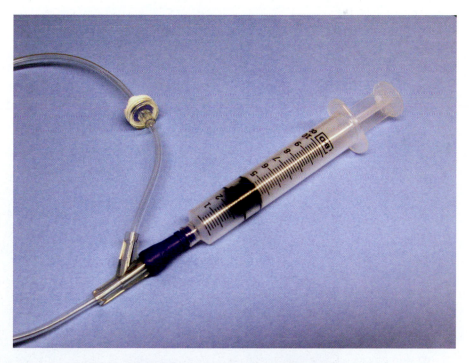

Figure 8-17   A needleless syringe is used to inject medication into existing IV tubing.

be added to IV infusions or administered IV push, therefore, syringes with 5, 6, 10, and 12 mL or even more are available (see Figure 8-18.) As with other syringes, volume is measured in milliliters, and the number of calibrations between numbered milliliters varies. Because of this you must look carefully at the marks to measure an accurate amount of medication.

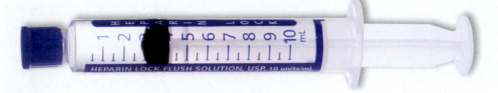

Figure 8-18 A large-capacity syringe.

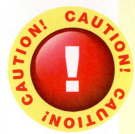

Ampules, Vials, and Cartridges

Parenteral medications may be packaged in ampules, vials, or cartridges (see Figure 8-19). **Cartridges** are prefilled containers shaped like syringe barrels. They generally hold one dose of medication and fit a reusable syringe. Tubex® and Carpuject are examples of cartridges. **Ampules** are glass containers and usually hold one dose of liquid medication. You snap them

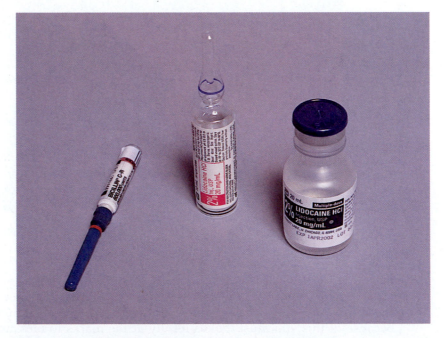

Figure 8-19 A cartridge (left), an ampule (center), and a vial (right).

open using care not to cut your fingers on the sharp edges. Sometimes a plastic protective sleeve is used when snapping the ampule, or an alcohol wipe package or 2 × 2 gauze is wrapped around the neck of the vial to avoid injury from the edge of the ampule. A filter needle (needle with a filter inside) should always be attached to the syringe to withdraw the medication from the ampule, and then the filter needle should be discarded and replaced by an appropriate needle for administration. By doing this, any glass fragments that may have been aspirated will be removed before patient use. **Vials** are containers covered with a rubber stopper, or diaphragm. They may hold more than a single dose of medication, in either liquid or powder form. If powder, then diluent is injected in the vial to reconstitute the medication. Vials are safer than ampules and used more commonly.

Preparing the Syringe

If you fill a syringe, you must label it with the contents, including the strength of the contents.

RULE 8-5	In most circumstances, the person who prepares a syringe for injection should deliver the injection. Exceptions include:

1. Pharmacy technicians who prefill syringes for nurses, medical assistants, or patients.

2. Nurses or medical assistants preparing a syringe for a physician.

3. Healthcare workers teaching a patient to administer his or her own medication.

This last exception occurs, for instance, when you teach a patient with diabetes how to administer insulin.

Needle Gauge and Length

When you administer an injection, you must choose a needle with an appropriate gauge. A needle's *gauge* is its interior diameter. Lower numbered gauges correspond to larger diameters; an 18-gauge needle is wider than a 22-gauge needle (see Figure 8-20). The gauge you use depends on the viscosity (thickness) of the medication as well as the injection site. More viscous drugs and deeper injections require larger needles (those with a lower gauge number), as seen in Table 8-1.

The injection site also determines the length of the needle. You should select a needle that is long enough to reach the area of tissue specified. However, the needle should not be so long that it penetrates beyond that area.

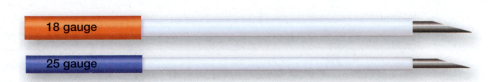

18 gauge

25 gauge

Figure 8-20 The gauge of the needle refers to the diameter. The larger the number the narrower the needle diameter.

TABLE 8-1 Suggested Needle Gauge, Length, Injection Amount and Location

TYPE	AGE	NEEDLE SIZE	NEEDLE LENGTH	MAXIMUM INJECTION AMOUNT	LOCATION
Intradermal (ID)					
ID	All ages	25 to 26 gauge	$\frac{1}{4}$ to $\frac{5}{8}$ inch	0.1 mL	Interior aspect of forearm (most common)
Subcutaneous (Subcut)					
Subcut	1 to 12 months	23 to 27 gauge	$\frac{5}{8}$ inch	0.5 mL	Fatty tissue over anterior lateral thigh muscle
Subcut	> 12 months to adults	23 to 27 gauge	$\frac{1}{2}$ to $\frac{3}{4}$; $\frac{5}{8}$ most common	0.5 to 1 mL	Fatty tissue over anterior lateral thigh muscle, triceps, or abdomen
Intramuscular (IM)					
IM	Infant to child	22 to 25 gauge	$\frac{5}{8}$ to 1 inch	0.5 to 1 mL	Vastus lateralis
IM	Adult	21 to 25 (very viscous medication may require 20 guage)	1 to $1\frac{1}{2}$ inch	2 to 3 mL	Ventroglueal
		23 to 25 guage		0.5 to 1 mL	Deltoid

CRITICAL THINKING ON THE JOB

Finishing What You Start

A healthcare professional prepares to deliver a single dose of Valium® by injection. He has a prefilled syringe containing 2.5 mL, but the prescribed dose is 1.5 mL. Before he can administer the injection, his pager goes off and he rushes to another patient's room. As he does, he asks another healthcare professional to administer the Valium.

She administers the Valium®, assuming that the prefilled syringe contains the appropriate dose. As a result of receiving more Valium® than was prescribed, the patient's blood pressure drops. The first healthcare professional does not ask if the correct dose has been administered, and the patient undergoes tests to find the cause of the drop in blood pressure.

Think! . . . Is It Reasonable? How could this error have been avoided?

 GO TO . . . Open the CD-ROM that accompanies your textbook and select Chapter 8, Prepare and Deliver Your Own Medication (LO 8.2). Review the animation and example problems, then complete the practice problems. Continue to the next section of the book once you have mastered the information presented.

REVIEW AND PRACTICE

8.2 Parenteral Medication Administration Devices

For Exercises 1–4, provide a brief answer.

1. What is the standard calibration of a 3-mL syringe?

2. What is the standard calibration of a 50-unit insulin syringe?

3. What is the standard calibration of a tuberculin syringe?

4. What is the standard calibration of a large-capacity syringe?

For Exercises 5–13, determine if the statement is true or false. If false, explain why it is incorrect.

5. Any extra medication in a syringe should be discarded before the injection is given.

6. The first calibration on any syringe is always zero (0).

7. When you are measuring a dose in a syringe, read the calibration that aligns with the trailing ring on the plunger.

8. Some prefilled syringes are overfilled with 0.1 to 0.2 mL of medication to allow for air expulsion from the needle.

9. Prefilled syringes and standard syringes do not have the same calibrations.

10. You can use an insulin syringe to measure 6 mL of medication.

11. A patient is punctured each time a syringe is used with an established intravenous line.

12. Safety syringes are a guaranteed way to avoid accidental needlestick injuries.

13. Tuberculin syringes are used to administer the subcutaneous PPD skin test.

For Exercises 14–25, identify the type of syringe and the volume of the dosage it contains. Identify the correct units of measurement.

    Example: Refer to the sample syringe below:

      Type: <u>tuberculin</u> Volume: <u>0.3 mL</u>

Sample

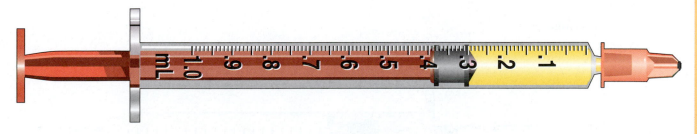

14. Refer to syringe A:

Type: _____ Volume: _____

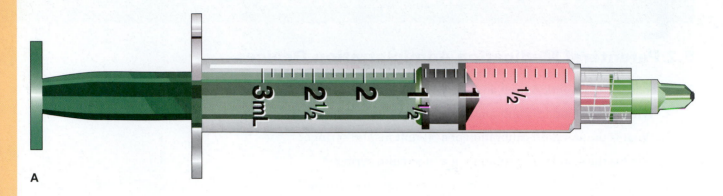

A

15. Refer to syringe B:

Type: _____ Volume: _____

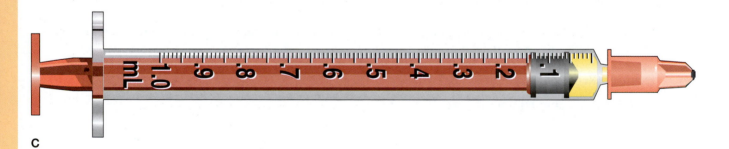

B

16. Refer to syringe C:

Type: _____ Volume: _____

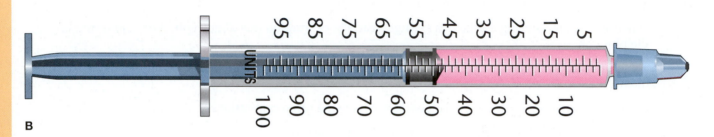

C

17. Refer to syringe D:

Type: _____ Volume: _____

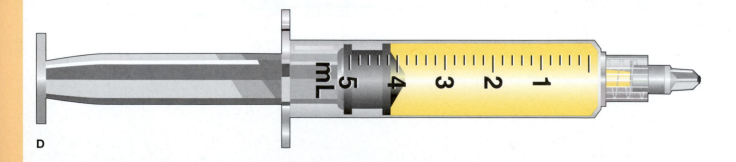

D

18. Refer to syringe E:

Type: _____ Volume: _____

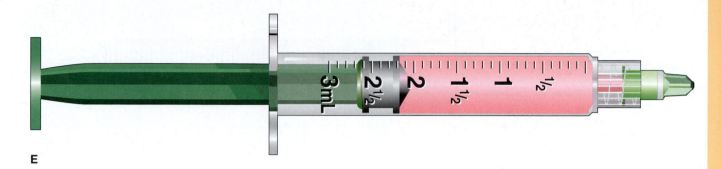

E

19. Refer to syringe F:

Type: _____ Volume: _____

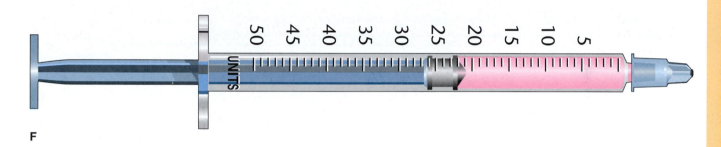

F

20. Refer to syringe G:

Type: _____ Volume: _____

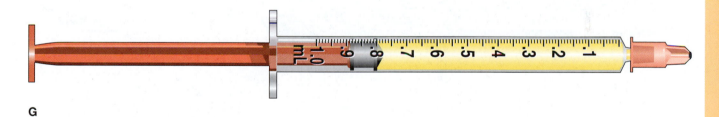

G

21. Refer to syringe H:

Type: _____ Volume: _____

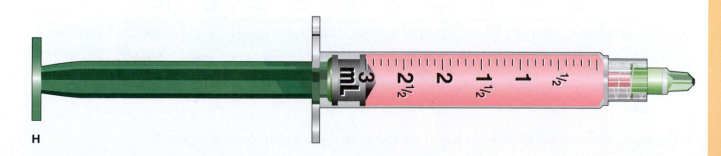

H

22. Refer to syringe I:

Type: _____ Volume: _____

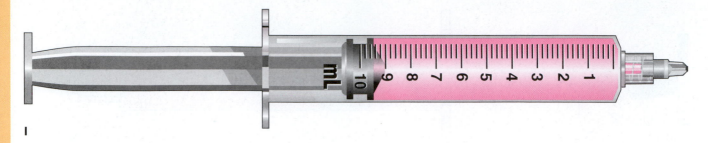

I

23. Refer to syringe J:

Type: _____ Volume: _____

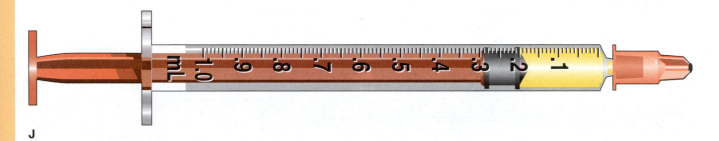

J

24. Refer to syringe K:

Type: _____ Volume: _____

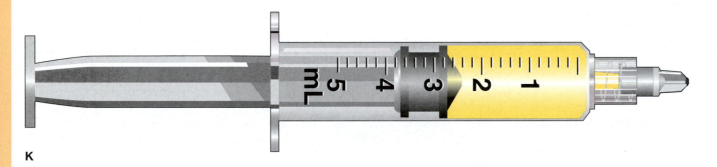

K

25. Refer to syringe L:

Type: _____ Volume: _____

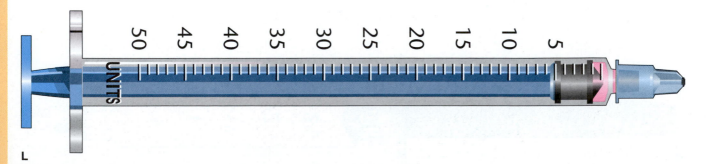

L

To check your answers, see the Answer Key at the end of the book, which starts on page A-1.

LEARNING OUTCOME	KEY POINTS
8.1 Recognize medication dosage volumes in different enteral equipment. Pages 133–139	Enteral devices are for medications absorbed through the GI Tract: *Medicine cup:* for liquids, measured at the bottom of the meniscus, easy administration; calibrations include mL (5 mL increments), tsp, tbs, oz ($\frac{1}{8}, \frac{1}{4}, \frac{1}{2}, \frac{3}{4}$) *Dropper:* for administering small amounts of liquids; calibrations vary; droppers may have different size openings – do not interchange droppers *Calibrated spoons:* used for small amounts of oral medication for pediatric and geriatric patients; calibrations include: mL (1 mL increments) and tsp ($\frac{1}{4}$ tsp increments) *Oral syringes:* for administering small amounts of *oral* medications; calibrations include: mL (in 0.1 mL increments) and tsp (in $\frac{1}{4}$ tsp increments); clean, not sterile – DO NOT USE for *parenteral* medication administration *Enteral tubes (NGT, GT, PEG, JT)* can become clogged by medications. Liquid medication is preferable; some solid medications can be crushed/opened and mixed with water. Some medications such as gel caps, enteric coated, and some capsules *should not be crushed.*
8.2 Recognize medication dosage volumes in different parenteral equipment. Pages 140–152	Parenteral devices are for medications given via the injection route: *3-mL syringe:* most commonly used for injections; calibrated to the tenths *1-mL/tuberculin syringe:* used to administer small doses; calibrated to the hundredths *Large capacity syringes:* deliver 5, 6, 10, 12 or more mL; calibration varies *Insulin syringes:* used to administer insulin only; 1-mL standard insulin syringe is calibrated by 1 or 2 unit markings, delivers up to 100 units; 0.5-mL/low-dose syringe is calibrated by 1 unit markings, delivers up to 50 units *Safety syringes:* has shield that covers the needle; various sizes, various calibrations. *Safety needle:* retracts, or has a device that caps the needle, keeping hands away from the tip *Prefilled syringe:* filled with single dose of medication *Syringe parts:* needle, hub, barrel, plunger, trailing ring (ring farthest from needle), leading ring (tip of plunger closest to needle)

Zero calibration: edge of the barrel closest to needle

Cartridge: prefilled contained shaped like syringe barrel

Ampule: glass single dose container that requires use of filtered needle to withdraw medication.

Vial: single or multiple dose container with rubber stopper or diaphragm through which medication is withdrawn

Needle gauge: interior diameter of a needle; 21–25 gauge for IM injections; 23–27 gauge for subcut injections; 25–26 gauge for intradermal injections;

Needle length: 1–2 inches for IM injections; $\frac{1}{2} - \frac{5}{8}$ inches for subcut injections; $\frac{3}{8} - \frac{5}{8}$ inches for intradermal injections

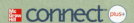

Determine if the statement is true or false. If false, explain what is incorrect about the statement.

1. Oral dosage forms are also called parenteral. (LO 8.1)

2. The leading ring is closer to the needle than the trailing ring. (LO 8.2)

3. Prefilled syringes can be used to give multiple injections as long as they are given to the same patient. (LO 8.2)

4. Tuberculin syringes have a capacity of 3 mL. (LO 8.2)

5. A vial can be used to give injections to multiple patients. (LO 8.2)

6. Syringes are always calibrated in milliliters. (LO 8.2)

Using the accompanying illustrations of equipment for the remaining questions, mark with a line or shading where you would measure the required dose. (LO 8.1, 8.2)

7. 30 mL

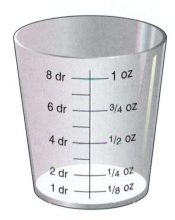

8. 0.7 mL

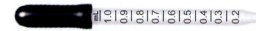

9. 2.4 mL

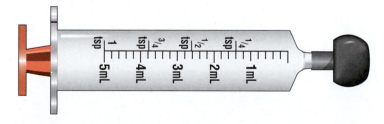

10. 2.4 mL

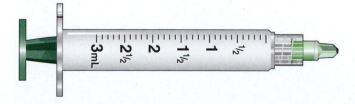

11. 18 units

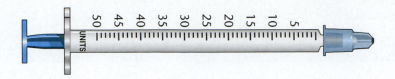

12. 0.38 mL

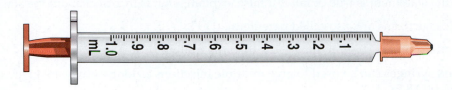

CHECK UP

For Exercises 1–10, answer the multiple-choice questions. More than one answer may be correct.

1. Which of the following equals 1 oz? (LO 8.1)

   a. 2 tbs   **b.** 20 mL   **c.** 30 mL   **d.** 22.5 mL as measured in an oral syringe tsp

2. A patient is supposed to receive 15 mL of Mylanta. A measuring cup cannot be found. What is an equivalent dose? (LO 8.1)

   a. 1 tsp   **b.** 2 tsp   **c.** 3 tsp   **d.** 5 tsp

3. The dose of a liquid medication for oral administration is $\frac{3}{4}$ oz. Which is the correct equivalent dose? (LO 8.1)

   a. 20 mL   **b.** 25 mL   **c.** 4.5 tsp   **d.** 1.5 tbs

4. The ordered dosage of a liquid medication for oral administration is 2.5 mL. What is the appropriate method of oral administration? (LO 8.1)

   a. $\frac{1}{8}$ oz as measured in a medicine cup   **b.** 1 oz as measured in a medicine cup

   c. $\frac{1}{2}$ tsp as measured in a calibrated spoon   **d.** 2.5 mL as measured in a calibrated dropper

5. The prescribed dosage of a medication is 5 drops. Which of the following is an appropriate method of administering the dose? (LO 8.1)

   a. 0.5 mL using only the calibrated dropper that accompanies the medicine bottle

   b. 5.0 mL using the calibrated dropper that accompanies the medicine bottle

   c. 5 drops using any calibrated dropper

   d. 5 drops using only the calibrated dropper that accompanies the medicine bottle

6. The ordered oral dosage of a medication is 5 mL. Which of the following is an appropriate method of administering the dose? (LO 8.1)

   a. 1 tsp using a calibrated spoon

   b. 5 mL using a syringe for parenteral administration with the needle removed

   c. 25 drops using a calibrated dropper

   d. 5 tsp using a calibrated spoon

7. The ordered dosage of a medication is 10 mg. The medication is mixed at a strength of 5 mg per milliliter. Using a 2.5-mL prefilled syringe, you should discard how much medication before administration? (LO 8.2)

   a. 0.2 mL   **b.** 1 mL   **c.** 0.5 mL   **d.** 2 mL

8. A tuberculin syringe is being used to administer 0.25 mL of a given medication. Which of the following is the equivalent dose? (LO 8.2)

   a. 2.5 hundredths of a milliliter   **b.** 25 hundredths of a milliliter

   c. 250 hundredths of a milliliter   **d.** 2.5 drops using a calibrated dropper

9. Which of the following can be used to administer a 7-mL dose via the parenteral route? (LO 8.2)

   a. A large-capacity syringe   **b.** A standard syringe

   c. A tuberculin syringe   **d.** An insulin syringe

10. Which of the following has the most precise and accurate calibrations? (LO 8.2)
   a. A 5-mL syringe to an established intravenous line
   b. A 3-mL syringe to an established intravenous line
   c. A 3-mL safety syringe
   d. A 1-mL tuberculin syringe

For Exercises 11–20, determine if the statement is true or false. If false, explain why it is incorrect. (LO 8.1, 8.2)

11. It is apparent from the calibrations on the medicine cups that 30 mL is equivalent to 1 oz. (LO 8.1)

12. If an ordered dose calls for 3 mL, a medicine cup may be used to measure it. (LO 8.1)

13. A calibrated dropper dispenses a standard drop of 3 mL. (LO 8.1)

14. The standard syringe can hold more than 1 mL. (LO 8.2)

15. The standard syringe is calibrated in tenths of a milliliter. (LO 8.2)

16. Prefilled, single-dose syringes can be used more than once. (LO 8.2)

17. The standard U-100 insulin syringe can hold up to 100 units or 1 mL. (LO 8.2)

18. The tuberculin syringe is used to measure doses of drugs larger than 3 mL. (LO 8.2)

19. The syringes used to deliver medication through already established intravenous systems are hypodermic syringes. (LO 8.2)

20. You may administer an oral medication by injecting it parenterally. (LO 8.1)

For Exercises 21–40, use the accompanying illustrations of equipment. For each question, mark with a line or with shading where you would measure the required dose:

21. 30 mL (Refer to medicine cup A.) (LO 8.1)

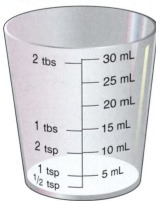

A

22. $\frac{1}{2}$ oz (Refer to medicine cup B.) (LO 8.1)

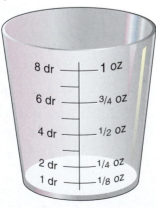

B

23. 1 mL (Refer to calibrated dropper C.) (LO 8.1)

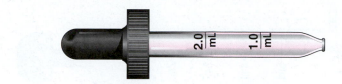

C

24. 0.6 mL (Refer to calibrated dropper D.) (LO 8.1)

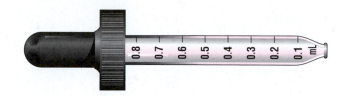

D

25. $\frac{3}{4}$ tsp (Refer to dropper E.) (LO 8.1)

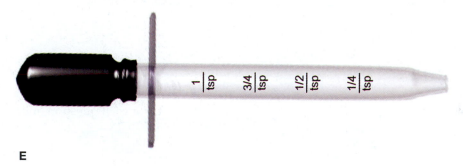

E

26. 0.5 mL (Refer to dropper F.) (LO 8.1)

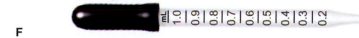

F

27. $\frac{1}{4}$ tsp (Refer to dropper G.) (LO 8.1)

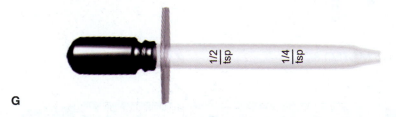

G

28. 0.32 mL (Refer to syringe H.) (LO 8.2)

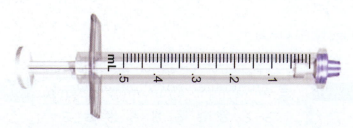

H

29. 2 mL (Refer to syringe I.) (LO 8.1)

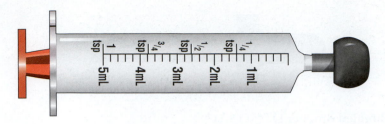

I

30. $1\frac{1}{2}$ tsp (Refer to syringe J.) (LO 8.1)

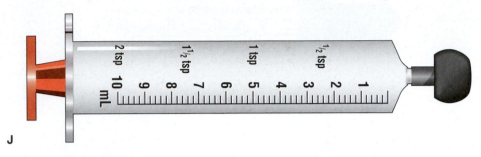

J

31. 1.5 mL (Refer to syringe K.) (LO 8.2)

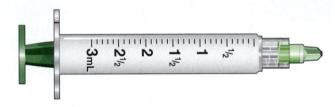

K

32. 2.3 mL (Refer to syringe L.) (LO 8.2)

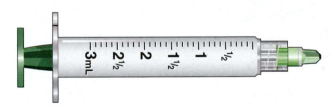

L

33. 80 units (Refer to syringe M.) (LO 8.2)

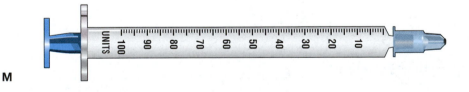

M

34. 45 units (Refer to syringe N.) (LO 8.2)

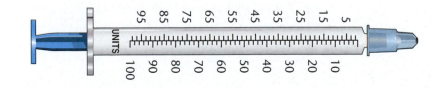

N

35. 35 units (Refer to syringe O.) (LO 8.2)

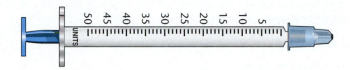

O

36. 27 units (Refer to syringe P.) (LO 8.2)

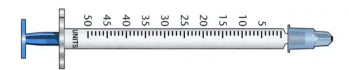

P

37. 0.5 mL (Refer to syringe Q.) (LO 8.2)

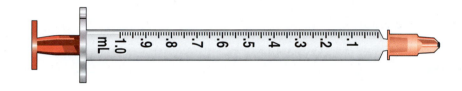

Q

38. 0.25 mL (Refer to syringe R.) (LO 8.2)

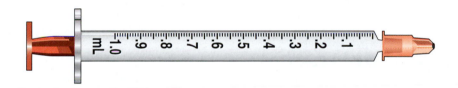

R

39. 5 mL (Refer to syringe S.) (LO 8.2)

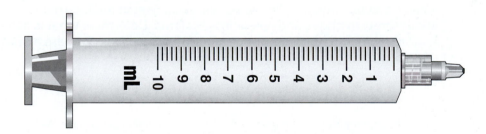

S

40. 7.2 mL (Refer to syringe T.) (LO 8.2)

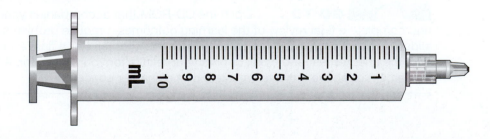

T

CRITICAL THINKING APPLICATIONS

What are the best utensils for measuring and administering the doses in each of the following situations? Choose from any of the equipment discussed in this chapter. (LO 8.1, 8.2)

1. 1.5 mL, to be delivered parenterally

2. 39 units of insulin, to be delivered parenterally

3. 0.3 mL, to be delivered parenterally

4. Oral liquid dose of 29 mL

5. Oral liquid dose of 1 tbs

6. Parenteral dose of 1.25 mL

7. Oral liquid dose of 2 tbs

8. 8 mL, to be administered parenterally

9. 0.3 mg, to be administered transdermally

10. 0.4 mL, to be administered orally

11. $\frac{3}{4}$ tsp to be administered orally

CASE STUDY

A healthcare professional must administer 10 drops of an oral medication. In attempting to administer the dose, the healthcare professional breaks the calibrated dropper. Instructions on the bottle say that 20 drops is equal to 1.5 tsp. What is the dose to be administered, and what is the best utensil for measuring it, now that the dropper is broken? (LO 8.1)

INTERNET ACTIVITY

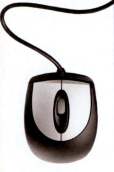

In the facility where you work, they want to implement the use of safety syringes and needleless systems for the protection of the healthcare employees. You have been asked to determine the types of syringes and systems available and to become familiar with their uses. Search the Internet for information about safety syringes and needleless systems. Determine what is available with regard to brand names, use, price, and safety statistics. Prepare a brief report or table comparing the items you have found.

To check your answers, see the Answer Key at the end of the book, which starts on page A-1.

GO TO . . . Open the CD-ROM that accompanies your textbook, and complete a final review of the learning outcomes, practice problems, games, slideshow, and other activities presented for this chapter. For a final evaluation, take the chapter test and email or print your results for your instructor. A score of 95 percent or above indicates mastery of the chapter concepts.

Interpreting Medication Orders

You must motivate yourself everyday!

—MATTHEW STASIOR

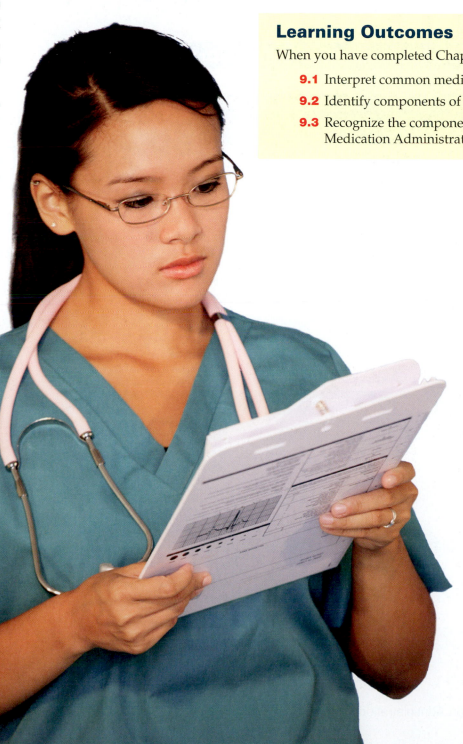

Learning Outcomes

When you have completed Chapter 9, you will be able to:

9.1 Interpret common medical abbreviations.

9.2 Identify components of a medication order.

9.3 Recognize the components of a medication order on the Medication Administration Record (MAR).

KEY TERMS

Authorized prescriber (AP)

Electronic Medication Administration Record (eMAR)

Frequency

Medication Administration Record (MAR)

Medication order

Prescription

Route

INTRODUCTION

To correctly calculate a medication dose, first you must be able to read and understand the drug order. To do this, you must learn and memorize common medical abbreviations. You must also recognize the components of a medication order. Motivate yourself for accuracy when completing this chapter about drug orders.

9.1 Medical Abbreviations

To promote efficiency in writing and interpreting medication orders, **authorized prescribers (AP's)** often use abbreviations for medication orders. AP's are licensed healthcare professionals that have the authority to write medication orders, also called **prescriptions**. The following table (Table 9-1) provides a list of commonly used medical abbreviations that pertain to medication administration. Table 9-1 is organized by abbreviation type

TABLE 9-1 Abbreviations Commonly Used in Drug Orders

General Abbreviations

ABBREVIATION	MEANING	ABBREVIATION	MEANING
aq	water	NPO, n.p.o.	nothing by mouth
$\bar{a}$	before	$\bar{p}$	after
BP	blood pressure	q, q.	every
$\bar{c}$	with	qs	quantity sufficient
d.c.*, D/C*	discontinue	$\bar{s}$	without
disp	dispense	sig, sig.	write on label
et	and	ss*, $\overline{ss}$*	one-half
iss*, $\overline{iss}$*	one and one-half	sys	systolic
NKA	no known allergies	tbsp, tbs, T	tablespoon
NKDA	no known drug allergies	tsp, t	teaspoon

Form of Medication

ABBREVIATION	MEANING	ABBREVIATION	MEANING
cap, caps	capsule	MDI	metered-dose inhaler
comp	compound	sol, soln.	solution
dil, dil.	dilute	SR	slow-release, sustained-release
EC	enteric-coated	supp, supp.	suppository
elix, elix.	elixir	susp, susp.	suspension
ext, ext.	extract	syr	syrup
fld., fl	fluid	syr	syringe
gt, gtt†	drop, drops	tab	tablet
LA	long-acting	tr, tinct, tinc.	tincture
liq	liquid	ung, oint	ointment

to include: general abbreviations, medication form abbreviations and abbreviations that pertain to route and frequency of medication administration. The medication **route** refers to the path by which a drug is brought into the body. For example, oral route indicates that the medication enters the body through the mouth while the rectal route means via the rectum. **Frequency** of medication administration refers to the time(s) of day and how often a medication is to be given.

TABLE 9-1 Continued

Route

ABBREVIATION	MEANING	ABBREVIATION	MEANING
ad*, A.D.*, AD*	right ear	NG, NGT, ng	nasogastric tube
as*, A.S.*, AS*	left ear	NJ	nasojejunal tube
au*, A.U.*, AU*	both ears	od*, O.D.*, OD*	right eye
GT	gastrostomy tube	os*, O.S.*, OS*	left eye
ID	intradermal	ou*, O.U.*, OU*	both eyes
IM, I.M.	intramuscular	per	per, by, through
IVPB	intravenous piggyback	po, p.o., PO, P.O.	by mouth; orally
IVSS	intravenous soluset	P.R., p.r., PR, pr	rectally
IV, I.V.	intravenous	subcut	subcutaneous, beneath the skin
IVP	intravenous push	SL, sl	sublingual, under the tongue
KVO, TKO	keep vein open, to keep open	top, TOP	topical, applied to skin surface

Frequency

ABBREVIATION	MEANING	ABBREVIATION	MEANING
a.c., ac, AC	before meals	p.r.n., prn, PRN	when necessary, when required
ad. lib., ad lib	as desired, freely	qam, q.a.m.	every morning
b.i.d., bid, BID	twice a day	qpm	every night
b.i.w.	twice a week	q.h., qh	every hour
h, hr	hour	q. _____ hrs, q_____h	every _____ hours
h.s.,* hs,* HS*	hour of sleep, at bedtime	qhs*, q.h.s.*	every night, at bedtime
LOS	length of stay	q.i.d., qid, QID	4 times a day
min	minute	rep	repeat
non rep	do not repeat	stat	immediately
noc, noct	night	t.i.d., tid, TID	3 times a day
p.c., pc, PC	after meals	t.i.w.*	3 times a week

*Indicates an "error-prone" abbreviation as established by the ISMP.
†commonly abbreviated at gtt and gtts

Memorize these abbreviations and have available a complete list of those accepted at your facility. Approved abbreviations vary among facilities. Abbreviations may be written in either uppercase or lowercase letters and with or without punctuation marks. AP's may also put a line over general and frequency abbreviations, such as *a, ac, c, p,* and *s,* when the abbreviations are lowercase. You may also notice slight differences in the way that the abbreviations are spelled.

Note the abbreviations with an asterisk * beside them in Table 9-1. Sometimes these abbreviations are still used by AP's; however, you need to recognize these abbreviations as those that should NOT be used as they are considered error-prone. Most electronic medical records allow practitioners to select from a list of standardized abbreviations when writing medication orders. This eliminates the use of error-prone abbreviations as well poor handwriting, thus helping to prevent medication errors. In Chapter 11, you will learn more about error-prone abbreviations and your role in promoting safe medication administration. Be certain to check abbreviations carefully when you read drug orders.

Roman Numerals

Roman numerals are sometimes used with drug orders written in the apothecary system, although this system is currently out of favor. The Institute for Safe Medication Practices (ISMP) recommends using the metric system for measuring medications. The ISMP will be discussed in more detail in Chapter 11. Since Roman numerals are still seen in practice you will need to understand how to change Roman numerals to Arabic numbers.

In the Roman numeral system, letters are used to represent numbers. Recall from Chapter 5 that lowercase letters are frequently used in pharmacy, especially for apothecary measurements. The Roman numerals that you are likely to encounter in a medical setting include ss ($\frac{1}{2}$), I (1), V (5), and X (10). These numerals may be written in either uppercase or lowercase, and a line is sometimes written above lowercase symbols. Thus, the number "one" can be written as I, i, or $\bar{\text{i}}$. The Roman numerals from 1 to 30 are the ones you are most likely to see in medication orders. Table 9-2 summarizes these numerals for you. Remember that "ss" could be added to the end of any of these expressions to add the value of $\frac{1}{2}$.

TABLE 9-2 Converting Roman Numerals

ROMAN NUMERAL*	ARABIC NUMBER	ROMAN NUMERAL	ARABIC NUMBER	ROMAN NUMERAL	ARABIC NUMBER
SS, $\overline{\text{ss}}$	$\frac{1}{2}$	XI, xi	11	XXII, xxii	22
I, i	1	XII, xii	12	XXIII, xxiii	23
II, ii	2	XIII, xiii	13	XXIV, xxiv	24
III, iii	3	XIV, xiv	14	XXV, xxv	25
IV, iv	4	XV, xv	15	XXVI, xxvi	26
V, v	5	XVI, xvi	16	XXVII, xxvii	27
VI, vi	6	XVII, xvii	17	XXVIII, xxviii	28
VII, vii	7	XVIII, xviii	18	XXIX, xxix	29
VIII, viii	8	XIX, xix	19	XXX, xxx	30
IX, ix	9	XX, xx	20		
X, x	10	XXI, xxi	21		

*Roman numerals written with small letters are also correctly written with a line over the top; for example, iv and $\overline{\text{iv}}$ are both correct.

COMBINING ROMAN NUMERALS Obviously, it is often necessary to write Roman numerals other than $\frac{1}{2}$, 1, 5, or 10. To do so, the letters are combined into a single expression. The expression can be translated to an Arabic number by following two simple steps.

RULE 9-1	When you read a Roman numeral containing more than one letter, follow these two steps: **1.** If any letter with a smaller value appears *before* a letter with a larger value, subtract the smaller value from the larger. **2.** Add the values of all the letters not affected by step 1 to those that were combined.
Example 1	**a.** IX = 10 − 1 = 9 **b.** iv = 5 − 1 = 4
Example 2	**a.** XIV = 10 + (5 − 1) = 14 **b.** VII = 5 + 2 = 7 **c.** ivss = (5 − 1) + $\frac{1}{2}$ = $4\frac{1}{2}$ **d.** VI = (5 + 1) = 6

It is important to note that there will never be more than three of the same Roman numerals in a row. If more than three need to be added to generate the new number, the convention is to subtract 1 from the larger number, rather than add 4 Roman numerals in a row. For example. The number 9 is written as ix, instead of viiii. Also, there will never be more than 1 subtracted from a larger number to generate a new number. For example the number 8 is written as viii, instead of iix.

CRITICAL THINKING ON THE JOB

Understanding the Order of Roman Numerals

A medication Administration Record lists a drug order of gr ix. (The abbreviation "gr" stands for grains. See Chapter 5.) A healthcare professional reading the order thinks, "The Roman numeral i equals 1 and x equals 10, so I should give 11 grains of the drug."

Think! . . . Is It Reasonable? What mistake did the healthcare professional make?

GO TO . . . Open the CD-ROM that accompanies your textbook, and select Chapter 9, Roman Numerals (LO 9.1). Review the animation then complete the practice problems. Continue to the next section of the book once you have mastered the information presented.

9.1 Medical Abbreviations

For Exercises 1-5, rewrite the medication order, interpreting the abbreviations.

1. Bactrim® (400 mg sulfamethoxazole and 80 mg trimethoprim) i tab po q 12h for 10 days.

2. Catapres® (clonidine hydrochloride, USP) 0.1 mg tablet po twice daily (morning and bedtime).

3. Lunesta® (eszopiclone) 1 mg tab i po qpm at bedtime prn insomnia.

4. Nitrostat® (Nitroglycerin) gr 1/150, tab i SL, prn chest pain; rep q 5 min prn continued pain, max 3 doses per episode.

5. Mevacor® (lovastatin) 20 mg tab ii po daily.

To check your answers, see the Answer Key at the end of the book, which starts on page A-1.

9.2 Components of a Medication Order

Always verify that a **medication order** contains all information needed to carry it out safely and accurately. Complete medication orders contain eight components to include: the full name of the patient, the patient's date of birth (DOB), the full name of the drug, the dose, the route, the time and frequency, the signature (electronic or written) of the authorized prescriber (AP), and the date of the order. See Figure 9-1 and Table 9-3. A prn order must include the reason for administering the medication. If an order is unclear or incomplete, contact the AP before you carry it out.

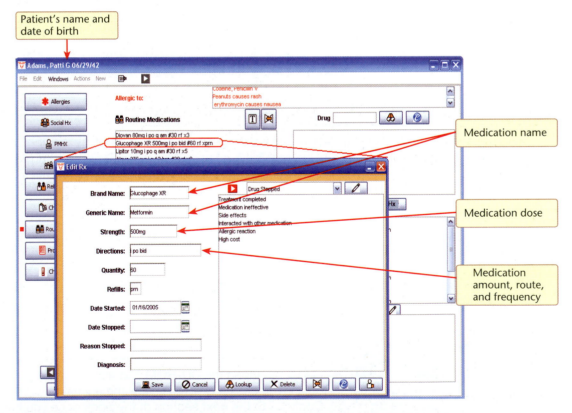

Figure 9-1 An electronic health record includes all parts of the medication order. In some cases a signature is not seen when an electronic signature is used, but will be shown on the printed or transmitted order.

Most facilities have a standard schedule for administering medication (see Table 9-4). To minimize errors, agencies frequently use the 24-hour clock (see Chapter 7). The person who verifies the transcription ensures that the times listed are appropriate for the medications. For example, some medications need to be given with food or after a meal; others, on an empty stomach. Times may need to be adjusted to accommodate a patient's meals. A patient may take two or more medications with conflicting schedules. Again, the timing may need to be adjusted.

TABLE 9-3 Components of a Medical Order

Patient's name	Should be full name with middle name or initial.
Date	Date the order was written. The time of the order is typically included for inpatient medication orders.
Date of birth (DOB)	Patient's date of birth (Note: A medical record number or bar code may also be included on the order.)
Name of medication	Full medication or drug name
Dose	Amount of medication to be administered at one time. (See Chapter 12)
Route	The path by which the drug enters the body (such as oral). (See Chapter 10.)
Frequency	The time of day and how often the medication is taken.
Authorized prescriber's (AP) signature	Handwritten or electronic signature from licensed MD (medical doctor), DO (osteopathic physician), DPM (podiatrist), DDS (dentists), PA (physician assistant), ARNP (advanced registered nurse practitioner) or other licensed healthcare professional with prescriptive authority.

TABLE 9-4 Sample Times for Medication Administration

FREQUENCY ORDERED	TIMES TO ADMINISTER
daily	0800
bid	0800, 2000
tid	0800, 1400, 2000
qid	0800, 1200, 1600, 2000
q 12 hrs	0800, 2000
q 8 hrs	2400, 0800, 1600
q 6 hrs	2400, 0600, 1200, 1800

CRITICAL THINKING ON THE JOB

When in Doubt, Check

A healthcare practitioner is preparing medications. An entry in the MAR calls for 600 mg of Lasix® IV, higher than what she usually administers. She checks a medication reference. It indicates that doses this high may be used for congestive

(Continued)

heart failure, the patient's diagnosis. Still, she is not comfortable with this level. She checks the original order on the medication order (See Figure 9-2).

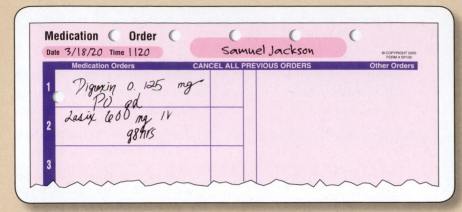

Figure 9-2 Medication order.

 Think! . . . Is It Reasonable? 1. What parts of the medication order are missing from figure 9-2?

2. What part of the medication order is the healthcare practitioner questioning?

3. What serious error did the healthcare practitioner prevent by checking the original medication order?

GO TO . . . Open the CD-ROM that accompanies your textbook, and select Chapter 9, Parts of a Medication Order (LO 9.2). Review the animation then complete the practice problems. Continue to the next section of the book once you have mastered the information presented.

REVIEW AND PRACTICE

9.2 Components of a Medication Order

For Exercises 1-8, match the eight components of a medication order to the corresponding order segments.

1. Patient's name	_____	a. *P. Sriker, MD*
2. Date	_____	b. Aricept (donepezil HCL)
3. Date of Birth (DOB)	_____	c. 4/12/56
4. Name of medication	_____	d. daily
5. Dose	_____	e. John M. Smith
6. Route	_____	f. 2/18/11
7. Frequency	_____	g. 5 mg
8. Authorized prescriber's signature	_____	h. po

To check your answers, see the Answer Key at the end of the book, which starts on page A-1.

9.3 | Medication Administration Records

Medication Administration Records (MARs) are legal documents that may be handwritten forms or electronic (see Figure 9-3). **Electronic Medication Administration Records (eMARs)** are viewed and completed on an electronic device and the authorized prescriber's signature is protected through a unique password. MARs contain the same information as a medication order and also specify the actual times to administer the medication. Additionally the MAR provides a place to document that each medication has been given. By law, when a medication is given, it must be documented.

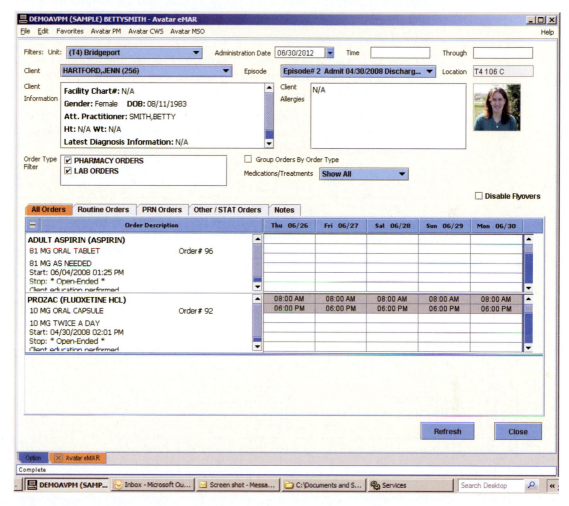

Figure 9-3 An electronic Medication Administration Record (eMAR) like this one allows the healthcare practitioner to document medication administration electronically.

Netsmart Technologies (www.ntst.com)

RULE 9-2

MARs must include the following information:

1. The full name of the medication, the dose, the route, and the frequency.

2. Times that accurately reflect the frequency specified.

3. The full name and date of birth (DOB) and/or other identification number of the patient.

4. The date the order was written. If no start date is listed, then the assumption is that the date of order is the start date. Orders for narcotics and antibiotics should include end dates, according to your facility's policies.

5. Any special instructions or information as required by your facility. This includes, but is not limited to, the patient's diagnosis and weight.

Example 1

Determine whether the MAR in Figure 9-4 is complete.

In Figure 9-4 all three orders are written correctly. In order A, the drug is Nitrobid® 2% cream, the dose is $\frac{1}{2}$ inch, the route is topical, and the frequency is every 6 hr. The scheduled times are 2400 (midnight), 0600 (6:00 a.m.), 1200 (12:00 p.m.), and 1800 (6:00 p.m.).

In order B, the drug is Vasotec®, the dose is 10 mg, the route is oral, and the frequency is twice a day. This order includes a special instruction to hold the medication if the systolic blood pressure is below 100

In order C, the drug is Glucophage®, the dose is 500 mg, the frequency is twice a day, and the route is oral. Glucophage® must be administered with meals. Therefore, the times have been adjusted to fit the facility's meal schedule.

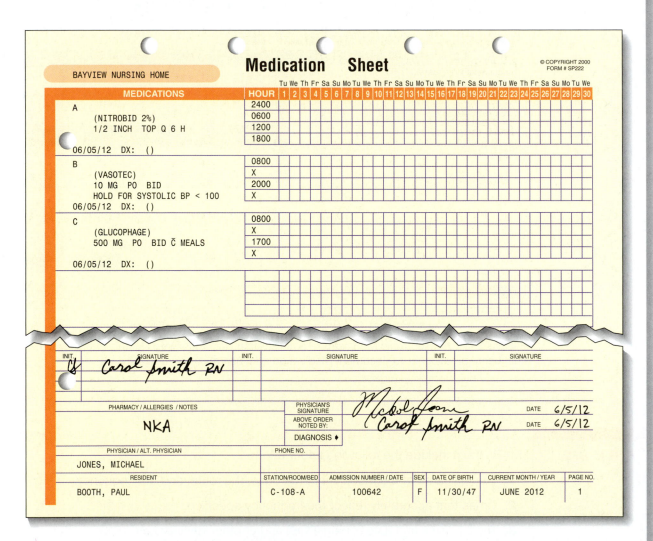

Figure 9-4 Medication Administration Record (MAR).

Example 2

Determine whether the MAR in Figure 9-5 is complete.

In Figure 9-5, order A is correct. The drug is Synthroid®, the dose is 50 mcg, the route is oral, and the frequency is daily.

Order B may seem to have all required information, but the dose—1 tablet—is not adequate. Erythromycin is available in several strengths. The order does not specify which dosage strength is intended. The times (0800, 2000) are for every 12 hours. Times should be listed as 0200, 0800, 1400, 2000. If the error is not corrected the patient will not receive a therapeutic level of the drug.

Order C contains an error in the times listed. Persantine® 75 mg is to be given q6h, or every 6 hours. The times (2400, 0800, 1600) are for every 8 hours. If the error is not recognized, then the patient will not receive a therapeutic level of the drug.

Order D does not include a route. Heparin can be administered either subcutaneously or intravenously. This order cannot be carried out as written.

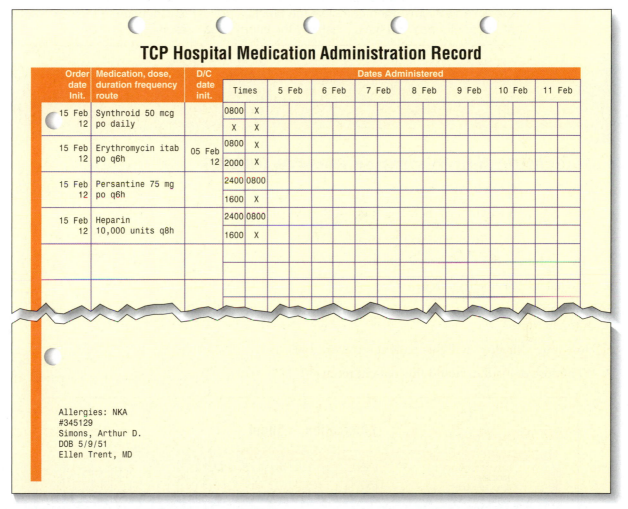

Figure 9-5 Medication Administration Record (MAR).

PATIENT EDUCATION

When administering medications, accurate and complete information should be given to patients.

1. Explain the purpose of a medication and its side effects.
2. Review the dose, route, frequency, and time that the physician has prescribed.

(Continued)

3. When appropriate, be certain that the patient understands how to self-administer the medication.

4. If the patient is taking liquid oral medications at home, emphasize the importance of using calibrated spoons and measuring cups.

5. When writing instructions for patients, do not use abbreviations; write the actual unit of measurement. For example, instead of writing "2 t PO t.i.d. prn cough", write "take two teaspoons by mouth three times a day as needed for cough."

GO TO . . . Open the CD-ROM that accompanies your textbook, and select Chapter 9, Medication Administration Record (LO 9.3). Review the animation and example problems, then complete the practice problems. Continue to the next section of the book once you have mastered the information presented.

REVIEW AND PRACTICE

9.3 Medication Administration Records (MARs)

For Exercises 1–7, refer to MAR 1 below.

1. What action must you take before administering Accupril®?

2. What dose of Accupril® should this patient receive?

3. At what time is the insulin to be given?

4. By what route is the insulin given?

5. This unit's schedule for QID medications is 0800, 1200, 1700, 2000. Why is Maalox® scheduled for different times?

6. How much Maalox® will this patient receive at 1400?

7. What dose of insulin should this patient receive?

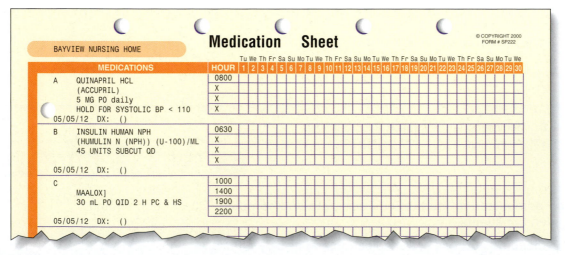

MAR 1

CHAPTER 9 SUMMARY

LEARNING OUTCOME	KEY POINTS
9.1 Interpret common medical abbreviations. Pages 164–168	See Table 9-1 for complete list. ▶ *General abbreviations:* $\bar{a}$ = before; $\bar{p}$ = after; q = every; qs = quantity sufficient; NKA = no known allergies; NKDA = no known drug allergies; NPO = nothing by mouth ▶ *Form:* cap = capsule; EC = enteric coated; gt = drop; MDI = metered-dose inhaler; tab = tablet ▶ *Route:* GT = gastrostomy tube; IM = intramuscular; IV = intravenous; IVP = intravenous push; IVPB = intravenous piggyback; KVO = keep vein open, NG = nasogastric tube, NJ = nasojejunal tube; po = by mouth; pr = per rectum; subcut = subcutaneous; SL = sublinguial; top = topical ▶ *Frequency:* ac = before meals; pc = after meals; BID = twice a day; h = hour; prn = as needed; qam = every morning; qpm = every night; qh = every hour; stat = immediately; tid = 3 times a day The error-prone abbreviations identified in Table 9.1 with an asterisk should not be used. Roman numerals are used to write medication dosages in the Apothecary System (see Table 9-2). The ISMP recommends using the metric system for writing medication dosages. Rule 9-1 When you read a Roman numeral containing more than one letter, follow these two steps: 1. If any letter with a smaller value appears *before* a letter with a larger value, subtract the smaller value from the larger. 2. Add the values of all the letters not affected by step 1 to those that were combined. No more than three of the same Roman numeral can follow (be added to) a numeral; No more than one Roman numeral can be subtracted from a numeral.

LEARNING OUTCOME	KEY POINTS
9.2 Identify components of a medication order. Pages 168–170	There are 8 components of a medication order: 1. Patient's name 2. Date 3. Date of birth (patient) 4. Name of medication 5. Dose 6. Route 7. Frequency 8. Authorized prescriber's signature For example, 5/11/2011 Peter Patient DOB 2/14/87 Tylenol 650 mg po q4h prn headache *A. Physician, MD*
9.3 Recognize the components of a medication order on the Medication Administration Record (MAR). Pages 171–174	Medication Administration Records (MAR) are transcriptions of the complete doctor's order, with an additional schedule of dates and times for the medication to be administered. A notation is made by the healthcare provider after a medication is administered. This is a legal document that can be hand written or computer generated (eMAR). Per Rule 9-2 MARs must include the following information: 1. The full name of the medication, the dose, the route, and the frequency. 2. Times that accurately reflect the frequency specified. 3. The full name and patient's date of birth or other identification number. 4. The date the order was written. If no start date is listed, then the assumption is that the date of order is the start date. Orders for narcotics and antibiotics should include end dates, according to your facility's policies. 5. Any special instructions or information as required by your facility. This includes, but is not limited to, the patient's diagnosis and weight.

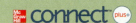
For Exercises 1–10, interpret the medical abbreviations in each order. (LO 9.1)

1. Ambien® (zolpidem tartrate) 10 mg po immediately before bedtime, prn insomnia

2. Sectral® (acebutolol hydrochloride) 400 mg po daily

3. Astelin® (azelastine hydrochloride) sprays ii each nostril BID

4. Bextra® (valdecoxib) 10 mg po daily

5. Wellbutrin XL® (bupropion hydrochloride extended-release) 300 mg po daily

6. Xigris® (drotrecogin alfa (activated)) 24 mcg/kg/hr IV for 96 hours

7. Zantac® Syrup (ranitidine hydrochloride) 150 mg/10 mL , tsp ii po BID

8. Serevent® Diskus® (salmeterol xinafoate) Inhalation Powder 50 mcg inhalation i po q 12h

9. Glucotrol® (glipizide) 5 mg tab i po daily ā breakfast

10. Lamisil® (terbinafine hydrochloride) 250 mg tab i po daily for 6 weeks

For examples 11–18, write the data that correspond with each medication order component (LO 9.2)

| RHODE ISLAND MEDICAL CENTER | Jane Doe   DOB 3/15/55 |
| Coventry, Rhode Island | 1534 Hopkins Trail Chepachet, RI 01222 |

| Diagnosis: Congestive Heart Failure | Allergies: NONE |

Date	Time	
1/3/11	8AM	tylenol 325 mg tab ii PO q4h prn fever > 101
		Mark Sanger, MD

11. Date/time _____

12. Patient's name _____

13. Patient's date of birth _____

14. Medication name _____

15. Dose _____

16. Route _____

17. Frequency _____

18. AP signature _____

Medication   Sheet

Order	Medication, dose, duration frequency route	D/C date init.	HOUR		1 Feb	2 Feb	3 Feb	4 Feb	5 Feb	6 Feb	7 Feb
A	NORMODYNE 100 MG PO BID		0800	X							
			2000	X							
B	HUMULIN N 24 UNITS before breakfast		0700	X							
			X	X							
C	DULCOLAX PR once a day PRN		X	X							
			X	X							
D	ATROVENT 2 PUFFS VIA MDI QID		0800	1200							
			1600	2000							
E	BUSPAR 15 MG PO TID		0800	1400							
			2000	X							

MAR 2

19. Why are no times marked beside the Dulcolax®?

20. Which medications should be given at 8 a.m.?

21. Which medication orders are not complete?

22. What is missing from the orders identified in the answer to question 21?

23. What is the route for the Buspar®?

24. What is the dose for the Atrovent®?

CHAPTER 9 REVIEW

CHECK UP

For Exercises 1–10 rewrite the medication order, interpreting the abbreviations. (LO 9.1)

1. Aldactone® (spironolactone) 25 mg tab i po daily.

2. Neurontin® (gabapentin) oral solution 250 mg/5 mL, 400 mg po TID.

3. Boniva® (ibandronate sodium) 150 mg tab i taken po ā breakfast q month.

4. Paxil® (paroxetine hydrochloride) oral susp 10 mg/5 mL, 20 mg po daily in a.m.

5. Singulair® (montelukast sodium) 5 mg tab, chew i po daily.

6. Aspirin gr v, tab ii po q4h prn headache.

7. Protonix® (pantoprazole sodium) 40 mg tab i po daily.

8. Nitrong® (nitroglycerin) 1 inch top q8h, remove for 8 hours at bedtime.

9. Naprosyn® (naproxen) 250 mg tab i po q8h.

10. Cozaar® (losartan potassium) 50 mg tab i po daily.

For Exercises 11 to 18 identify each of the components of the electronic medication order below. (LO 9.2)

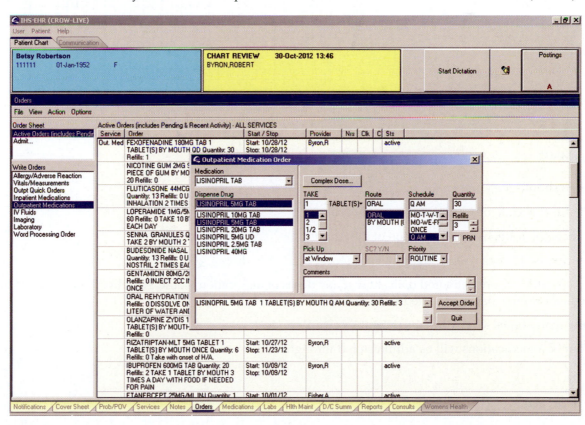

Electronic medication order

11. Date   _____

12. Medication   _____

13. Frequency   _____

14. Route   _____

15. AP   _____

16. Dose   _____

17. Patient   _____

18. DOB   _____

For Exercises 19-25, refer to MAR 3 below (LO 9.3)

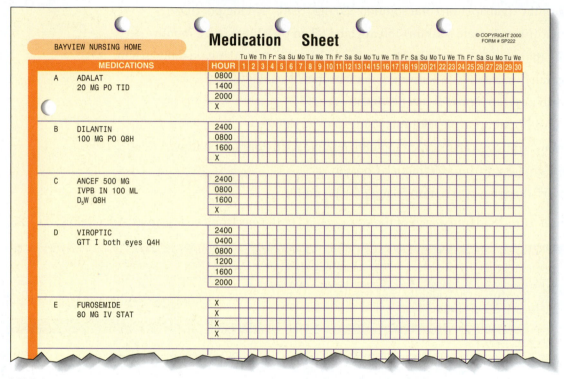

MAR 3

19. When should the Furosemide be given?

20. What is the route of administration of the Viroptic?

21. What is the route of administration of the Ancef®?

22. Which medications will be given at 4 p.m.?

23. If medications were delivered daily, how many doses of medication would be delivered for each of the medications this patient is scheduled to receive?

24. How many times a day does the patient receive Viroptic?

25. What two medications will be administered through an IV?

CRITICAL THINKING APPLICATION

For Exercises 1-3, refer to the medication order below. (LO 9.2)

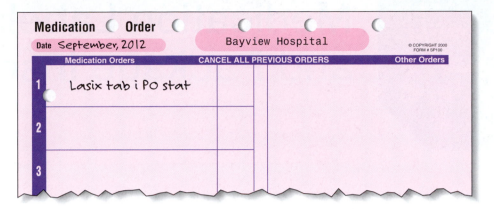

Medication (Order (

Date September, 2012

Bayview Hospital

© COPYRIGHT 2000
FORM # SP100

	Medication Orders	CANCEL ALL PREVIOUS ORDERS	Other Orders
1	Lasix tab i PO stat		
2			
3			

1. Interpret the medical abbreviations in this order.

2. What components of the medication order are missing?

3. Describe the importance of knowing the eight components of the medication order.

CASE STUDY

Katherine Drexel, born 20 years ago today, is complaining of pain and discomfort after the delivery of her baby. The midwife, Louise Pingree, has ordered on this date, at this hour, eight hundred milligrams of Motrin® (ibuprofen) to be given orally every eight hours as needed for pain. Write a medication order using appropriate medical abbreviations and identify each of the eight components of the order. (LO 9.1)

INTERNET ACTIVITY

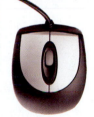

Go to the Internet site Quia at http://www.quia.com/mc/405408.html and practice matching the medical terminology with the correct abbreviations.

To check your answers, see the Answer Key at the end of the book, which starts on page A-1.

GO TO . . . Open the CD-ROM that accompanies your textbook, and complete a final review of the learning outcomes, practice problems, games, slideshow, and other activities presented for this chapter. For a final evaluation, take the chapter test and email or print your results for your instructor. A score of 95 percent or above indicates mastery of the chapter concepts.

10
CHAPTER

Interpreting Medication Labels and Package Inserts

Read in order to live.

—HENRY FIELDING

Learning Outcomes

When you have completed Chapter 10, you will be able to:

10.1 Differentiate information on a medication label and within a package insert.

10.2 Distinguish information related to administration routes for medications.

KEY TERMS

Bar code
Dosage strength
Generic name
ID—intradermal
IM—intramuscular
IV—intravenous
Package insert
Reconstitute
Subcut—subcutaneous
Trade name
Transdermal

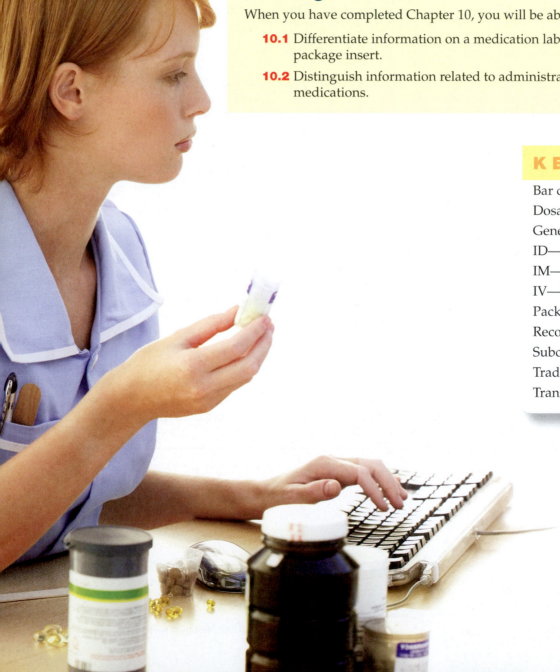

INTRODUCTION

Now that you have learned basic math (Chapters 1 to 4), other systems of measurement (Chapter 5), conversions (Chapters 6 and 7), equipment (Chapter 8), and drug orders (Chapter 9), it is time to learn a little bit about drug packaging. The drug label and package insert contain the information you need to perform dosage calculations, and they must be read carefully. Make sure you know exactly what is found on a drug label, and do not forget to read the fine print. Very essential information is located there.

10.1 Information on Medication Labels and Package Inserts

To prepare and administer drugs, you must understand information that appears on drug labels, including the drug name, form, dosage strength, total amount in the container, route of administration, warnings, storage requirements, and manufacturing information.

Drug Name

Every drug has an official name—its **generic name.** By law, this name must appear on the drug's label. It is also recorded with a national listing of drugs: the *United States Pharmacopeia* (USP) and the *National Formulary* (NF). In Figures 10-1, 10-2, 10-3, and 10-4 each drug's generic name has been identified. If USP appears on the label, it indicates that this drug's name is recorded with the *United States Pharmacopeia.*

Many drug labels include the **trade,** or *brand,* **name** used to market the drug. In Figures 10-1 and 10-2 note that the trade name is listed before the generic name. However, some drug labels list only a generic name (see Figures 10-3 and 10-4). A trade name is the property of a specific drug company. The registered mark® indicates the name has been legally registered with the U.S. Patent and Trademark Office. Several companies may manufacture a drug but market it under different trade names.

Authorized prescribers can write drug orders using either generic or trade names. Some companies produce drugs under their generic names and market them at a lower cost than that of the trade name equivalents. For example, ibuprofen is sold under its generic name as well as trade names such as Advil® and Motrin®.

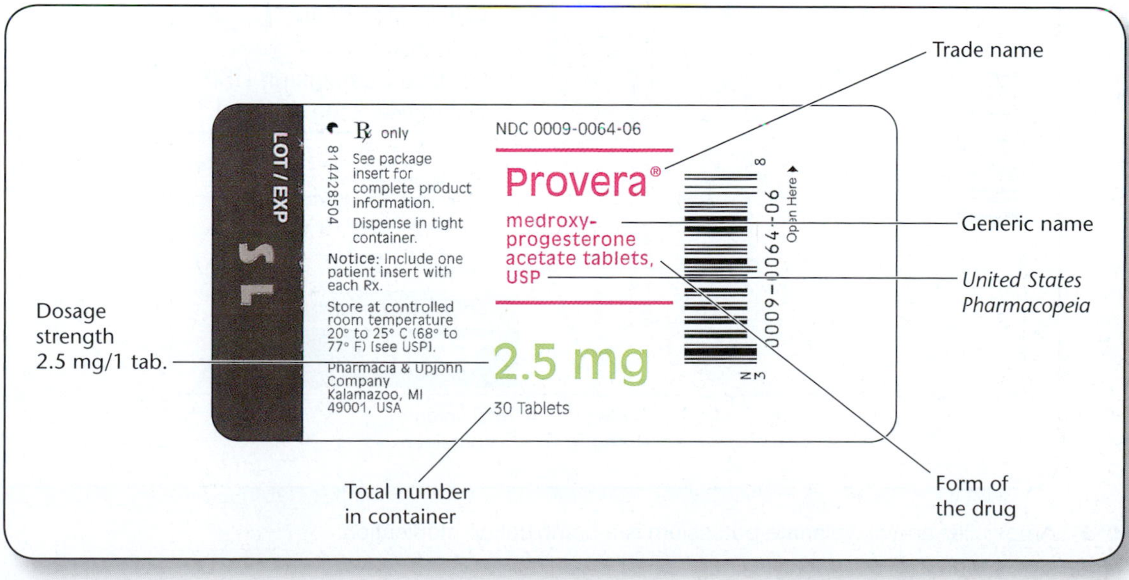

Trade name
Generic name
United States Pharmacopeia
Form of the drug
Total number in container
Dosage strength 2.5 mg/1 tab.
LOT / EXP
814428504
℞ only
See package insert for complete product information.
Dispense in tight container.
Notice: Include one patient insert with each Rx.
Store at controlled room temperature 20° to 25° C (68° to 77° F) [see USP].
Pharmacia & Upjohn Company Kalamazoo, MI 49001, USA
NDC 0009-0064-06
Provera®
medroxy-progesterone acetate tablets, USP
2.5 mg
30 Tablets
Open Here

Figure 10-1 A ® beside the trade name indicates it is legally registered with the U.S. Patent and Trademark Office.

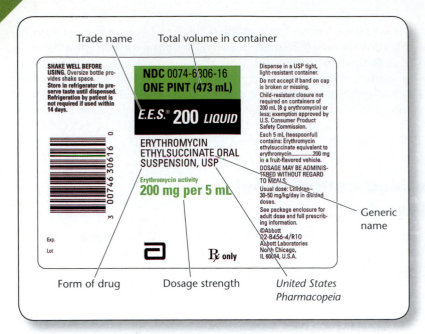

Figure 10-2 E.E.S.® 200 Liquid is the trade name.

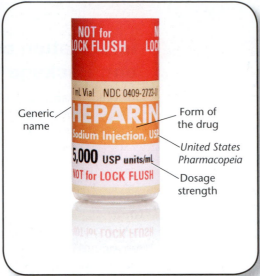

Figure 10-3 Some medications are generic only and have no trade name.

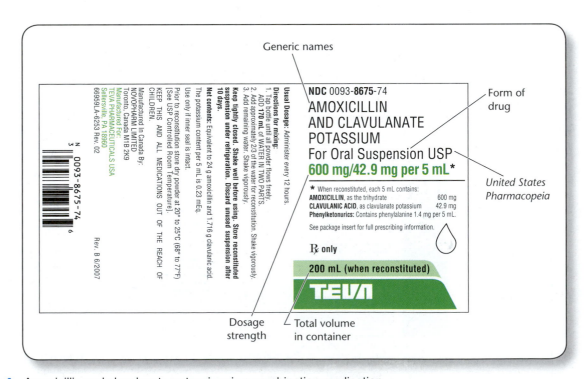

Figure 10-4 Amoxicillin and clavulanate potassium is a combination medication.

RULE 10-1	You must know both the generic and trade names of drugs.
Example	Suppose a patient is allergic to Vicodin®, a narcotic painkiller. The generic drugs in Vicodin®—hydrocodone bitartrate and acetaminophen—are also found in the trade name drugs Anexsia®, Lortab®, and Zydone®. If you administer one of these drugs or any drug containing hydrocodone bitartrate or acetaminophen as an alternative to Vicodin®, the patient may have a similar allergic reaction. When you record a patient's drug allergy, include both the trade and generic names. Resources such as the PDR (*Physicians' Desk Reference*) provide information about a drug's ingredients.

GO TO . . . Open the CD-ROM that accompanies your textbook, and select Chapter 10, Generic and Trade Names (LO 10.1). Review the animation and example problems, then complete the practice problems. Continue to the next section of the book once you have mastered the information presented.

Form of the Drug

Manufacturers may offer the same drug in different forms. For example, penicillin is available as a tablet, a capsule, a liquid for oral administration, and an injection. Every label indicates the drug's form. Solid oral medications come in the form of tablets, capsules, gelcaps, and caplets. Liquid forms include oral, injections, inhalants, drops, sprays, and mists. Other forms of medication include ointments, creams, lotions, patches, suppositories, and shampoos. See Figures 10-1, 10-2, 10-3, and 10-4.

Dosage Strength

Drug labels include information about the amount of the drug present. This amount, combined with information about the form of the drug, identifies the drug's **dosage strength** (supply dose). On the label, the dosage strength is stated as the amount of drug per dosage unit. In most cases, the amount of the drug is listed in grams (g), milligrams (mg), micrograms (mcg), or possibly grains (gr). In certain cases, such as insulin, the amount is listed in units. Certain liquid drugs, such as hydrogen peroxide and glycerin, may list the amount in milliliters (mL). Some medications are also listed as milliequivalents (mEq).

For solid medications, the dosage strength is the amount of drug present per tablet, capsule, or other form. In Figure 10-1, note the amount of Provera® (2.5 mg) present in a tablet, the form of medication. The dosage strength is 2.5 mg per tablet. *Note: For most solid medications, if the unit is not listed, assume it is one tablet, one capsule, one gelcap, and so forth.*

For liquid medications, the dosage strength is the amount of the drug present in a certain quantity of solution. For example in Figure 10-2, the dosage strength of EES is 200 mg/5 mL. In Figure 10-3 the dosage strength of heparin sodium is 5000 units/1 mL.

Pharmaceutical companies manufacture medications with dosage strengths corresponding to commonly prescribed doses. This practice along with the practice of packaging unit doses (discussed further in this chapter) reduces the risk of medical error by reducing the number of dosage calculations.

Combination Drugs

The generic names and dosage strengths of all components of a combination drug must appear on the label. The label in Figure 10-4 lists the components amoxicillin and clavulanate. It also provides information about the individual drugs' dosage strengths. The line 600 mg/42.9 mg per 5 mL indicates that this medication contains 600 mg of amoxicillin and 42.9 mg of clavulanate in every 5 mL. Combination drugs sometimes have a trade name, which may be used in physician orders. For example, for the drug Lortab® 5/500 (trade name), which includes 5 mg of hydrocodone bitratrate and 500 mg of acetaminophen (generic names), the order might read Lortab® 5/500 1 tab q 4-6h PRN for pain. The order would *not* read hydrocodone bitartrate 5 mg, acetaminophen 500 mg, q 4–6h PRN for pain.

Total Number or Volume in Container

Many oral medications are packaged separately in *unit doses*. These packages may contain a single dosage unit, for example, a single tablet or a vial with 2 mL of solution for injection. If the container holds more than one dosage unit, the total number or volume must be listed on the label. See Figures 10-1, 10-2, 10-3, and 10-4. Prescription and nonprescription medications are often packaged in multiple-dose containers. Figure 10-5 indicates that prescription-strength Ritalin® is available in containers of 100 tablets, each tablet with 5 mg of drug.

Figure 10-6 shows the label for a dose pack of Azithromycin, a prescription medication. The container has 6 tablets taken over 5 days. Two tablets are taken on the first day. Each tablet is packaged as a unit dose. In Figure 10-7, the container of Rocephin® has 15 mL and provides a unit dose of 1 g/15 mL in a single-use vial. The label's directions indicate that you reconstitute the drug, administer it intravenously or intramuscularly, and discard any unused portion. Single-use vials are preservative-free and should be used for one dose and then discarded.

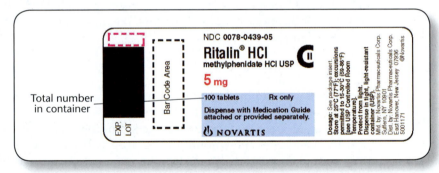

Figure 10-5   This container of Ritalin® contains 100 tablets and each tablet has 5 mg of medication.

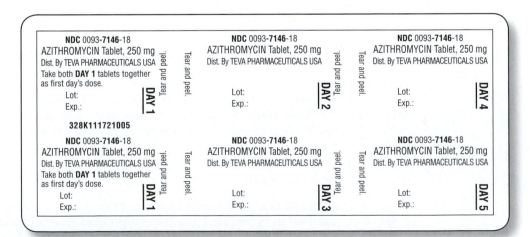

Figure 10-6   A five-day dose pack of Azithromycin has one tablet in each package.

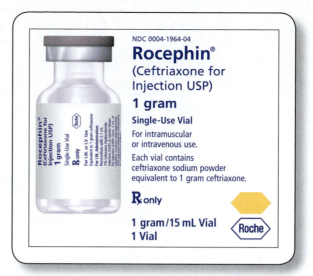

Figure 10-7 Unit-dose package of Rocephin® for IV or IM administration.

RULE 10-2	Do not confuse the total amount of drug in the container with the dosage strength.
Example 1	According to Figure 10-1, the Provera® container holds 30 tablets, with a dosage strength of 2.5 mg per tablet. The entire container holds 30 × 2.5 mg, or 75 mg, of drug whereas an individual tablet holds 2.5 mg of drug.
Example 2	According to Figure 10-2, each 5 mL of E.E.S.® solution contains 200 mg of drug. The entire amount of solution is one pint or 473 mL*, not 5 mL. The entire container, therefore, holds 473 mL ÷ 5 mL = 94.6 or 94 complete doses. Even though the entire contents of the container is one pint (473 mL*), you will only administer a small portion (5 mL) of it at a time.
	*For practical purposes, household (pint) to metric (mL) conversions are approximate. The conversion factor 1 oz = 30 mL will yield 480 mL in 1 pint. This is an approximate conversion. When the manufacturer gives you an exact metric amount, the math is based on that number.

GO TO . . . Open the CD-ROM that accompanies your textbook, and select Chapter 10, Total Amount of Drug VS Dosage Strength (LO 10.1). Review the animation and example problems, then complete the practice problems. Continue to the next section of the book once you have mastered the information presented.

Route of Administration

Directions for the route of administration may be specified on the label. This information may not be included for oral medications. However, if a tablet or a capsule is not to be swallowed, additional information will be provided. For example, the label for Nitrostat® (Figure 10-8) shows it is administered sublingually, under the tongue. Chewable tablets will be labeled as such. Medications for topical use only will also be marked on the label (Figure 10-9).

Liquid medications may be given orally or injected. Labels will indicate whether an injection is given **intradermally** (ID), **intravenously** (IV), **intramuscularly** (IM), or **subcutaneously** (subcut) (see Figures 10-10 and 10-11). Labels will indicate other routes as well. For example, Aerobid-M is a solution for oral inhalation only (see Figure 10-12).

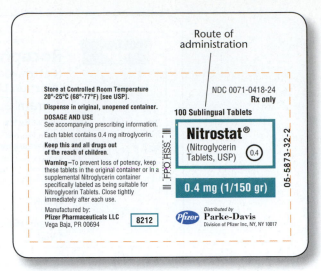

Figure 10-8 Sublingual tablets should be placed only under the tongue.

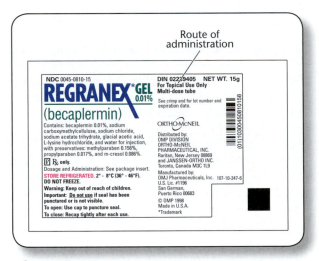

Figure 10-9 Regranex® is a topical gel.

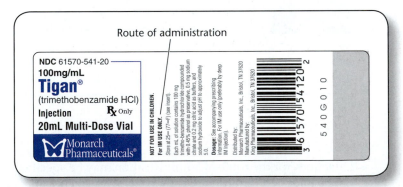

Figure 10-10 For intramuscular (IM) administration only.

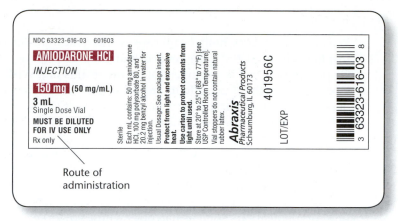

Figure 10-11 For intravenous (IV) administration only.

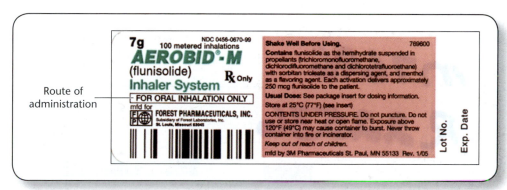

Figure 10-12 For oral inhalation only.

ERROR ALERT!

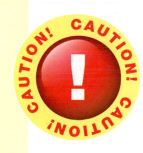

Read the Label Carefully!

Certain medications are available in a variety of forms, including an antibacterial suspension for otic (ear) use and an antimicrobial suspension for ophthalmic (eye) use. (See label A and B below.) The product label indicates the route. The usual dosage of the otic suspension is 4 drops instilled 3 to 4 times a day into the affected ear. The usual dosage of the ophthalmic suspension is 1 or 2 drops instilled into the affected eye every 3 or 4 h. If you were to carry out an order for the otic suspension by administering it to the patient's eye, you would not only fail to provide appropriate care for the ear, but also cause considerable irritation to the eye. *The bottom line: do not administer drugs by any route other than intended, as described on the drug label and on the order.*

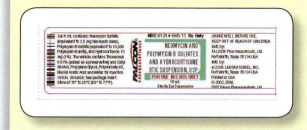

A

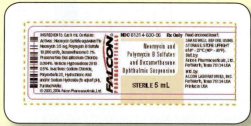

B

Warnings

Warnings on labels help healthcare workers administer drugs safely. They include statements such as "It is recommended that drug dispensing should not exceed weekly supply. Dispensing should be contigent upon the results of a WBC count." (See Figure 10-13.) Other labels indicate that the contents are poisonous. Labels may carry warnings for specific groups of patients. For example a label may caution that you should find out what medications may not be taken with the medication (See Figure 10-14) or that a medication may not be safe for pregnant women or for children. Controlled substances may contain a warning that says "May be habit forming." Other labels describe harmful effects resulting from combinations with other products.

Every facility follows guidelines for disposing of drugs that are not used. The guidelines for medications that carry warnings are especially strict. For example, in some cases, you dispose of medications such as narcotics with a coworker as witness, then provide appropriate documentation.

Storage Information

Some drugs must be stored under specific conditions to maintain their potency and effectiveness. Storage information will appear on the drug's label. The label may have information

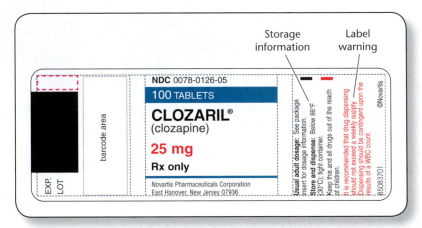

Figure 10-13 Always read label warnings and storage information.

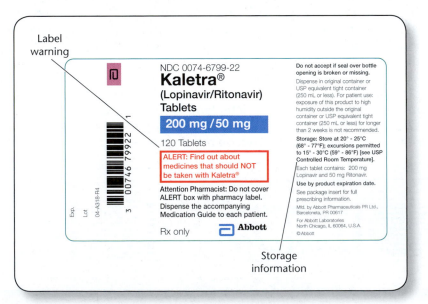

Figure 10-14 Always read label warnings and storage information.

about storage temperature, exposure to light, or the length of time the drug will remain potent after the container has been opened. Storage at the wrong temperature or exposure to light can trigger a chemical reaction that makes the drug unusable. (See Figures 10-13 and 10-14 for storage information.)

Manufacturing Information

Pharmaceutical manufacturers are strictly regulated by the U.S. Food and Drug Administration (FDA). FDA regulations state that every drug label must include the name of the manufacturer; an expiration date, abbreviated EXP, after which the drug may no longer be used; and the lot number (see Figure 10-15).

Medications are produced in batches, known as *lots*. The lot number is a code that indicates when and where a drug was produced. It allows the manufacturer to trace problems linked to a particular batch. If a manufacturer has to remove an entire lot from the market because of contamination, suspected tampering, or unexpected side effects, the lot number helps identify which batch to recall. **Bar codes** on medication labels are used to electronically identify the drug. This information is useful to ensure that an individual receives the correct medication. Bar coding has reduced medication administration and dispensing errors (see Figure 10-15). NDC on a label indicates the National Drug Code.

Drug manufacturers assign a specific identification number to each of their drug products, called an *NDC (National Drug Code)* number. Each NDC number has 10 digits and is divided into three groups of numbers. The first group of numbers identifies the manufacturer; the second group identifies the medication, its strength, and its dosage form; and the third group identifies the package size. If any the three groups of numbers begin with zeros, the manufacture may omit the zeros when printing the numbers on the product label. When ordering drugs and comparing NDC numbers on the drug label on the drug bottle, all 10 digits are used (see Figure 10-15).

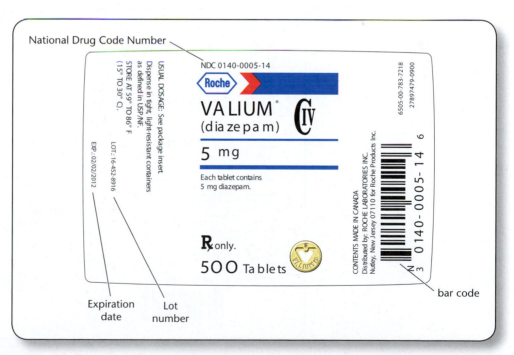

Figure 10-15 The lot number, expiration date and bar code are stamped on the drug label during manufacturing.

RULE 10-3	Never use a drug after the expiration date has passed.
Example	Older drugs may become chemically unstable or altered. As a result, they may not provide the correct dosage strength. Worse, they could have an effect different from the intended one. Advise patients to check the expiration dates on all drug labels. If patients have not used a product by the date listed, they should discard it. At an inpatient setting, the medication may need to be returned to the pharmacy, depending on the facility's policy.

GO TO . . . Open the CD-ROM that accompanies your textbook, and select Chapter 10, Expiration Dates (LO 10.1). Review the animation and example problems, then complete the practice problems. Continue to the next section of the book once you have mastered the information presented.

Information About Reconstituting Drugs

Some drugs, such as antibiotics, are packaged in powder form. You **reconstitute** the drug (add liquid to the powder) shortly before administering it. Reconstituted medications remain potent for only a short time. The label indicates the time period within which they can be safely administered (see Figures 10-16 and 10-17). Other drugs must be diluted before they are administered; they, too, must be used within a limited time. Directions for reconstituting or diluting a drug appear on the label (see Figures 10-16 and 10-17). Additional information can be found in the package insert, discussed in the next section.

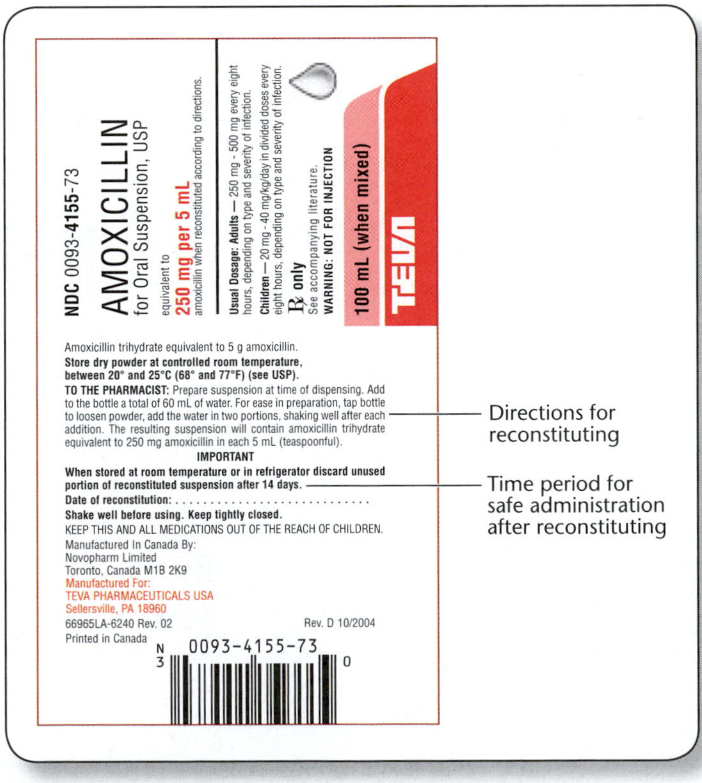

Figure 10-16 To reconstitute a drug, you add liquid to a powder.

Copyright © 2012 by The McGraw-Hill Companies, Inc.

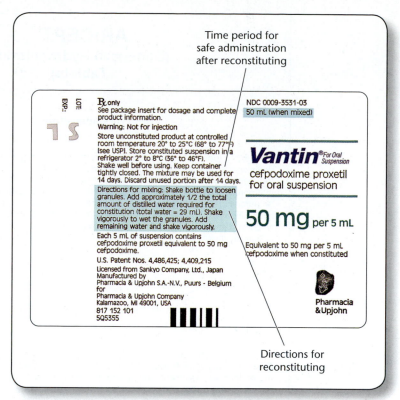

Time period for safe administration after reconstituting

Directions for reconstituting

Rx only
See package insert for dosage and complete product information.

Warning: Not for injection

Store unconstituted product at controlled room temperature 20° to 25°C (68° to 77°F) [see USP]. Store constituted suspension in a refrigerator 2° to 8°C (36° to 46°F). Shake well before using. Keep container tightly closed. The mixture may be used for 14 days. Discard unused portion after 14 days.

Directions for mixing: Shake bottle to loosen granules. Add approximately 1/2 the total amount of distilled water required for constitution (total water = 29 mL). Shake vigorously to wet the granules. Add remaining water and shake vigorously.

Each 5 mL of suspension contains cefpodoxime proxetil equivalent to 50 mg cefpodoxime.

U.S. Patent Nos. 4,486,425; 4,409,215
Licensed from Sankyo Company, Ltd., Japan
Manufactured by
Pharmacia & Upjohn S.A.-N.V., Puurs - Belgium
for
Pharmacia & Upjohn Company
Kalamazoo, MI 49001, USA
817 152 101
5Q5355

NDC 0009-3531-03
50 mL (when mixed)

Vantin®For Oral Suspension
cefpodoxime proxetil for oral suspension

50 mg per 5 mL

Equivalent to 50 mg per 5 mL cefpodoxime when constituted

Pharmacia & Upjohn

Figure 10-17 Follow the information about reconstituting a drug carefully.

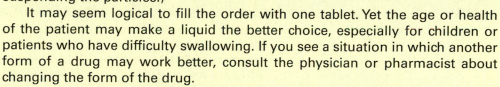

ERROR ALERT!

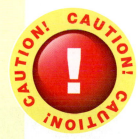

Consider the Age and Health Needs of Your Patient When You Administer a Drug

Suppose the drug order reads Biaxin® 250 mg po b.i.d. Biaxin®, an antibiotic, is available in 250-mg tablets and as an oral suspension with a reconstituted dosage strength of 125 mg/5 mL. (An *oral suspension* is a liquid that contains solid particles of medication. You shake the medication before administering it, suspending the particles.)

It may seem logical to fill the order with one tablet. Yet the age or health of the patient may make a liquid the better choice, especially for children or patients who have difficulty swallowing. If you see a situation in which another form of a drug may work better, consult the physician or pharmacist about changing the form of the drug.

Package Inserts

Package inserts provide complete and authoritative information about a medication. The information in package inserts can also be found in the PDR and other guides. Figure 10-18 shows a portion of a package insert. Table 10-1 summarizes the sections of a package insert.

ARICEPT®
(Donepezil Hydrochloride Tablets)

DESCRIPTION

ARICEPT® (donepezil hydrochloride) is a reversible inhibitor of the enzyme acetylcholinesterase, known chemically as (±)-2,3-dihydro-5,6-dimethoxy-2-[[1-(phenylmethyl)-4-piperidinyl]methyl]-1H-inden-1-one hydrochloride. Donepezil hydrochloride is commonly referred to in the pharmacological literature as E2020. It has an empirical formula of $C_{24}H_{29}NO_3HCl$ and a molecular weight of 415.96. Donepezil hydrochloride is a white crystalline powder and is freely soluble in chloroform, soluble in water and in glacial acetic acid, slightly soluble in ethanol and in acetonitrile and practically insoluble in ethyl acetate and in n-hexane.

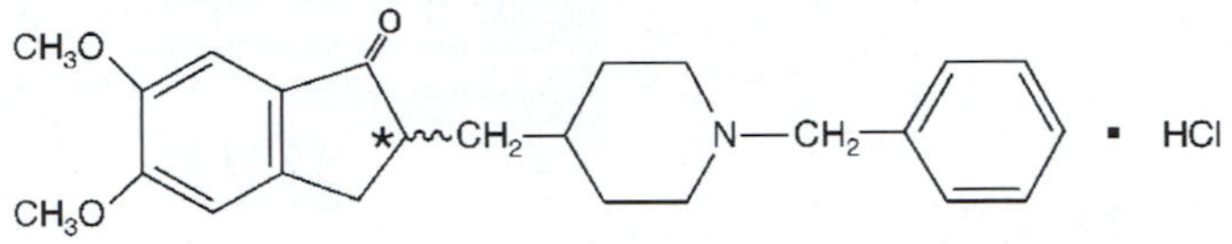

ARICEPT® is available for oral administration in film-coated tablets containing 5 or 10 mg of donepezil hydrochloride. Inactive ingredients are lactose monohydrate, corn starch, microcrystalline cellulose, hydroxypropyl cellulose, and magnesium stearate. The film coating contains talc, polyethylene glycol, hypromellose and titanium dioxide. Additionally, the 10 mg tablet contains yellow iron oxide (synthetic) as a coloring agent.

CLINICAL PHARMACOLOGY

Current theories on the pathogenesis of the cognitive signs and symptoms of Alzheimer's Disease attribute some of them to a deficiency of cholinergic neurotransmission.

Figure 10-18 The top portion of a typical package insert.

TABLE 10-1 Sections of a Package Insert

SECTION	DESCRIPTION	EXAMPLE INFORMATION
Description	Chemical and physical description of the drug	Aricept® (donepezil hydrochloride) is a reversible inhibitor of the enzyme acetylcholinesterase, known chemically as (±)-2,3-dihydro-5, 6-dimethoxy-2-[[1-(phenylmethyl)-4-piperidinyl]methyl]-1H-inden-1-one hydrochloride. 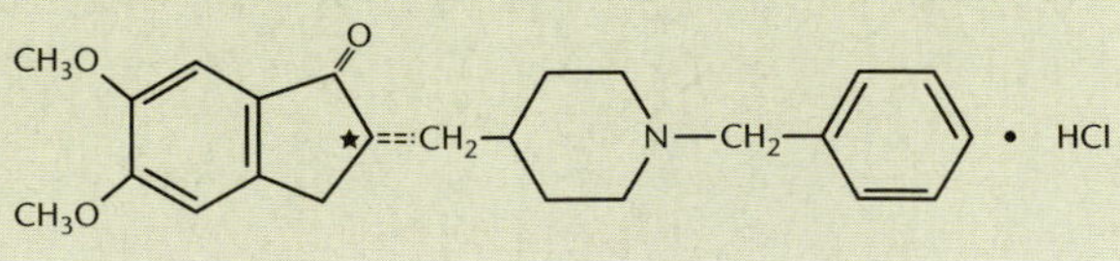
Clinical pharmacology	Description of the actions of the drug	Current theories on the pathogenesis of the cognitive signs and symptoms of Alzheimer's Disease attribute some of them to a deficiency of cholinergic neurotransmission.

TABLE 10-1 Continued

SECTION	DESCRIPTION	EXAMPLE INFORMATION
Indications and usage	Medical conditions in which the drug is safe and effective; instructions for use	Aricept® is indicated for the treatment of mild to moderate dementia of the Alzheimer's type.
Contraindications	Conditions and situations under which the drug should not be administered	Aricept® is contraindicated in patients with known hypersensitivity to donepezil hydrochloride or to piperidine derivatives.
Warnings	Information about serious, possibly fatal, side effects	*Gastrointestinal conditions:* Through their primary action, cholinesterase inhibitors may be expected to increase gastric acid secretion due to increased cholinergic activity.
Precautions	Information about drug interactions and other conditions that may cause unwanted side effects	*Use with anticholinergics:* Because of their mechanism of action, cholinesterase inhibitors have the potential to interfere with the activity of anticholinergic medications.
Adverse reactions	Less serious, anticipated side effects that can be caused by the drug	These include nausea, diarrhea, insomnia, vomiting, muscle cramps, fatigue, and anorexia. These adverse events were often of mild intensity and transient, resolving during continued Aricept® treatment without the need for dose modification.
Overdosage	Effects of overdoses and instructions for treatment	As in any case of overdose, general supportive measures should be utilized. Overdosage with cholinesterase inhibitors can result in cholinergic crisis characterized by severe nausea, vomiting, salivation, sweating, bradycardia, hypotension, respiratory depression, collapse, and convulsions.
Dosage and administration	Recommended dosages under various conditions and recommendations for administration routes	The dosages of Aricept® shown to be effective in controlled clinical trials are 5 mg and 10 mg administered once per day.
Preparation for administration	Directions for reconstituting or diluting the drug, if necessary	Aricept® should be taken in the evening, just prior to retiring. Aricept® can be taken with or without food.
Manufacturer supply	Information on dosage strengths and forms of the drug available	Aricept® is supplied as film-coated, round tablets containing either 5 mg or 10 mg of donepezil hydrochloride.

CRITICAL THINKING ON THE JOB

Read Labels Carefully

A healthcare professional is filling the order Synthroid® 0.05 mg p.o. daily. Synthroid® is available in tablets of 11 different strengths, each in a different color. The healthcare professional has access to tablets in 0.025-mg (orange), 0.05-mg (white), 0.125-mg (brown), and 0.15-mg (blue) doses.

Looking quickly at two labels (see Figures 10-19 and 10-20), the healthcare professional sees a Synthroid® label with "5" on it. Without realizing it is for 0.15 mg, he removes a tablet. When he tries to administer it, the patient tells him that her usual pill is white, not blue.

(Continued)

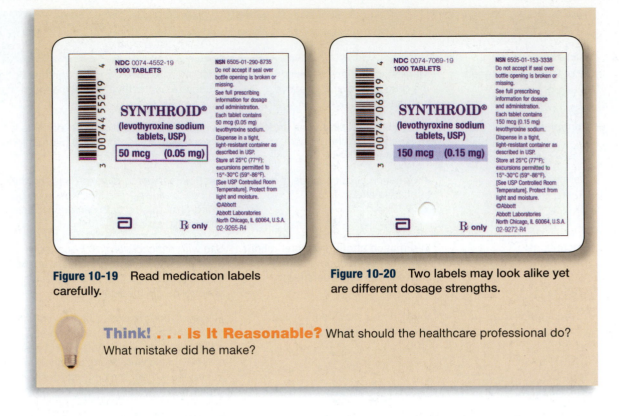

Figure 10-19 Read medication labels carefully.

Figure 10-20 Two labels may look alike yet are different dosage strengths.

Think! . . . Is It Reasonable? What should the healthcare professional do? What mistake did he make?

REVIEW AND PRACTICE

10.1 Locating Information on Medication Labels and Package Inserts

For Exercises 1–6, refer to label A.

1. What is the trade name of the drug?

2. What is the generic name of the drug?

3. Does this container hold multiple doses or a unit dose? How do you know?

4. What is the name of the manufacturer?

5. What is the dosage strength?

6. What is the NDC code?

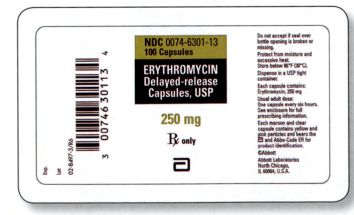

A

For Exercises 7–12, refer to label B.

7. What is the generic name of the drug?

8. What is the trade name of the drug?

9. What is the dosage strength?

10. What type of tablets are in this bottle?

11. What is the bar code number?

12. What are the storage requirements for this drug?

For Exercises 13–18, refer to label C.

13. What is the trade name of the drug?

14. Is this medication packaged in an ampule or a vial?

15. What is the dosage strength?

16. How would you administer this drug?

17. What is the total volume?

18. Where would you find the typical adult dose of this medication?

For Exercises 19–24, refer to label D.

19. What is the generic name of the drug?

20. By what route is this drug administered?

21. What is the usual dose?

22. What is the dosage strength?

23. If you had a drug order for 200 mg of Zithromax®, how many teaspoons would you administer to the patient?

24. How long would two bottles last if you administered 1 dose of 10 mL daily?

For Exercises 25–30, refer to label E.

25. What is the generic name of the drug?

26. What is the trade name of the drug?

27. By what route is this drug administered?

28. What special storage information is provided on the label?

29. How much medication is in one vial?

30. How many doses are in one vial?

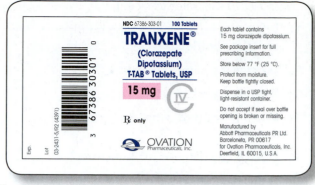

B

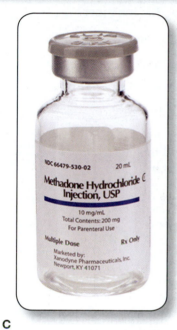

C

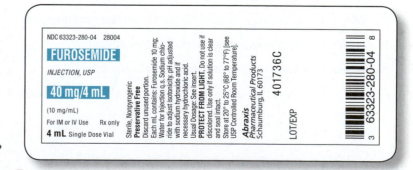

D

E

For Exercises 31–36, refer to label F.

31. When it is mixed, how many milliliters are in the bottle?

32. What is the name of the drug?

33. What is the form of the drug?

34. When it is mixed, what is the dosage strength?

35. What is the name of manufacturer?

36. If the usual dose is 5 mL, how many doses are in this container?

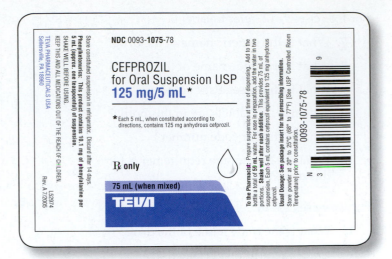

F

For Exercises 37–43, refer to label G.

37. What is the trade name of the drug?

38. What is the generic name of the drug?

39. What is the dosage strength?

40. How should this medication be stored?

41. Through what route is this drug administered?

42. How many prescriptions could be filled from this bottle if each prescription's quantity was 30 tablets?

43. What is the name of the manufacturer?

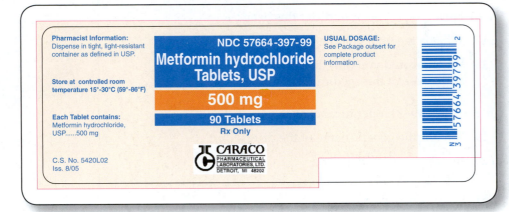

G

For Exercises 44–50, refer to labels A through (labels may be used more than once).

44. Which of these drugs are tablets?

45. Which of these drugs are given orally?

46. Which of these is delayed release drug?

47. Which of these drugs are oral suspensions?

48. Which of these drugs would be administered parenterally?

49. Which medication(s) must be mixed before using?

50. Which medication(s) do not include a trade name?

To check your answers, see the Answer Key at the end of the book, which starts on page A-1.

Oral Medications

Medications labels contain unique information related to the route by which the medication is to be administered. You must read each label carefully and identify this information when calculating doses, administering or dispensing medications.

Oral medications are available in either solid or liquid form. Tablets are the most common form. They may be scored, chewable, or enteric-coated. Scored tablets can be broken into equal portions so that you can administer a partial dosage, if necessary. Chewable tablets must be chewed to be effective. Enteric-coated tablets must be swallowed whole as they are covered with a substance that prevents absorption of the medication until it reaches the small intestine. Chewing them or dividing them breaks the seal provided by their coating, allowing the drug to be absorbed sooner than intended.

Capsules have a gelatin shell that contains the drug. In most cases, they should be swallowed whole. In some cases, capsules may be opened and mixed with food. *Controlled-release capsules,* also called *sustained-release* or *extended-release capsules,* release the drug over a long time. If these capsules are not swallowed whole, they may release too much of the drug too quickly for absorption. See Chapter 13 for more information about solid oral medications.

RULE 10-4

You may break tablets to give a partial dose *only* when the tablets are scored. Enteric-coated, controlled-release, extended-release, and sustained-release medications should *never* be crushed or broken.

GO TO . . . Open the CD-ROM that accompanies your textbook, and select Chapter 10, Breaking Tablets Properly (LO 10.2). Review the animation and example problems, then complete the practice problems. Continue to the next section of the book once you have mastered the information presented.

Abbreviations such as SR, CR, ER, and XL listed after the drug name indicate a special drug action. The SR following the brand name means the drug is designed for *sustained release;* CR means that a drug is *controlled release;* and ER or XL following the brand name means the drug has an *extended-release* mechanism (Figure 10-21).

Liquid oral medications are described as oral solutions, syrups, elixirs, oral suspensions, and simply liquids (see Figures 10-22 and 10-23). In liquid medications, the dosage strength corresponds to a specific volume of the solution, for example, 250 mg/5 mL.

If a medication needs to be reconstituted, the instructions will be on the label.

RULE 10-5

When you reconstitute a drug that is to be used for more than one dose, you must write your initials as well as the time and date of reconstitution on the label. Reconstituted medications will be usable only for a certain length of time. So the date and time will document when the medication will expire. Your initials document who reconstituted the medication in case a question arises.

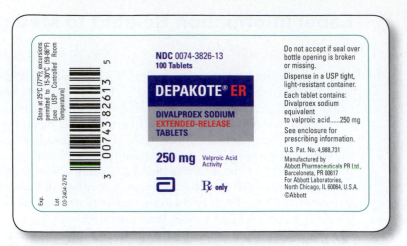

Figure 10-21 Do not break this tablet.

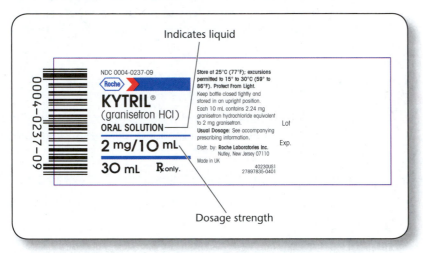

Indicates liquid

Dosage strength

Figure 10-22 For liquid medications the dosage strength corresponds to a number of milligrams per a specific volume of solution.

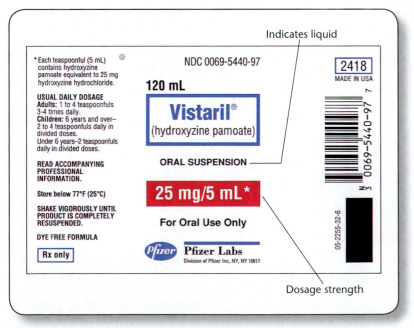

Indicates liquid

Dosage strength

Figure 10-23 The dosage strength is 25 mg per 5 mL volume for this medication.

GO TO . . . Open the CD-ROM that accompanies your textbook, and select Chapter 10, Labeling Reconstituted Medications (LO 10.2). Review the animation and example problems, then complete the practice problems. Continue to the next section of the book once you have mastered the information presented.

LEARNING LINK Recall from Chapter 8 that liquids may be measured in droppers, calibrated spoons, medicine cups, or oral syringes. Calibrated cups and spoons are available at most pharmacies and sometimes come with the medication. Advise patients who take oral liquid medications at home to use a medicine cup or baking measuring spoon—not a household cup or spoon—if they do not have calibrated cups or spoons.

PATIENT EDUCATION

Healthcare workers often educate patients about the proper way to take drugs at home. This responsibility may be the duty of the pharmacy technician, the nurse, or the certified medical assistant. If you are authorized to provide patient education, you should take the following steps:

1. Ensure there is no language barrier. If a language barrier exists, obtain a healthcare interpreter.
2. Be sure the patient or caretaker can read and understand the label. Some patients cannot see the fine print on labels. Others do not have the necessary literacy skills.
3. Ask the patient about drug allergies and any medications that he or she may be taking. Check the label or the package insert for drug interactions. Also check with the patient about any over-the-counter medications and herbal remedies being taken.
4. Review the dose, frequency, and length of time the drug is to be taken. Have the patient or caretaker repeat this information to you.
5. Review any special written instructions. Have the patient or caretaker repeat this to you.
6. Describe any adverse effects of the drug that are serious enough to warrant prompt medical attention. Encourage the patient to seek help immediately if these side effects occur. Also discuss side effects that are considered normal.
7. Remind the patient to refer to the label when needed. Emphasize that the patient should call the pharmacy or physician with any questions that cannot be answered from the label or additional written instructions that are provided by the pharmacy.

Parenteral Medications

Parenteral drugs may be packaged in single-use ampules or vials, single-use prefilled syringes, or multiuse vials. These small containers have small labels that have limited space for providing comprehensive information (Figure 10-24). You must read these labels with extra care. You will often need to review the package insert to obtain complete drug information.

Parenteral drugs can be injected intradermally (ID), intramuscularly (IM), intravenously (IV), or subcutaneously (subcut). Parenteral drugs can also be inhalants and **transdermal** (through the skin) medications or any mode of administration other than through the gastrointestinal tract. For example, a medication can be administered into the vagina (see Figure 10-24). The drug label specifies the appropriate route. Tigan® is made for IM intramuscular use only (see Figure 10-10). Primaxin® is a drug that can be administered either intramuscularly or intravenously. Figure 10-25 indicates Camptosar for IV (intravenous) use only.

Recall from earlier in this chapter that of the label of medications the dosage strength may be labeled as the amount of drug per dosage unit or in units per mL. This is also true for parenteral medication (Figure 10-25). In some cases the label is marked with milligrams and micrograms. Dosage strength may also be expressed in milliequivalents per milliliter or as a percent, which is grams per 100 mL.

Look at the labels for insulin in Figures 10-26 and 10-27. In addition to the standard components, these labels contain information about the origin of the medication and how quickly the insulin takes effect. Insulin can be made from human sources (recombinant DNA origin, or rDNA) or animal sources (beef or pork). Animal insulin has been phased out in the United States. Different types of insulin take effect over different time periods. NPH insulin (Figure 10-26) is an intermediate-acting insulin. Regular insulin (Figure 10-27) is shorter acting. See Chapter 18 for more information about insulin.

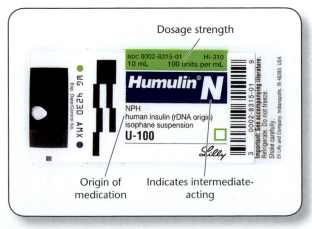

Figure 10-24 The NuvaRink delivers hormones through vaginal use only. It releases 0.120 mg/day of etonogestrel and 0.015 mg/day of ethinyl estradiol over three weeks of use.

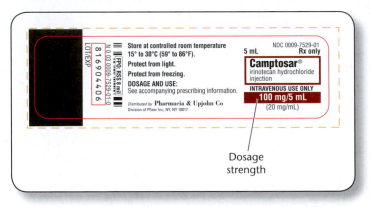

Dosage strength

Figure 10-25 This dosage strength is expressed in milligrams per milliliter 100 mg/5 mL.

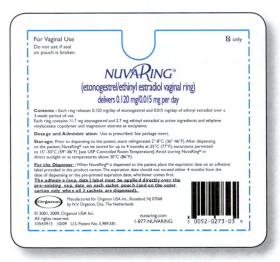

Dosage strength

Origin of medication

Indicates intermediate-acting

Figure 10-26 Insulin dosage strength is expressed in units per milliliter.

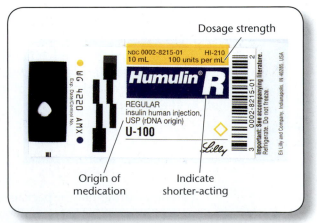

Dosage strength

Origin of medication

Indicate shorter-acting

Figure 10-27 Shorter-acting Humulin® R insulin has a dosage strength of 100 units/mL.

Medications Administered by Other Routes

In addition to the oral and injection routes, there are several other routes of medication administration. They include sublingual (under the tongue), buccal (between the gums and cheek), rectal, and vaginal. Drugs may also be administered as topical ointments (used on the skin); eye or ear drops; patches applied to the skin (transdermal delivery); or nasal, oral, and throat inhalants (see Figures 10-28, 10-29, and 10-30).

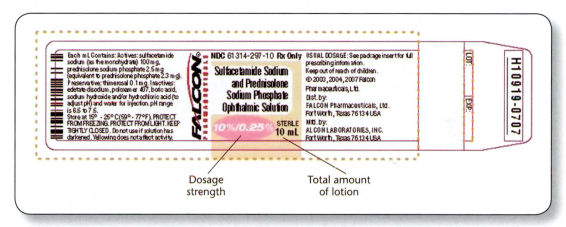

Dosage strength

Total amount of lotion

Figure 10-28 This drug is used in the eyes (opthalmic solution).

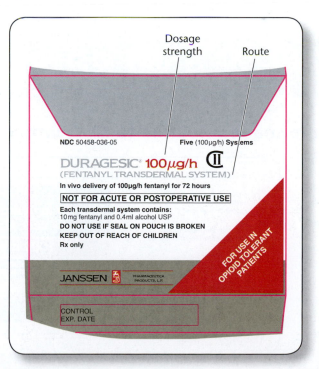

Figure 10-29 Transdermal medications deliver medication through the skin at a dosage rate.

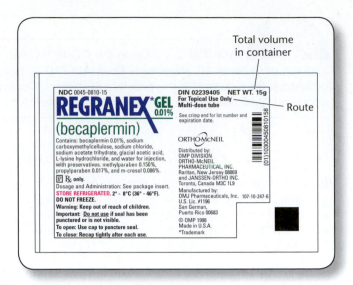

Total volume in container

Route

Figure 10-30 This medication is for topical use only.

The dosage strength is expressed slightly differently on these labels. In Figure 10-28, the dosage strength is the percentage of the active ingredients in the solution. Sulfacetamide 10% and prednisolone 0.25% are found in this ophthalmic medication. In Figure 10-29, the dosage rate is given as 100 mcg/h; this drug is absorbed over time through the skin. Thus the dosage rate indicates 100 mcg are delivered each hour. In Figure 10-30, the medication is also measured in a percentage. Regranex® has 0.01% becaplermin in a gel base.

GO TO . . . Open the CD-ROM that accompanies your textbook, and select Chapter 10, Other Routes (LO 10.2). Review the animation and example problems, then complete the practice problems. Continue to the next section of the book once you have mastered the information presented.

REVIEW AND PRACTICE

10.2 Label Information Related to Medication Routes

For Exercises 1–4, refer to label A.

1. What is the NDC number?

2. What is the dosage strength?

3. Can you store this drug on a shelf in the storeroom?

4. How many tablets are in the container?

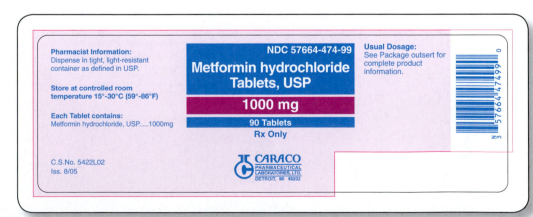

A

For Exercises 5–8, refer to label B.

    5. What is the trade name of this drug?

    6. Who is the manufacturer?

    7. What is the dosage strength?

    8. How many tablets are in the container?

For Exercises 9–12, refer to label C.

    9. What is the generic name of this drug?

    10. How is this medication administered?

    11. What is the dosage strength?

    12. How many doses are in this vial?

For Exercises 13–16, refer to label D.

    13. How many milliliters of water should be used to reconstitute this drug?

    14. What is the dosage strength when the drug is mixed?

    15. What is the total volume in the container when the drug is mixed?

    16. How long can this drug be stored after it is reconstituted?

For Exercises 17–20, refer to label E.

    17. What is the generic name of this drug?

    18. What is the dosage strength?

    19. What is the trade name of this medication?

    20. How should this drug be stored?

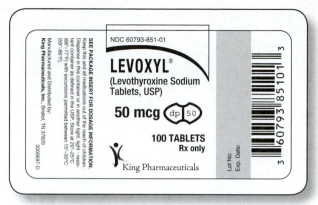

B

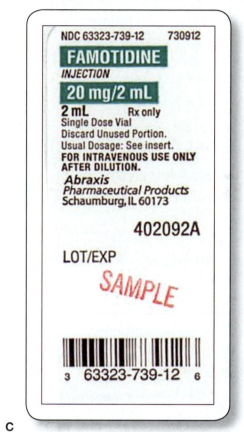

C

D

For Exercises 21–25, refer to labels A through E.

21. Which of these medication labels indicate that there are 100 tablets in the bottle?

22. Which of these drugs could be divided to give a partial dose? Why?

23. Which labels are on multiple dose containers?

24. Which of these drugs are to be given via the oral route?

25. Which medication is to be given by injection?

For Exercises 26–29, refer to label F.

26. What is the dosage strength?

27. By what route of administration is this drug given?

28. What color is this medication?

29. What is the total volume of medication in this bottle?

For Exercises 30–33, refer to label G.

30. What is the dosage strength of this drug?

31. Who manufactures this medication?

32. What is the generic name of this medication?

33. If you were not familiar with this drug, would you be able to administer it with only the information on the label? Why?

For Exercises 34–37, refer to label H.

34. What are the storage requirements for this medication?

35. What is the dosage strength?

36. By what route of administration is this drug given?

37. If the dose was 50 mg (2 capsules), how many doses does the container hold?

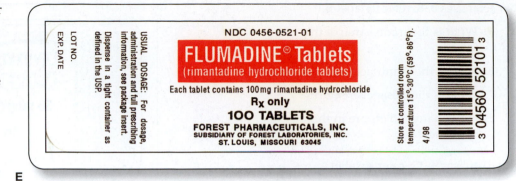

E

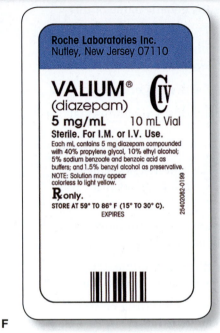

F

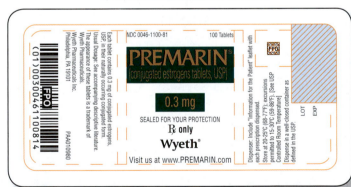

G

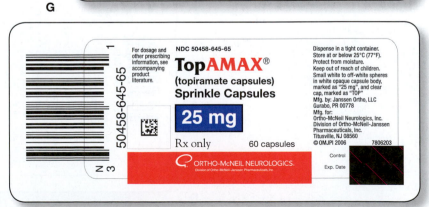

H

For Exercises 38–41, refer to label I.

38. What is the origin of this insulin?

39. What is the dosage strength of the insulin?

40. What is the generic name of this insulin?

41. What is the total volume in this container

For Exercises 42–45, refer to label J.

42. What is the dosage strength?

43. What is the generic name of this medication?

44. How many 100-mg doses does this container hold?

45. What are the storage requirements for this drug?

For Exercises 46–49, refer to label K.

46. What is the generic name?

47. What is the route of administration?

48. What instructions for administration are indicated on the label?

49. How would this medication be stored?

For Exercises 50–53, refer to label L.

50. By what route is this drug to be administered?

51. What are the drug's storage requirements?

52. What is the dosage strength?

53. What is the generic name of the drug?

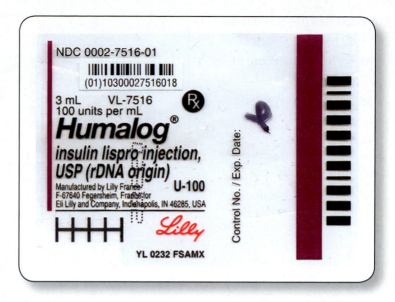

I

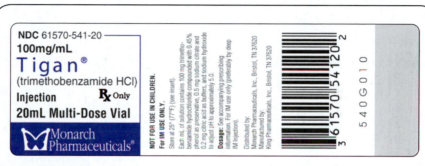

J

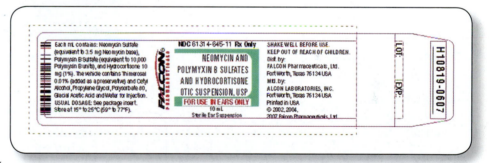

K

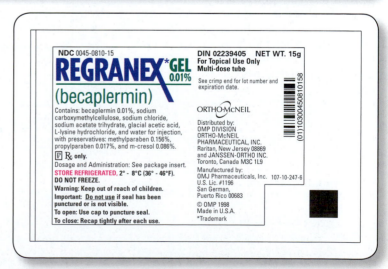

L

For Exercises 54–57, refer to label M.

54. What is the route of administration?

55. What is the generic name of the drug?

56. What is the total volume in the container?

57. What is the name of the manufacturer?

For Exercises 58–61, refer to label N.

58. By what route is this drug delivered?

59. What is the dosage strength?

60. What type of patients should use this medication?

61. How many doses are in this box?

For Exercises 62–65, refer to label O.

62. What is the generic name?

63. What is the dosage strength?

64. By what route is this drug to be administered?

65. How many doses are in this container?

To check your answers, see the Answer Key at the end of the book, which starts on page A-1.

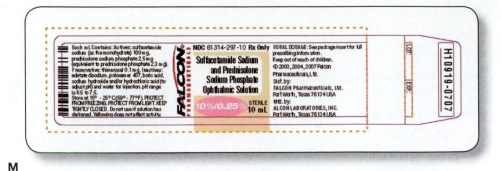

M

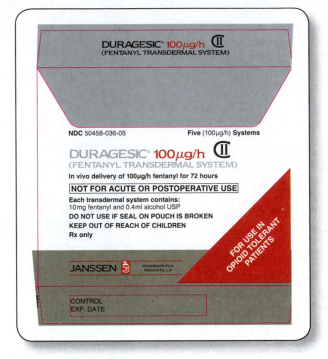

N

O

LEARNING OUTCOME	KEY POINTS
10.1 Differentiate information on a medication label and within a package insert. Pages 183–198	Drug Name ▸ Generic–official name recorded in the *US Pharmacopeia* (USP) and *National Formulary* (NF) ▸ Trade–brand name identified as such with registered trademark Form of Drug ▸ Solid–tablet, capsule, caplet, gelcap ▸ Liquid–oral liquid, injectable liquid, inhalant, drop, spray, mist ▸ Other–ointment, cream, lotion, patches, suppositories, shampoo Dosage Strength–amount of drug per dosage unit, e.g. 1 g/tablet or 500 mg/5 mL Combination Drugs–must list the generic name and the dosage strength of each medication in the combination, e.g. Lortab 5/500 = 5 mg of hydrocodone bitartrate with 500 mg of acetaminophen Total Volume Route of Administration Warnings Storage Information Manufacturing Information–pharmaceutical company, expiration date, lot number, bar code, and National Drug Code (NDC) Reconstitution Information–directions for mixing the medication Package Insert Information–complete drug information to include: chemical description, clinical pharmacology, indication and usage, contraindications, warnings, precautions, adverse reactions, effects of overdosage, recommended dosages, recommendations for administration routes, preparation for administration, manufacturer supply information

LEARNING OUTCOME	KEY POINTS
10.2 Distinguish information related to administration routes for medications. Pages 199–208	Oral Medications–medications given via the gastrointestinal (GI) tract

Oral Medications–medications given via the gastrointestinal (GI) tract

▶ Tablets

- Scored tablets may be divided for partial dosing
- Chewable tablets must be chewed to be effective
- Enteric-coated (EC) tablets must be swallowed whole to protect coating that prevents absorption of medication until it reaches the small intestine
- RULES: Do not break a tablet unless it is scored. Do not break or crush EC tablets.

▶ Capsules

- Usually swallowed whole; some may be opened and mixed with food
- Controlled-release capsules release drug over a long period of time are identified as sustained release (SR) or extended release (ER, XL)
- RULE: Do not crush or break ER, SR, XL capsules.

▶ Liquids

- Available in syrups, elixirs, suspensions, solutions
- Reconstituted solutions should be labeled with initials as well as the date and time medication was mixed.
- Calibrated equipment should be used for administration.

Parenteral Medications–medications given outside the GI tract

▶ Injection routes–intradermal (ID), intramuscular (IM), intravenous (IV), subcutaneous (subcut)

▶ Other routes–inhalant, transdermal, sublingual (SL), buccal (between the gum and the cheek), rectal, vaginal, topical, eye or ear drops

Use the identified drug labels to answer the following questions: (LO 10.1, 10.2)

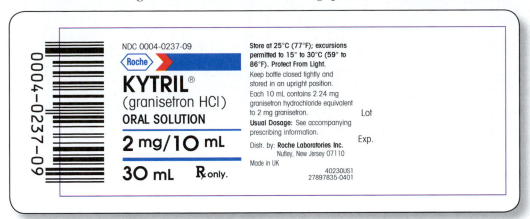

A

Label A

1. What is the generic name of this drug?

2. List three items of storage information on this label?

3. What is the total drug volume of the container?

4. 2 mg of the drug is equal to how many milliliters?

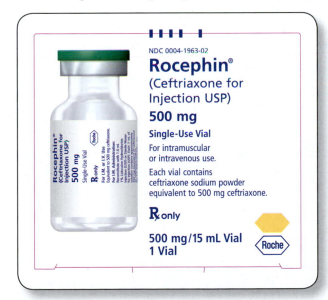

B

Label B

5. What is the brand name of this drug?

6. What two routes of administration are listed on this label?

7. What are the reconstitution directions for an IM injection?

8. How many times may this vial be used?

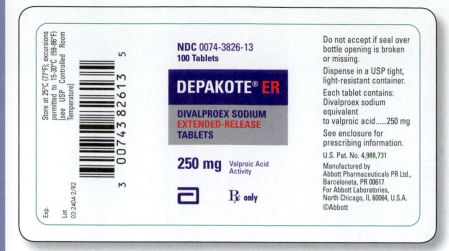

C

Label C

9. What is the brand name of this drug?

10. What does ER after the drug name mean?

11. How many tablets are in the container?

12. What is name of the manufacturer?

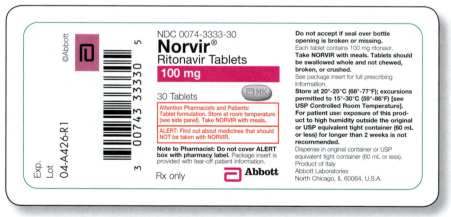

D

Label D

13. What is the generic name of this drug?

14. If the usual dose is one tablet, how many doses are available in this container?

15. Can this medication be crushed?

16. At what temperature should this medication be stored?

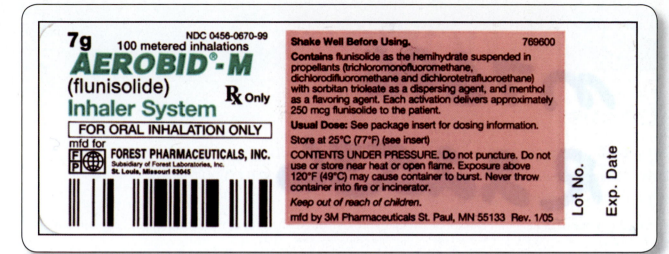

E

Label E

17. What is the route of administration for this drug?

18. Approximately how much medication is delivered with each inhalation?

19. How many inhalations are in this container?

20. What are the before-use instructions for this drug?

CHECK UP

1. Distinguish a drug's trade name from its generic name. (LO 10.1)

2. Which name, generic or trade name, is followed by this symbol, ®? (LO 10.1)

3. Explain the difference between IM and IV. (LO 10.2)

4. List the types of tablets that cannot be divided, broken, or crushed for administration, and explain why. (LO 10.2)

5. Describe when you would use a package insert. (LO 10.1)

6. Explain the importance of a lot number. (LO 10.1)

In Exercises 7–10, refer to label A. (LO 10.1)

7. What is the dosage strength of the drug?

8. How many tablets of medication are in this container?

9. What is the name of the manufacturer of the drug?

10. How is it administered?

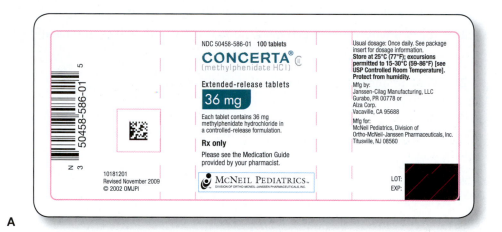

A

In Exercises 11–14, refer to label B. (LO 10.1)

11. What is the generic name of this drug?

12. How is this drug administered?

13. What is the dosage strength?

14. How many doses are in the container?

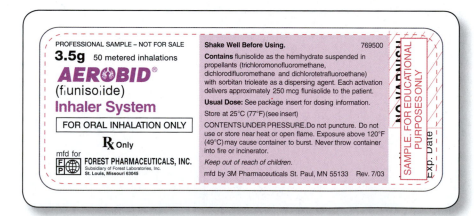

B

In Exercises 15–18, refer to label C.
(LO 10.1)

15. How is this drug administered?

16. What is the dosage strength?

17. What is the drug name?

18. How many capsules are in the
container?

In Exercises 19–22, refer to label D.
(LO 10.1)

19. What is the origin of this insulin?

20. What word on the label describes
the time frame in which this insulin
acts?

21. How is this drug administered?

22. What is the dosage strength?

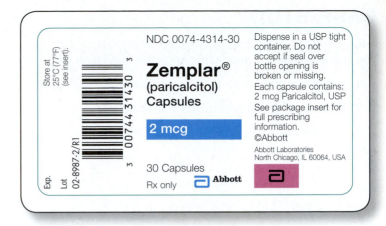

C

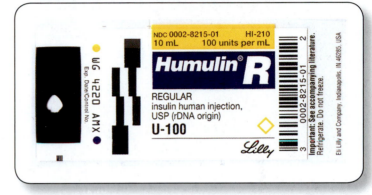

D

CRITICAL THINKING APPLICATION

You are working in a clinic that serves many adult homeless people. Two forms of Erythromycin are available
(see labels below). If the patient needs to take Erythromycin for 5 days, which form of the medication would be
better and why? (LO 10.2)

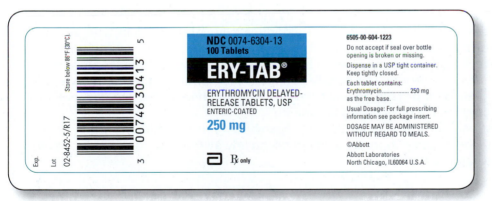

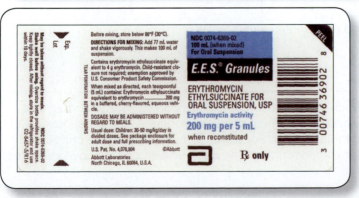

CASE STUDY

A drug order reads Gentamicin 5 mg IV now. (LO 10.2)
You have available a drug with the following label:

1. What would you do to prepare for administering this drug?

2. How would you administer the drug?

3. What would you do with the vial after administering a dose of the drug?

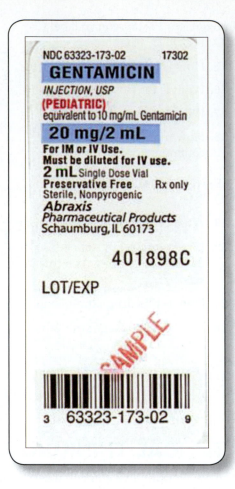

NDC 63323-173-02   17302

GENTAMICIN

INJECTION, USP

(PEDIATRIC)
equivalent to 10 mg/mL Gentamicin

20 mg/2 mL

For IM or IV Use.
Must be diluted for IV use.
2 mL Single Dose Vial
Preservative Free   Rx only
Sterile, Nonpyrogenic
Abraxis
Pharmaceutical Products
Schaumburg, IL 60173

401898C

LOT/EXP

SAMPLE

3 63323-173-02 9

INTERNET ACTIVITY

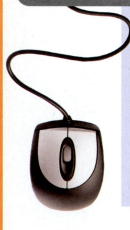

Mr. Liu is about to be discharged from the hospital with instructions to take Coumadin® 1 mg bid. Mr. Liu is an elderly, easily confused man who will be cared for by his daughter who also has difficulty with instructions. Although you have reviewed his medication instructions with him and his daughter several times, you are not completely confident they understand that he should not drink alcohol or take any self-prescribed, over-the-counter medications or herbal cures while he is taking Coumadin®.

Assignment: Conduct an Internet search to find information in plain language regarding the importance of not taking any over-the-counter medications while taking Coumadin®.

To check your answers, see the Answer Key at the end of the book, which starts on page A-1.

GO TO . . . Open the CD-ROM that accompanies your textbook, and complete a final review of the learning outcomes, practice problems, games, slideshow, and other activities presented for this chapter. For a final evaluation, take the chapter test and email or print your results for your instructor. A score of 95 percent or above indicates mastery of the chapter concepts.

Safe Medication Administration

"It is better to be safe than sorry."

—AMERICAN PROVERB

Learning Outcomes

When you have completed Chapter 11, you will be able to:

11.1 Recall the eight required elements of a prescription/medication order.

11.2 Apply The Joint Commission steps to receiving and writing a verbal order.

11.3 Execute safe transcription practices.

11.4 Identify error-prone abbreviations and symbols.

11.5 Identify the three checks in the medication administration procedure.

11.6 Implement the "rights" of medication administration.

11.7 Recognize the importance of observation in safe medication administration.

11.8 Describe the appropriate use of patient teaching as it relates to safe drug administration.

KEY TERMS

Institute for Safe Medication Practice (ISMP)

Electronic Medication Administration Record (eMAR)

Physicians' Desk Reference (PDR)

The Joint Commission (TJC)

Transcription

Verbal order

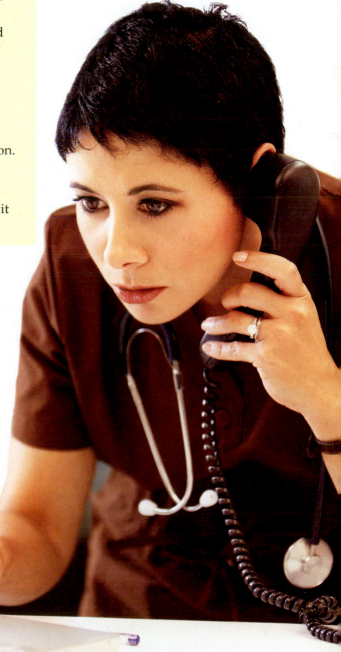

INTRODUCTION

Research by the Institute of Medicine reveals that patients in the United States experience at least 1.5 million preventable injuries due to medication errors and these errors drive up healthcare costs by more than 3.5 billion dollars! [Source: Schneider, M: The cost of medication errors. *BNET (CBS Business Network)* August 15, 2006.] The importance of safe medication administration cannot be overstated. Medication administration is a complex process that may involve several individuals (the authorized prescriber, the pharmacist, and the healthcare practitioner who administers the medication), often from several departments. The elements of safe medication administration include prescription, transcription, three "checks" of medication administration, "rights of medication administration," observation, and patient teaching. This chapter will focus on the vital role of the healthcare practitioner in preventing medication errors by attending to the elements of safe medication administration.

11.1 Prescription/Medication Order

The first step in the medication delivery process is prescription. The prescription is the medication order. It can be written on a prescription tablet (pad) or printed through an electronic health record for medication procurement in the outpatient setting, or it can be written or added electronically to patient's chart for administration by healthcare practitioners.

 LEARNING LINK Recall the components of a medication order addressed in Chapter 9: name of patient, patient's date of birth, date and time the order is written, drug name, drug dose, route, time and/or frequency of medication administration, and signature of authorized prescriber (AP). (See Table 9-3.)

Only licensed healthcare professionals with prescriptive authority, i.e., MDs (medical doctors), DOs (osteopathic physicians), DPMs (podiatrists), DDSs (dentists), PAs (physician assistants), and ARNPs (advanced practice registered nurse practitioners) are permitted to write prescriptions. These are typical authorized prescribers (APs). It is important to note that those authorized to write prescriptions may differ according to state law.

Authorized prescribers (APs) use abbreviations when prescribing medications. Review Table 9-1 in Chapter 9 for "Abbreviations Commonly Used in Drug Orders." Approved abbreviations may vary among healthcare facilities. It is important to memorize these commonly used abbreviations and to have available a complete list of abbreviations accepted at your facility.

In outpatient settings, for medication procurement, medication orders are given as *prescriptions* that are filled at an outpatient pharmacy. These prescriptions are written on a prescription tablet, telephoned in to the pharmacist, or written electronically and communicated through a computerized system to the pharmacist. Prescriptions must include all eight components of a medication order, plus the prescriber number, the quantity to be dispensed, the number of refills permitted, and instructions for the label of the container. These instructions are preceded by the word *sig* (see Figure 11-1). Sig is an abbreviation for the Latin term *signetur* which means "let it be labeled." Some APs write instructions without the use of "sig."

Note in figure 11-1 that the patient is Arthur Simons. His date of birth (DOB) is September 29, 1949. The drug is Doxycycline. The dose is 100 mg. From the **sig** line, the instructions on the label should read, "Take one capsule twice a day after meals" or one capsule (1 cap), twice a day (BID), by mouth (po), after meals (pc). Form, number, route, frequency, and timing are all shown. The quantity, sometimes abbreviated quan, of capsules is 20. The prescription cannot be refilled. The physician's name, prescriber number, and signature are present. This order contains all the necessary components.

When medications are administered by a healthcare practitioner the prescription will be in the form of a medication order in the patient's chart. This order will be either handwritten or entered electronically into the patient's chart. An order or group of orders will

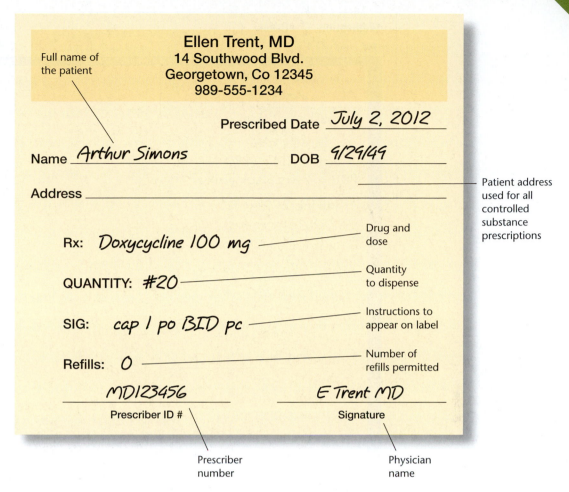

Ellen Trent, MD
14 Southwood Blvd.
Georgetown, Co 12345
989-555-1234

Full name of
the patient

Prescribed Date _July 2, 2012_

Name _Arthur Simons_   DOB _9/29/49_

Patient address
used for all
controlled
substance
prescriptions

Address _____

Rx: _Doxycycline 100 mg_ ——— Drug and
dose

QUANTITY: _#20_ ——————— Quantity
to dispense

SIG: _cap 1 po BID pc_ ——— Instructions to
appear on label

Refills: _0_ ——————— Number of
refills permitted

_MD123456_   _E Trent MD_
Prescriber ID #   Signature

Prescriber
number

Physician
name

Figure 11-1 A typical outpatient prescription.

include the current *date/time* and *signature* of the AP with each order entry on an electronic or paper form marked with the *patient's name* and date of birth (DOB) comprising four of the eight medication order components. The remaining four components should be identified for every medication ordered: *drug name*, *dose*, *route*, and *frequency/time*. Additional instructions are provided as needed.

The form in Figure 11-2 shows several medication orders; some are correct and others have errors.

- Order 1 contains all necessary components. The drug is Lasix, the dose is 20 mg, the route is oral (po), and the frequency is once a day (daily).
- Order 2, for KCl (potassium chloride) elixir, is not complete. The order lists 1 tsp as the amount, but KCl elixir is available in strengths of 10, 20, 30, or 40 mEq per 15 mL. Each strength provides a different dose per teaspoon.
- Order 3 is correct. The drug is Motrin®, the dose is 200 mg, the route is oral (po), and the frequency is whenever necessary (PRN) every 4 hours (q 4 h). For PRN drugs, the AP must specify how often it may be given. In this order, an authorized prescriber verbalized directly, in person or via the telephone, to a nurse or other practitioner. Motrin® may not be administered more often than every 4 h.
- Order 4 is not complete because it does not include a frequency.
- In Order 5, the physician has included instructions for "holding" (not administering) the medication. Inderal should not be given if the patient's apical pulse is below 50. However, the dose ordered includes number of tablets, but not number of milligrams, thus it is incomplete. Because Inderal is available in 10-, 20-, 40-, 60-, and 90-mg tablets, this order is unsafe.

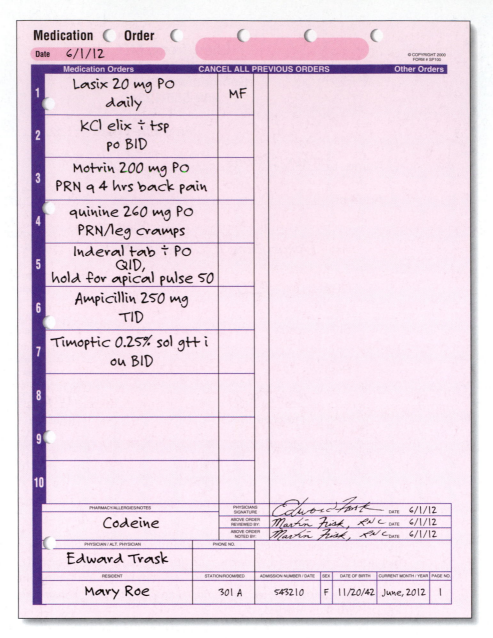

Figure 11-2 Medication order form. Do you see any errors?

- Order 6 does not specify the route for 250 mg Ampicillin, which is available in oral, intramuscular, and intravenous forms. The order writer should be consulted for clarification of this order.
- Order 7 is complete. The physician specified the number of drops as well as the strength of Timoptic® desired.

GO TO . . . Open the CD-ROM that accompanies your textbook, and select Chapter 11, Parts of a Prescription (LO 11.1). Review the animation and example problems, then complete the practice problems. Continue to the next section of the book once you have mastered the information presented.

11.1 Prescription/Medication Order

For Exercises 1–5, refer to prescription A.

Alan Capsella, MD
Westtown Medical Clinic
989-555-1234

Prescribed Date _July 9, 2012_

Name _Ann Pechin_   DOB _5/30/60_

Address _____

Rx: _Lopressor 50 mg_

QUANTITY: _#90_

SIG: _tab i po tid_

Refills: _5_

_MD398475_   _Alan Capsella MD_
Prescriber ID #   Signature

Prescription A

1. What components, if any, are missing from prescription A?
2. How many Lopressor® tablets should the pharmacy technician dispense?
3. How often should the patient take Lopressor®?
4. What strength tablets should be dispensed?
5. If the patient gets all the refills permitted, how long will the medication covered by this prescription last?

For Exercises 6–10, refer to prescription B on the next page.

6. What components, if any, are missing from prescription B?
7. How much Amoxil® should the pharmacy technician dispense?
8. How much Amoxil® should the patient take at one time?
9. How many times can this prescription be refilled?
10. How often should the patient take Amoxil®?

Prescribed Date _April 10, 2012_

Name _Mark Ward_   DOB _8/12/10_

Address _____

Rx: _Amoxil – oral susp_

QUANTITY: _100 mL_

SIG: _i tsp po q8h_

Refills: _O_

_MD398475_   _Alan Capsella MD_

Prescriber ID #   Signature

Prescription B

For Exercises 11-12, refer to Medication Order Form C.

Rhode Island Medical Center
Coventry, Rhode Island
Medication Order Form

Jane Doe   DOB 3/15/55
1534 Hopkins Trail Chepachet, RI 01222
MR # 345466610

Diagnosis: Congestive Heart Failure   Allergies: NONE

Date	Time		
1/3/10	8AM	A	tylenol PO q4h prn fever > 101
		B	furosemide 10 mg b.i.d
		C	valproic acid 250 mg by mouth
		D	10,000 units subcut q am

Mark Sanger, MD

Medication Order From C

11. List the eight components of a medication order.

12. Refer to prescription B and identify the missing component of orders A–D.

To check your answers, see the Answer section at the end of the book, which starts on page A-1.

Usually, orders must be written and/or personally signed by the licensed prescribing practitioner. However, if the authorized prescriber is not able to write an order that must be carried out quickly, verbal orders may be permitted. This may occur, for example, when a physician is performing a sterile procedure on the patient, and verbally orders that the patient receive a sedative, to facilitate the safe completion of the procedure.

Verbal orders are orders from an authorized prescriber stated directly, in person, or via the telephone to a nurse or other practitioner whose scope of practice includes the authorization to receive and document such orders. State laws govern which personnel may accept such orders and how soon the prescriber must countersign them. Accepting verbal orders is a serious task, since it can readily lead to medication errors. Most healthcare agencies limit the use of verbal orders, so learn the agency's policy before accepting a verbal order. To minimize errors when receiving verbal orders, **The Joint Commission (TJC)**, the accrediting body for healthcare organizations, has identified three guidelines for verbal orders:

1. **Write the order.** If you are legally permitted to accept a telephone order, write it carefully and legibly *as* you receive it, *not after* the call. In some cases, you may write the order on the physician's order form, identifying it as a verbal order. Verify that all components of the medication order are included. For example, if the AP forgets to include the route, ask "by what route would you like that medication administered?"
2. **Read the order.** Read the order back to the prescribing practitioner to verify that you have transcribed it correctly. If you are not certain of the spelling of the drug name, ask the prescriber to spell it. Many drugs have names that are pronounced or spelled similarly.
3. **Confirm the order.** Get confirmation from the prescriber that the order is correct.

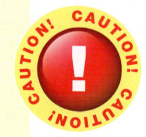

ERROR ALERT!

Always Be Certain That You Are Dispensing the Correct Medication

Many drugs have names that are very similar. Read the order carefully and, when in doubt, contact the authorized prescriber. The following list gives just a few examples of how similar the names of different drugs can look and sound. It is especially easy to confuse them when they are written rather than printed.

Acular®—Ocular	Iodine—Lodine®
Benadryl®—Bentyl®	Nicobid—Nitrobid®
Cafergot®—Carafate®	Pavabid—Pavased
Darvon®—Diovan®	Phenaphen—Phenergan®
Digitoxin—digoxin	Quinidine—Quinine
Eurax—Urex®	Uracel—Uracil

For example, Nurse Jones is receiving a telephone order from Dr. Smith for patient Robert Brown. After physician and nurse have identified themselves, and then identified the patient by double identifier, the order would proceed as follows:

Step 1: The *authorized prescriber* states the order:
"Acetaminophen every four hours as needed for fever greater than 101."
The *receiver* writes the order as stated:

Acetaminophen   *q4h prn fever greater than 101*

The *receiver* asks:

"How much acetaminophen and by what route should it be administered?"

The *authorized prescriber* states:

"650 mg po"

The *receiver* fills in the blanks as the order is stated:

Acetaminophen 650 mg po q4h prn fever greater than 101

Step 2: The *receiver* reads the order back to the prescriber, as written:

"OK, that is: acetaminophen 650 mg po q4h prn fever greater than 101."

Step 3: The *receiver* continues on to confirm the order:

"Is that correct?"

The *authorized prescriber* answers "yes."

The order would have the date and time recorded, and the signature would begin: T.O. (for telephone order), and have the AP's name and license printed, followed by the receiver's professional signature.

Date/time   *Acetaminophen 650 mg po q4h prn fever greater than 101*

T.O. S. Smith, MD / J. Jones, RN

ERROR ALERT!

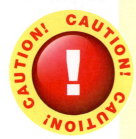

Never Guess What the Prescriber Meant

If an order is not legible, always contact the authorized prescriber to clarify the order.

In Figure 11-3, the physician intended to order Zyrtec® 10 mg po qd. However, the order is illegible, and you could read Zantac®. The loop on the m in mg could be an extra zero, or 100 mg. A small extra loop in qd makes it hard to tell if the order is *qd* (once every day) or *qod* (every other day).

Note: The abbreviations qd and qod are on the "Do not use" list by TJC. The physician should not use them. Instead she or he should have written *daily.*

Because you bear the responsibility of administering the correct dose at the correct frequency, you must contact the physician to clarify the order. Also contact the physician if any part of the order is missing.

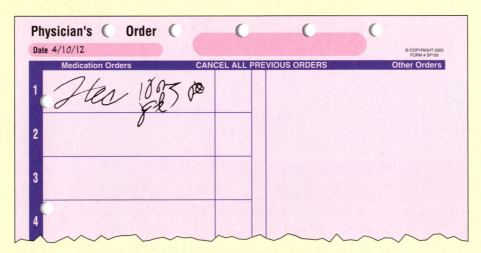

Figure 11-3 Handwritten Physician's orders can be difficult to read.

GO TO . . . Open the CD-ROM that accompanies your textbook, and select Chapter 11, Receiving and Writing Verbal Orders (LO 11.2). Review the animation and example problems, then complete the practice problems. Continue to the next section of the book once you have mastered the information presented.

REVIEW AND PRACTICE

11.2 Verbal Orders

Complete the steps the receiver will take during a verbal order:
The nurse is receiving a telephone order from the physician. The physician and nurse have identified themselves, and then identified the patient by double identifier.

Step 1: The *authorized prescriber* states the order: "cefixime 200 mg every 12 hours for 10 days"

    The receiver writes: _____

    The receiver asks: _____

    The *authorized prescriber* states: "by mouth"

    The receiver fills in the blanks as the order is stated: cefixime 200 mg po q12h for 10 days

Step 2: *The receiver* states: _____

Step 3: *The receiver* continues on to confirm the order: _____

To check your answers, see the Answer section at the end of the book, which starts on page A-1.

11.3 Safe Medication Order Transcription

Transcription of a medication order is the process of taking the information from the prescribing practitioner's order (prescription) and transferring it to the prescription label for outpatient settings (done by a pharmacist) or to the Medication Administration Record (MAR) (done by a nurse or pharmacist) for inpatient settings. *Incorrect transcription is one of the main causes of medication errors.* Although the transcription process may not be the responsibility of the person who is administering medications, it is the duty of the registered nurse in the inpatient setting to ensure that a transcribed order is accurate and complete before signing off an order for implementation. It is important that the transcriber is familiar with medical terminology and abbreviations. If the medication order is not written neatly and is difficult to interpret, the nurse must contact the authorized prescriber for clarification. An entry on the order sheet should be written, reflecting the clarification. If the medicating practitioner does not understand an abbreviation, or any part of a medication order as it is written or transcribed, the authorized prescriber or pharmacist, or registered nurse, should be contacted for clarification.

The following four orders are transcribed on the Medication Administration Record, Figure 11-4.

- Dilantin 125 mg orally twice per day around the clock
- Cleocin 225 mg intravenously every six hours
- Digoxin 0.125 mg by mouth every other day on the even days
- Probanthine 15 mg orally three times a day

Medication Administration Record (MAR)

MO/YR: 2/2009 Start/Stop Date				1	2	3	4	5	6	7	8	9	10	11	12	13	14	15	16	17	18	19	20	21	22	23	24	25	26	27	28	29	30	31
Medication			Hour																																
Dilantin 125 mg PO q12h	Start		0800																																
			2000																																
	Stop																																		
Cleocin 225 mg IV q6h	Start		0600																																
			1200																																
			1800																																
			2400																																
	Stop																																		
Digoxin 0.125 mg PO every other day; even days	Start		0800	X		X		X		X		X		X		X		X		X		X		X		X		X		X		X		X
	Stop																																		
Probanthine 15 mg PO tid	Start		0600																																
			1400																																
			2200																																
	Stop																																		
	Start																																		
	Start																																		
	Start																																		
	Stop																																		

Diagnosis:

DIET (Special instructions. e.g. Texture, Bite Size, Position, etc.)

Comments

Allergies:

Physician Name

Phone Number

A. Put initials in appropriate box when medication is given.
B. Circle initials when not given.
C. State reason for refusal / omission on back of form.
D. PRN Medications: Reason given and results must be noted on back of form.
E. Legend: S = School; H = Home visit; W = Work; P = Program.

NAME:

Record #

Date of Birth:

Sex:

VITAL SIGNS	1	2	3	4	5	6	7	8	9	10	11	12	13	14	15	16	17	18	19	20	21	22	23	24	25	26	27	28	29	30	31
TEMPERATURE																															
PULSE																															
RESPIRATION																															
WEIGHT																															

PRN AND MEDICATIONS NOT ADMINSTERED							Initials	Staff Signature
Date	Hour	Initials	Medication	Reason	Result			
						1		
						2		
						3		
						4		
						5		

Figure 11-4 Medication Administration Record sample.

GO TO . . . Open the CD-ROM that accompanies your textbook, and select Chapter 11, Safe Transcription Practices (LO 11.3). Review the animation and example problems, then complete the practice problems. Continue to the next section of the book once you have mastered the practice presented.

11.3 Safe Medication Order Transcription

Use the information below to complete Exercises 1–3 on the Medication Administration Record. Transcribe orders E, F, and G on the Medication Order Form to the Medication Administration Record (MAR).

- t.i.d. = 6 a.m.–2 p.m–10 p.m.

- daily = 10 a.m.

- bedtime = 10 p.m.

To check your answers, see the Answer section at the end of the book, which starts on page A-1.

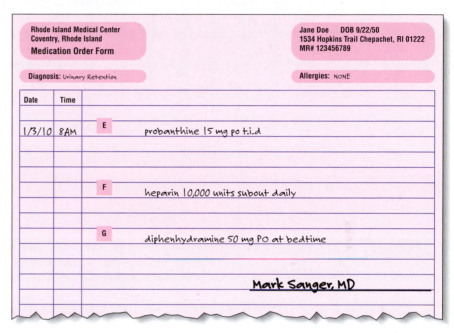

Rhode Island Medical Center
Coventry, Rhode Island
Medication Order Form

Jane Doe   DOB 9/22/50
1534 Hopkins Trail Chepachet, RI 01222
MR# 123456789

Diagnosis: Urinary Retention

Allergies: NONE

Date	Time		
1/3/10	8AM	E	probanthine 15 mg po t.i.d
		F	heparin 10,000 units subout daily
		G	diphenhydramine 50 mg PO at bedtime

Mark Sanger, MD

Medication Administration Record (MAR)

MO/YR:	Start/Stop Date		Facility Name:																															
Medication			Hour	1	2	3	4	5	6	7	8	9	10	11	12	13	14	15	16	17	18	19	20	21	22	23	24	25	26	27	28	29	30	31
Exercise 1: Order E	Start																																	
	Stop																																	
Exercise 1: Order F	Start																																	
	Stop																																	
Exercise 1: Order G	Start																																	
	Stop																																	

Diagnosis:	DIET (Special instructions. e.g. Texture, Bite Size, Position, etc.)	Comments
Allergies:	Physician Name	A. Put initials in appropriate box when medication is given. B. Circle initials when not given. C. State reason for refusal / omission on back of form.
	Phone Number	D. PRN Medications: Reason given and results must be noted on back of from. E. Legend: S = School; H = Home visit; W = Work; P = Program.
NAME:	Record #	Date of Birth:	Sex:

11.4 Error-Prone Abbreviations and Symbols

Some abbreviations, symbols, and acronyms are prone to misinterpretation and have resulted in a significant number of medications errors. For this reason, The Joint Commission (TJC) and the **Institute for Safe Medication Practice (ISMP)** have identified abbreviations that should not be used. An example of an error-prone abbreviation is U (for unit). When handwritten, U can be mistaken for a zero, potentially leading to a drug overdose. Other error-prone abbreviations include: IU (international unit), QD (every day), QOD (every other day), and MS (morphine sulfate). The Joint Commission (TJC) and the Institute for Safe Medication Practice (ISMP) are two healthcare organizations whose mission includes promotion of patient safety. These organizations have identified frequently misinterpreted abbreviations and symbols that have contributed to harmful medication errors. To reduce transcription errors, TJC, in 2005, published the *Official "Do Not Use" List*, a standardized list of abbreviations, acronyms, and symbols (U, IU, QD, QOD, trailing zero, MS, MSO_4 $MgSO_4$) that are not to be used on prescriptions and medication orders. In 2006, the The ISMP published a more comprehensive *"ISMP's List of Error-Prone Abbreviations, Symbols, and Dose Designations in 2006, and updated it in 2010."* This list includes all of the abbreviations on TJC's "Do Not Use" list, denoting them with a double asterisk (**). The ISMP, through its Medication Errors Reporting Program has compiled this table of error-prone abbreviations that should NOT be used in the processes of prescription and transcription (see Table 11-1). Although you may see these on preprinted order sheets, *do not use* the error-prone abbreviations when transcribing an order.

TABLE 11-1 ISMP's List of Error-Prone Abbreviations, Symbols, and Dose Designations

ABBREVIATIONS	INTENDED MEANING	MISINTERPRETATION	CORRECTION
μg	Microgram	Mistaken as "mg"	Use "mcg"
AD, AS, AU	Right ear, left ear, each ear	Mistaken as OD, OS, OU (right eye, left eye, each eye)	Use "right ear," "left ear," or "each ear"
OD, OS, OU	Right eye, left eye, each eye	Mistaken as AD, AS, AU (right ear, left ear, each ear)	Use "right eye," "left eye," or "each eye"
BT	Bedtime	Mistaken as "BID" (twice daily)	Use "bedtime"
cc	Cubic centimeters	Mistaken as "u" (units)	Use "mL"
D/C	Discharge or discontinue	Premature discontinuation of medications if D/C (intended to mean "discharge") has been misinterpreted as "discontinued" when followed by a list of discharge medications	Use "discharge" and "discontinue"
IJ	Injection	Mistaken as "IV" or "intrajugular"	Use "injection"
IN	Intranasal	Mistaken as "IM" or "IV"	Use "intranasal" or "NAS"
HS hs	Half-strength At bedtime, hours of sleep	Mistaken as bedtime Mistaken as half-strength	Use "half-strength" or "bedtime"
IU**	International unit	Mistaken as IV (intravenous) or 10 (ten)	Use "units"

TABLE 11-1 Continued

ABBREVIATIONS	INTENDED MEANING	MISINTERPRETATION	CORRECTION
o.d. or OD	Once daily	Mistaken as "right eye" (OD-oculus dexter), leading to oral liquid medications administered in the eye	Use "daily"
OJ	Orange juice	Mistaken as OD or OS (right or left eye); drugs meant to be diluted in orange juice may be given in the eye	Use "orange juice"
Per os	By mouth, orally	The "os" can be mistaken as "left eye" (OS-oculus sinister)	Use "PO," "by mouth," or "orally"
q.d. or QD**	Every day	Mistaken as q.i.d., especially if the period after the "q" or the tail of the "q" is misunderstood as an "i"	Use "daily"
qhs	Nightly at bedtime	Mistaken as "qhr" or every hour	Use "nightly"
qn	Nightly or at bedtime	Mistaken as "qh" (every hour)	Use "nightly" or "at bedtime"
q.o.d. or QOD**	Every other day	Mistaken as "q.d." (daily) or "q.i.d." (four times daily) if the "o" is poorly written	Use "every other day"
q1d	Daily	Mistaken as q.i.d. (four times daily)	Use "daily"
q6PM, etc.	Every evening at 6 PM	Mistaken as every 6 hours	Use "daily at 6 PM" or "6 PM daily"
SC, SQ, sub q	Subcutaneous	SC mistaken as SL (sublingual); SQ mistaken as "5 every;" the "q" in "sub q" has been mistaken as "every" (e.g., a heparin dose ordered "sub q 2 hours before surgery" misunderstood as every 2 hours before surgery)	Use "subcut" or "subcutaneously"
ss	Sliding scale (insulin) or $\frac{1}{2}$ (apothecary)	Mistaken as "55"	Spell out "sliding scale;" use "one-half" or "$\frac{1}{2}$"
SSRI	Sliding scale regular insulin	Mistaken as selective-serotonin reuptake inhibitor	Spell out "sliding scale (insulin)"
SSI	Sliding scale insulin	Mistaken as Strong Solution of Iodine (Lugol's)	
i/d	One daily	Mistaken as "tid"	Use "1 daily"
TIW or tiw (also BIW or biw)	TIW: 3 times a week BIW: 2 times a week	TIW mistaken as "3 times a day" or "twice in a week" BIW mistaken ad "2 times a day"	Use "3 times weekly" Use "2 times weekly"

(Continued)

TABLE 11-1 Continued

ABBREVIATIONS	INTENDED MEANING	MISINTERPRETATION	CORRECTION
U or u**	Unit	Mistaken as the number 0 or 4, causing a 10-fold overdose or greater (e.g., 4U seen as "40" or 4u seen as "44"); mistaken as "cc" so dose given in volume instead of units (e.g., 4u seen as 4cc)	Use "unit"
UD	As directed ("ut dictum")	Mistaken as unit dose (e.g., diltiazem 125 mg IV infusion "UD" misinterpreted as meaning to give the entire infusion as a unit [bolus] dose)	Use "as directed"

DOSE DESIGNATIONS AND OTHER INFORMATION	INTENDED MEANING	MISINTERPRETATION	CORRECTION
Trailing zero after decimal point (e.g., 1.0 mg)**	1mg	Mistaken as 10 mg if the decimal point is not seen	Do not use trailing zeros for doses expressed in whole numbers
No leading zero before a decimal point (e.g., .5 mg)**	0.5 mg	Mistaken as 5 mg if the decimal point is not seen	Use zero before a decimal point when the dose is less than a whole unit
Drug name and dose run together (especially problematic for drug names that end in "l" such as Inderal40 mg; Tegretol300 mg)	Inderal 40 mg Tegretol 300 mg	Mistaken as Inderal 140 mg Mistaken as Tegretol 1300 mg	Place adequate space between the drug name, dose, and unit of measure
Numerical dose and unit of measure run together (e.g., 10mg, 100mL)	10 mg 100 mL	The "m" is sometimes mistaken as a zero or two zeros, risking a 10- to 100-fold overdose	Place adequate space between the dose and unit of measure
Abbreviations such as mg. or mL. with a period following the abbreviation	mg mL	The period is unnecessary and could be mistaken as the number 1 if written poorly	Use mg, mL, etc. without a terminal period
Large doses without properly placed commas (e.g., 100000 units; 1000000 units)	100,000 units 1,000,000 units	100000 has been mistaken as 10,000 or 1,000,000; 1000000 has been mistaken as 100,000	Use commas for dosing units at or above 1,000, or use words such as 100 "thousand" or 1 "million" to improve readability

DRUG NAME ABBREVIATIONS	INTENDED MEANING	MISINTERPRETATION	CORRECTION
ARA A	vidarabine	Mistaken as cytarabine (ARA C)	Use complete drug name
AZT	zidovudine (Retrovir)	Mistaken as azathioprine or aztreonam	Use complete drug name

TABLE 11-1 Continued

DRUG NAME ABBREVIATIONS	INTENDED MEANING	MISINTERPRETATION	CORRECTION
CPZ	Compazine (prochlorperazine)	Mistaken as chlorpromazine	Use complete drug name
DPT	Demerol-Phenergan-Thorazine	Mistaken as diphtheria-pertussis-tetanus (vaccine)	Use complete drug name
DTO	Diluted tincture of opium, or deodorized tincture of opium (Paregoric)	Mistaken as tincture of opium	Use complete drug name
HCl	hydrochloric acid or hydrochloride	Mistaken as potassium chloride (The "H" is misinterpreted as "K")	Use complete drug name unless expressed as a salt of a drug
HCT	hydrocortisone	Mistaken as hydrochlorothiazide	Use complete drug name
HCTZ	hydrochlorothiazide	Mistaken as hydrocortisone (seen as HCT250 mg)	Use complete drug name
MgSO4**	magnesium sulfate	Mistaken as morphine sulfate	Use complete drug name
MS, MSO4**	morphine sulfate	Mistaken as magnesium sulfate	Use complete drug name
MTX	methotrexate	Mistaken as mitoxantrone	Use complete drug name
PCA	procainamide	Mistaken as patient controlled analgesia	Use complete drug name
PTU	propylthiouracil	Mistaken as mercaptopurine	Use complete drug name
T3	Tylenol with codeine No. 3	Mistaken as liothyronine	Use complete drug name
TAC	triamcinolone	Mistaken as tetracaine, Adrenalin, cocaine	Use complete drug name
TNK	TNKase	Mistaken as "TPA"	Use complete drug name
ZnSO4	zinc sulfate	Mistaken as morphine sulfate	Use complete drug name
STEMMED DRUG NAMES	**INTENDED MEANING**	**MISINTERPRETATION**	**CORRECTION**
"Nitro" drip	nitroglycerin infusion	Mistaken as sodium nitroprusside infusion	Use complete drug name
"Norflox"	norfloxacin	Mistaken as Norflex	Use complete drug name
"IV Vanc"	intravenous vancomycin	Mistaken as Invanz	Use complete drug name

(Continued)

TABLE 11-1 **Continued**

SYMBOLS	INTENDED MEANING	MISINTERPRETATION	CORRECTION
ʒ	Dram	Symbol for dram mistaken as "3"	Use the metric system
ℳ	Minim	Symbol for minim mistaken as "mL"	
x3d	For three days	Mistaken as "3 doses"	Use "for three days"
> and <	Greater than and less than	Mistaken as opposite of intended; mistakenly use incorrect symbol; "< 10" mistaken as "40"	Use "greater than" or "less than"
/ (slash mark)	Separates two doses or indicates "per"	Mistaken as the number 1 (e.g., "25 units/10 units" misread as "25 units and 110" units)	Use "per" rather than a slash mark to separate doses
@	At	Mistaken as "2"	Use "at"
&	And	Mistaken as "2"	Use "and"
+	Plus or and	Mistaken as "4"	Use "and"
°	Hour	Mistaken as a zero (e.g., q2° seen as q 20)	Use "hr," "h," or "hour"
Ø	zero, null sign	Mistaken as the numerals 4, 6, or 9	Use the number "0" or the word "zero"

ISMP's List of Error-Prone Abbreviations, Symbols, and Dose Designation, copyright 2010, Institute for Safe Medication Practices.
**These abbreviations are included on The Joint Commission's "minimum list" of dangerous abbreviations, acronyms, and symbols that must be included on an organization's "Do Not Use" list, effective January 1, 2004. Visit www.jcaho.org for more information about this Joint Commission requirement.

GO TO . . . Open the CD-ROM that accompanies your textbook, and select Chapter 11, Error-Prone Abbreviations (LO 11.4). Review the animation and example problems, then complete the practice problems. Continue to the next section of the book once you have mastered the information presented.

REVIEW AND PRACTICE

11.4 Error-Prone Abbreviations and Symbols

For Exercises 1-5, refer to Medication Order shown on the next page.

1. Identify the error-prone abbreviations transcribed on this medication order form.

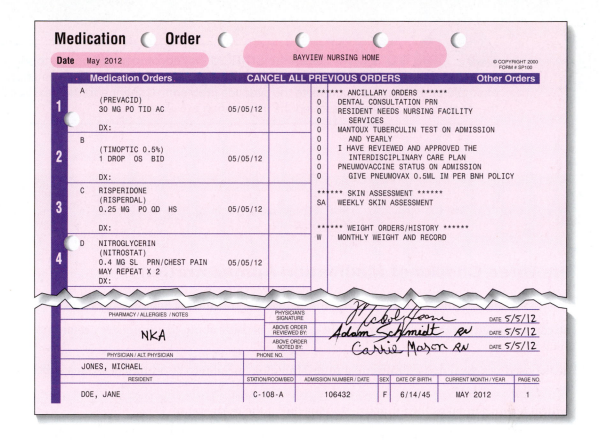

Medication ○ **Order** ○

Date May 2012   BAYVIEW NURSING HOME   © COPYRIGHT 2000 FORM # SP100

Medication Orders	CANCEL ALL PREVIOUS ORDERS	Other Orders

A
1   (PREVACID)
    30 MG PO TID AC   05/05/12
    DX:

B
2   (TIMOPTIC 0.5%)
    1 DROP OS BID   05/05/12
    DX:

C RISPERIDONE
3   (RISPERDAL)
    0.25 MG PO QD HS   05/05/12
    DX:

D NITROGLYCERIN
4   (NITROSTAT)
    0.4 MG SL PRN/CHEST PAIN   05/05/12
    MAY REPEAT X 2
    DX:

****** ANCILLARY ORDERS ******
O   DENTAL CONSULTATION PRN
O   RESIDENT NEEDS NURSING FACILITY
O   SERVICES
O   MANTOUX TUBERCULIN TEST ON ADMISSION
O   AND YEARLY
O   I HAVE REVIEWED AND APPROVED THE
O   INTERDISCIPLINARY CARE PLAN
O   PNEUMOVACCINE STATUS ON ADMISSION
O   GIVE PNEUMOVAX 0.5ML IM PER BNH POLICY

****** SKIN ASSESSMENT ******
SA   WEEKLY SKIN ASSESSMENT

****** WEIGHT ORDERS/HISTORY ******
W   MONTHLY WEIGHT AND RECORD

PHARMACY / ALLERGIES / NOTES		PHYSICIAN'S SIGNATURE	*Nichol Hearn*	DATE 5/5/12
NKA		ABOVE ORDER REVIEWED BY:	*Adam Schmidt RN*	DATE 5/5/12
		ABOVE ORDER NOTED BY:	*Carrie Mason RN*	DATE 5/5/12
PHYSICIAN / ALT. PHYSICIAN		PHONE NO.		
JONES, MICHAEL				

RESIDENT	STATION/ROOM/BED	ADMISSION NUMBER / DATE	SEX	DATE OF BIRTH	CURRENT MONTH / YEAR	PAGE NO.
DOE, JANE	C-108-A	106432	F	6/14/45	MAY 2012	1

For Exercises 2–5, correct the medication orders, using the published list from the ISMP (Table 11-1). Hint: See items marked with a double-asterisk.

2. Give Coumadin® 5.0 mg p.o. QD.

3. MS 4 mg sc q4h prn pain.

4. Vitamin D 1000 IU QOD

5. Digoxin .125 mg (125 μ) p.o. q.d.

To check your answers, see the Answer section at the end of the book, which starts on page A-1.

11.5 The Three Checks of Medication Administration

To promote accuracy and safety with medication administration, the drug label should be checked three times (see Rule 11-1).

RULE 11-1

Check medication three times:

1st check—when you take it from the storage container and match it to the MAR

2nd check—when you prepare it

3rd check—before you close the storage container or just before you administer the medication to the patient.

Check the medication three times even if the dose is prepackaged, labeled, and ready to be administered.

GO TO . . . Open the CD-ROM that accompanies your textbook, and select Chapter 11, Check Medication Three Times (LO 11.5). Review the animation and example problems, then complete the practice problems. Continue to the next section of the book once you have mastered the information presented.

REVIEW AND PRACTICE

11.5 The Three Checks of Medication Administration

In Scenarios 1–5, identify which check (1, 2, or 3) the healthcare practitioner demonstrates.

1. The certified medication technician is at the patient's bedside about to administer acetaminophen tablets. _____

2. The licensed practical nurse draws up 4 units Humalog® insulin to be administered via subcutaneous route. _____

3. Medical technician takes the influenza vaccine out of the refrigerator. _____

4. The registered nurse reads the medication label on the intravenous (IV) medication bag before connecting the IV to the patient. _____

5. The physician retrieves epinephrine from the emergency cart. _____

To check your answers, see the Answer section at the end of the book, which starts on page A-1.

11.6 The Rights of Medication Administration

The rights of medication administration are a set of safety checks the practitioner follows to prevent a medication administration error. When administering medications, the healthcare practitioner should observe the rights of medication administration (see Table 11-2) to avoid errors and ensure patient safety. The six basic rights of medication administration include right patient, right drug, right dose, right route, right time, and right documentation. A violation of any of the six basic rights constitutes a medication error. Additional rights include right reason, right to refuse, right to know, and right technique.

TABLE 11-2 The Rights of Medication Administration	
1. Right patient	6. Right documentation
2. Right drug	7. Right reason
3. Right dose	8. Right to know
4. Right route	9. Right to refuse
5. Right time	10. Right technique

RIGHT PATIENT   Before you give a medication to a patient you must check two identifiers: the full name and another identifier such as the patient's date of birth, social security number, or medical record number. Check that the name on the medication order is exactly the same as the name of the patient. Two patients with the same last name may have the same first initials, or even the same first names. Ask the patient to state his or her full name and date of birth or other identifying information. If the patient is unable to do so, ask the parent or caregiver to state the patient's full name. In outpatient settings, you may be required to ask for photographic identification, such as a driver's license. In an inpatient setting, check the patient's name and date of birth. In many facilities you may be required to scan the bar code on the patient's identification bracelet as well as the medication you will be administering. Remember, you are not only identifying that you have the right patient, you are also identifying that you are using the *right patient's MAR.* This is why recognizing the patient is not good enough, but a comparison of double identifiers from the patient to the MAR must be completed before medication administration.

RIGHT DRUG   Be certain that a patient receives the *right drug.* Administer only drugs you have prepared yourself or that are clearly and completely labeled. Carefully check the medication label at least three times (see Rule 11-1) before administering the medication. Check that the drug/order has not expired. (See Chapter 10 for more details on drug labels.) If a patient questions a medication, recheck the original order. Patients are often familiar with their medications. Listening to them may prevent an error.

CRITICAL THINKING ON THE JOB

The Importance of the Right Drug

A patient is brought to the hospital with a severe thumb laceration. The attending physician verbally orders lidocaine 1% solution 2 mL as a local anesthetic. The healthcare professional picks up a vial labeled lidocaine 1% with epinephrine and draws up 2 mL. He then says, "This is lidocaine 1% solution 2 mL," but neither mentions the epinephrine nor shows the physician the label.

A while later, the patient expresses concern about continuing numbness in his thumb. After locating the vial, the staff member realized that the patient received epinephrine, a vasoconstricting drug, in addition to the lidocaine. The patient is reassured that feeling will return to his thumb, although not quite as quickly as was first anticipated.

 Think! . . . Is It Reasonable? What could have been done to prevent the patient from losing feeling in his thumb?

RIGHT DOSE   The patient must be given the *right dose* of medication. In later chapters, you will learn to calculate the *amount to administer* to a patient, factoring in the strength of the medication and the equipment you are using. Use extreme caution with dosage calculations. Pay special attention to decimal points. They can easily be placed in the wrong location or missed altogether when an order is copied. If you misread a decimal point, the patient could receive a dose significantly different from the one ordered.

The Importance of the Right Dose

A medication order reads Compazine® supp i pr q4h PRN/nausea. The health-care professional interprets this order as "administer 1 Compazine® supposi-tory rectally every four hours as necessary for nausea."

He assumes that the patient is an adult and dispenses 25 mg suppositories, the normal adult dose. In turn another healthcare professional, who does not notice that the dose is not specified in the order, administers the 25 mg sup-pository to the patient, a 6-year-old boy.

The usual dose of Compazine® for children is a 2.5 mg suppository. The pediatrician who wrote the order did not include the dose, assuming the staff would know this information. The child receives 10 times the normal dose of Compazine®. He has a seizure and develops fever, respiratory distress, severe hypotension, and tachycardia because of drug toxicity. He is admitted to the intensive care unit for treatment.

 Think! . . . Is It Reasonable? What could have been done to prevent this problem?

RIGHT ROUTE You must give patients drugs by the *right route*. A drug intended for one route is often not safe if administered via another route. For example, only drugs labeled *for ophthalmic use* should be instilled (applied with a dropper) into the eye. Some medications are produced in different versions for different routes. The drug label (see Chapter 10) will indi-cate the intended route. For example, Compazine® is available as a suppository, a tablet, and an injection. Always check that the route listed on the drug label matches the route ordered.

RIGHT TIME Give medications at the *right time*. In most cases, to be "on time," you must administer medications within 30 minutes of the scheduled time. The right time may refer to an absolute time, such as 6:00 p.m., or to a relative time, such as "before breakfast." Some medications, such as insulin, antibiotics, and antidysrhythmic drugs, must be given at spe-cific times because of how they interact with food or the patient's body. Other medications may be spaced over waking hours without changing their effectiveness. The drug order must identify special timing considerations to be followed. If a medication is ordered PRN (when-ever necessary), a time interval and/or condition should be specified (e.g., q4h for tempera-ture ≥ 101). Before you administer a PRN drug, check that enough time has passed since the previous dose was given. Otherwise, the patient could receive the medication too soon, leading to severe consequences.

RIGHT DOCUMENTATION Medication administration should be followed by the *right doc-umentation* on the patient's Medication Administration Record (MAR). The MAR is a paper form or electronic record that tracks the medication that a patient receives. A computerized record is sometimes used as the ongoing working document that records medications as they are administered. These are called **electronic Medication Administration Records (eMARs).** Users of these systems must log in to the computer, entering their names and secure passwords. With some electronic medication administration systems, both the medi-cation bar code and the patient's identification band are scanned. This information is docu-mented directly into the patient's eMAR. This system allows medication administration to be tracked electronically to help reduce errors. (See Figure 11-5) If medication administration is not documented, it is not considered complete. If the patient declines the medication, con-sumes only part of the dose, or vomits shortly after taking the medication, this information must be documented, as well.

RIGHT REASON The healthcare professional who administers the medication should know the reason the drug is ordered and ensure that it is given for the right reason. Knowing why a medication is ordered also helps the practitioner know when not to give (hold) a medication. For example, if a medication is ordered to slow down a rapid heart rate and the patient's heart rate is slower than normal (less than 60 beats/ minute), the drug should be held until the prescriber is notified of the situation.

RIGHT TO KNOW All patients have the right to be educated about the medications they are receiving. Information that patients should receive includes: dose, schedule, reason, effect and side effects of medications.

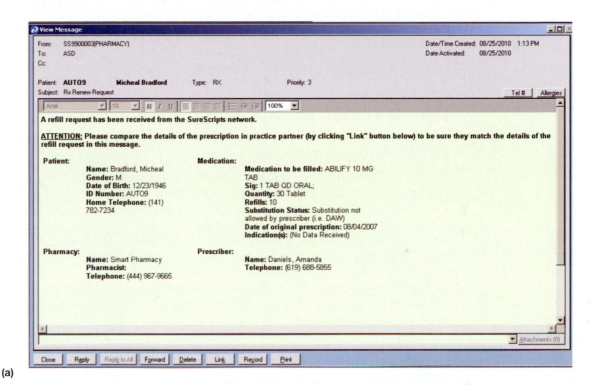

(a)

(b)

Figure 11-5 With electronic health records, the nurse in an outpatient practice can verify that the medication refill requested electronically by the pharmacy through Sure Scripts is the same medication as the original medication ordered on the patient chart.
(a) An order for Abilify is received and viewed and then the Link button is selected; (b) Once the Link button is selected, the patient's medication record with the original order is viewed and compared to the refill request. In this case the order is for aripiprazole, the generic equivalent of Abilify.

Patient education, although not one of the six basic rights of medication administration, is critical to the patient's right to know. Patients should always be provided with basic information regarding their medications.

1. Explain the purpose of a medication and its side effects.
2. Review the dose, route, frequency, and time that the physician has prescribed.
3. When appropriate, be certain that the patient understands how to self-administer the medication.
4. If the patient is taking liquid oral medications at home, emphasize the importance of using calibrated spoons and measuring cups.

RIGHT TO REFUSE   Every patient has the *right to refuse* a medication. If a patient refuses a medication, the physician should be notified and this information should be documented in the patient's medical record.

RIGHT TECHNIQUE   Be familiar with the *right technique* to administer a medication. For example, both buccal and sublingual medications are applied to the mucous membranes of the mouth. A buccal medication, such as Fentanyl® tablets, is placed between the cheek and the gum, whereas a sublingual medication, such as nitroglycerin, is placed under the tongue. If you are not familiar with the correct technique to use, check resources such as the ***Physicians' Desk Reference* (PDR),** a current drug reference book, the facility policy and procedure manual, or a valid Internet resource for more information.

Following the "rights" of medication administration needs to become automatic, just like looking both ways before crossing the street. Following the "rights" of medication administration will avert a dangerous medication error.

GO TO . . . Open the CD-ROM that accompanies your textbook, and select Chapter 11, Rights of Medication Administration (LO 11.6). Review the animation and example problems, then complete the practice problems. Continue to the next section of the book once you have mastered the information presented.

REVIEW AND PRACTICE

11.6 The Rights of Medication Administration

Match the rights of drug administration with an example of how that right can be violated.

a. Right patient   **b.** Right drug   **c.** Right dose   **d.** Right route

e. Right time   **f.** Right documentation   **g.** Right reason   **h.** Right to know

i. Right to refuse   **j.** Right technique

1. The medication bottle said *for optic use,* and the medication was instilled into the patient's ears.

2. A patient with a bleeding disorder is scheduled to be given an anticoagulant (blood thinner).

3. James F. Jones received James E. Jones' medication.

4. The nurse charted a medication on the medication record before the patient had taken the medication.

5. A patient asks why she is getting a medication and although the nurse knows why, she does not answer and administers the medication anyway.

6. The dose to be administered was ½ tsp, and the patient received 5 mL.

7. The medication was ordered at bedtime, and the patient took it at 9 a.m.

8. The physician ordered Uracel, and the patient received uracil.

9. The medication was to be given under the tongue, and the patient was told to swallow it.

To check your answers, see the Answer section at the end of the book, which starts on page A-1.

CRITICAL THINKING ON THE JOB

The Importance of the Right Drug and Right Reason

Over the course of several days, a staff nurse administered quinidine to a patient whose order was for quinine. Quinine is usually ordered to treat malaria, while quinidine is typically ordered to treat altered heart rhythms. The patient had no documented heart problems. The nurse assumed that the order writer must have intended to order quinidine as it was a typical medication ordered for many patients on this particular medical unit. The nurse also rationalized that quinine must be an alternate name or brand name for quinidine. The consequence to the patient was a critical drop in blood pressure, a side effect of quinidine.

 Think! . . . Is It Reasonable? What went wrong?

11.7 Observation

Observation refers to observing that the medication will be, or was, safely received. Observation is an essential part of medication administration. Observation takes place before, during, and after medication administration. Before preparing medications to be administered, the healthcare practitioner should assess the patient's allergy status, condition, and ability to take medications via the prescribed route, which might include checking the intravenous site and available equipment. Before administering the medication, the healthcare professional observes the patient to determine if it is safe or appropriate to administer the medication: Has the patient's condition changed so that the route or the medication itself is no longer indicated? Is there sufficient access to administer the medication: Is the IV functional? Is the nasogastric tube (NGT) in place? If the authorized prescriber (AP) is present, such as in a doctor's office or a clinic, the AP, who just ordered the medication, will perform this observation. If the AP has not just examined the patient, the practitioner should inform the RN or question the AP as to whether the medication should be given as ordered.

During medication administration the practitioner observes that the medication is received and retained. Did the patient swallow the medication? Was the suppository retained?

Did the infusion enter the vein, or did the IV infiltrate? The practitioner also observes for any untoward reactions that may occur during administration.

After medication administration the practitioner observes for any untoward reactions. The AP and the nurse also observe to see if the medication has had the desired effect.

GO TO . . . Open the CD-ROM that accompanies your textbook, and select Chapter 11, Observation in Safe Medication Administration (LO 11.7). Complete the practice problems. Continue to the next section of the book once you have mastered the information presented.

REVIEW AND PRACTICE

11.7 Observation

For Questions 1–5 write the observation that would occur during this phase of medication administration.

1. The patient is scheduled to receive an IV antibiotic
2. The patient is receiving eye drops
3. The patient has just received an IM injection
4. The patient is about to receive an oral medication
5. The patient is about to receive a medication through a nasogastric tube

To check your answers, see the Answer section at the end of the book, starting on page A-1.

11.8 Patient Teaching

Patient teaching refers to teaching the patient and/or caregiver how to procure the medication, administer the medication, and what to look for when administering a medication outside of the healthcare setting. If the patient/family will be administering the medication, the patient must be informed of all the steps in medication administration, including observation. Additionally, patients have the right to know about the medications they receive as well as the right to refuse medications. This basic right to know is an essential right of all patients' rights. The medicating practitioner, after assessing the patient's knowledge and literacy level, should ensure all patients have this basic information regarding their drugs:

1. Name of the medication, including generic and brand name
2. Purpose of the medication
3. Dose and use of calibrated equipment for liquid medications
4. Route and self-administration guidelines, as needed
5. Medication schedule, related to food intake

6. Drug-drug interactions
7. Side effects and other reportable concerns
8. Where to procure the medication
9. Additional instructions, as needed

Proper patient education promotes accuracy and compliance with the medication regime. Patients should maintain a complete and up-to-date list of medications to provide for any AP they encounter.

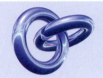 **GO TO . . .** Open the CD-ROM that accompanies your textbook, and select Chapter 11, Patient Teaching (LO 11.8). Complete the practice problems. Continue to the next section of the book once you have mastered the information presented.

Medication Reference Materials

In order to provide patient teaching when you dispense or administer medications, you are responsible for knowing their effects. Hundreds of drugs exist. New ones are produced and approved all the time. You cannot memorize all the information you might need to know. Therefore, you need to be familiar with drug information sources.

LEARNING LINK Recall from Chapter 10, package inserts provided by the manufacturers with each medication are important reference tools. They describe intended effects, possible side effects, typical doses, dosage forms available, conditions under which the drug should not be used, and special precautions to be taken while using the drug.

Information from package inserts is also available in print or electronically in the *Physicians' Desk Reference* (PDR). The PDR is an authoritative, current drug reference containing comprehensive information from the drug manufacturer regarding prescription drugs. Some versions feature nonprescription medications and herbal medications. A new volume is produced each year. Many physicians' offices, pharmacies, and healthcare facilities have the PDR available for employee use.

Many other guides are available for healthcare professionals, including the *United States Pharmacopeia/National Formulary,* found in most pharmacies. Most are updated every year or two. Other books have titles suggesting they are for nurses, but they are useful to all healthcare professionals. Their information is similar to that of the PDR, but they often have easy-to-understand language.

Internet users can access information about the 200 most commonly prescribed drugs at www.rxlist.com. This site provides information about the most frequently prescribed drugs. For each drug listed, the site lists appropriate doses of the drug for specific indications, available dosages and dosage forms, descriptions of the pills or liquids, and the drug's effects. Another Internet site, www.druginfonet.com, lists drug information, allows searches by brand or generic names, and provides many other useful features.

Also available are software programs that can run on a handheld computer, known as a personal digital assistant (PDA) or smart phone. One such program is called Epocrates. This program is updated regularly and is a handy resource for any healthcare professional needing the latest medication information. When an electronic health record (EHR) system is used, medication database software programs are frequently linked and can be accessed easily while working within the EHR programs.

11.8 Patient Teaching

For Exercises 1–5 match the patient teaching, a-e, to the situation, 1-5.

Patient Teaching:

   a. Procedure for administering an injection

   b. Use of calibrated equipment

   c. Medication schedule, related to food intake

   d. Drug-drug interactions

   e. Side effects and reportable concerns

Situation:

   1. The patient has been ordered an ACE-inhibitor. If the patient develops a nonproductive cough related to this medication, the AP will discontinue the medication. _____

   2. The patient has been newly prescribed subcutaneous insulin. _____

   3. The patient has been prescribed a medication that interacts with several over-the-counter medications. _____

   4. The patient has been prescribed a medication to take before meals. _____

   5. The patient has been prescribed a liquid cough syrup. _____

To check your answers, see the answer section at the end of the book, which stars on page A-1.

CHAPTER 11 SUMMARY

LEARNING OUTCOME	KEY POINTS
11.1 Recall the eight required elements of a prescription. Pages 218–222	▶ Name of patient ▶ Date of birth (DOB) ▶ Date and time the order is written ▶ Drug name ▶ Dose ▶ Route ▶ Time and/or frequency of medication administration ▶ Signature of authorized prescriber (AP)

LEARNING OUTCOME	KEY POINTS
11.2 Apply The Joint Commission steps to receiving and writing a verbal order. Pages 223–225	Step 1: Write the order Step 2: Read the order Step 3: Confirm the order
11.3 Execute safe transcription practices. Pages 225–227	▶ Transfer information from the AP's order to the prescription label or to the Medication Administration Record (MAR) ▶ Accurate ▶ Legible ▶ Contact AP if order is not clear

11.4 Identify error-prone abbreviations and symbols. Pages 228–233	▶ Result in death or injury when misinterpreted
	▶ TJC's Do Not Use List:
	  • U (write unit)
	  • IU (write international unit)
	  • qd, QD, OD, or q1d (write daily)
	  • QOD (write every other day)
	  • MS or MSO4 (write morphine sulfate)
	  • MgSO4 (write magnesium sulfate)
	▶ Include leading zeros (write 0.4 mg not .4 mg)
	▶ Omit trailing zeros (write 4 mg not 4.0 mg)
	▶ ISMP's Error-Prone Abbreviations:
	  • μg (write mcg)
	  • AD, AS, AU (write right ear, left ear, both ears)
	  • OD, OS, OU (write right eye, left eye, both eyes)
	  • cc (write mL)
	  • d/c (write discontinue or discharge)
	  • HS (write half-strength or hour of sleep/bedtime)
	  • qhs (write nightly or bedtime)
	  • SC or sq (write subcut)
	  • ss (write sliding scale or one-half)

11.5 Identify the three checks in the medication administration procedure. Pages 233–234	1: When you take it from the storage container and match it to the MAR. 2: When you prepare it. 3: Before closing the storage container or just before you administer the medication to the patient.

LEARNING OUTCOME	KEY POINTS
11.6 Implement the "rights" of medication administration. Pages 234–239	▶ Right patient ▶ Right drug ▶ Right dose ▶ Right route ▶ Right time/frequency ▶ Right documentation ▶ Also right reason, right to know, right to refuse, and right technique
11.7 Recognize the importance of observation in safe medication administration. Pages 239–240	Observe that the medication will be, or was, safely received ▶ Before medication administration ▶ During medication administration ▶ After medication administration
11.8 Describe the appropriate use of patient teaching as it relates to safe drug administration. Pages 240–242	Teach patient or caregiver: ▶ How to procure the medication ▶ How to administer the medication ▶ Reportable side effects and concerns

For Exercises 1–3, refer to Prescription 1. (LO 11.1)

1. What instructions should be printed for the patient?

2. By what route is the medication to be administered?

3. How many refills may the patient be given?

Mark DeSantis
123 Baker Drive
Owosso, MI 48867
989-555-1234

Prescribed Date _1/23/2012_

Name _Jeannies Kucharek_   DOB _8/10/1939_

Address _____

Rx: _Synthroid 0.1 mg_

QUANTITY: _#30_

SIG: _tab i po tid_

Refills: _0_

_MD1234567_   _Mark Desantis, MD_
Prescriber ID #   Signature

Prescription 1

For Exercises 4 and 5, refer to Prescription 2. (LO 11.1)

4. What information must be obtained before this order can be filled?

5. What instructions should be printed for the patient?

Mark DeSantis
123 Baker Drive
Owosso, MI 48867
989-555-1234

Prescribed Date _1/23/2012_

Name _Jeannies Kucharek_   DOB _8/10/1939_

Address _____

Rx: _Amoxil 250 mg/5ml_

QUANTITY:

SIG: _1 tsp. p.o. q8h until gone_

Refills: _0_

_MD1234567_   _Mark Desantis, MD_
Prescriber ID #   Signature

Prescription 2

For Exercise 6, refer to Prescription 3. (LO 11.1)

6. What action must be taken before this prescription can be filled?

Mark DeSantis
123 Baker Drive
Owosso, MI 48867
989-555-1234

Prescribed Date 1/23/2012

Name Jeannies Kucharek   DOB 8/10/1939

Address

Rx: Cortisporin Otic Drops

QUANTITY: 5 ml

SIG: gtts. ii os quid

Refills: 0

MD1234567   Mark Desantis, MD

Prescriber ID #   Signature

Prescription 3

For Exercises 7–11, refer to MAR 4. (LO 11.1)

TCP Hospital Medication Administration Record

Order date	Medication, dose, duration frequency route	D/C date	Times	22 Feb	23 Feb	24 Feb	25 Feb	26 Feb	27 Feb	28 Feb
5/21/12	heparin 5,000 units subcut q12h		0900							
			2100							
5/22/12	Procan SR 500 mg tab po q6h	05 Feb 12	0600 1200							
			1800 2400							
5/22/12	digoxin [Lanoxin] 125 mg tab po daily		0900							
5/22/12	furosemide [Lasix] 40 mg tab po daily		0900							

MAR 4

7. By what route will the heparin be given?

8. How many times a day will the patient receive Procan?

9. Will Lanoxin® be administered in the morning or at night?

10. How many oral medications is the patient receiving?

11. If the patient has a dose of Procan at 6 p.m., when should he receive the next dose?

For Exercise 12, apply The Joint Commission steps to receiving and writing a verbal order. (LO 11.2)

12. The nurse is receiving a telephone order from the physician. The physician and nurse have identified themselves, and then identified the patient by double identifier.

Step 1: The *authorized prescriber* states the order: "fentanyl 100 mcg now, may repeat once in 30 minutes if pain is not relieved."
The receiver writes:
The receiver asks:
The *authorized prescriber* states: "buccal"
The receiver fills in the blanks as the order is stated:
Step 2: *The receiver* states:
Step 3: *The receiver* continues on to confirm the order:

For Exercises 13–14, transcribe the following orders onto MAR 5. (LO 11.3)

Medication Administration Record (MAR)

MO/YR:	Start/Stop Date		Facility Name:																															
Medication			Hour	1	2	3	4	5	6	7	8	9	10	11	12	13	14	15	16	17	18	19	20	21	22	23	24	25	26	27	28	29	30	31
		Start																																	
		Stop																																	
		Start																																	
		Stop																																	

Diagnosis:	DIET (Special instructions. e.g. Texture, Bite Size, Position, etc.)	Comments	
Allergies:	Physician Name	A. Put initials in appropriate box when medication is given. B. Circle initials when not given.	
	Phone Number	C. State reason for refusal / omission on back of form. D. PRN Medications: Reason given and results must be noted on back of from. E. Legend: S = School; H = Home visit; W = Work; P = Program.	
NAME:	Record #	Date of Birth:	Sex:

MAR 5

13. Keflex 250 mg p.o. every six hours starting at midnight

14. Docusate sodium 100 mg p.o. twice a day in the morning and at bedtime

For Exercises 15–16, rewrite the orders, correcting the error-prone abbreviations. (LO 11.4)

15. MS 4.0 mg sc QD prn pain.

16. Tylenol with codeine 5 cc p.o. QHS

For Exercise 17, name which check in the three-check medication administration procedure is described. (LO 11.5)

17. The RN withdraws the narcotic from the vial.

For Exercises 18–19, identify which "right" of medication administration is violated. (LO 11.6)

18. The 6 p.m. dose of propanol is given at 1930.

19. "Hydromorphone 2 mg subcut now" is ordered. Hydromorphone 2 mg is administered intramuscularly from a pre-filled syringe with a 1.5 inch pre-attached needle.

For Exercises 20–21, describe which observation should be made to promote safe medication administration. (LO 11.7)

20. The patient is about to receive the first dose of a newly prescribed medication.

21. The patient has received a medication.

For Exercise 22, indicate the appropriate patient teaching to be provided. (LO 11.8)

22. The patient has just been order an Epi-Pen® for subcutaneous injection

CHECK UP

1. What action should you take when you receive this drug order? Dilaudid® tab 2 mg po PRN for pain q4h. (LO 11.5, 11.6)

2. What action should you take when you receive this drug order? Codeine tab 30 mg po qid. (LO 11.5, 11.6)

For Exercises 3–6, refer to Prescription 1. (LO 11.1)

Alan Capsella, MD
Westtown Medical Clinic
989-555-1234

Prescribed Date _July 8, 2012_

Name _Maria Ortiz_   DOB _____

Address _____

Rx: _Timoptic 0.5%_

QUANTITY: _5 mL_

SIG: _gtts ii right eye QID_

Refills: _2_

_MD398475_   _Alan Capsella MD_
Prescriber ID #   Signature

Prescription 1

3. What instructions should be printed for the patient?

4. How many times can this prescription be refilled?

5. By what route should this medication be administered?

6. What information should be on the drug label to verify that this medication is appropriate for the ordered route?

For Exercises 7–12, refer to Medication Order Form 2. (LO 11.3)

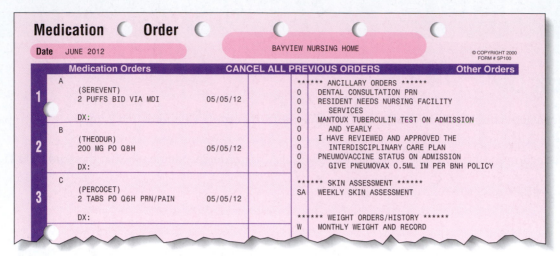

Medication Order Form 2

7. How often should Theodur® be given?

8. By what route is Serevent® administered?

9. If the patient receives Percocet® for pain at 4:00 a.m., when can the next dose be given?

10. If medications are delivered to this unit once daily, how many Percocet® tablets should be dispensed at one time?

11. What dose of Theodur® should be given?

12. How often should Serevent® be given?

For Exercises 13–18, refer to MAR 3 for Arthur Simmons. (LO 11.3, 11.4, 11.6)

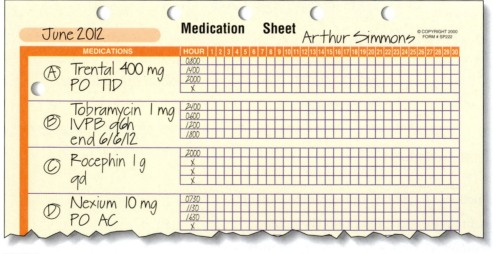

MAR 3

13. By what route is the tobramycin to be given?

14. What dose of Nexium® does Arthur Simmons receive?

15. What medications does Arthur Simmons receive at 8:00 p.m.?

16. How frequently does Arthur Simmons receive Trental®?

17. Should Arthur Simmons be served breakfast at 7:00 a.m., 7:30 a.m., or 8:00 a.m.?

18. Which orders do *not* have all the essential elements for a MAR order? State what is missing from each.

19. Identify and correct the error-prone abbreviation in order C.

For Exercises 20–30, refer to MAR 4 for Carrie Kay Smith. (LO 11.1, 11.3, 11.4, 11.6)

TCP Hospital Medication Administration Record

Order date	Medication, dose, duration frequency route	D/C date	Times		5 Feb	6 Feb	7 Feb	8 Feb	9 Feb	10 Feb	11 Feb
5 Feb 12	heparin 5000 units subcut on MAR 4 q8h		2400	0800							
			1600	X							
5 Feb 12	Bleph-10 OD q6h	05 Feb 12	0800	1400							
			2000	0200							
5 Feb 12	Premarin 1.25 mg daily		0800								
5 Feb 12	Proventil 2 mg PO bid		0800	X							
			1600	X							
5 Feb 12	Sinemet 25/100 tab i PO tid		0800	1400							
			2000								
5 Feb 12	Benadryl 25 mg PO q4h PRN/ITCH										

MAR 4

20. By what route will the heparin be given?

21. What dose of Premarin® will be given to Carrie Kay Smith?

22. At what times should Carrie Smith receive her Sinemet®?

23. Which medications will be administered at 1600?

24. If Carrie Smith has a dose of Benadryl® at 0200, when can she have her next dose?

25. How often should Carrie Smith receive heparin?

26. If the Proventil® were to be given TID instead of BID, how would the MAR be changed?

27. Which two medication orders are not complete, and what elements are missing?

28. Identify and correct the error-prone abbreviation in the Bleph-10 order.

29. At 1:30 p.m., you are preparing medications for patients who have just returned from lunch. Describe some precautions you might take to ensure that you administer the right dose.

30. You have just started your shift on a unit with geriatric and pediatric patients. You are scheduled to administer drugs to several elderly patients with Alzheimer's as well as to several children. What steps should you take to ensure that you administer the right drugs to the right patients?

For Exercise 31, apply The Joint Commission steps to receiving and writing a verbal order. (LO 11.2)

31. The nurse is receiving a telephone order from the physician. The physician and nurse have identified themselves, and then identified the patient by double identifier.

Step 1: The *authorized prescriber* states the order:
"Tylenol 650 mg pr"
The receiver writes:
The receiver asks:
The *authorized prescriber* states:
"every 4 hours as needed for headache."
The receiver fills in the blanks as the order is stated:
Tylenol 650 mg pr *q4h prn headache*
Step 2: *The receiver* states:
Step 3: *The receiver* continues on to confirm the order:

For Exercises 32–33, identify which of the three checks in the medication administration procedure is indicated. (LO 11.5)

32. The medication technician is about to hand the medication to the patient.

33. The medical assistant takes the bronchodilator out of the cabinet.

For Exercises 34–35, identify what observation should be made to promote safe medication administration. (LO 11.7)

34. The nurse is about to administer a subcutaneous injection.

35. The patient has received a medication.

36. If "yellow vision" is a sign of toxicity due to the drug digoxin, describe the appropriate patient teaching for this medication. (LO 11.8)

For Exercises 37–39, using international time and the following information, transcribe the orders to the blank MAR 5 on the next page. (LO 11.3)

- Daily refers to 8 a.m.
- Three times per day refers to 0600, 1400, 2200.
- Every six hours should be initiated at midnight.

37. Give Lasix 40 mg orally every day.

38. Give nifedipine 10 mg orally three times each day.

39. Give ampicillin 1 g intravenously every six hours.

Medication Administration Record (MAR)

MO/YR:	Start/Stop Date		Facility Name:																														
Medication		Hour	1	2	3	4	5	6	7	8	9	10	11	12	13	14	15	16	17	18	19	20	21	22	23	24	25	26	27	28	29	30	31
	Start																																	
	Stop																																	
	Start																																	
	Stop																																	
	Start																																	
	Stop																																	
	Start																																	
	Stop																																	
	Start																																	
	Stop																																	
	Start																																	
	Stop																																	

Diagnosis:	DIET (Special instructions. e.g. Texture, Bite Size, Position, etc.)	Comments
Allergies:	Physician Name	A. Put initials in appropriate box when medication is given. B. Circle initials when not given. C. State reason for refusal / omission on back of form. D. PRN Medications: Reason given and results must be noted on back of from.
	Phone Number	E. Legend: S = School; H = Home visit; W = Work; P = Program.
NAME:	Record #	Date of Birth:	Sex:

MAR 5

CRITICAL THINKING APPLICATIONS

What action should you take with the following drug order? (LO 11.1)

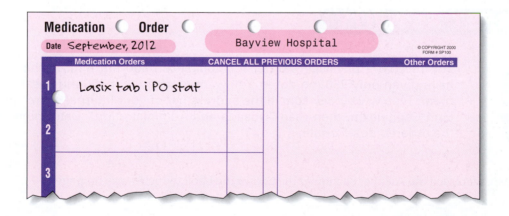

CASE STUDY

A physician gives a patient the following prescription. (LO 11.1, 11.8)

Alan Capsella, MD
Westtown Medical Clinic
989-555-1234

Prescribed Date *January 6, 2012*

Name *Martin Burke*   DOB *2/22/57*

Address *105 North Main, Bolivia, KS 88807*

Rx: *Xanax 0.5 mg*

QUANTITY: *120*

SIG: *tab i po tid with meals*

Refills: *1*

MD398475   *Alan Capsella MD*
Prescriber ID #   Signature

---

1. One of your jobs is to instruct patients on how to take prescription drugs. What should you tell Martin Burke?

2. If you are filling the prescription, how many tablets will you dispense to the patient? Will you refill the prescription?

INTERNET ACTIVITY

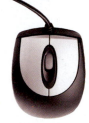

You receive a physician's order for Cephalexin 500 mg q6h. In the past, you have given only 250 mg doses. You want to verify that 500 mg is safe. *Assignment:* Type www.rxlist.com in the address bar of your Internet search program. Find Cephalexin, then read "Dosage and Administration." Determine whether the ordered dose is safe.

To check your answers, see the Answer section at the end of the book, which starts on page A-1.

GO TO . . . Open the CD-ROM that accompanies your textbook and complete a final review of the learning outcomes, practice problems, games, slideshow, and other activities presented for this chapter. Review your results then email or print them for your instructor. A score of 95 percent or above indicates mastery of the chapter learning outcomes.

For examples 1 and 2, rewrite the medication order interpreting the abbreviations.

1. Montelukast 10 mg tab i po q evening.

2. Morphine sulfate 10 mg supp pr q4h prn pain

For Examples 3 and 4, Identify which component of the medication order is missing.

3.

> Paul Mayor, DOB 8/27/53
>
> 5/4/2012 Paroxetine 25 mg po
>
> *T. Holmes, MD*

4.

> Carolyn Flynn, DOB 2/28/80
>
> 9/14/2011 Rifaximin po TID for 3 days.
>
> *Y. Xong, MD*

5. Which medications will be administered at 9:00 a.m. on 6/2, according to the following MAR?

Robert Reams, DOB 4/12/48		Allergies : iodine		Room 412				
Order	Time	6/1	6/2	6/3	6/4	6/5	6/6	6/7
Rosuvastatin 10 mg PO daily	0900	GF						
Cefuroxime Sodium 500 mg IV q12h	0900	GF						
	2100	SS						
Phenytoin 100 mg Po TID	0800	GF						
	1400	GF						
	2200	SS						

6. What is the volume of medicine in the cup?

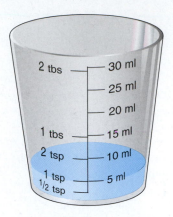

7. What is the volume of medicine in the dropper?

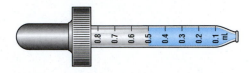

8. What is the dose of insulin in the following syringe?

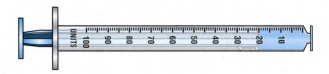

9. What is the dose of insulin in the following syringe?

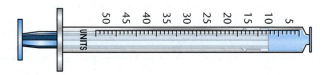

10. What is the volume of medicine in the following syringe?

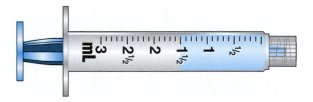

11. Answer the following questions about medication label A.

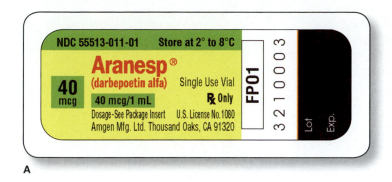

A

    a. Differentiate the brand name and the generic name of the drug.

    b. What is the dosage strength?

    c. Where are the lot number and expiration date located?

    d. How many doses are in this vial?

    e. List the storage instructions.

12. Explain the following medication administration routes.

    a. PO

    b. IM

    c. IV

    d. Subcut

    e. SL

13. Describe three types of information found on a medication package insert.

14. List eight components of a medication order and identify each component that is also considered a "Right of Medication Administration."

15. How will the medication technician ensure that the "right patient" is given the "right medication"?

16. Give an example of patient teaching that might accompany medication administration.

17. What important observation will the nurse make after administration of ibuprofen for pain?

18. Correct the following error-prone abbreviations and indicate why the abbreviation is no longer used.

    a. OD

    b. qhs

    c. QD

    d. SC

    e. U

19. What potential transcription error may occur from this order: Coumadin 5.0 mg PO daily? How can this error be avoided?

20. Identify three guidelines from The Joint Commission (TJC) regarding verbal orders.

To check your answers, see the Answer section at the end of the book, which starts on page A-1.

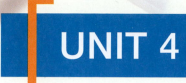

UNIT 4

Basic Dosage Calculations

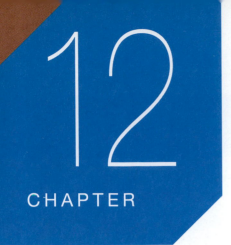

12 CHAPTER

Methods of Dosage Calculations

Each problem that I solved became a rule, which served afterwards to solve other problems.

—RENÉ DESCARTES

KEY TERMS

Amount to administer
Conversion factor
Desired dose
Dosage ordered
Dosage strength
Dosage unit
Dose on hand

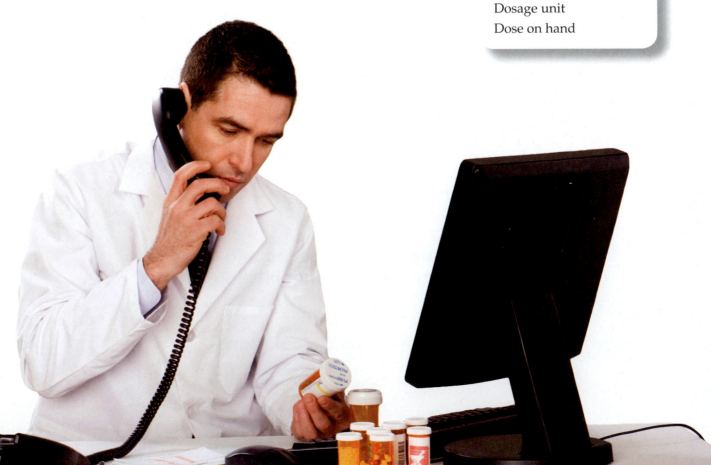

INTRODUCTION

It is time to bring together all the information you have learned in previous chapters to calculate the amount of medication to administer to a patient. You will bring together basic math, information from the physician's order and drug labels, and methods of converting quantities from one unit of measurement to another. Do not hesitate to refer to previous rules to help you solve the problems presented here.

12.1 Information Needed to Perform Dosage Calculations

Before you calculate the **amount to administer,** it is first necessary to determine the **desired dose.** The desired dose (the amount of drug given at one time) or "*D,*" is simply the ordered dose converted to the same unit of measurement as the dose on hand (found on the drug label) or "*H.*" The **dosage ordered** (desired dose), "*D,*" will not always be written in the same units as are found on the drug label. For example, an order may be written in grams while the drug is supplied in milligrams. When this occurs, it is necessary to convert grams to milligrams. This is done by using a **conversion factor** that identifies the equivalent amounts of each unit, in this case gram and milligrams.

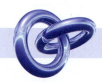

LEARNING LINK   Recall from Chapter 6 Rule 6-1, Writing Conversion Factors.

In order to calculate the amount to administer you will also need to know the **dosage unit** (*Q*), which is the quantity of solid or liquid in which the dose is supplied. See Figure 12-1 and Table 12-1.

This section reviews two methods that can be used to convert the desired dose into the same units of measurement as the dose on hand: the proportion method and dimensional analysis. Remember, each will give you the same result, and the method you use is a matter of personal preference. Once you identify the method you prefer, follow the color coding of that method.

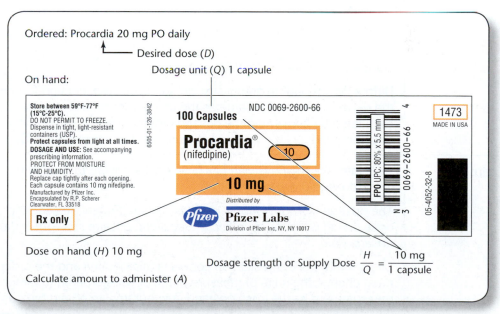

Figure 12-1   The language of dosage calculations.

TABLE 12-1 The Language of Dosage Calculations

TERM	ABBREVIATION	DEFINITION	EXAMPLES REFER TO FIGURE 12-1
Dosage ordered	O	The amount of drug to be given to the patient and how often it is to be given *This value will be found on the drug order or prescription.*	40 mg bid (twice a day)
Desired dose	D	The amount of drug to be given at a single time	This amount might require conversion to the same unit of measurement as the dose on hand.
Dosage unit	Q	The quantity of solid or liquid in which the dose is supplied. *This value will be found on the drug label.*	In Figure 12-1 this is capsules. Other examples include: tablets, 1 mL, 5 mL, drops, or units.
Dose on hand	H	The amount of drug contained in each dosage unit *This value will be found on the drug label.*	In Figure 12-1 this is 20 mg.
Amount to administer	A	The volume of a liquid or the number of solid dosage units that contains the desired dose *This value is found with a calculation.*	If the desired dose is 40 mg and the dosage strength is 20 mg per capsule, the amount to administer is 2 capsules.
Dosage strength, also called **supply dose**	$\dfrac{H}{Q}$	Dose on hand per dosage unit *This value can be determined from the drug label.*	In Figure 12-1 this is 10 mg per capsule.

RULE 12-1	Converting to Like Units of Measurement
	Before the amount to administer can be calculated, convert the unit of measure of the desired dose to the same as the unit of measurement of the dose on hand. This is calculated by converting the dosage ordered into the same unit of measurement as the dose on hand; once converted, it becomes the desired dose (*D*).
Example	Consider that the physician has ordered the patient to receive 0.2 mg of medication. This is the dosage ordered.
	The dosage strength (supply dose) is 100 mcg/tablet, making the unit of measure of the dose on hand micrograms (mcg). *Recall the dosage strength is the dose on hand per dosage unit.*
	Since the bottle of medication comes in micrograms and the order is for milligrams, you must change the units of measure of the dosage ordered (0.2 mg) to the same unit of measurement as the dose on hand (micrograms) to obtain the desired dose.

GO TO . . . Open the CD-ROM that accompanies your textbook, and select Chapter 12, Converting to Like Units of Measurement (LO 12.1). Review the animation and example problems, then complete the practice problems. Continue to the next section of the book once you have mastered the information presented.

PROPORTION METHOD

You can use proportions to convert from one unit of measure to another. The ratio of the units you have to the units you desire can be written two ways: $A:B = C:D$ (read as "A is to B as C is to D") or as a fraction $\frac{A}{B} = \frac{C}{D}$ (read as "A is to B as C is to D"). As a ratio multiply the means to equal the extremes ($B \times C = A \times D$). As a fraction, cross multiply the numerators with the denominators ($A \times D = B \times C$).

LEARNING LINK   Recall Chapter 6, Procedure Checklist 6-1.

Procedure Checklist 6-1

Converting by the Proportion Method

1. Write a conversion factor with the units that you are converting to as *A* (numerator) and the units you are converting from as *B* (denominator).

   $A:B$ or $\frac{A}{B}$

2. Write a proportion with the unknown *x* as *C* (numerator) and the number that you need to convert as *D* (denominator). *(The unknown is the desired dose D).*

   $x:D$ or $\frac{x}{D}$

3. Set up the proportion.

   $\frac{A}{B} = \frac{C}{D}$ or $A:B = C:D$

4. Cancel units.

5. Cross-multiply or multiply the means and extremes and then solve for the unknown value.

EXAMPLE 1

The dosage ordered is 0.2 mg once a day.

The dosage strength is 100 mcg per tablet.

Find the desired dose.

In this case, the drug is measured in milligrams on the drug order and micrograms on the drug label. The units for the desired dose must match those found on the drug label, which means that we must convert 0.2 mg to micrograms.

Follow the steps of Procedure Checklist 6-1.

1. Since we are converting to micrograms, micrograms must appear in the numerator of our conversion factor. Our conversion factor is $\frac{1000 \text{ mcg}}{1 \text{ mg}}$.

2. The other fraction for our proportion has the unknown D for a numerator. The value that is being converted, 0.2 mg or the dosage ordered, must appear as the denominator. Our conversion factor is $\frac{D}{0.2 \text{ mg}}$.

3. Setting the two fractions into a proportion gives us the following equation:

$$\frac{D}{0.2 \text{ mg}} = \frac{1000 \text{ mcg}}{1 \text{ mg}}$$

4. Cancel units.

$$\frac{D}{0.2 \text{ m\cancel{g}}} = \frac{1000 \text{ mcg}}{1 \text{ m\cancel{g}}}$$

5. Cross-multiply and then solve for the unknown.

$$1 \times D = 1000 \text{ mcg} \times 0.2$$

$$D = 200 \text{ mcg} = \text{desired dose}$$

EXAMPLE 2

Ordered: 500 mg q6h

Dosage strength available: 250 mg per tablet

Find the desired dose.

In this case the unit for the dose ordered is the same as that for the dose on hand. No calculation is needed. The drug is measured in milligrams on both the order and the drug label, so the desired dose D = 500 mg.

EXAMPLE 3

Ordered: Nitrostat® 800 mcg sublingually PRN chest pain

On hand: See Figure 12-2.

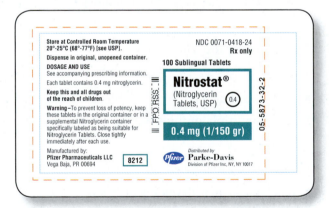

Figure 12-2

In this case, the drug is measured in micrograms on the drug order and in milligrams on the drug label. The units for the *desired dose* must match those found on the drug label, which means that we will convert 800 mcg to milligrams.

Follow the steps of Procedure Checklist 6-1.

1. Conversion factor 1 mg = 1000 mcg. Since we are converting to milligrams, our first fraction is:

$$\frac{1 \text{ mg}}{1000 \text{ mcg}}$$

2. The other fraction is:

$$\frac{D}{800 \text{ mcg}}$$

3. Set up the fractions.

$$\frac{D}{800 \text{ mcg}} = \frac{1 \text{ mg}}{1000 \text{ mcg}}$$

4. Cancel units.

$$\frac{D}{800 \text{ \cancel{mcg}}} = \frac{1 \text{ mg}}{1000 \text{ \cancel{mcg}}}$$

5. Cross-multiply and then solve for the unknown.

$$D \times 1000 = 800 \times 1 \text{ mg}$$

$$D \times \frac{1000}{1000} = \frac{800}{1000} \times 1 \text{ mg}$$

$$D = \frac{800}{1000} = 0.8 \text{ mg} = \text{desired dose}$$

DIMENSIONAL ANALYSIS

Recall from Chapter 6 that the dimensional analysis (DA) method is a modification of the proportion method. When we are using DA, the unknown value stands alone on one side of an equation. In this case, the unknown is the desired dose. The conversion factor is placed on the other side of the equation, and the number being converted is placed over 1.

Procedure Checklist 6-2

Converting Using the Dimensional Analysis Method

1. Determine the unit of measure for the answer, and place it as the unknown on one side of the equation.

2. On the other side of the equation, write a conversion factor with the units of measure for the answer on top and the units you are converting from on the bottom.

3. Multiply the conversion factor by the number that is being converted over 1.

4. Cancel units on the right side of the equation. The remaining unit of measure on the right side of the equation should match the unknown unit of measure on the left side of the equation.

5. Solve the equation.

EXAMPLE 1

The dosage ordered is 0.2 mg once a day.

The dosage strength is 100 mcg per tablet.

Find the desired dose.

The drug is measured in milligrams on the drug order and in micrograms on the drug label. The units for the desired dose must match the units of the dose on hand. We must determine how many micrograms is equivalent to 0.2 mg.

Follow the steps of Procedure Checklist 6-2.

1. The unit of measure for the answer is micrograms. Place this on the left side of the equation.

$$D \text{ mcg} =$$

(D represents the desired dose, which is the unknown.)

2. Since we are converting to micrograms, micrograms must appear in the numerator of our conversion factor. Our conversion factor is $\frac{1000 \text{ mcg}}{1 \text{ mg}}$. This will go on the other side of the equation.

3. Multiply the numerator of the conversion factor by the number that is being converted, the dosage ordered over 1.

$$D \text{ mcg} = \frac{1000 \text{ mcg}}{1 \text{ mg}} \times \frac{0.2 \text{ mg}}{1}$$

4. Cancel units. The remaining unit on both sides is micrograms.

$$D \text{ mcg} = \frac{1000 \text{ mcg}}{1 \text{ mg}} \times \frac{0.2 \text{ mg}}{1}$$

5. Solve the equation.

$$D = 1000 \text{ mcg} \times 0.2 = 200 \text{ mcg} = \text{desired dose}$$

EXAMPLE 2

Ordered: 500 mg q6h

Dosage strength available: 250 mg per tablet

Find the desired dose.

In this case the unit for the dose ordered is the same as that for the dose on hand. No calculation is needed. The drug is measured in milligrams on both the order and the drug label, so the desired dose $D = 500$ mg.

EXAMPLE 3

Ordered: Nitrostat 800 mcg sublingually PRN chest pain

On hand: Nitrostat 0.4 mg sublingual tablets. (Refer to Figure 12-2.)

In this case, the drug is measured in micrograms on the drug order and in milligrams on the drug label. The units for the desired dose must match those found on the drug label, which means that we will convert 800 mcg into milligrams.

Follow the steps of Procedure Checklist 6-2.

1. The unit of measure for the answer is milligrams. Place this on the left side of the equation.
   $$D \text{ mg} =$$

2. Since we are converting to milligrams, milligrams must appear in the numerator of our conversion factor. Our conversion factor is $\frac{1 \text{ mg}}{1000 \text{ mcg}}$.

3. Multiply the numerator of the conversion factor by the number that is being converted, the dosage ordered over 1.

$$D \text{ mg} = \frac{1 \text{ mg}}{1000 \text{ mcg}} \times \frac{800 \text{ mcg}}{1}$$

4. Cancel units.

$$D \text{ mg} = \frac{1 \text{ mg}}{1000 \text{ mcg}} \times \frac{800 \text{ mcg}}{1}$$

5. Solve the equation.

$$D = \frac{800 \text{ mg}}{1000} = 0.8 \text{ mg} = \text{desired dose}$$

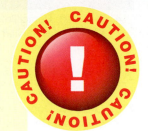

In Dimensional Analysis, Units Can Be Canceled Only When They Are Found in Both the Numerator and the Denominator of the Fraction

In an earlier example, the dosage ordered was in milligrams and the dosage strength was measured in micrograms. Suppose that you had used the conversion factor $\frac{1 \text{ mg}}{1000 \text{ mcg}}$ instead of $\frac{1000 \text{ mcg}}{1 \text{ mg}}$. Your equation would then have been:

$$D = \frac{1 \text{ mg}}{1000 \text{ mcg}} \times \frac{0.2 \text{ mg}}{1}$$

You may cancel units within a fraction only when they are found in both the numerator and the denominator. Here, the common unit (milligrams) is found in the numerator only and cannot be canceled. You should immediately realize that the conversion factor is incorrect because the units cannot be canceled. If you had not included the units when setting up the equation, the error might have gone unnoticed. *Always include the units when you are performing calculations.*

REVIEW AND PRACTICE

12.1 Information Needed to Perform Dosage Calculations

For Exercises 1–20, for each order: identify the dose on hand, dosage unit, desired dose, and if necessary identify the conversion factor and convert to like units of measurement. Use conversion tables from Chapter 4 and 5 as needed. For Exercises 8-20, use Labels A-M located below the table.

medication order	dose on hand	dosage unit	conversion factor	desired dose
1. Ordered: Amoxicillin 0.25 g On hand: Amoxicillin 125 mg capsules				
2. Ordered: Erythromycin 0.5 g On hand: Erythromycin 500 mg tablets				
3. Ordered: Phenobarbital 30 mg On hand: Phenobarbital 15 mg tablets				

(Continued)

medication order	dose on hand	dosage unit	conversion factor	desired dose
4. Ordered: Penicillin VK 0.25 g On hand: Penicillin VK 500 mg tablet				
5. Ordered: Levoxyl 0.15 mg On hand: Levoxyl 300 mcg tablets				
6. Ordered: Docusate 100 mg On hand: Docusate sodium elixir 150 mg/15 mL Available measuring device is marked in teaspoons				
7. Ordered: Robitussin 2 tsp Available measuring device is marked in mL				
8. Ordered: Biaxin 1 g PO daily On hand: Refer to label A.				
9. Ordered: Tranxene 30 mg On hand: Refer to label B.				
10. Ordered: Synthroid 0.05 mg On hand: Refer to label C.				
11. Ordered: Synthroid 0.088 mg On hand: Refer to label D.				
12. Ordered: Depakote 0.5 g On hand: Refer to label E.				
13. Ordered: Synthroid 250 mcg On hand: Refer to label F.				
14. Ordered: $1\frac{1}{2}$ teaspoon Zinthromax 200 mg/5mL PO q6h On hand: Refer to label G. (Only available measuring device is marked in mL.)				
15. Ordered: 7.5 mL clarithromycin PO q4h On hand: Refer to label H. (Available measuring device is a teaspoon.)				
16. Ordered: Levothroid 0.137 mg PO daily On hand: Refer to label I.				
17. Ordered: Levothroid 0.112 mg On hand: Refer to label J.				
18. Ordered: Risperdal 250 mcg On hand: Refer to label K.				
19. Ordered: Prandin 750 mcg On hand: Refer to label L.				
20. Ordered: Metformin 1 g On hand: Refer to label M.				

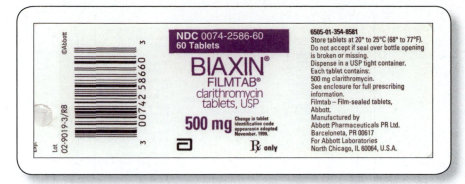

A

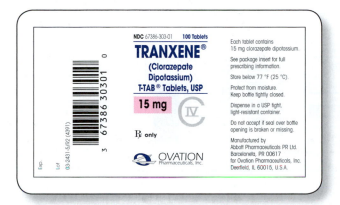

B

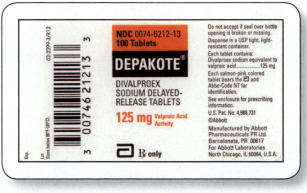

C

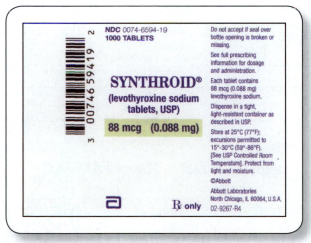

D

E

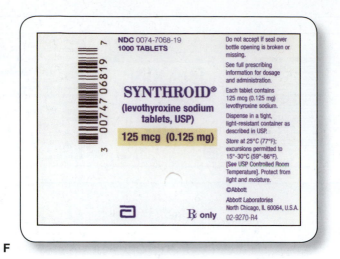

F

NDC 0074-7068-19
1000 TABLETS

SYNTHROID®
(levothyroxine sodium
tablets, USP)

125 mcg (0.125 mg)

Do not accept if seal over
bottle opening is broken or
missing.

See full prescribing
information for dosage
and administration.

Each tablet contains
125 mcg (0.125 mg)
levothyroxine sodium.

Dispense in a tight,
light-resistant container as
described in USP.

Store at 25°C (77°F);
excursions permitted to
15°-30°C (59°-86°F).
[See USP Controlled Room
Temperature]. Protect from
light and moisture.

©Abbott

Abbott Laboratories
North Chicago, IL 60064, U.S.A.

℞ only

02-9270-R4

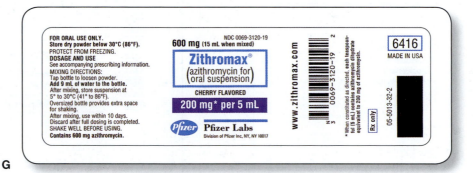

G

FOR ORAL USE ONLY.
Store dry powder below 30°C (86°F).
PROTECT FROM FREEZING.
DOSAGE AND USE
See accompanying prescribing information.
MIXING DIRECTIONS:
Tap bottle to loosen powder.
Add 9 mL of water to the bottle.
After mixing, store suspension at
5° to 30°C (41° to 86°F).
Oversized bottle provides extra space
for shaking.
After mixing, use within 10 days.
Discard after full dosing is completed.
SHAKE WELL BEFORE USING.
Contains 600 mg azithromycin.

NDC 0069-3120-19
600 mg (15 mL when mixed)

Zithromax®
(azithromycin for
oral suspension)

CHERRY FLAVORED

200 mg* per 5 mL

Pfizer **Pfizer Labs**
Division of Pfizer Inc, NY, NY 10017

www.zithromax.com

6416
MADE IN USA

* When constituted as directed, each teaspoonful (5 mL) contains azithromycin dihydrate
equivalent to 200 mg of azithromycin.

℞ only
05-5013-32-2

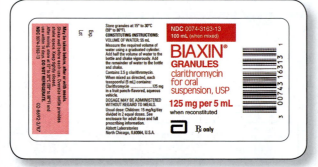

H

Store granules at 15° to 30°C
(59° to 86°F).
CONSTITUTING INSTRUCTIONS:
VOLUME OF WATER: 55 mL
Measure the required volume of
water using a graduated cylinder.
Add half the volume of water to the
bottle and shake vigorously. Add
the remainder of water to the bottle
and shake.
Contains 2.5 g clarithromycin.
When mixed as directed, each
teaspoonful (5 mL) contains
Clarithromycin ....125 mg
in a fruit punch-flavored, aqueous
vehicle.
DOSAGE MAY BE ADMINISTERED
WITHOUT REGARD TO MEALS.
Usual dose: Children: 15 mg/kg/day
divided in 2 equal doses. See
enclosure for adult dose and full
prescribing information.
Abbott Laboratories
North Chicago, IL 60064, U.S.A.

NDC 0074-3163-13
100 mL (when mixed)

**BIAXIN®
GRANULES**
clarithromycin
for oral
suspension, USP

125 mg per 5 mL
when reconstituted

℞ only

Exp.
Lot

May be taken before, after or with meals.
Shake well before each use. Oversize bottle provides
After mixing, store at 15° to 30°C (59° to 86°F) and
use within 14 days. DO NOT REFRIGERATE.
NDC 0074-3163-13

02-8692-3/R7

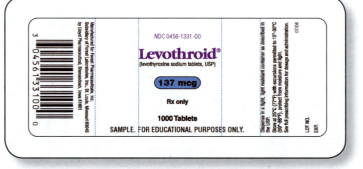

I

Manufactured for Forest Pharmaceuticals, Inc.
Subsidiary of Forest Laboratories, Inc.
by Lloyd Pharmaceutical, Shenandoah, Iowa 51601

NDC 0456-1331-00

Levothroid®
(levothyroxine sodium tablets, USP)

137 mcg

℞ only

1000 Tablets

SAMPLE. FOR EDUCATIONAL PURPOSES ONLY.

Dispense in a tight, light resistant container as described in
the USP.
Store at 25°C (77°F) with excursions permitted to 15°-30°C
(59°-86°F); protect from moisture and light.
See full prescribing information for dosage and administration.

07/04

LOT NO.
EXP.

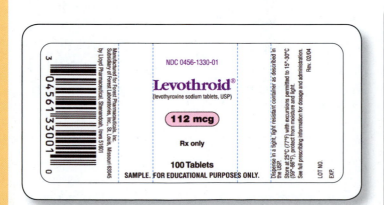

J

Manufactured for Forest Pharmaceuticals, Inc.
Subsidiary of Forest Laboratories, Inc. St. Louis, Missouri 63045
by Lloyd Pharmaceutical, Shenandoah, Iowa 51601

NDC 0456-1330-01

Levothroid®
(levothyroxine sodium tablets, USP)

112 mcg

℞ only

100 Tablets

SAMPLE. FOR EDUCATIONAL PURPOSES ONLY.

Dispense in a tight, light resistant container as described in
the USP.
Store at 25°C (77°F) with excursions permitted to 15°-30°C
(59°-86°F); protect from moisture and light.
See full prescribing information for dosage and administration.

Rev. 02/04

LOT NO.
EXP.

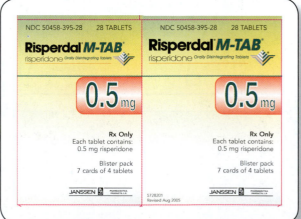

K

NDC 50458-395-28   28 TABLETS

Risperdal M-TAB®
risperidone Orally Disintegrating Tablets

0.5 mg

℞ Only
Each tablet contains:
0.5 mg risperidone

Blister pack
7 cards of 4 tablets

JANSSEN   PHARMACEUTICA
PRODUCTS, L.P.

5728201
Revised Aug 2005

NDC 50458-395-28   28 TABLETS

Risperdal M-TAB®
risperidone Orally Disintegrating Tablets

0.5 mg

℞ Only
Each tablet contains:
0.5 mg risperidone

Blister pack
7 cards of 4 tablets

JANSSEN   PHARMACEUTICA
PRODUCTS, L.P.

L

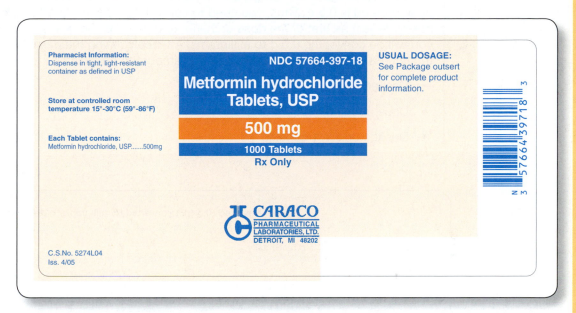

M

To check your answers, see the Answer section at the end of the book, which starts on page A-1.

12.2 Methods of Dosage Calculation

Once you have converted the desired dose to the same unit of measurement as the dosage ordered, you are ready to calculate the amount to administer. In this section, you will be presented three methods of dosage calculation: proportion method, dimensional analysis, and the formula method. Regardless of which method you use, always follow these steps:

Step A: Convert to like units of measurement.
Step B: Calculate the dosage.
Step C: Think! . . . Is It Reasonable?

RULE 12-2

Calculating the Amount to Administer
Step A: Convert
Convert desired dose to the same unit of measurement as the dose on hand (if applicable). NOTE: When using the dimensional analysis method introduced later in this chapter, step A will be to determine the conversion factor.

Step B: Calculate
Perform the dosage calculation using the method of your choice: proportion method, dimensional analysis, or the formula method.

Example

Ordered: Erythromycin 0.5 g PO twice daily.

On hand: See label (Figure 12-3).

Step A: Convert

In this case the dose on hand is 250 mg and the dosage unit is one capsule. The dose ordered is 0.5 g. Thus, you need to convert the dose ordered to the same unit of measurement as that of the dose on hand, to determine the desired dose. In this case you will be converting 0.5 g to milligrams. After calculating the desired dose, you have all the necessary information to calculate the amount to administer.

- Desired dose = 500 mg

- Dose on hand = 250 mg

- Dosage unit = 1 capsule

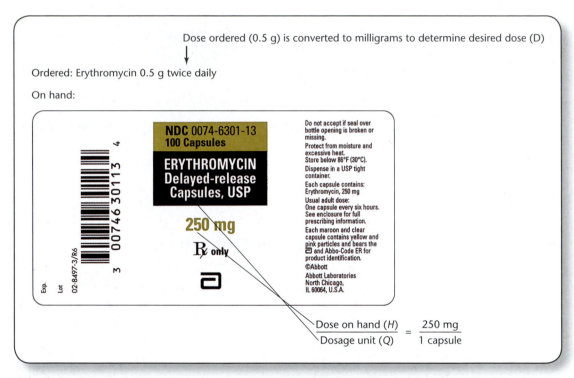

Figure 12-3 Information necessary to calculate the amount to administer. In this case the dose ordered must be converted to milligrams to obtain the desired dose.

GO TO . . . Open the CD-ROM that accompanies your textbook, and select Chapter 12, Amount to Administer (LO 12.2). Review the animation and example problems, then complete the practice problems. Continue to the next section of the book once you have mastered the information presented.

Procedure Checklist 12-1

Calculating the Amount to Administer by Proportion Method

1. The proportion will be set up as follows:

$$\frac{\text{Dosage on hand}}{\text{Dose unit}} = \frac{\text{Desired dose}}{\text{Amount to administer}} \quad \text{or} \quad \frac{H}{Q} = \frac{D}{A} \quad \text{or} \quad H{:}Q = D{:}A$$

2. Cancel units.

3. Cross-multiply the fractions, or multiply the means and the extreme, and then solve for the unknown value.

EXAMPLE 1

Find the amount to administer.

Ordered: Famvir® 500 mg PO q8h

On hand: See label in Figure 12-4.

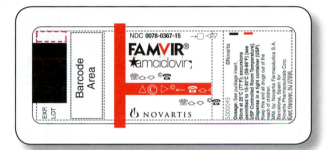

Figure 12-4

STEP A: CONVERT

The drug is ordered in milligrams, which is the same unit used on the label. Therefore, the dosage ordered is the same as the desired dose (500 mg), so no conversion is needed. By reading the label we find that the dosage unit is 1 tablet and the dose on hand is 250 mg. Therefore,

$$D = 500 \text{ mg}$$

$$Q = 1 \text{ tablet}$$

$$H = 250 \text{ mg}$$

STEP B: CALCULATE

Follow the Procedure Checklist 12-1.

1. Fill in the proportion.

$$\frac{250 \text{ mg}}{1 \text{ tablet}} = \frac{500 \text{ mg}}{A}$$

2. Cancel units.

$$\frac{250 \text{ mg}}{1 \text{ tablet}} = \frac{500 \text{ mg}}{A}$$

3. Cross-multiply and solve for the unknown.

$$250 \times A = 1 \text{ tablet} \times 500$$

$$A = \frac{500}{250} \text{ tablets}$$

$$A = 2 \text{ tablets} = \text{amount to administer}$$

If 1 tablet equals 250 mg, then how many tablets equals 500 mg? Do I need more or less than the dose on hand. (500 is greater than 250; therefore, more than 1 tablet is administered.)

What is the relationship between the dose on hand and the ordered dose?

(The ordered dose is twice a large as the dose on hand and 2 tablets is twice as many as 1 tablet, so it is reasonable.)

EXAMPLE 2

Find the amount to administer.

Ordered: Norvir® 200 mg PO now

On hand: See label in Figure 12-5.

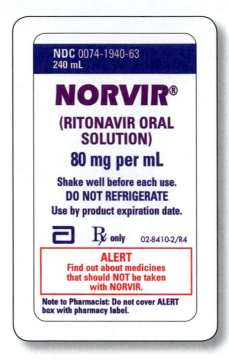

Figure 12-5

STEP A: CONVERT

Again, the drug order and the drug label use the same units, so no conversion is necessary. Our desired dose is 200 mg. Reading the label tells us that the dosage unit is 1 mL and the dose on hand is 80 mg. Therefore,

$D = 200$ mg

$Q = 1$ mL

$H = 80$ mg

STEP B: CALCULATE

Follow the Procedure Checklist 12-1.

1. Fill in the proportion.

$$\frac{80 \text{ mg}}{1 \text{ mL}} = \frac{200 \text{ mg}}{A}$$

2. Cancel units.

$$\frac{80 \text{ mg}}{1 \text{ mL}} = \frac{200 \text{ mg}}{A}$$

3. Solve for the unknown.

$$80 \times A = 1 \text{ mL} \times 200$$

$$A = 2.5 \text{ mL} = \text{amount to administer}$$

STEP C: THINK! . . . IS IT REASONABLE?

If 80 mg is in 1 mL, is it reasonable that 40 mg would be in 0.5 mL? (*80 is two times 40 and 1 is two times 0.5, so it is reasonable.*)

EXAMPLE 3

Find the amount to administer.

Ordered: 250 mg Ampicillin IM now

On hand: Ampicillin 0.5 g/mL

In this case, the order is written in milligrams, and the drug is labeled in grams. Before we can determine the amount to administer, we must calculate a desired dose that is in grams.

STEP A: CONVERT

Follow the Procedure Checklist 6-1.

1. Recall that 1 gr = 1000 mg. Since we are converting to grams, our conversion factor is $\dfrac{1\text{ g}}{1000\text{ mg}}$.

2. The other fraction for our proportion is $\dfrac{D}{250\text{ mg}}$.

3. Setting the two fractions into a proportion gives us the following equation:

$$\frac{D}{250\text{ mg}} = \frac{1\text{ g}}{1000\text{ mg}}$$

4. Cancel units.

$$\frac{D}{250\text{ m\!\!\!/g}} = \frac{1\text{ g}}{1000\text{ m\!\!\!/g}}$$

5. Solve for the unknown.

$$1000 \times D = 250 \times 1\text{ g}$$

$$D = 0.25\text{ g} = \text{desired dose}$$

STEP B: CALCULATE

Follow the Procedure Checklist 12-1.

1. Fill in the proportion.

$$\frac{0.5\text{ g}}{1\text{ mL}} = \frac{0.25\text{ g}}{A}$$

2. Cancel units.

$$\frac{0.5\text{ g\!\!\!/}}{1\text{ mL}} = \frac{0.25\text{ g\!\!\!/}}{A}$$

3. Cross-multiply and solve for the unknown.

$$0.5 \times A = 1\text{ mL} \times 0.25$$

$$A = 0.5\text{ mL} = \text{amount to administer}$$

STEP C: THINK! . . . IS IT REASONABLE?

If 0.5 g are is 1 mL, is it reasonable that there is 0.25 g in 0.5 mL? (Yes, it is reasonable; 0.25 is one half of 0.5 and 0.5 is one half of 1.)

EXAMPLE 4

Find the amount to administer.

Ordered: Metformin 2 g PO daily

On hand: See label in Figure 12-6 on the next page.

In this case, the order is written in grams, and the drug is labeled in milligrams. Before we can determine the amount to administer, we must calculate a desired dose that is in milligrams.

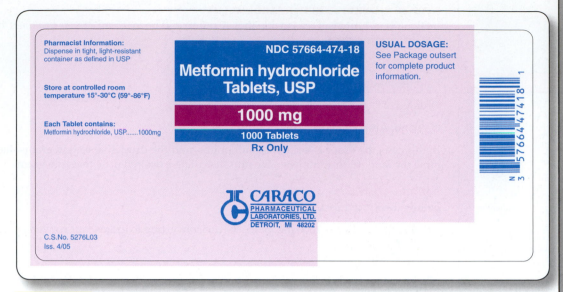

Figure 12-6

STEP A: CONVERT
Follow the Procedure Checklist 6-1.

1. Recall that 1 g = 1000 mg. Since we are converting to milligrams, our conversion factor is $\frac{1000 \text{ mg}}{1 \text{ g}}$.

2. The other fraction for our proportion is $\frac{D}{2 \text{ g}}$.

3. Set up the proportion equation.

$$\frac{D}{2 \text{ g}} = \frac{1000 \text{ mg}}{1 \text{ g}}$$

4. Cancel units.

$$\frac{D}{2 \cancel{\text{g}}} = \frac{1000 \text{ mg}}{1 \cancel{\text{g}}}$$

5. Solve for the unknown.

$$1 \times D = 1000 \text{ mg} \times 2$$

$$D = 2000 \text{ mg} = \text{desired dose}$$

$$D = 2000 \text{ mg} \qquad Q = 1 \text{ tablet} \qquad H = 1000 \text{ mg}$$

STEP B: CALCULATE
Follow the Procedure Checklist 12-1.

1. Fill in the proportion.

$$\frac{1000 \text{ mg}}{1 \text{ tablet}} = \frac{2000 \text{ mg}}{A}$$

2. Cancel units.

$$\frac{1000 \cancel{\text{mg}}}{1 \text{ tablet}} = \frac{2000 \cancel{\text{mg}}}{A}$$

3. Cross-multiply and solve for the unknown.

$$1000 \times A = 1 \text{ tablet} \times 2000$$

$$A = \frac{2000}{1000} = 2 \text{ tablets} = \text{amount to administer}$$

STEP C: THINK! . . . IS IT REASONABLE?

If 1000 mg is in 1 tablet, is it reasonable that there is 2000 mg in 2 tablets? (Yes it is reasonable, 1000 is one-half of 2000 and 1 is half of 2.)

GO TO . . . Open the CD-ROM that accompanies your textbook, and select Chapter 12. Determine *A* using the Proportion Method (LO 12.2). Review the animation and example problems, then complete the practice problems. Continue to the next section of the book once you have mastered the information presented.

DIMENSIONAL ANALYSIS

Procedure Checklist 12-2
Calculating the Amount to Administer using Dimensional Analysis

With dimensional analysis you will not need to calculate the desired dose and amount to administer separately. You will place your unknown (amount to administer) on one side of the equation and then multiply a series of factors on the right side of the equation. Canceling units will help you determine that the equation has been set up correctly.

1. Determine the unit of measure for the answer, and place it as the unknown on one side of the equation. (In this case the answer would be the amount to administer. The unit of measure will be the same unit of measure as that of the dosage unit.)

2. If the desired dose (dose ordered) is a different unit of measure than the dose on hand, use a conversion factor as your first factor. The conversion factor should have the same unit of measure as the dose on hand on the left side or top and the same unit of measure as the dose ordered on the right side or bottom.

3. Multiply the conversion factor by a second factor—the dosage unit over the dose on hand.

4. Multiply by a third factor—dose ordered over the number 1.

5. Cancel units on the right side of the equation. The remaining unit of measure on the right side of the equation should match the unknown unit of measure on the left side of the equation.

6. Solve the equation.

EXAMPLE 1

Ordered: Famvir® 500 mg PO q8h

On hand: Famvir® 250 mg per tablet. See Figure 12-4 on page 273.

Find the amount to administer.

STEP A: CONVERT
The unit of measurement for the desired dose and the dose on hand are both milligrams. No conversion factor needed.

STEP B: CALCULATE
Follow Procedure Checklist 12-2.

1. The unit of measure for the amount to administer will be tablets. This is the dosage unit.

   A tablets =

2. No conversion factor needed.

3. The dosage unit is 1 tablet. The dosage strength is 250 mg. This is our first factor.

$$A \text{ tablets} = \frac{1 \text{ tablet}}{250 \text{ mg}}$$

4. The dose ordered is 500 mg. Place this quantity over the number 1 for the next factor.

$$A \text{ tablets} = \frac{1 \text{ tablet}}{250 \text{ mg}} \times \frac{500 \text{ mg}}{1}$$

5. Cancel the units.

$$A \text{ tablets} = \frac{1 \text{ tab}}{250 \text{ \cancel{mg}}} \times \frac{500 \text{ \cancel{mg}}}{1}$$

6. Solve the equation.

$$A \text{ tablets} = \frac{1 \text{ tablet}}{250 \text{ \cancel{mg}}} \times \frac{500 \text{ \cancel{mg}}}{1}$$

$$A = 2 \text{ tablets} = \text{amount to administer}$$

STEP C: THINK! . . . IS IT REASONABLE?

If 1 tablet equals 250 mg, then how many tablets equals 500 mg? Do I need more or less than the dose on hand. (500 is greater than 250, therefore, more than 1 tablet is administered.)

Consider the relationship between the dose on hand and the ordered dose.

(The ordered dose is twice a large as the dose on hand and 2 tablets is twice as many as 1 tablet, so it is reasonable.)

EXAMPLE 2

Ordered: Norvir® liquid 40 mg PO daily

On hand: Norvir® 80 mg/1 mL. See Figure 12-5 page 274.

Find the amount to administer.

STEP A: CONVERT

The unit of measurement for the desired dose and the dose on hand are both milligrams. No conversion factor needed.

STEP B: CALCULATE

Follow Procedure Checklist 12-2.

1. The amount to administer will be in milliliters. This is the dosage unit or how the medication is supplied.

$$A \text{ mL} =$$

2. No conversion factor needed.

3. The dosage unit is 1 mL. The dose on hand is 80 mg. This is our first factor.

$$A \text{ mL} = \frac{1 \text{ mL}}{80 \text{ mg}}$$

4. The dose ordered is 40 mg. Place this over 1

$$A \text{ mL} = \frac{1 \text{ mL}}{80 \text{ mg}} \times \frac{40 \text{ mg}}{1}$$

5. Cancel units on the right side of the equation.

$$A \text{ mL} = \frac{1 \text{ mL}}{80 \text{ \cancel{mg}}} \times \frac{40 \text{ \cancel{mg}}}{1}$$

6. Solve the equation.

$$A = \frac{40 \text{ mL}}{80} = 0.5 \text{ mL} = \text{amount to administer}$$

STEP C: THINK! . . . IS IT REASONABLE?

If 80 mg is in 1 mL, is it reasonable that 40 mg would be in 1 mL? (80 is two times greater than 40, so it is reasonable.)

| **EXAMPLE 3** | Ordered: 250 mg Ampicillin IM now |

On hand: Ampicillin 0.5 g/mL

Find the amount to administer.

STEP A: CONVERT

The unit of measure for the dose on hand is grams. The unit of measure for the dose ordered is milligrams. Determine the conversion factor grams to milligrams.

STEP B: CALCULATE

Follow Procedure Checklist 12-2.

1. The unit of measure for the amount to administer will be milliliters.

   A mL =

2. Use the conversion factor.

   $A = \dfrac{1\ g}{1000\ mg}$

3. The dosage unit is 1 mL, and the dose on hand is 0.5 g. This is our second factor.

   A mL $= \dfrac{1\ g}{1000\ mg} \times \dfrac{1\ mL}{0.5\ g}$

4. The dose ordered is 250 mg. Place this over 1.

   A mL $= \dfrac{1\ g}{1000\ mg} \times \dfrac{1\ mL}{0.5\ g} \times \dfrac{250\ mg}{1}$

5. Cancel units to check your equation.

   A mL $= \dfrac{1\ \cancel{g}}{1000\ \cancel{mg}} \times \dfrac{1\ mL}{0.5\ \cancel{g}} \times \dfrac{250\ \cancel{mg}}{1}$

6. Solve the equation.

   A mL $= \dfrac{250\ mL}{500}$ (Reduce the fraction to its lowest terms.)

   $A = 0.5$ mL = amount to administer

STEP C: THINK! . . . IS IT REASONABLE?

If 0.5 g are is 1 mL, is it reasonable that there is 0.25 g in 0.5 mL? (Yes, it is reasonable; 0.25 is one half of 0.5 and 0.5 is one half of 1.)

| **EXAMPLE 4** | Ordered: Metformin 2 g PO daily |

On hand: Metformin hydrochloride 1000 mg. See Figure 12-6 on page 276.

Find the amount to administer.

STEP A: CONVERT

The unit of measure for the dose on hand is milligrams. The unit of measure for the dose ordered is grams. Determine the conversion factor grams to milligrams.

STEP B: CALCULATE

Follow Procedure Checklist 12-2.

1. The unit of measure for the amount to administer will be tablets.

   A tablets =

2. Use the conversion factor.

   A tablets $= \dfrac{1000\ mg}{1\ g}$

3. The dosage unit is 1 tablet, and the dose on hand is 1000 mg. This is our second factor.

   A tablets $= \dfrac{1000\ mg}{1\ g} \times \dfrac{1\ tablet}{1000\ mg}$

4. The dose ordered is 2 g. Place this over 1.

   A tablets $= \dfrac{1000\ mg}{1\ g} \times \dfrac{1\ tablet}{1000\ mg} \times \dfrac{2\ g}{1}$

5. Cancel units.

$$A \text{ tablets} = \frac{1000 \text{ mg}}{1 \text{ g}} \times \frac{1 \text{ tablet}}{1000 \text{ mg}} \times \frac{2 \text{ g}}{1}$$

6. Solve the equation.

$$A \text{ tablets} = \frac{2000}{1000} \quad \text{(Reduce the fraction to its lowest terms.)}$$

$$A = 2 \text{ tablets} = \text{amount to administer}$$

STEP C: THINK! . . . IS IT REASONABLE?
If 1000 mg are in 1 tablet, is it reasonable that there is 2000 mg in 2 tablets? (Yes it is reasonable, 1000 is one half of 2000 and 1 is half of 2.)

GO TO . . . Open the CD-ROM that accompanies your textbook, and select Chapter 12, Determine *A* Using Proportion Method (LO 12.2). Review the animation and example problems, then complete the practice problems. Continue to the next section of the book once you have mastered the information presented.

FORMULA METHOD

Procedure Checklist 12-3
Calculating the Amount to Administer by the Formula Method

1. Determine the components of the formula method, *D, H, Q,* and *A.*

2. Fill in the formula:

$$\frac{D}{H} \times Q = A$$

where *D* = desired dose (this is the dose ordered changed to the same unit of measure as the dose on hand).

H = dose on hand—the amount of drug contained in each unit.

Q = dosage unit—how the drug will be administered, such as tablets or milliliters.

A = unknown or amount to administer.

3. Cancel the units.

4. Solve for the unknown.

EXAMPLE 1

Ordered: Famvir® 500 mg PO q8h

On hand: Famvir® 250 mg per tablet. See Figure 12-4 on page 273.

Find the amount to administer.

STEP A: CONVERT
The drug is ordered in milligrams, which is the same unit used on the label. No conversion needed.

STEP B: CALCULATE
Follow Procedure Checklist 12-3.

1. *D* (desired dose) = 500 mg
   Q (dosage unit) = 1 tablet
   H (dose on hand) = 250 mg

2. Fill in the formula.

$$\frac{500 \text{ mg}}{250 \text{ mg}} \times 1 \text{ tablet} = A$$

3. Cancel units.

$$\frac{500 \text{ m\cancel{g}}}{250 \text{ m\cancel{g}}} \times 1 \text{ tablet} = A$$

4. Solve for the unknown.

A = 2 tablets = amount to administer

STEP C: THINK! . . . IS IT REASONABLE?

If 1 tablet equals 250 mg, then how many tablets equals 500 mg? Do I need more or less than the dose on hand. (500 is greater than 250, therefore, more than 1 tablet is administered.)

What is the relationship between the dose on hand and the ordered dose?

(The ordered dose is twice a large as the dose on hand and 2 tablets is twice as many as 1 tablet, so it is reasonable.)

EXAMPLE 2

Ordered: Norvir® liquid 40 mg PO daily

On hand: Norvir® 8 mg/1 mL. See Figure 12-5 on page 274.

Calculate the amount to administer.

STEP A: CONVERT

The drug order and the drug label use the same units. No conversion necessary.

STEP B: CALCULATE

Follow Procedure Checklist 12-3.

1. D (desired dose) = 40 mg

Q (dosage unit) = 1 mL

H (dose on hand) = 80 mg

2. Insert the numbers and units into the formula.

$$\frac{40 \text{ mg}}{80 \text{ mg}} \times 1 \text{ mL} = A$$

3. Cancel units.

$$\frac{40 \text{ m\cancel{g}}}{80 \text{ m\cancel{g}}} \times 1 \text{ mL} = A$$

4. Solve for the unknown.

0.5 mL = A = amount to administer

STEP C: THINK! . . . IS IT REASONABLE?

If 80 mg is in 1 mL, is it reasonable that 40 mg would be in 0.5 mL? (*80 is two times greater than 40 and 1 is two times greater than 0.5, so it is reasonable.*)

EXAMPLE 3

Ordered: Ampicillin 250 mg IM now

On hand: Ampicillin 0.5 g/mL

Find the amount to administer.

STEP A: CONVERT

In this case, the order is written in milligrams, and the drug is labeled in grams. Before we can determine the amount to administer, we must calculate a desired dose that is in grams. (In this example we will use proportion method Procedure Checklist 6-1.)

1. Recall that 1 g = 1000 mg. Since we are converting to grams, our conversion factor is:

$$\frac{1 \text{ g}}{1000 \text{ mg}}.$$

2. The other fraction for our proportion is $\frac{D}{250 \text{ mg}}$.

3. Setting the two fractions into a proportion gives us the following equation:

$$\frac{D}{250 \text{ mg}} = \frac{1 \text{ g}}{1000 \text{ mg}}$$

4. Cancel units.

$$\frac{D}{250 \text{ m\cancel{g}}} = \frac{1 \text{ g}}{1000 \text{ m\cancel{g}}}$$

5. Solve for the unknown.

$$1000 \times D = 250 \times 1 \text{ g}$$
$$D = 0.25 \text{ g} = \text{desired dose}$$

STEP B: CALCULATE

Follow Procedure Checklist 12-3.

1. D (desired dose) = 0.25 g

   Q (dosage unit) = 1 mL

   H (dose on hand) = 0.5 g

2. Insert the numbers and units into the formula.

$$\frac{0.25 \text{ g}}{0.5 \text{ g}} \times 1 \text{ mL} = A$$

3. Cancel units.

$$\frac{0.25 \text{ \cancel{g}}}{0.5 \text{ \cancel{g}}} \times 1 \text{ mL} = A$$

4. Solve for the unknown.

$$0.5 \text{ mL} = A = \text{amount to administer}$$

STEP C: THINK! . . . IS IT REASONABLE?

If 0.5 g are is 1 mL, is it reasonable that there is 0.25 g in 0.5 mL? (Yes, it is reasonable; 0.25 is one half of 0.5 and 0.5 is one half of 1.)

EXAMPLE 4

Ordered: Metformin 2 g PO daily

On hand: Metformin hydrochloride 1000 mg. See Figure 12-6 on page 276.

Calculate the amount to administer.

STEP A: CONVERT

In this case, the order is written in grams, and the drug is labeled in milligrams. Before we can determine the amount to administer, we must calculate a desired dose that is in milligrams. (In this example we will use the proportion method, Procedure Checklist 6-1.)

1. Recall that 1 g = 1000 mg. Since we are converting to milligrams, our conversion factor is:

   1000 mg : 1 g

2. The other ratio in our proportion is:

   D : 2 g

3. Set up the ratio proportion equation.

   1000 mg:1 g = D:2 g

4. Cancel units.

   1000 mg:1 $\cancel{g}$ = D:2 $\cancel{g}$

5. Multiply the means and extremes and solve the equation.

$$1 \times D = 1000 \text{ mg} \times 2$$
$$D = 2000 \text{ mg} = \text{desired dose}$$

STEP B: CALCULATE

Follow Procedure Checklist 12-3.

1. D (desired dose) = 2000 mg

   Q (dosage unit) = 1 tablet

   H (dose on hand) = 1000 mg

2. Insert the numbers and units into the formula.

$$\frac{2000 \text{ g}}{1000 \text{ g}} \times 1 \text{ tablet} = A$$

3. Cancel units.

$$\frac{2000 \text{ g}}{1000 \text{ g}} \times 1 \text{ tablet} = A$$

4. Solve for the unknown.

   2 tablets = A = amount to administer

STEP C: THINK! . . . IS IT REASONABLE?

If 1000 mg is in 1 tablet, is it reasonable that there is 2000 mg in 2 tablets? (Yes it is reasonable, 1000 is one-half of 2000 and 1 is half of 2.)

GO TO . . . Open the CD-ROM that accompanies your textbook, and select Chapter 12, Determine A Using the Formula Method (LO 12.2). Review the animation and example problems, then complete the practice problems. Continue to the next section of the book once you have mastered the information presented.

CRITICAL THINKING ON THE JOB

When in Doubt, Check

Jorge was working in the emergency room when a patient arrived with life-threatening internal bleeding. The physician in charge told Jorge, "Aminocaproic acid 5 grams STAT! You'd better give him liquid, I don't think he's able to swallow pills." Jorge repeated the order, "Aminocaproic acid liquid 5 grams STAT."

On hand, Jorge had Amicar Syrup (aminocaproic acid) 25%, 1.25 g/5 mL (see Figure 12-7). Jorge determined the amount to administer by using the ratio proportion method.

$$\frac{1.25 \text{ g}}{5 \text{ mL}} = \frac{5 \text{ g}}{A}$$

$$\frac{1.25 \text{ g}}{5 \text{ mL}} = \frac{5 \text{ g}}{A}$$

$$1.25 \times A = 5 \text{ mL} \times 5$$

$$A = \frac{25 \text{ mL}}{1.25}$$

$$A = 20 \text{ mL} = 4 \text{ tsp}$$

(Continued)

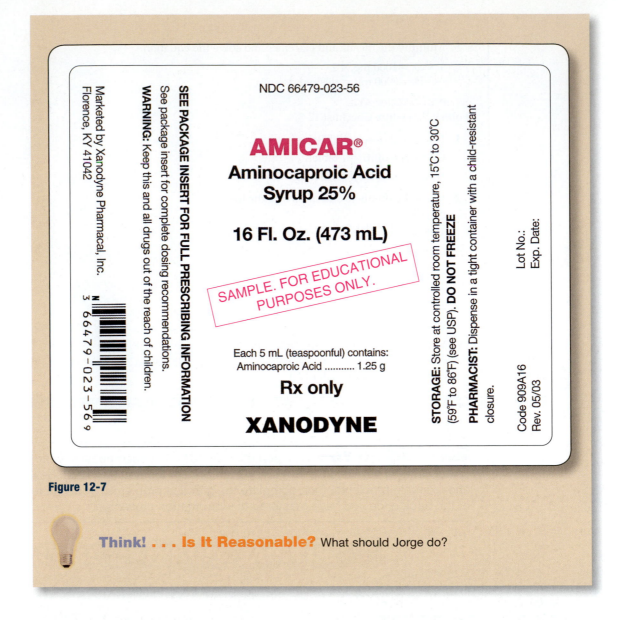

Figure 12-7

Think! . . . Is It Reasonable? What should Jorge do?

REVIEW AND PRACTICE

12.2 Dosage Calculations

In Exercises 1–20, calculate the amount to administer.

1. Ordered: Thorazine® 20 mg PO tid
   On hand: Thorazine® 10 mg tablets

2. Ordered: Ranitidine hydrochloride 150 mg PO bid
   On hand: Zantac® syrup 15 mg ranitidine hydrochloride per mL

3. Ordered: Ceclor® 0.375 g PO bid
   On hand: Ceclor® Oral Suspension 187 mg per 5 mL

4. Ordered: Nitroglycerin gr $\frac{1}{100}$ SL stat
   On hand: Nitroglycerin 0.3-mg tablets

5. Ordered: Amoxicillin 250 mg PO tid
   On hand: Refer to label A.

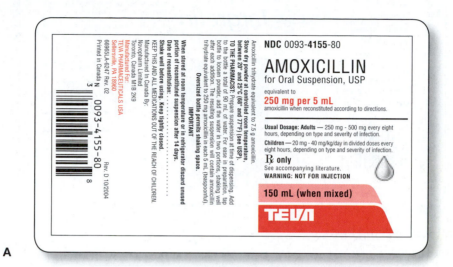

A

6. Ordered: Tricor® 108 mg PO daily
   On hand: Refer to label B.

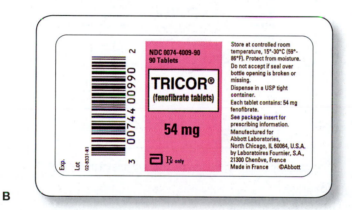

B

7. Ordered: Procardia® 20 mg PO tid
   On hand: Refer to label C.

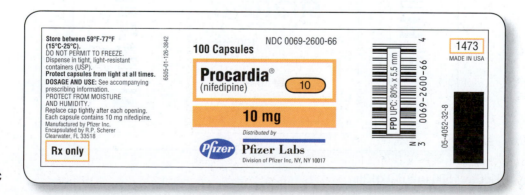

C

8. Ordered: Targretin® 150 mg PO daily a.c.

On hand: Refer to label D.

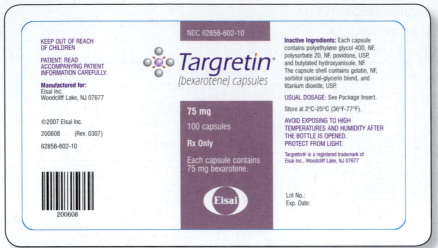

D

9. Ordered: Synthroid® 0.3 mg PO daily

On hand: Refer to label E.

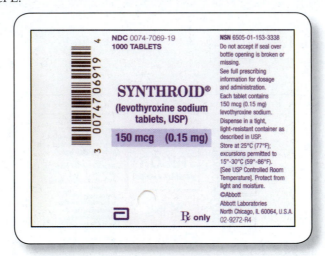

E

10. Ordered: Strattera® 0.1 g PO bid

On hand: Refer to label F.

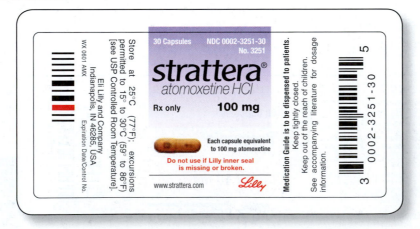

F

11. Ordered: Keflex® 500 mg PO q12h

On hand: Keflex® 250 mg per 5 mL

12. Ordered: Decadron® 6 mg IM q.i.d.
    On hand: Decadron® 4 mg per mL

13. Ordered: Ketoconazole® 100 mg PO daily.
    On hand: Ketoconazole® 200-mg scored tablets

14. Ordered: Dilaudid® 2 mg IM prn for pain q6h
    On hand: Dilaudid® for injection, 4 mg per mL

15. Ordered: Erythromycin Oral Suspension 150 mg PO bid
    On hand: Refer to label G.

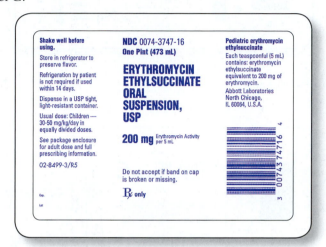

G

16. Ordered: Tranxene® 30 mg PO nightly before bedtime
    On hand: Refer to label H.

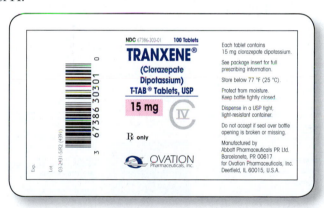

H

17. Ordered: Depakene® 150 mg po.
    On hand: Refer to label I.

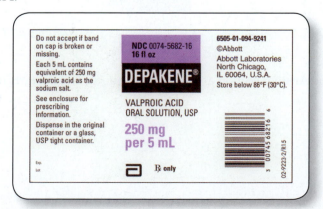

I

18. Ordered: Humulin® R 28 units subcut stat
    On hand: Refer to label J.

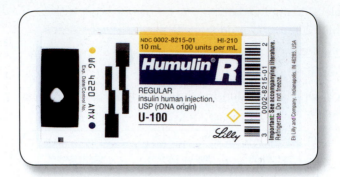

J

19. Ordered: Ritalin® 15 mg PO bid ac
    On hand: Refer to label K.

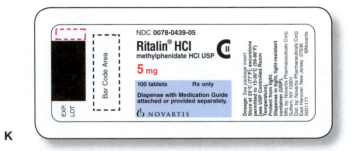

K

20. Ordered: Targretin® 75 mg PO q am ac
    On hand: Refer to label L.

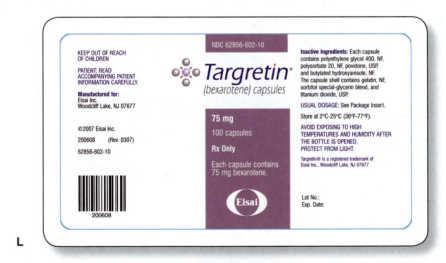

L

To check your answers, see the Answer section at the end of the book, which starts on page A-1.

LEARNING OUTCOME	KEY POINTS
12.1 Determine information needed to perform dosage calculation. Pages 261–271	*Dose ordered:* found on order or prescription, or MAR or eMAR *Dosage strength:* found on medication label as dosage unit (Q) per dose on hand (H) If the dose ordered is in a different unit of measurement from the dose on hand, convert them to the same unit of measurement. For example, if the dose ordered is 500 mg and the dose on hand is 1 g, convert 500 mg to grams using the Proportion Method (Procedure Checklist 6-1) or Dimensional Analysis (Procedure 6-2). **Proportion Method:** $$\frac{1 \text{ g}}{1000 \text{ mg}} = \frac{D}{500 \text{ mg}}$$ $$D = 0.5 \text{ g}$$ **Dimensional Analysis:** $$D = \frac{1 \text{ g}}{1000 \text{ mg}} \times \frac{500 \text{ mg}}{1}$$ $$D = 0.5 \text{ g}$$
12.2 Utilize three methods of dosage calculation. Pages 271–288	*Remember, D = desired dose, H = dose on hand, Q = dosage unit, A = amount to administer, Conversion factor = Units of measurement on hand/units of measurement ordered* **Proportion Method:** The proportion of the units you have to the units you desire can be written two ways: *Ratio $H : Q = D : A$* As a ratio multiply the means to equal the extremes ($Q \times D = H \times A$) *Fraction* $\dfrac{H}{Q} = \dfrac{D}{A}$ As a fraction, cross multiply the numerators with the denominators ($H \times A = Q \times D$). Use the Procedure Checklist 12-1 to convert to units using a ratio and a fraction.

Dimensional Analysis Method:

Step A: Convert

Determine if a conversion factor is needed

Step B: Calculate

Amount to administer

$$= \text{conversion factor} \times \frac{Q}{H} \times \frac{D}{1}$$

Step C: Think . . . Is It Reasonable? Example: Ordered: Metformin 2 g po daily On hand: Metformin hydrochloride 1000 mg per 1 tablet.

Step A: Convert A conversion factor is needed since the tablet strength is measured in mg, and the order calls for g.

Step B: Calculate

$$A = \frac{1000 \text{ mg}}{1 \text{ g}} \times \frac{1 \text{ tablet}}{1000 \text{ mg}} \times \frac{2 \text{ g}}{1}$$

Cancel and reduce

$$2 \text{ tablets} = 1 \text{ tablet} \times 2$$

Step C: Think! . . . Is It Reasonable? We know we will need more than 1 tablet since 2 g is more than the amount in 1 tablet (the amount in 1 tablet is 1 g, since 1000 mg = 1 g).

We also know that we need twice the amount found in 1 tablet, since 2 g is twice as much as 1 g. 2 tablets is twice as much as 1 tablet, so the answer is reasonable

Formula Method:`

$$\frac{D}{H} \times Q = A$$

Example: Ordered: Metformin 2 g po daily

On hand: Metformin hydrochloride 1000 mg per 1 tablet

Step A: Convert

$$\frac{1000 \text{ mg}}{1 \text{ g}} \times 2 \text{ g} = 2000 \text{ mg}$$

Step B: Calculate

$$\frac{2000 \text{ mg}}{1000 \text{ mg}} \times 1 \text{ tablet} = A$$

Cancel units and reduce

$$2 \times 1 \text{ tablet} = 2 \text{ tablets}$$

Step C: Think! . . . Is It Reasonable? (see above answer)

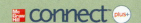
Answer the following questions. (LO 12.1)

1. Define the term desired dose.

2. Define the term dosage unit.

3. Define the term dose on hand.

4. Define the term amount to administer.

5. Define the term conversion factor and tell when it is used.

For Exercises 6–10, for each order: identify the dose on hand, dosage unit, desired dose, and if necessary identify the conversion factor and convert to like units of measurement. Use conversion tables from Chapter 4 as needed. (LO 12.1)

medication order	dose on hand	dosage unit	conversion factor	desired dose
6. Ordered: Flagyl 0.50 g po tid On hand: Flagyl 500 mg tablets				
7. Ordered: Synthroid 0.05 mg po daily On hand: Synthroid 25 mcg tablets				
8. Ordered: Tolbutamide 250 mg po tid On hand: Tolbutamide 0.5 g tablets				
9. Ordered: Dexamethasone 1000 mcg po now On hand: Dexamethasone 1 mg tablets				
10. Ordered: Erythromycin 0.5 g po q6h On hand: Erythromycin 250 mg tablets				

Select the appropriate label (pp. 292–293) for the following drug orders and indicate the number of tablets/capsules/milliliters that will be required to administer the dosage ordered. Labels may be used for more than one example. (LO 12.2)

Assume that all tablets are scored. Notice that both generic and brand names are used for the orders.

11. Ordered: 2 grams amoxicillin liquid. Label _____

Amount to administer: _____

12. Ordered: Zemplar® 1 mcg. Label _____

Amount to administer: _____

13. Ordered: Gleevec® 300 mg.

Label _____

Amount to administer: _____

14. Ordered: Nifedipine 10 mg.

Label _____

Amount to administer: _____

15. Ordered: Cefprozil 500 mg liquid.

Label _____

Amount to administer: _____

16. Ordered: Valproic acid 250 mg.

Label _____

Amount to administer: _____

17. Ordered: Sertraline HCL 75 mg.

Label _____

Amount to administer: _____

18. Ordered: Aranesp® 0.02 mg.

Label _____

Amount to administer: _____

19. Ordered: Amoxicillin 300 mg liquid.

Label _____

Amount to administer: _____

20. Ordered: Risperidone 1 mg.

Label _____

Amount to administer: _____

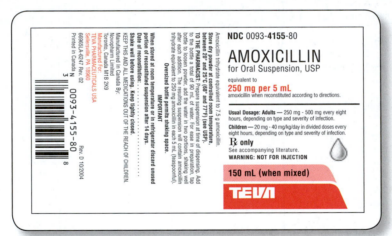

LABEL A

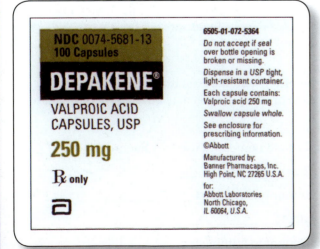

LABEL B

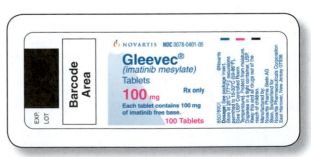

LABEL C

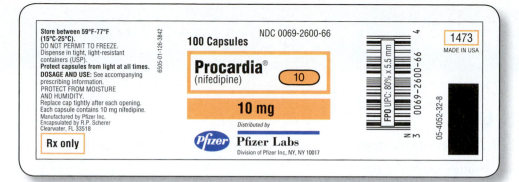

LABEL D

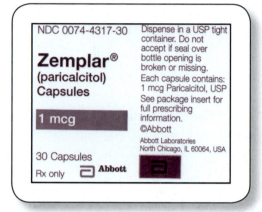

LABEL E

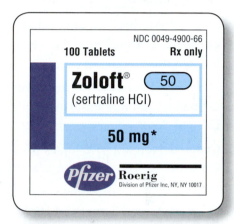

LABEL F

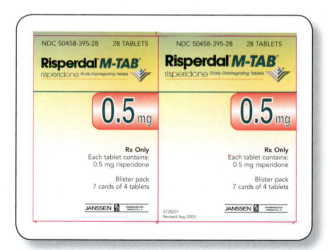

LABEL G

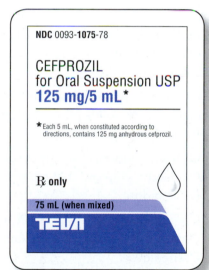

LABEL H

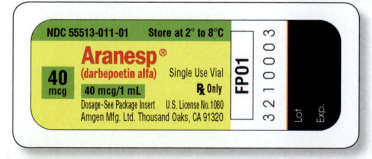

LABEL I

CHECK UP

For Exercises 1–23, calculate the desired dose. Then calculate the amount to administer. (LO 12.1, 12.2)

1. Ordered: Valium® 5 mg PO tid
   On hand: Valium® 2-mg scored tablets
   Desired dose: _____   Amount to administer: _____

2. Ordered: Atacand® 16 mg PO bid
   On hand: Atacand® 8-mg tablets
   Desired dose: _____   Amount to administer: _____

3. Ordered: Cimetidine 400 mg PO qid
   On hand: Cimetidine 200 mg tablets
   Desired dose: _____   Amount to administer: _____

4. Ordered: Noroxin® 800 mg PO daily ac $\bar{c}$ H$_2$O
   On hand: Noroxin® 400-mg tablets
   Desired dose: _____   Amount to administer: _____

5. Ordered: Tenex® 2 mg PO nightly at bedtime
   On hand: Tenex® 1-mg tablets
   Desired dose: _____   Amount to administer: _____

6. Ordered: Tranxene® 7.5 mg PO nightly at bedtime
   On hand: Tranxene® 3.75-mg tablets
   Desired dose: _____   Amount to administer: _____

7. Ordered: Pergolide mesylate 100 mcg PO tid
   On hand: Pergolide mesylate 0.05-mg tablets
   Desired dose: _____   Amount to administer: _____

8. Ordered: Zyloprim® 0.25 g PO bid
   On hand: Zyloprim® 100-mg scored tablets
   Desired dose: _____   Amount to administer: _____

9. Ordered: Zaroxolyn® 7.5 mg PO daily
   On hand: Zaroxolyn® 2.5-mg tablets
   Desired dose: _____   Amount to administer: _____

10. Ordered: Ciprofloxacin hydrochloride 500 mg PO q12h

On hand: Refer to label A.

Desired dose: _____   Amount to administer: _____

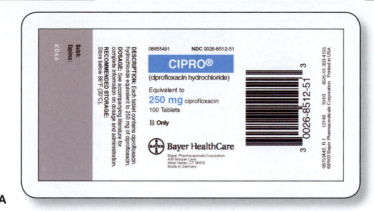

A

11. Ordered: Lexapro® 20 mg PO daily

On hand: Refer to label B.

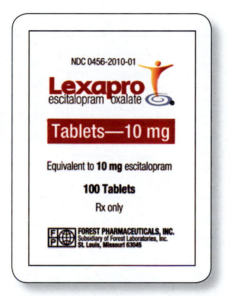

B

12. Ordered: Erythromycin 500 mg PO BID

On hand: Refer to label C.

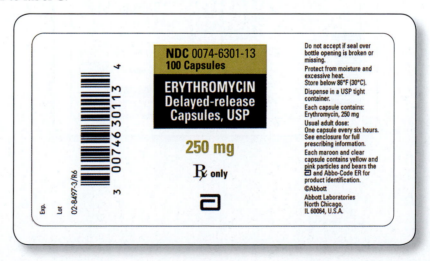

C

13. Ordered: Depakene® 250 mg PO bid
On hand: Refer to label D.

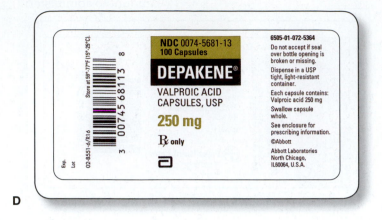

D

14. Ordered: Dilantin® 60 mg PO daily
On hand: Refer to label E.

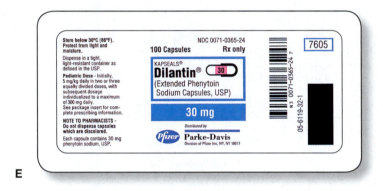

E

15. Ordered: Lisinopril 40 mg PO daily
On hand: Refer to label F.

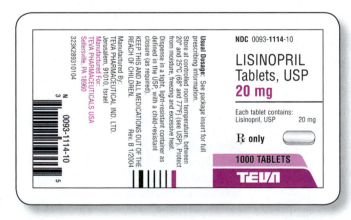

F

16. Ordered: Biaxin® 125 mg PO tid
On hand: Refer to label G.

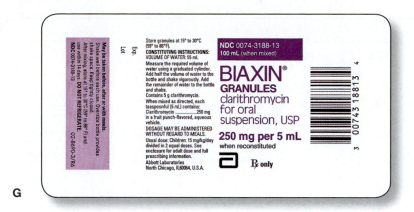

G

17. Ordered: Amoxicillin 1 gram PO bid
On hand: Refer to label H.

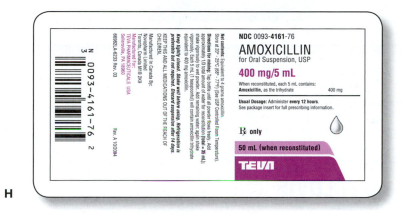

H

18. Ordered: Clarinex® 5 mg PO daily
On hand: Refer to label I.

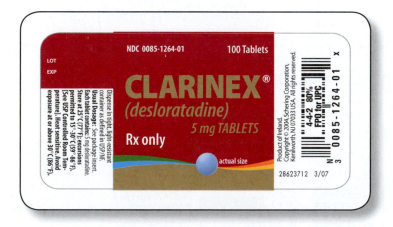

I

19. Ordered Cefprozil 200 mg PO q8h
On hand: Refer to label J.

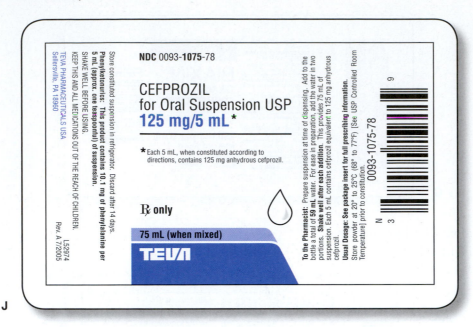

J

20. Ordered: Acyclovir 0.5 g IV now.
On hand: Refer to label K.

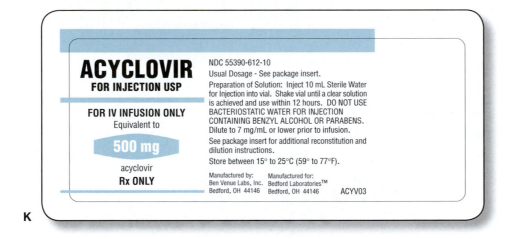

K

21. Ordered: Kytril® Oral Solution 4 mg PO tid
On hand: Refer to label L.

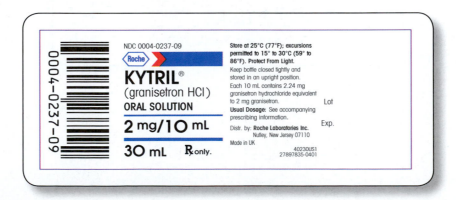

L

22. Ordered: Furosemide 100 mg IM now
On hand: Refer to label M.

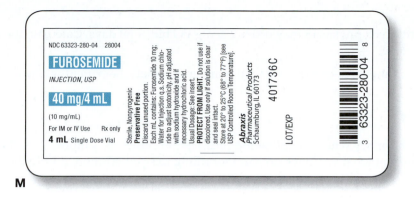

M

23. Ordered: Lipitor® 20 mg PO now
On hand: Refer to label N.

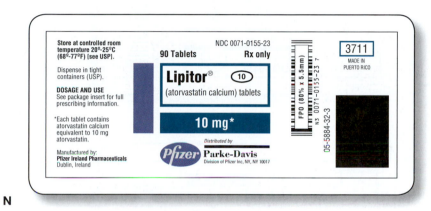

N

CRITICAL THINKING APPLICATIONS

Use the following label to answer the questions on the next page (LO 12.1, 12.2)

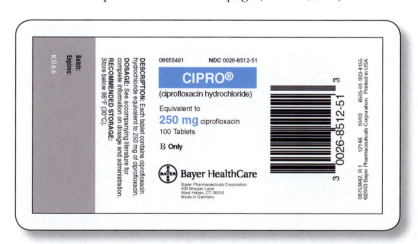

1. A physician's order reads Cipro® 250 mg q12 hr PO × 3 days. Calculate the amount to administer.

2. In some cases, the patient may receive 500 mg q12 hours × 10 days. Calculate the amount to administer for this dose.

3. For cutaneous anthrax a physician may order 250 mg PO bid × 60 days. Calculate the amount to administer for 1 dose.

4. In each of the cases above, determine the total number of tablets the patient will need.

CASE STUDY

You are working in a pharmacy when the following prescription comes in: Valium® 7 mg PO tid for 7 days. The drug labels below represent what you have on hand for filling this prescription. (LO 12.2)

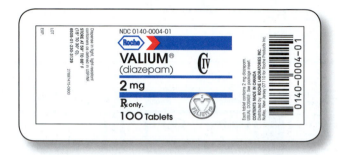

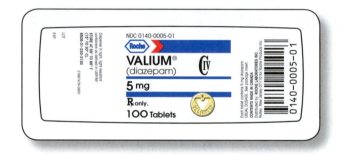

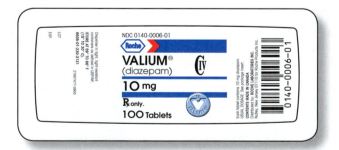

1. What is the amount to administer?

2. How many total tablets will the patient need?

3. What changes would you make in filling the order if the prescription read Valium 15 mg PO tid for 7 days? How many tablets will the patient need for this new order?

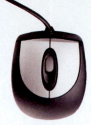

Many times medications come in different dosage strengths. (Recall the dosage strength is the dose on hand per dosage unit.) If you do not look at the label carefully, you can easily select the wrong medication and/or calculate the amount to administer incorrectly. Search the Internet for at least three medications, other than ones found in this chapter, that come in different dosage strengths. List each medication and its various dosage strengths.

To check your answers, see the Answer section at the end of the book, which starts on page A-1.

GO TO . . . Open the CD-ROM that accompanies your textbook, and complete a final review of the learning outcomes, practice problems, games, slideshow, and other activities presented for this chapter. For a final evaluation, take the chapter test and email or print your results for your instructor. A score of 95 percent or above indicates mastery of the chapter concepts.

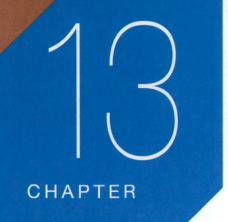

13

CHAPTER

Oral Dosages

If you want to achieve excellence, you can get there today. As of this second, quit doing less-than-excellent work.

—THOMAS JOHN WATSON, JR.

Learning Outcomes

When you have completed Chapter 13, you will be able to:

13.1 Demonstrate administration of solid oral medications.

13.1a. Calculate dosages for solid oral medications.

13.1b. Explain principles related to administration of solid oral medications.

13.2 Demonstrate administration of liquid oral medications.

13.2a. Calculate dosages for liquid oral medications.

13.2b. Explain principles related to administration of liquid oral medications.

KEY TERMS

Caplet
Capsule
Enteric-coated
Gelcap
Reconstitution
Scored
Spansules
Sustained release
Tablet

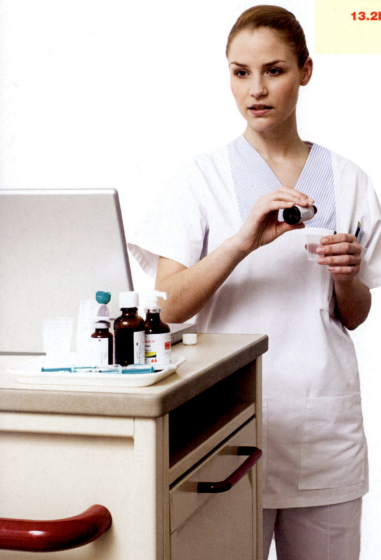

INTRODUCTION

You have learned the proportion, formula, and dimensional analysis methods for simple calculations. In this chapter you will apply these methods to oral dosages including solids and liquids. By now you may have chosen one method with which you are most comfortable. If so, follow that method throughout this chapter, using the corresponding color coding in the examples given; then complete the practice problems, using your method of choice. In this chapter you will also apply the principles of label reading learned in Chapter 10. Many practice problems in this chapter will require you to carefully read medication labels. While you are practicing these problems, remember that excellence is a *must* with dosage calculations.

13.1 Solid Oral Medications

Solid oral medications come in several forms, including tablets, caplets, capsules, and gelcaps (see Figure 13-1).

The **tablet** is the most common form of solid oral medication. It combines an amount of drug with inactive ingredients such as starch or talc to form a solid disk or cylinder that is convenient for swallowing. Certain tablets are specially designed to be administered sublingually (under the tongue) or buccally (between the cheek and gum). Sublingual and buccal tablets release medication into an area rich in blood vessels, where it can be quickly absorbed for rapid action. Some tablets are designed to be chewed; others dissolve in water to make a liquid that the patient can drink. Always check the drug label to determine how a tablet is meant to be administered.

Caplets are similar to tablets. Oval-shaped, they have a special coating that makes them easy to swallow. **Capsules** are usually oval-shaped gelatin shells that contain medication in powder or granule form. The gelatin shell usually has two pieces that fit together. These pieces may sometimes be separated to remove the medication when the patient cannot swallow a pill. **Gelcaps** consist of medication, usually liquid, in gelatin shells that are not designed to be opened.

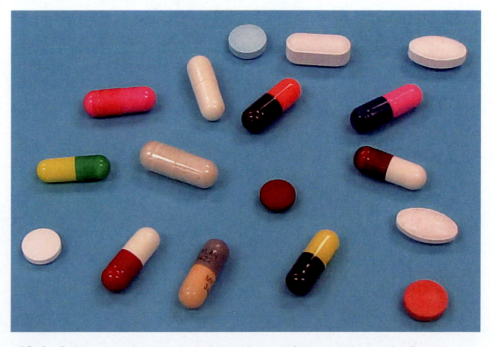

Figure 13-1 Solid oral medications including tablets, caplets, capsules, and gelcaps.

Calculating Dosages for Solid Oral Medications

Tablets are sometimes **scored** so that they can be divided when smaller doses are ordered. Most often, scored tablets divide into halves (see Figure 13-2), but some are scored to divide into thirds or quarters. The medication in scored tablets is evenly distributed throughout the tablet, allowing the dose to be divided evenly when the tablet is broken. Tablets may be broken into parts *only if they are scored,* and they must be broken only along the line of the scoring. Gloves must be worn when handling medication to prevent absorption of medication through the skin. Unscored tablets *must not* be broken into parts. Remember, breaking scored tablets to administer an ordered dosage is permitted but not optimal. Determine if another dosage strength is available before you break scored tablets.

RULE 13-1	Always question and/or verify when your calculation indicates to give a portion of a tablet when the tablet is not scored.
Example 1	Do not administer $\frac{1}{2}$ of an unscored tablet.
Example 2	Do not administer $\frac{1}{3}$ or $\frac{1}{4}$ of a tablet scored for division in two.

GO TO . . . Open the CD-ROM that accompanies your textbook, and select Chapter 13, Scored Tablets (LO 13.1). Review the animation and example problems, then complete the practice problems. Continue to the next section of the book once you have mastered the information presented.

RULE 13-2	Question and recheck any calculation that indicates that you should administer more than 3 tablets or capsules.

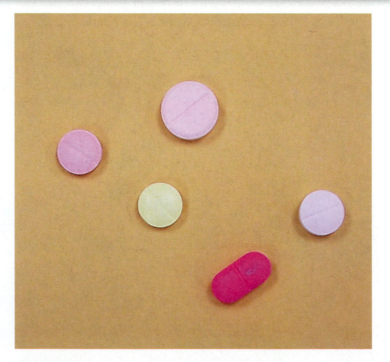

Figure 13-2 Scored tablets.

If the situations in Rules 13-1 and 13-2 arise, recheck your calculations. If you are confident that your calculations are correct, then check with the physician or pharmacist, or your drug reference book, to be sure there is no error in the order or the dosage strength you are using.

GO TO . . . Open the CD-ROM that accompanies your textbook, and select Chapter 13, Multiple Tablets (LO 13.1). Review the animation and example problems, then complete the practice problems. Continue to the next section of the book once you have mastered the information presented.

To calculate the *amount to administer,* you must know the *desired dose* and the dosage strength. The dosage strength is the amount of medication (dose on hand "*H*") per unit dose (dosage unit "*Q*"). This information should be clearly marked on the medication label. The desired dose and the dose on hand must be in the same unit of measurement.

RULE 13-3	Follow these steps when you are determining the amount of oral medication to administer to a patient.

Step A: Convert
If necessary, convert the *dosage ordered O* to the *desired dose D* that has the same unit of measure as the *dose on hand H.*

Step B: Calculate
Calculate: perform the dosage calculation using the method of your choice and round the volume for liquid medications according to the calibration of the equipment used for administration.

- The proportion method (using Procedure Checklist 12-1)

- Dimensional analysis (using Procedure Checklist 12-2)

- The formula method (using Procedure Checklist 12-3)

Step C: Think! . . . Is It Reasonable?
Apply critical thinking skills to determine whether the amount you have calculated is reasonable, keeping in mind both Rules 13-1 and 13-2. Recheck your calculation, if necessary.

PROPORTION METHOD

EXAMPLE 1   The order is to give the patient 15 mg codeine PO now. You have 30 mg scored tablets available.

STEP A: CONVERT
The desired dose (*D*) is 15 mg. The dose on hand *H* is 30 mg, and the dosage unit *Q* is 1 tablet. Because the desired dose and the dose on hand have the same units, no conversion needed.

STEP B: CALCULATE
Follow Procedure Checklist 12-1.

1. Fill in the proportion.

$$\frac{H}{Q} = \frac{D}{A} \quad \text{or} \quad \frac{\text{Dose on hand}}{\text{Dosage unit}} = \frac{\text{Desired dose}}{\text{Amount to administer}}$$

$$\frac{30 \text{ mg}}{1 \text{ tablet}} = \frac{15 \text{ mg}}{A}$$ or $$30 \text{ mg} : 1 \text{ tablet} = 15 \text{ mg} : A$$

2. Cancel units.

$$\frac{30 \text{ m\cancel{g}}}{1 \text{ tablet}} = \frac{15 \text{ m\cancel{g}}}{A}$$ or $$30 \text{ m\cancel{g}} : 1 \text{ tablet} = 15 \text{ m\cancel{g}} : A$$

3. Cross-multiply or multiply the means and extremes and solve for the unknown.

$$30 \times A = 1 \text{ tablet} \times 15$$

$$A = 1 \text{ tablet} \times \frac{15}{30}$$

$$A = 0.5 \text{ tablet}$$

STEP C: THINK! . . . IS IT REASONABLE?

Because 15 mg is one-half of 30 mg, $\frac{1}{2}$ tablet is a reasonable answer since the tablets are scored.

EXAMPLE 2   The order is Inderal 80 mg PO qid. You have 40 mg tablets available.

STEP A: CONVERT

The desired dose D is 80 mg. The dose on hand H is 40 mg, and the dosage unit Q is 1 tablet. Because the dosage ordered and the dose on hand have the same units, no conversion is needed.

STEP B: CALCULATE

Follow Procedure Checklist 12-1.

1. Fill in the proportion.

$$\frac{40 \text{ mg}}{1 \text{ tablet}} = \frac{80 \text{ mg}}{A}$$ or $$40 \text{ mg} : 1 \text{ tablet} = 80 \text{ mg} : A$$

2. Cancel units.

$$\frac{40 \text{ m\cancel{g}}}{1 \text{ tablet}} = \frac{80 \text{ m\cancel{g}}}{A}$$ or $$40 \text{ m\cancel{g}} : 1 \text{ tablet} = 80 \text{ m\cancel{g}} : A$$

3. Cross-multiply or multiply the means and extremes and solve for the unknown.

$$40 \times A = 1 \text{ tablet} \times 80$$

$$A = 1 \text{ tablet} \times \frac{80}{40}$$

$$A = 2 \text{ tablets}$$

STEP C: THINK! . . . IS IT REASONABLE?

80 is twice 40 so this dose requires twice 1 tablet. The calculated dosage does not call for more than 3 tablets, so this answer seems reasonable.

EXAMPLE 3   Refer to Figures 13-3 and 13-4.

STEP A: CONVERT

Apply Rule 12-2

Convert desired dose to same unit of measurement as the dose on hand, if necessary. The desired dose (D) is 0.5 g. The dose on hand H is 250 mg, and the dosage unit Q is 1 tablet. Because the dosage ordered and the dose on hand are in different units, you need to convert the dosage ordered to milligrams.

Follow Procedure Checklist 6-1.

1. Fill in the proportion, recalling that 1 g = 1000 mg.

$$\frac{1000 \text{ mg}}{1 \text{ g}} = \frac{x}{0.5 \text{ g}}$$ or $$1000 \text{ mg} : 1 \text{ g} = x \text{ mg} : 0.5 \text{ g}$$

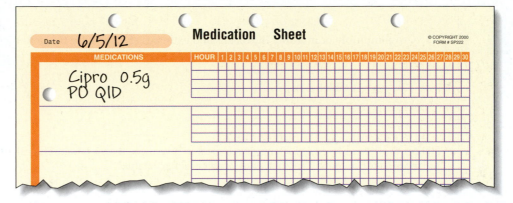

Figure 13-3 Medication ordered.

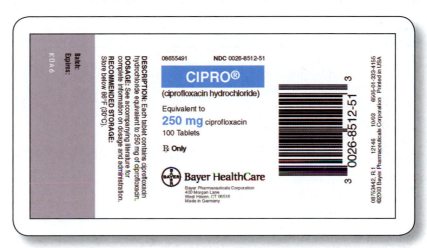

Figure 13-4 Medication on hand.

2. Cancel units.

$$\frac{1000 \text{ mg}}{1 \, g} = \frac{x}{0.5 \, g} \qquad \text{or} \qquad 1000 \text{ mg} : 1 \, g = x \text{ mg} : 0.5 \, g$$

3. Cross-multiply or multiply the means and extremes and solve for the unknown.

$$1 \times x = 0.5 \times 1000 \text{ mg}$$

$$x = 500 \text{ mg}$$

STEP B: CALCULATE

Follow Procedure Checklist 12-1.

1. Fill in the proportion.

$$\frac{250 \text{ mg}}{1 \text{ tablet}} = \frac{500 \text{ mg}}{A} \qquad \text{or} \qquad 250 \text{ mg} : 1 \text{ tablet} = 500 \text{ mg} : A$$

2. Cancel units.

$$\frac{250 \text{ mg}}{1 \text{ tablet}} = \frac{500 \text{ mg}}{A} \qquad \text{or} \qquad 250 \text{ mg} : 1 \text{ tablet} = 500 \text{ mg} : A$$

3. Cross-multiply or multiply the means and extremes and solve for the unknown.

$$250 \times A = 1 \text{ tablet} \times 500$$

$$A = 1 \text{ tablet} \times \frac{500}{250}$$

$$A = 2 \text{ tablets}$$

STEP C: THINK! . . . IS IT REASONABLE?

500 mg is twice as large as 250 mg. It is logical to give more than 1 tablet. The calculation does not call for more than 3 tablets. The answer of 2 tablets is reasonable.

DIMENSIONAL ANALYSIS

EXAMPLE 1

The order is to give the patient 15 mg codeine PO now. You have 30 mg scored tablets available.

STEP A: CONVERT

The unit of measurement for the desired dose and the dose on hand are both milligrams. No conversion factor needed.

STEP B: CALCULATE

Follow Procedure Checklist 12-2.

1. The unit of measure for the amount to administer will be tablets.

$$A \text{ tablets} =$$

2. No conversion factor needed.

3. The dosage unit is 1 tablet. The dosage on hand is 30 mg.

$$A \text{ tablets} = \frac{1 \text{ tablet}}{30 \text{ mg}}$$

4. The dosage ordered is 15 mg.

$$A \text{ tablets} = \frac{1 \text{ tablet}}{30 \text{ mg}} \times \frac{15 \text{ mg}}{1}$$

5. Cancel units.

$$A \text{ tablets} = \frac{1 \text{ tablet}}{30 \cancel{\text{ mg}}} \times \frac{15 \cancel{\text{ mg}}}{1}$$

6. Solve the equation.

$$A \text{ tablets} = \frac{1 \text{ tablet}}{30} \times \frac{15}{1}$$

$$A = 0.5 \text{ tablet} = \frac{1}{2} \text{ tablet}$$

STEP C: THINK! . . . IS IT REASONABLE?

Because 15 mg is one-half of 30 mg, $\frac{1}{2}$ tablet is an appropriate answer since the tablets are scored.

EXAMPLE 2

The order is Inderal® 80 mg PO qid. You have 40 mg tablets available.

STEP A: CONVERT

The unit of measurement for the desired dose and the dose on hand are both milligrams. No conversion factor needed.

STEP B: CALCULATE

Follow Procedure Checklist 12-2.

1. The unit of measure for the amount to administer will be tablets.

   A tablets =

2. No conversion factor needed.

3. The dosage unit is 1 tablet. The dose on hand is 40 mg.

   $$A \text{ tablets} = \frac{1 \text{ tablet}}{40 \text{ mg}}$$

4. The dosage ordered is 80 mg.

   $$A \text{ tablets} = \frac{1 \text{ tablet}}{40 \text{ mg}} \times \frac{80 \text{ mg}}{1}$$

5. Cancel units.

   $$A \text{ tablets} = \frac{1 \text{ tablet}}{40 \text{ \cancel{mg}}} \times \frac{80 \text{ \cancel{mg}}}{1}$$

6. Solve the equation.

   $$A \text{ tablets} = \frac{1 \text{ tablet}}{40 \text{ mg}} \times \frac{80}{1}$$

   $$A = 2 \text{ tablets}$$

STEP C: THINK! . . . IS IT REASONABLE?

80 is 40 × 2, so this dose requires twice 1 tablet. The calculated dosage does not call for more than 3 tablets.

EXAMPLE 3

Refer to Figures 13-3 and 13-4 on page 307.

STEP A: CONVERT

The unit of measure for the dose on hand is milligrams. The unit of measure for the dose ordered is grams. Determine the conversion factor milligrams to grams.

STEP B: CALCULATE

Follow Procedure Checklist 12-2.

1. The unit of measure for the amount to administer will be tablets.

   A tablets =

2. The unit of measure for the dosage ordered is grams. The unit of measure for the dose on hand is milligrams. Recall that 1 g = 1000 mg. Because we wish to convert to milligrams (the units of the dose on hand), our first factor must have milligrams on top.

   $$A \text{ tablets} = \frac{1000 \text{ mg}}{1 \text{ g}}$$

3. The dosage unit is 1 tablet. The dose on hand is 250 mg. This is the second factor.

   $$A \text{ tablets} = \frac{1000 \text{ mg}}{1 \text{ g}} \times \frac{1 \text{ tablet}}{250 \text{ mg}}$$

4. The dosage ordered is 0.5 g. Place this over 1 and set up the equation.

   $$A \text{ tablets} = \frac{1000 \text{ mg}}{1 \text{ g}} \times \frac{1 \text{ tablet}}{250 \text{ mg}} \times \frac{0.5 \text{ g}}{1}$$

5. Cancel units.

   $$A \text{ tablets} = \frac{1000 \text{ \cancel{mg}}}{1 \text{ \cancel{g}}} \times \frac{1 \text{ tablet}}{250 \text{ \cancel{mg}}} \times \frac{0.5 \text{ \cancel{g}}}{1}$$

6. Solve the equation.

$$A \text{ tablets} = \frac{1000}{1} \times \frac{1 \text{ tablet}}{250} \times \frac{0.5}{1}$$

$$A = 2 \text{ tablets}$$

STEP C: THINK! . . . IS IT REASONABLE?

500 mg is larger than 250 mg. It is logical to give more than 1 tablet. The calculation does not call for more than 3 tablets. The answer of 2 tablets is reasonable.

FORMULA METHOD

EXAMPLE 1

The order is to give the patient 15 mg codeine PO now. You have 30 mg scored tablets available.

STEP A: CONVERT

The drug is ordered in milligrams, which is the same unit of measure as that for the dose on hand. No conversion needed.

STEP B: CALCULATE

Follow Procedure Checklist 12-3.

1. Determine the components of the formula method.

$$D = 15 \text{ mg}$$

$$Q = 1 \text{ tablet}$$

$$H = 30 \text{ mg}$$

2. Fill in the formula.

$$\frac{D}{H} \times Q = A$$

$$\frac{15 \text{ mg}}{30 \text{ mg}} \times 1 \text{ tablet} = A$$

3. Cancel units.

$$\frac{15 \, \cancel{\text{mg}}}{30 \, \cancel{\text{mg}}} \times 1 \text{ tablet} = A$$

4. Solve for the unknown.

$$\frac{1}{2} \times 1 \text{ tablet} = A$$

$$A = 0.5 \text{ tablet} = \frac{1}{2} \text{ tablet}$$

STEP C: THINK! . . . IS IT REASONABLE?

Because 15 mg is one-half of 30 mg, $\frac{1}{2}$ tablet is a reasonable answer since the tablets are scored.

EXAMPLE 2

The order is Inderal® 80 mg PO qid. You have 40 mg tablets available.

STEP A: CONVERT

The drug is ordered in milligrams, which is the same unit of measure as that for the dose on hand. No conversion needed.

STEP B: CALCULATE

Follow Procedure Checklist 12-3.

1. Determine the components of the formula method.

    $D = 80$ mg

    $Q = 1$ tablet

    $H = 40$ mg

2. Fill in the formula.

    $$\frac{80 \text{ mg}}{40 \text{ mg}} \times 1 \text{ tablet} = A$$

3. Cancel units.

    $$\frac{80 \text{ mg}}{40 \text{ mg}} \times 1 \text{ tablet} = A$$

4. Solve for the unknown.

    2×1 tablet $= A$

    $A = 2$ tablets

STEP C: THINK! . . . IS IT REASONABLE?

80 is 40 × 2, so this dose requires twice 1 tablet. The calculated dosage does not call for more than 3 tablets.

EXAMPLE 3   Refer to Figures 13-3 and 13-4 on page 307.

STEP A: CONVERT

The desired dose, 0.5 g, to the same unit of measurement as the dose on hand, milligrams. Recall that 1 g = 1000 mg, therefore, convert by setting up the proportion:

$$\frac{1 \text{ g}}{1000 \text{ mg}} = \frac{0.5 \text{ g}}{D}$$

$D = 500$ mg

STEP B: CALCULATE

Follow Procedure Checklist 12-3

1. Determine the components of the formula method.

    $D = 500$ mg

    $Q = 1$ tablet

    $H = 250$ mg

2. Fill in the formula.

    $$\frac{500 \text{ mg}}{250 \text{ mg}} \times 1 \text{ tablet} = A$$

3. Cancel units.

    $$\frac{500 \text{ mg}}{250 \text{ mg}} \times 1 \text{ tablet} = A$$

4. Solve for the unknown.

    2×1 tablet $= A$

    2 tablets $= A$

STEP C: THINK! . . . IS IT REASONABLE?

500 mg is larger than 250 mg. It is logical to give more than 1 tablet. The calculation does not call for more than 3 tablets. The answer of 2 tablets is reasonable.

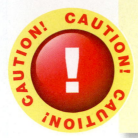 **GO TO . . .** Open the CD-ROM that accompanies your textbook, and select Chapter 13, Determining the Amount to Administer (LO 13.1). Review the animation and example problems, then complete the practice problems. Continue to the next section of the book once you have mastered the information presented.

ERROR ALERT!

Observe Patients as They Take Their Medications

Medications left at the bedside lead to errors because patients may:

- Forget to take the medication or may consume it at an incorrect time.
- Inadvertently spill or drop medication.
- Encounter difficulty when swallowing leading to potential aspiration.

Crushing Tablets or Opening Capsules

For patients who have difficulty swallowing pills, you may crush certain tablets and open certain capsules. However, in many settings such as nursing homes, you must first get a physician's order. Check with your facility about these policies before you crush tablets. See Figure 13-6.

Sometimes you can mix a crushed tablet or an opened capsule with soft food or liquid. First check for interactions between the medication and the food or fluid being mixed with it or other medications that are being administered (Table 13-1). For example, tetracycline is inactivated by milk. It must not be dissolved in foods that contain milk. In addition, it should not be given with either antacids or vitamin and mineral supplements.

Oral forms of medication are also ordered for patients with nasogastric, gastrostomy, or jejunostomy tubes. See Chapter 8, Figure 8-6. Before administering medication through the tube, you first dissolve the contents from a crushed tablet or opened capsule in a small amount of warm water.

Some medications cannot be crushed. If these medications are ordered for a patient with a feeding tube or one who cannot swallow pills, determine whether an alternative form of the medication exists. Consult a drug reference or pharmacist for information, then ask the physician if the medication could be ordered in one of these forms. Always follow the policy of the facility where you are employed regarding substituting forms of medications.

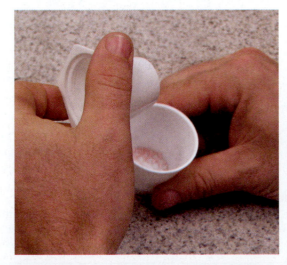 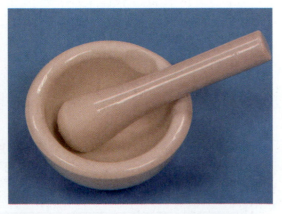

Figure 13-6 A pill crusher or mortar and pestle may be used to crush tablets when necessary.

TABLE 13-1 Examples of Food and Drug Interactions

DRUG	FOOD	INTERACTION
Antipsychotics	Coffee and tea	Reduced effectiveness of drug
Bronchodilators	Caffeine	Stimulation of the nervous system
Central nervous system (CNS) depressants	Black cohosh, ginseng kava kava, St. John's Wort, valerian, ETOH	Intensified sedative effects of CNS depressant
Erythromycin	Acidic fruits or juices, carbonated beverages	Decreased antimicrobial activity
Ferrous sulfate	Tea	Decreased absorption
Haloperidol	Coffee and tea	Decreased absorption
Insulin	Coffee	Stimulated excretion
Monoamine oxidase inhibitors	Foods containing tyramine, such as hard cheeses, chocolate, red wine, and beef or chicken liver	Headache, nosebleed, chest pain, severe hypertension
Tetracyclines	Dairy products	Reduced effectiveness of drug
Antihistamines, cholesterol lowering agents, calcium channel blockers	Grapefruit and grapefruit juice	Muscle aches, fatigue, fever, increased side effects

Enteric-coated tablets have a coating that dissolves only in an alkaline environment, such as the small intestine. These tablets deliver medication that would be destroyed by stomach acid or that could injure the stomach lining. Enteric-coated tablets often look like candies that have a soft center and a hard shell. Some aspirins are enteric-coated, as are certain iron tablets such as ferrous gluconate. Enteric-coated tablets must *never* be crushed, broken, or chewed. A patient must swallow them with their coating intact (see Figure 13-7).

Some medications are available in **sustained-release** forms. They allow the drug to be released slowly into the bloodstream over a period of several hours. If the medication is scored, you may break it at the scored line. Otherwise you must not break it. Crushing or dissolving sustained-release tablets would allow more than the intended amount of medication to be absorbed at one time, causing overdose or toxicity of the drug.

Special capsules, often called **spansules,** contain granules of medication with different coatings that delay release of some of the medication. You may open spansules and gently mix the granules in soft food, but you must not crush or dissolve the granules. (See Figure 13-8.)

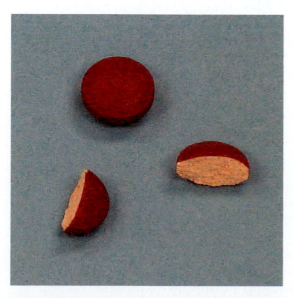

Figure 13-7 Enteric-coated tablet. One tablet has been split for visualization only. Enteric-coated tablets should never be split when given to patients.

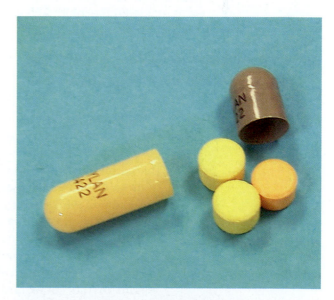

Figure 13-8 This sustained-release capsule has three smaller tablets inside that release medication into the bloodstream over a period of several hours.

RULE 13-4	To prevent an incorrect dose of medication do not crush or otherwise alter any of the following:
	• Enteric-coated tablets.
	• Sustained-release forms of medication.
	• Any tablet with a hard shell or coating.
	• Any tablet with layers or speckles of different colors.
	• Tablets for sublingual or buccal use.
	• Capsules with seals that prevent separating the two parts.
Example	The following lists indicate some medications that should not be crushed or altered. Crushing or altering these medications could cause an inaccurate dose of the medication to be administered.

• Names that indicate sustained-release such as:

-Bid	LA	Tempule
-Dur	CR	Chronotab
Plateau cap	XL	Repetab
Span	Sequel	Tembid
SA	Spansule	
SR	Extentab	

• Names that indicate enteric-coated such as:
EC
Enseal

GO TO . . . Open the CD-ROM that accompanies your textbook, and select Chapter 13, Do Not Crush (LO 13.1). Review the animation and example problems, then complete the practice problems. Continue to the next section of the book once you have mastered the information presented.

PATIENT EDUCATION

Review with patients the following guidelines for taking tablets and capsules:

1. Perform all necessary calculations, so that you can tell patients how many pills to take.
2. Tell patients whether they need to take a medication with food. Encourage them to drink at least 8 oz of water with any medication.
3. Tell patients who need to divide tablets that pharmacists can provide this service on request. If the patients will be dividing the tablets, demonstrate and advise them as follows:
   a. Wash hands before you handle tablets.
   b. Grasp the tablet with the scored line between your fingers. Exert pressure in the same direction—downward or upward—with both hands, until the tablet breaks along the scored line.

c. You may use a knife or pill cutter to break the tablet. Place the tablet on a clean surface, place the blade in the scored line, and press directly downward until the tablet breaks.

4. For patients who have difficulty swallowing, offer the following suggestions:

a. Drink water before taking pills, so your mouth is moist.

b. Place whole tablets or capsules in a small amount of food, such as applesauce or pudding. The pill will go down when the food is swallowed. *Note:* Also tell patients which foods should **not** be used.

c. Crush tablets by placing them on a spoon and pressing another spoon down on top of them or use a pill crusher. **Note:** Warn patients not to crush any medication without first checking with the pharmacist or physician.

REVIEW AND PRACTICE

13.1 Solid Oral Medications

For Exercises 1–20, calculate the amount to administer. Unless otherwise noted, all scored tablets are scored in half.

1. Ordered: Tegretol® 400 mg PO bid
   On hand: Tegretol® 200 mg unscored tablets
   Administer: _____

2. Ordered: Seroquel® 75 mg PO tid
   On hand: Seroquel® 25 mg unscored tablets
   Administer: _____

3. Ordered: Tolectin® 300 mg PO tid
   On hand: Tolectin® 200 mg scored tablets
   Administer: _____

4. Ordered: Isordil® Titradose 15 mg PO now
   On hand: Isordil® Titradose 10 mg deep-scored tablets
   Administer: _____

5. Ordered: Felbatol® 600 mg PO qid
   On hand: Felbatol® 400 mg scored tablets
   Administer: _____

6. Ordered: Decadron® 1.5 mg PO daily
   On hand: Decadron® 0.75 mg unscored tablets
   Administer: _____

7. Ordered: Coumadin® 5 mg PO daily
   On hand: Coumadin® 2 mg scored tablets
   Administer: _____

8. Ordered: Cardizem® 90 mg PO tid
   On hand: Cardizem® 60 mg scored tablets
   Administer: _____

9. Ordered: Tambocor® 150 mg PO q12h
   On hand: Tambocor® 100 mg scored tablets
   Administer: _____

10. Ordered: Clozaril® 50 mg PO daily   Administer: _____

   On hand: Refer to label A. Tablets are unscored.

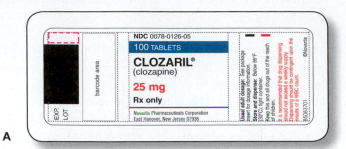

A

11. Ordered: Alprazolam 0.5 mg PO tid   Administer: _____

   On hand: Refer to label B. Tablets are scored into fourths.

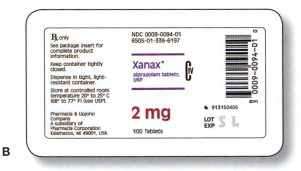

B

12. Ordered: Valium® 10 mg PO q12h   Administer: _____

   On hand: Refer to label C.

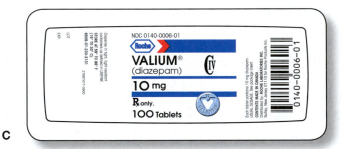

C

13. Ordered: Famvir® 250 mg PO bid   Administer: _____

   On hand: Refer to label D. Tablets are unscored.

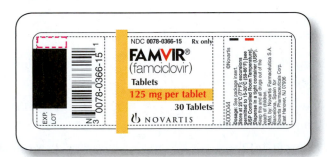

D

14. Ordered: Aricept® 10 mg PO daily   Administer: _____

On hand: Refer to label E. Tablets are unscored.

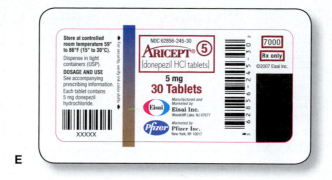

E

15. Ordered: Prandin 1 mg PO bid   Administer: _____

On hand: Refer to labels F and G. Tablets are unscored.   Dosage strength: _____

Determine dosage strength to use.

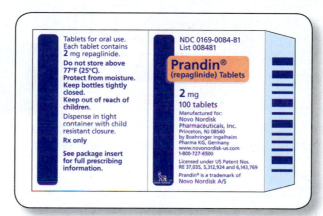

F

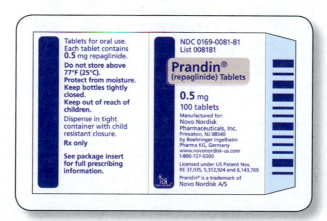

G

16. Ordered: Pioglitazone HCl 60 mg PO daily   Administer: _____

On hand: Refer to label H. Tablets are unscored.

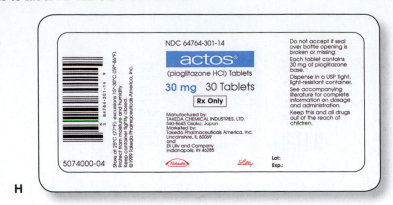

H

17. Ordered: Lipitor® 30 mg PO daily   Administer: _____

On hand: Refer to label I. Tablets are unscored.

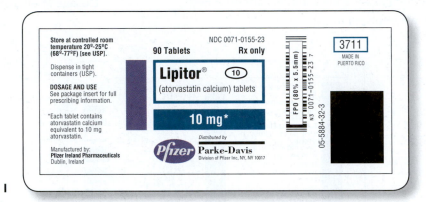

I

18. Ordered: Zoloft® 50 mg PO daily   Administer: _____

On hand: Refer to label J. Tablets are scored.

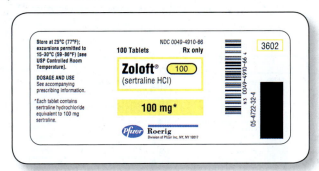

J

19. Ordered: Gleevec® 200 mg PO daily   Administer: _____

On hand: Refer to label K. Tablets are not scored.

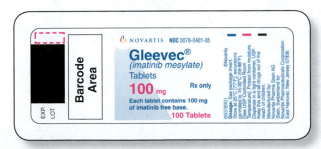

K

20. Ordered: Clonazepam 1 mg PO tid   Administer: _____

On hand: Clonazepam 2 mg scored tablets

For Exercises 21–24, match the term to the description:

    a. tablet   **b.** spansule   **c.** gelcap   **d.** enteric coating   **e.** capsule

21. Contains granules that delay the release of the medication   _____

22. Hard shell that is absorbed in the small intestine, not the stomach   _____

23. Most common form of oral medication   _____

24. Liquid medication in a gelatin shell   _____

25. Differentiate the rationale for splitting and crushing pills.   _____

To check your answers, see the Answer section at the end of the book, which starts on page A-1.

13.2 Liquid Oral Medications

Many medications are available in liquid form. Liquids can be measured in small units of volume; thus, a greater range of dosages can be ordered and administered. Because they are easier to swallow than tablets and capsules, they are often used for children and elderly patients. Liquids can also be administered easily through feeding tubes.

Liquids may be less stable than solid forms of drugs. Many medications that are intended to be administered as liquids are provided as powders because they rapidly lose their power once they are mixed into a solution. These drugs will then have to be **reconstituted,** or mixed with a liquid, before they can be administered. Many liquids, especially antibiotics, require refrigeration.

The directions for reconstitution are located on the medication label (or package insert.) If clarification of reconstitution information is needed, contact the pharmacist who dispensed the medication.

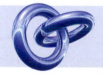

LEARNING LINK Recall from Chapter 10, Information on Medication Labels and Package Inserts, that directions for reconstituting or diluting a drug appear on the label or in the package insert.

RULE 13-5   When reconstituting liquid medications:

- Use only the liquid specified on the drug label.

- Use the exact amount of liquid specified on the drug label.

- Check the label to determine whether the medication should be shaken before administering.

- Check the label to determine whether the reconstituted medication must be refrigerated.

- Write on the label the date and time you reconstitute the medication. Also, write your initials. Check the label to determine how long the reconstituted medication may be stored. Discard any medication left after this time period has passed.

- When medication can be reconstituted in different strengths, write on the label the strength that you choose.

- When medication can be reconstituted in different strengths, select the strength that will allow the desired dose to be administered in the smallest volume.

Example 1

How would you reconstitute the following medication? Find the amount to administer.

Ordered: Kytril® 5 mg PO now

On hand: Refer to Figure 13-9.

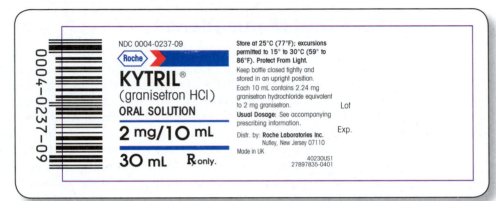

NDC 0004-0237-09

Roche

KYTRIL®
(granisetron HCl)
ORAL SOLUTION

2 mg/10 mL

30 mL   ℞ only.

Store at 25°C (77°F); excursions permitted to 15° to 30°C (59° to 86°F). Protect From Light.
Keep bottle closed tightly and stored in an upright position.
Each 10 mL contains 2.24 mg granisetron hydrochloride equivalent to 2 mg granisetron.
Usual Dosage: See accompanying prescribing information.
Distr. by: **Roche Laboratories Inc.**
    Nutley, New Jersey 07110
Made in UK

Lot

Exp.

40230US1
27897835-0401

Figure 13-9

According to the label, this medication is already in liquid form as a solution, so no reconstitution is necessary.

Calculate the amount to administer. The dosage ordered is 5 mg. The dosage strength is 2 mg/10 mL, which makes the dose on hand 2 mg and the dosage unit 10 mL.

PROPORTION METHOD

EXAMPLE 1

Calculate the amount of Kytril to administer (refer to Figure 13-9).

Ordered: Kytril® 5 mg PO now
Dosage strength: 2 mg/10 mL

STEP A: CONVERT
No conversion needed.

STEP B: CALCULATE
Follow Procedure Checklist 12-1.

1. Fill in the proportion.

$$\frac{H}{Q} = \frac{D}{A} \quad \text{or} \quad \frac{\text{Dose on hand}}{\text{Dosage unit}} = \frac{\text{Desired dose}}{\text{Amount to administer}}$$

$$\frac{2\ \text{mg}}{10\ \text{mL}} = \frac{5\ \text{mg}}{A} \quad \text{or} \quad 2\ \text{mg} : 10\ \text{mL} = 5\ \text{mg} : A$$

2. Cancel units.

$$\frac{2 \text{ mg}}{10 \text{ mL}} = \frac{5 \text{ mg}}{A} \qquad \text{or} \qquad 2 \text{ mg} : 10 \text{ mL} = 5 \text{ mg} : A$$

3. Cross-multiply and solve for the unknown.

$$2 \times A = 10 \text{ mL} \times 5$$

$$A = \frac{10 \text{ mL} \times 5}{2}$$

$$A = \frac{50 \text{ mL}}{2}$$

$$A = 25 \text{ mL}$$

STEP C: THINK! . . . IS IT REASONABLE?

Since 2 mg of medication is in 10 mL of liquid, it is reasonable that 5 mg of medication would be in 25 mL of liquid.

DIMENSIONAL ANALYSIS

EXAMPLE 1

Calculate the amount of Kytril to administer (refer to Figure 13-9 on page 320).

Ordered: Kytril® 5 mg PO now
Dosage strength: 2 mg/10 mL

STEP A: CONVERT

The unit of measurement for the desired dose and the dose on hand is milligrams. No conversion needed.

STEP B: CALCULATE

Follow Procedure Checklist 12-2.

1. The unit of measure for the amount to administer will be milliliters.

$$A \text{ mL} =$$

2. No conversion factor is needed.

3. The dosage unit is 10 mL. The dose on hand is 2 mg. This is the first factor.

$$A \text{ mL} = \frac{10 \text{ mL}}{2 \text{ mg}}$$

4. The dosage ordered is 5 mg. Place this over 1 for the second factor.

$$A \text{ mL} = \frac{10 \text{ mL}}{2 \text{ mg}} \times \frac{5 \text{ mg}}{1}$$

5. Cancel units.

$$A \text{ mL} = \frac{10 \text{ mL}}{2 \text{ mg}} \times \frac{5 \text{ mg}}{1}$$

6. Solve the equation.

$$A \text{ mL} = \frac{50 \text{ mL}}{2}$$

$$A = 25 \text{ mL}$$

STEP C: THINK! . . . IS IT REASONABLE?

Since 2 mg of medication is in 10 mL of liquid, it is reasonable that 5 mg of medication would be in 25 mL of liquid.

FORMULA METHOD

EXAMPLE 1

Calculate the amount of Kytril to administer (refer to Figure 13-9 on page 320).

Ordered: Kytril® 5 mg PO now
Dosage strength: 2 mg/10 mL

STEP A: CONVERT

The drug is ordered in milligrams, which is the same unit used on the label. No conversion needed.

STEP B: CALCULATE

Follow Procedure Checklist 12-3.

1. Determine the components of the formula method.

   $D = 5$ mg

   $Q = 10$ mL

   $H = 2$ mg

2. Fill in the formula.

   $$\frac{D}{H} \times Q = A$$

   $$\frac{5 \text{ mg}}{2 \text{ mg}} \times 10 \text{ mL} = A$$

3. Cancel units.

   $$\frac{5 \cancel{\text{ mg}}}{2 \cancel{\text{ mg}}} \times 10 \text{ mL} = A$$

4. Solve for the unknown.

   $$\frac{50 \text{ mL}}{2} = A$$

   $$A = 25 \text{ mL}$$

STEP C: THINK ABOUT IT! . . . IS IT REASONABLE?

Since 2 mg of medication is in 10 mL of liquid, it is reasonable that 5 mg of medication would be in 25 mL of liquid.

EXAMPLE 2

How would you reconstitute the following medication? Calculate the amount to administer.

Ordered: E.E.S.® susp 400 mg PO q6h
On hand: Refer to Figure 13-10.

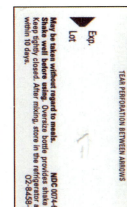

6505-00-080-0653

Before mixing, store below 86°F (30°C).
DIRECTIONS FOR MIXING: Add 154 mL water and shake vigorously. This makes 200 mL of suspension.

Contains erythromycin ethylsuccinate equivalent to 8 g erythromycin. Child-resistant closure not required; exemption approved by U.S. Consumer Product Safety Commission.

When mixed as directed, each teaspoonful (5 mL) contains: Erythromycin ethylsuccinate equivalent to erythromycin ....200 mg in a buffered, cherry-flavored, aqueous vehicle.

DOSAGE MAY BE ADMINISTERED WITHOUT REGARD TO MEALS.

Usual dose: Children: 30-50 mg/kg/day in divided doses. See package enclosure for adult dose and full prescribing information.

U.S. Pat. No. 4,076,804   ©Abbott

Abbott Laboratories
North Chicago, IL 60064, U.S.A.

NDC 0074-6369-10
200 mL (when mixed)
For Oral Suspension

E.E.S.® Granules

ERYTHROMYCIN ETHYLSUCCINATE FOR ORAL SUSPENSION, USP

Erythromycin activity
200 mg per 5 mL
when reconstituted

℞ only

May be taken without regard to meals.
Shake well before using. Oversize bottle provides shake space.
Keep tightly closed. After mixing, store in the refrigerator and use within 10 days.

Exp.
Lot

NDC 0074-6369-10
02-8458-5/R15

TEAR PERFORATION BETWEEN ARROWS

Figure 13-10

According to the label, you add 154 mL of water to the bottle of granules and shake vigorously. You then have a total of 200 mL of oral suspension that must be stored in the refrigerator for up to 10 days.

Calculate the amount to administer. The dosage ordered is 400 mg. The dosage strength is 200 mg/5 mL which makes the dose on hand 200 mg and the dosage unit 5 mL.

PROPORTION METHOD

EXAMPLE 2

Calculate the amount of E.E.S.® to administer.

Ordered: E.E.S.® susp 400 mg PO q6h
On hand: Refer to Figure 13.10, page 322

STEP A: CONVERT
The dose on hand is the same unit of measure as the dose ordered. No conversion needed.

STEP B: CALCULATE
Follow Procedure Checklist 12-1.

1. Fill in the proportion.

$$\frac{H}{Q} = \frac{D}{A} \quad \text{or} \quad \frac{\text{Dose on hand}}{\text{Dosage unit}} = \frac{\text{Desired dose}}{\text{Amount to administer}}$$

$$\frac{200 \text{ mg}}{5 \text{ mL}} = \frac{400 \text{ mg}}{A} \quad \text{or} \quad 200 \text{ mg} : 5 \text{ mL} = 400 \text{ mg} : A$$

2. Cancel units

$$\frac{200 \cancel{\text{ mg}}}{5 \text{ mL}} = \frac{400 \cancel{\text{ mg}}}{A}$$

3. Cross-multiply and solve for the unknown.

$$200 \times A = 5 \text{ mL} \times 400$$

$$A = 5 \text{ mL} \times \frac{400}{200}$$

$$A = 5 \text{ mL} \times 2$$

$$A = 10 \text{ mL}$$

STEP C: THINK! . . . IS IT REASONABLE?
If 5 mL of liquid contain 200 mg of medication, it is reasonable that 10 mL of liquid contains 400 mg of medication.

DIMENSIONAL ANALYSIS

EXAMPLE 2

Calculate the amount of E.E.S.® to administer.

Ordered: E.E.S.® susp 400 mg PO q6h
On hand: Refer to Figure 13-10, page 322

STEP A: CONVERT
The unit of measurement for the desired dose and the dose on hand are both milligrams. No conversion factor needed.

STEP B: CALCULATE
Follow Procedure Checklist 12-2.

1. The unit of measure for the amount to administer will be milliliters.

$$A \text{ mL} =$$

2. No conversion factor needed.

3. The dosage unit is 5 mL. The dose on hand is 200 mg. This is your first factor.

$$\frac{5\ \text{mL}}{200\ \text{mg}}$$

4. The dosage ordered is 400 mg. Place this over 1 for the second factor.

$$A\ \text{mL} = \frac{5\ \text{mL}}{200\ \text{mg}} \times \frac{400\ \text{mg}}{1}$$

5. Cancel units.

$$A\ \text{mL} = \frac{5\ \text{mL}}{200\ \cancel{\text{mg}}} \times \frac{400\ \cancel{\text{mg}}}{1}$$

6. Solve the equation.

$$A\ \text{mL} = \frac{2000\ \text{mL}}{200}$$

$$A = 10\ \text{mL}$$

STEP C: THINK! . . . IS IT REASONABLE?

If 5 mL of liquid contain 200 mg of medication, it is reasonable that 10 mL of liquid contains 400 mg of medication.

FORMULA METHOD

EXAMPLE 2

Calculate the amount of E.E.S.® to administer.

Ordered: E.E.S.® susp 400 mg PO q6h
On hand: Refer to Figure 13.10, page 322

STEP A: CONVERT

The dose on hand is the same unit of measure as the dose ordered. No conversion needed.

STEP B: CALCULATE

Follow Procedure Checklist 12-3.

1. Determine the components of the formula method.

   $D = 400\ \text{mg}$

   $Q = 5\ \text{mL}$

   $H = 200\ \text{mg}$

2. Fill in the formula.

   $$\frac{D}{H} \times Q = A$$

   $$\frac{400\ \text{mg}}{200\ \text{mg}} \times 5\ \text{mL} = A$$

3. Cancel units.

   $$\frac{400\ \cancel{\text{mg}}}{200\ \cancel{\text{mg}}} \times 5\ \text{mL} = A$$

4. Solve for the unknown.

   $$\frac{2000\ \text{mL}}{200} = A$$

   $$A = 10\ \text{mL}$$

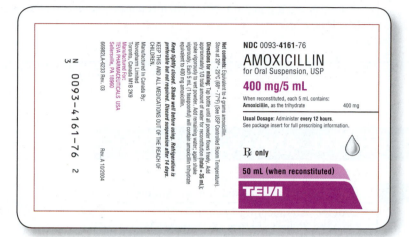

STEP C: THINK! . . . IS IT REASONABLE?

If 5 mL of liquid contain 200 mg of medication, it is reasonable that 10 mL of liquid contains 400 mg of medication.

EXAMPLE 3

How would you reconstitute the following medication? Find the amount to administer.

Ordered: Amoxicillin 500 mg PO q8h
On hand: Refer to Figure 13-11.

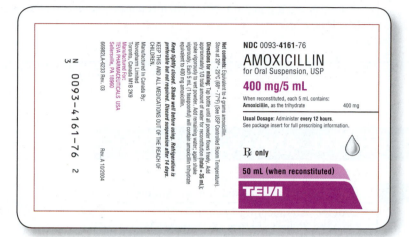

NDC 0093-4161-76

AMOXICILLIN
for Oral Suspension, USP

400 mg/5 mL

When reconstituted, each 5 mL contains:
Amoxicillin, as the trihydrate   400 mg

Usual Dosage: Administer **every 12 hours.**
See package insert for full prescribing information.

℞ only

50 mL (when reconstituted)

TEVA

Figure 13-11

Tap bottle until all powder flows freely. Add approximately $\frac{1}{3}$ the total amount of water for reconstitution. The total amount of water to add is 35 mL. Shake vigorously to wet the powder. Add remaining water, again shake vigorously.

When it is reconstituted, you will have total of 50 mL of oral suspension.

Calculate the amount to administer. The dosage ordered is 500 mg. The dosage strength is 400 mg/ 5 mL which makes the dose on hand 400 mg and the dosage unit 5 mL.

PROPORTION METHOD

EXAMPLE 3

Calculate the amount of amoxicillin to administer.

Ordered: amoxicillin 500 mg PO q8h
On hand: Refer to Figure 13-11.

STEP A: CONVERT
The dose on hand is the same unit of measure as the dose ordered. No conversion needed.

STEP B: CALCULATE
Follow Procedure Checklist 12-1.

1. Fill in the proportion.

$$\frac{H}{Q} = \frac{A}{D} \quad \text{or} \quad \frac{\text{Dose on hand}}{\text{Dosage unit}} = \frac{\text{Desired dose}}{\text{Amount to administer}}$$

$$\frac{400 \text{ mg}}{5 \text{ mL}} = \frac{500 \text{ mg}}{A} \quad \text{or} \quad 400 \text{ mg} : 5 \text{ mL} = 500 \text{ mg} : A$$

2. Cancel units.

$$\frac{400 \cancel{\text{ mg}}}{5 \text{ mL}} = \frac{500 \cancel{\text{ mg}}}{A}$$

3. Cross-multiply and solve for the unknown.

$$400 \times A = 5 \text{ mL} \times 500$$

$$A = 5 \text{ mL} \times \frac{500}{400}$$

$$A = 6.25 \text{ or } 6.3 \text{ mL}$$

STEP C: THINK! . . . IS IT REASONABLE?

If there is 400 mg in 5 mL of liquid, it is reasonable that 500 mg would be in 6.25, rounded to 6.3 mL (see Rule 13-5).

DIMENSIONAL ANALYSIS

EXAMPLE 3

Find the amount of amoxicillin to administer.

Ordered: Amoxicillin 500 mg PO q8h
On hand: Refer to Figure 13-11, page 325.

STEP A: CONVERT

The unit of measurement for the desired dose and the dose on hand are both milligrams. No conversion factor needed.

STEP B: CALCULATE

Follow Procedure Checklist 12-2.

1. The unit of measure for the amount to administer will be milliliters.

$$A \text{ mL} =$$

2. No conversion factor needed.

3. The dosage unit is 5 mL. The dose on hand is 400 mg.

$$A \text{ mL} = \frac{5 \text{ mL}}{400 \text{ mg}}$$

4. The dosage ordered is 500 mg.

$$A \text{ mL} = \frac{5 \text{ mL}}{400 \text{ mg}} \times \frac{500 \text{ mg}}{1}$$

5. Cancel units.

$$A \text{ mL} = \frac{5 \text{ mL}}{400 \text{ \cancel{mg}}} \times \frac{500 \text{ \cancel{mg}}}{1}$$

6. Solve the equation.

$$A \text{ mL} = \frac{2500 \text{ ml}}{400}$$

$$A = 6.25 \text{ or } 6.3 \text{ mL}$$

STEP C: THINK! . . . IS IT REASONABLE?

If there is 400 mg in 5 mL of liquid, it is reasonable that 500 mg would be in 6.25 mL, rounded to 6.3 mL (see Rule 13-5).

FORMULA METHOD

EXAMPLE 3   Calculate the amount of amoxicillin to administer.

Ordered: Amoxicillin 500 mg PO q8h
On hand: Refer to Figure 13-11, page 325.

STEP A: CONVERT
The dose on hand is the same unit of measure as the dose ordered. No conversion needed.

STEP B: CALCULATE
Follow Procedure Checklist 12-3.

1. Determine the components of the formula method.

   $D = 500$ mg

   $Q = 5$ mL

   $H = 400$ mg

2. Fill in the formula.

   $$\frac{D}{H} \times Q = A$$

   $$\frac{500 \text{ mg}}{400 \text{ mg}} \times 5 \text{ mL} = A$$

3. Cancel units.

   $$\frac{500 \text{ mg}}{400 \text{ mg}} \times 5 \text{ mL} = A$$

4. Solve for the unknown.

   $$\frac{2500 \text{ mL}}{400} = A$$

   $A = 6.25$ or 6.3 mL

STEP C: THINK! . . . IS IT REASONABLE?
If there is 400 mg in 5 mL of liquid, it is reasonable that 500 mg would be in 6.25 mL, rounded to 6.3 mL (see Rule 13-5).

GO TO . . . Open the CD-ROM that accompanies your textbook, and select Chapter 13, Reconstituting Liquid Medications (LO 13.2). Review the animation and example problems, then complete the practice problems. Continue to the next section of the book once you have mastered the information presented.

PATIENT EDUCATION

Review with patients who are taking medications in a home environment the steps for reconstituting liquid medications. Follow Rule 13-5. If necessary, copy the rule for them, then discuss. If you are dispensing medications, give the patients the same information that the pharmacist would, if you are allowed to do so. Give patients the following information about handling liquid medication:

(Continued)

1. Read the label to learn how to store the medication.
2. Use the measuring device provided or a device purchased specifically to measure medications. Household teaspoons and tablespoons do not measure liquid accurately.
3. Do not store medication longer than the label indicates. Medication used after its expiration date may have lost potency, or its chemical composition may have changed.
4. Wash the measuring device with hot water and a dishwashing detergent after each use. Dry it thoroughly. Store it in a clean container such as a plastic sandwich bag.
5. Keep liquid medication in its original container. Do not transfer it to other containers.

CRITICAL THINKING ON THE JOB

Reconstituting Powders

A healthcare professional is preparing a bottle of Amoxicillin suspension for this order: Amoxicillin 500 mg PO q8h × 5 days. The pharmacy has available 100-mL bottles and 150-mL bottles containing 250 mg/5 mL (see Figures 13-12 and 13-13).

After calculating as follows:

$$\frac{500 \text{ mg}}{250 \text{ mg}} \times 5 \text{ mL} = A$$

$$\frac{500 \text{ mg}}{250 \text{ mg}} \times 5 \text{ mL} = A = 2 \times 5 \text{ mL} = 10 \text{ mL}$$

the healthcare professional determines that the patient will receive 10 mL for each dose and 3 doses each day. This will require 30 mL of suspension each day for 5 days, or a total of 150 mL. The reconstituted medication can be refrigerated for 14 days.

The healthcare professional selects the 150-mL bottle and adds 150 mL of water to it. However, the liquid overflows from the bottle.

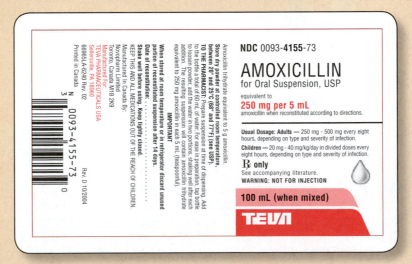

Figure 13-12

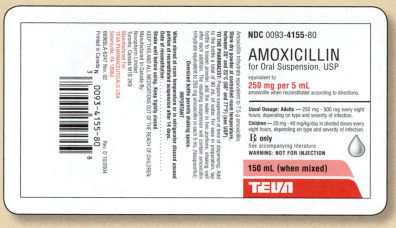

Figure 13-13

Think! . . . **Is It Reasonable?** What went wrong? How will this problem affect the patient's care?

REVIEW AND PRACTICE

13.2 Liquid Oral Medications

For Exercises 1–20, calculate the amount to administer.

1. Ordered: Trilisate® 400 mg PO tid
   On hand: Trilisate® liquid labeled 500 mg/5 mL

   Administer: _____

2. Ordered: MSIR sol 15 mg PO q4h
   On hand: MSIR solution labeled 10 mg/5 mL

   Administer: _____

3. Ordered: Megace® 200 mg PO qid
   On hand: Megace® solution labeled 40 mg/mL

   Administer: _____

4. Ordered: Norvir® 60 mg PO bid
   On hand: Norvir® solution labeled 80 mg/mL

   Administer: _____

5. Ordered: Zofran® 8 mg PO q12h
   On hand: Zofran® liquid labeled 4 mg/5 mL

   Administer: _____

6. Ordered: Motrin® 600 mg PO tid
   On hand: Motrin® liquid labeled 100 mg/5 mL

   Administer: _____

7. Ordered: E.E.S.® 500 mg via NGT bid   Administer: _____
On hand: Refer to label A.

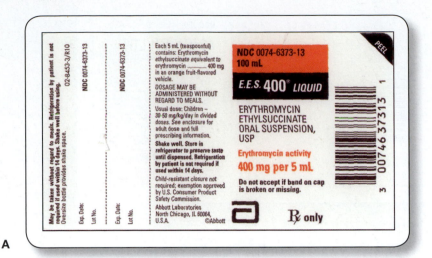

A

8. Ordered: Amoxicillin 270 mg PO q8h   Administer: _____
On hand: Refer to label B.

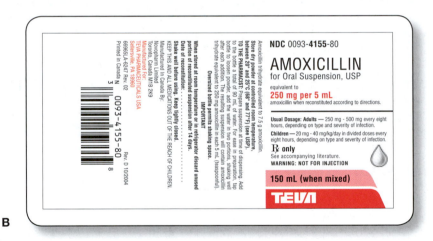

B

9. Ordered: Zithromax® 250 mg PO daily   Administer: _____
On hand: Refer to label C.

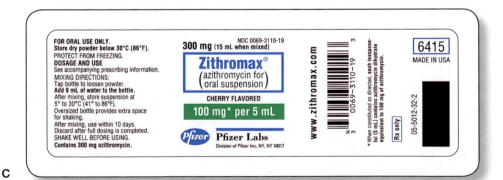

C

10. Ordered: Depakene® 125 mg via NGT bid   Administer: _____
On hand: Refer to label D.

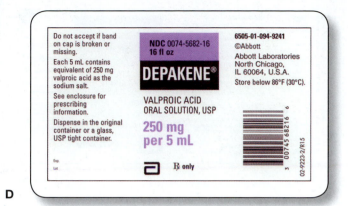

D

11. Ordered: Kytril 1 mg PO bid   Administer: _____
On hand: Refer to label E.

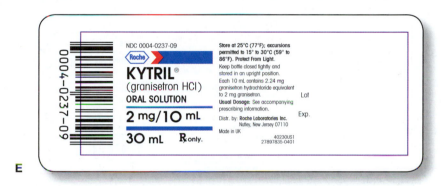

E

12. Ordered: CellCept® 500 mg PO bid   Administer: _____
On hand: Refer to label F.

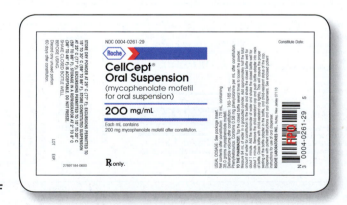

F

13. Ordered: EES Granules® 250 mg PO q12h   Administer: _____

On hand: Refer to label G.

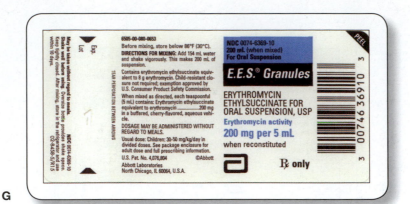

G

14. Ordered: Cefzil® 500 mg PO q24h   Administer: _____

On hand: Cefzil® 125 mg/5 mL oral suspension

15. Ordered: Flumadine® 100 mg via NGT bid   Administer: _____

On hand: Refer to label H.

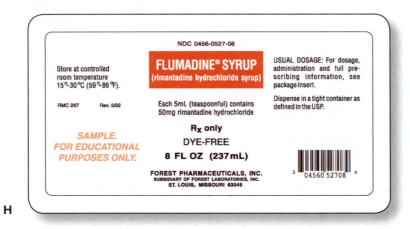

H

16. Ordered: Zithromax® 500 mg PO daily   Administer: _____

On hand: Refer to label I.

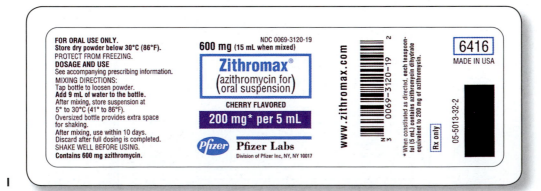

I

17. Ordered: Griseofulvin 500 mg PO daily   Administer: _____

On hand: Griseofulvin 125 mg/5 mL suspension

18. Ordered: Depakene® 500 mg PO daily
On hand: Refer to label J.

Administer: _____

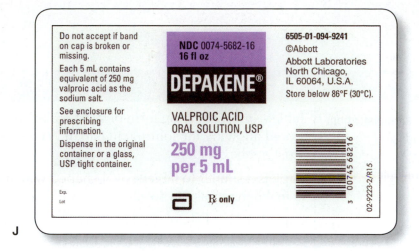

J

19. Ordered: Trileptal® 75 mg PO q6h
On hand: Refer to label K.

Administer: _____

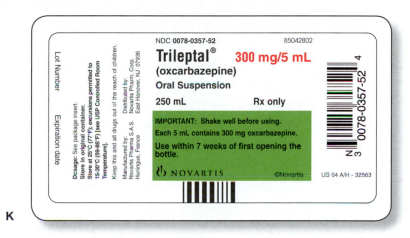

K

20. Ordered: Prozac® 60 mg PO daily
On hand: Prozac® 20 mg/5 mL oral solution

Administer: _____

To check your answers, see the Answer section at the end of the book, which begins on page A-1.

LEARNING OUTCOME	KEY POINTS
13.1 Demonstrate administration of solid oral medications: a. Calculate dosages. b. Explain related principles. Pages 303–319	Tablet—most common form of solid oral medication; may be scored allowing for splitting in half, if needed; unscored tablets must not be divided Caplets—similar to tablets; oval-shaped with a special coating to make them easy to swallow Capsules—oval-shaped gelatin shells that contain medication in powder or granule form NOTE: For patients with difficulty swallowing, some tablets and caplets may be crushed and capsules may be opened and mixed with food (or dissolved in liquid and given via NGT); to determine which medications can be crushed, consult a drug reference or pharmacist. Gelcaps—liquid medication in gelatin shells that are not designed to be opened Enteric coated tablets—have a coating that dissolves in the small intestine (not the stomach); these tablets should never be split or crushed Spansules—capsules with granules that delay the release of the medication Dosage Calculation: Give 650 mg Tylenol from a supply dose of 325 mg tablets. **Proportion Method:** **Step A: Convert** Determine no conversion step is necessary because the desired dose is mg and the supply dose is mg. **Step B: Calculate** Set up the ratio-proportion with the supply dose on the left and the desired dose on the right: $$\frac{325\text{ mg}}{1\text{ tablet}} = \frac{650\text{ mg}}{A}$$ Cancel units and cross multiply: $325\,A = 650$ $A = 2$ tablets **Step C: Think! . . . Is It Reasonable?** Since the desired dose (650 mg) is twice the amount of the dose on hand (325 mg), then the amount to administer should be twice the dosage unit (1 tablet), so 2 tablets is a reasonable answer.

Dimensional Analysis:

Step A: Convert Determine that there is no conversion factor needed.

Step B: Calculate Set up the equation:

$$A \text{ tablets} = \frac{\text{dosage unit}}{\text{dose on hand}} \times \frac{\text{desired dose}}{1}$$

$$A \text{ tablets} = \frac{1 \text{ tablet}}{325 \text{ mg}} \times \frac{650 \text{ mg}}{1}$$

$$A \text{ tablets} = \frac{650}{325} = 2 \text{ tablets}$$

Step C: Think! . . . Is It Reasonable? (see above)

Formula Method:

Step A: Convert Determine that no conversion step is needed.

Step B: Calculate Determine D, H, Q, A and set up the equation:

$$\frac{D}{H} \times Q = A$$

$$\frac{650 \text{ mg}}{325 \text{ mg}} \times 1 \text{ tablet} = A$$

Cancel units: $\frac{650}{325} = 2$ tablets

Step C: Think! . . . Is It Reasonable? (see above)

13.2 Demonstrate administration of liquid oral medications:
a. Calculate dosages
b. Explain related principles.
Pages 319–333

Liquids—can be measured in small units of volume; thus, a greater range of dosages can be ordered and administered; may be less stable than solid forms of drugs because they rapidly lose their power once they are mixed into a solution—these drugs will then have to be reconstituted, or mixed with a liquid, before they can be administered

Dosage Calculation: Add 40 mL of water to a 2 gram bottle of Amoxicillin. The dosage strength after reconstitution $\frac{0.25 \text{ g}}{5 \text{ mL}}$. Give Amoxicillin 100 mg from a supply dose of $\frac{0.25 \text{g}}{5 \text{ mL}}$.

Proportion Method:

Step A: Convert Convert 0.25 g to 250 mg

Step B: Calculate Set up the ratio-proportion with the supply dose on the left and the desired dose on the right:

$$\frac{250 \text{ mg}}{5 \text{ mL}} = \frac{100 \text{ mg}}{A}$$

Cancel units and cross multiply:

$$250 \, A = 500 \text{ mL}$$

$$A = 2 \text{ mL}$$

Step C: Think! . . . Is It Reasonable? Since the desired dose (100 mg) is less than half of the dose on hand (250 mg), then the amount to administer should be less than half of the dosage unit (5 mL); since 2 is less than half of 5, this answer is reasonable.

Dimensional Analysis:

Step A: Convert Determine the conversion factor: $\dfrac{1 \text{ g}}{1000 \text{ mg}}$

(unit of msmt on hand/unit of msmt ordered)

Step B: Calculate Set up the equation:

$$A \text{ mL} = \text{Conversion factor} \times \frac{\text{dosage unit}}{\text{dose on hand}} \times \frac{\text{desired dose}}{1}$$

$$A \text{ mL} = \frac{1 \cancel{\text{g}}}{1000 \text{ mg}} \times \frac{5 \text{ mL}}{0.25 \cancel{\text{g}}} \times \frac{100 \text{ mg}}{1}$$

$$A \text{ mL} = \frac{500}{250} = 2 \text{ mL}$$

Step C: Think! . . . Is It Reasonable? (see above)

Formula Method:

Step A: Convert Convert 0.25 g to 250 mg

Step B: Calculate Determine D, H, Q, A; $D = 100$ mg; $H = 250$ mg; $Q = 5$ mL; A is unknown

Set up the equation: $\dfrac{D}{H} \times Q = A$

$$\frac{100 \text{ mg}}{250 \text{ mg}} \times 5 \text{ mL} = A$$

Cancel units: $\dfrac{500}{250} = 2 \text{ mL} = A$

Step C: Think! . . . Is It Reasonable? (see above)

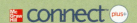
Answer the following questions.

1. Define each of the following terms: scored tablet, sublingual, buccal, capsule, spansule. (LO 13.1b)

2. List four solid forms of medications that may not be crushed and explain why. (LO 13.1b)

3. Explain one technique for preparing a solid medication for administration through a nasogastric, gastrostomy, or jejunostomy tube. (LO 13.1b, 13.2b)

4. List three techniques that may be suggested to a patient who complains of difficulty swallowing a tablet. (LO 13.1b, 13.2b)

5. Children or elderly patients who require medication that is easily swallowed are often prescribed what form of medication? (LO 13.2b)

6. Define the term *reconstitution*. (LO 13.2b)

7. List four things to be written on the label of a reconstituted medication. (LO 13.2b)

Use the identified drug labels to answer the following questions:

8. In Label A, what are the brand name and the form of this drug? (LO 13.1b)

9. If the order was for 50 mg of this drug, what amount would you administer? (LO 13.1a)

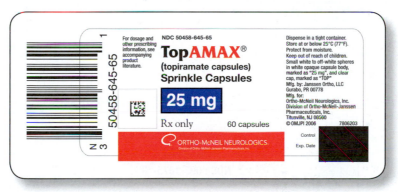

Label A

10. In Label B, what are the generic name and the form of this drug? (LO 13.1b)

11. Is it acceptable to crush this drug? (LO 13.1b)

12. If the order was for 40 mg of this drug, what amount would you administer? (LO 13.1a)

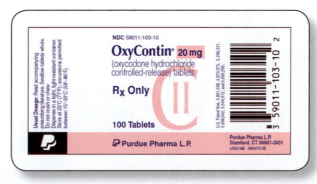

Label B

13. In Label C, what are the generic name and the form of this drug? (LO 13.1b)

14. If the order was for 150 mg of this drug what action would you take? (LO 13.1b)

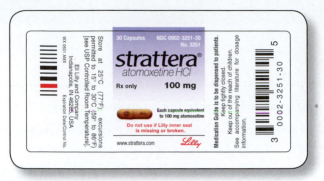

Label C

15. In Label D, what are the brand name and the form of this drug? (LO 13.2b)

16. If the order was for 15 mg of this drug what amount would you administer? (LO 13.2a)

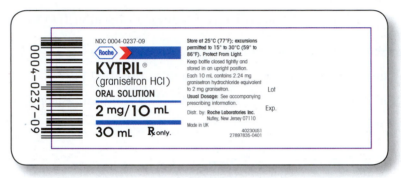

Label D

17. In Label E, how many milliliters of water would you add to reconstitute this drug to a 75 mL suspension? (LO 13.2b)

18. How are you instructed to reconstitute this drug? (LO 13.2b)

19. What is the warning on the label? (LO 13.2b)

20. If the order was for 200 mg of this drug what amount would you administer? (LO 13.2a)

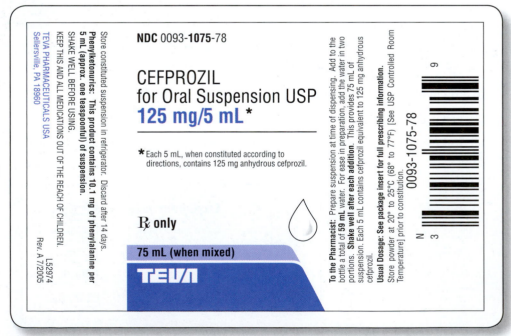

Label E

CHECK UP

For Exercises 1–17, calculate the amount to administer and the daily dose. Unless otherwise noted, tablets are scored in half.

1. Ordered: Dilaudid® 4 mg PO q6h
   On hand: Dilaudid® 8 mg scored tablets

   Administer: _____ (LO 13.1a)
   Daily dose: _____

2. Ordered: DiaBeta® 2.5 mg PO qam ac
   On hand: DiaBeta® 1.25 mg scored tablets

   Administer: _____ (LO 13.1a)
   Daily dose: _____

3. Ordered: Biltricide 450 mg PO q8h
   On hand: Biltricide 600 mg tablets scored in quarters

   Administer: _____ (LO 13.1a)
   Daily dose: _____

4. Ordered: Amoxicillin 300 mg PO q12h
   On hand: Amoxicillin suspension labeled 50 mg/mL

   Administer: _____ (LO 13.2a)
   Daily dose: _____

5. Ordered: Artane® 3 mg PO daily
   On hand: Artane® solution labeled 2 mg/5 mL

   Administer: _____ (LO 13.2a)
   Daily dose: _____

6. Ordered: Fosamax® 10 mg PO qam 30 min ac with water
   On hand: Fosamax® 5 mg unscored tablets

   Administer: _____ (LO 13.1a)
   Daily dose: _____

7. Ordered: Biaxin® liquid 62.5 mg via NGT q12h
   On hand: Biaxin® liquid labeled 125 mg/5 mL

   Administer: _____ (LO 13.2a)
   Daily dose: _____

8. Ordered: Isoptin® 270 mg PO qam
   On hand: Isoptin® 180 mg scored tablets

   Administer: _____ (LO 13.1a)
   Daily dose: _____

9. Ordered: Duricef® 0.5 g PO bid
   On hand: Duricef® suspension labeled 250 mg/5 mL

   Administer: _____ (LO 13.2a)
   Daily dose: _____

10. Ordered: Levoxyl® 0.45 mg PO daily
    On hand: Levoxyl® 300 mcg scored tablets

    Administer: _____ (LO 13.1a)
    Daily dose: _____

11. Ordered: Hivid 750 mcg PO q8h
    On hand: Hivid 0.375 mg unscored tablets

    Administer: _____ (LO 13.1a)
    Daily dose: _____

12. Ordered: Duricef® 500 mg PO bid
    On hand: Duricef® 1 g scored tablets

    Administer: _____ (LO 13.1a)
    Daily dose: _____

13. Ordered: Famvir 750 mg PO q12h
    On hand: Famvir 250 tablets

    Administer: _____ (LO 13.1a)
    Daily dose: _____

14. Ordered: Felbatol® 400 mg via NGT tid
    On hand: Felbatol® liquid labeled 600 mg/5 mL

    Administer: _____ (LO 13.2a)
    Daily dose: _____

15. Ordered: Synthroid® 0.175 mg PO daily
Administer: _____ (LO 13.1a)
On hand: Refer to label A. Tablets are unscored.
Daily dose: _____

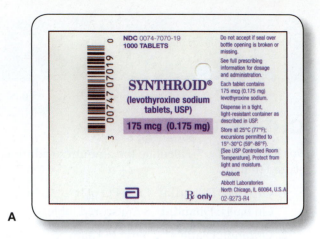

A

16. Ordered: Metformin 0.5 g po daily
On hand: Refer to label B.

Administer: _____ (LO 13.1a)
Daily dose: _____

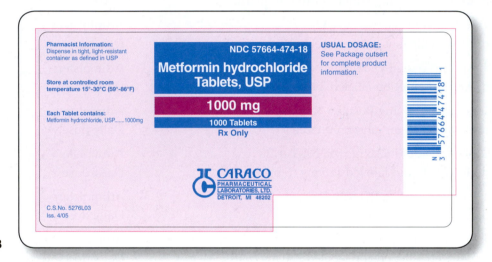

B

17. Ordered: Cefprozil 125 mg via NGT tid
On hand: Refer to label C.

Administer: _____ (LO 13.2a)
Daily dose: _____

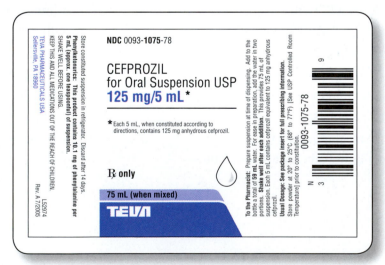

C

18. What combination will provide the desired dose with the fewest tablets? (LO 13.1b)
Ordered: Hytrin® 5 mg PO qpm
On hand: Hytrin® 1 mg unscored tablets and Hytrin 2 mg unscored tablets

19. A patient receives 15 mL of Lortab® elixir every 6 h. Lortab® elixir contains 7.5 mg hydrocodone and 500 mg acetaminophen in each 15 mL. How much acetaminophen will this patient receive in 24 h? (LO 13.1a)

20. How would you reconstitute the following medication? Find the amount to administer. (LO 13.2a, b)
Ordered: Cephalexin 375 mg PO bid
On hand: Refer to label D.

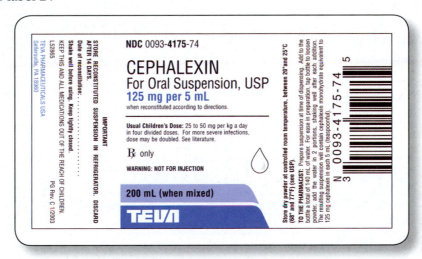

D

Each of the following sets of exercises provides a medication administration record (MAR) listing several medication orders and a variety of drug labels. Select the correct label for each medication order. Then calculate the amount to administer.

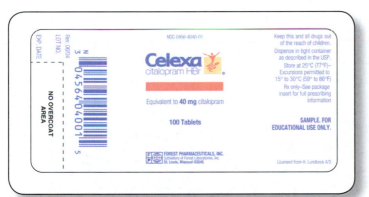

E Tablets are scored

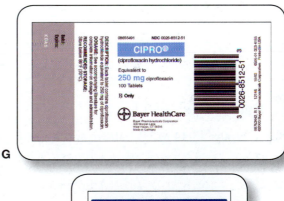

G

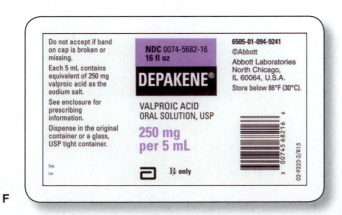

F

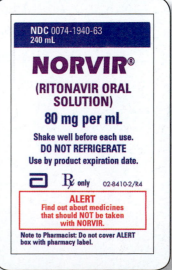

H

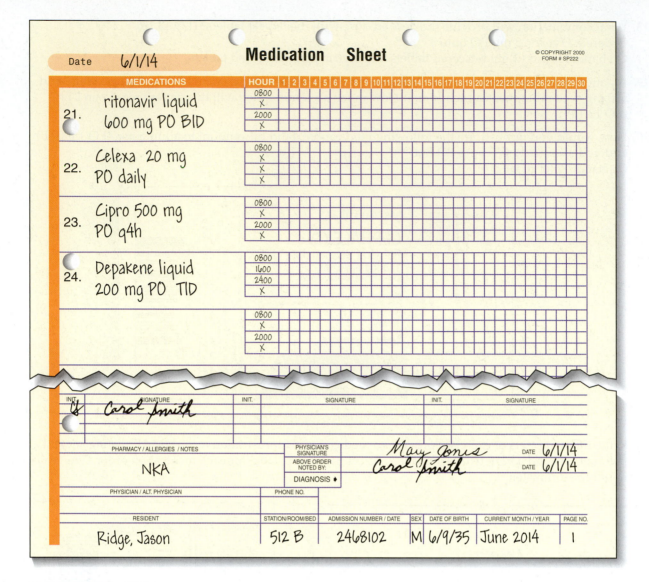

Figure 13-14 MAR 1

Refer to Figure 13-14 MAR 1 above and labels E to H on the previous page.

21. Use: _____   Administer: _____ (LO 13.2a)

22. Use: _____   Administer: _____ (LO 13.1a)

23. Use: _____   Administer: _____ (LO 13.1a)

24. Use: _____   Administer: _____ (LO 13.2a)

Refer to Figure 13-15 MAR 2 below and labels I to O on the next page.

25. Use: _____   Administer: _____ (LO 13.1a)

26. Use: _____   Administer: _____ (LO 13.1a)

27. Use: _____   Administer: _____ (LO 13.2a)

28. Use: _____   Administer: _____ (LO 13.1a)

29. Use: _____   Administer: _____ (LO 13.1a)

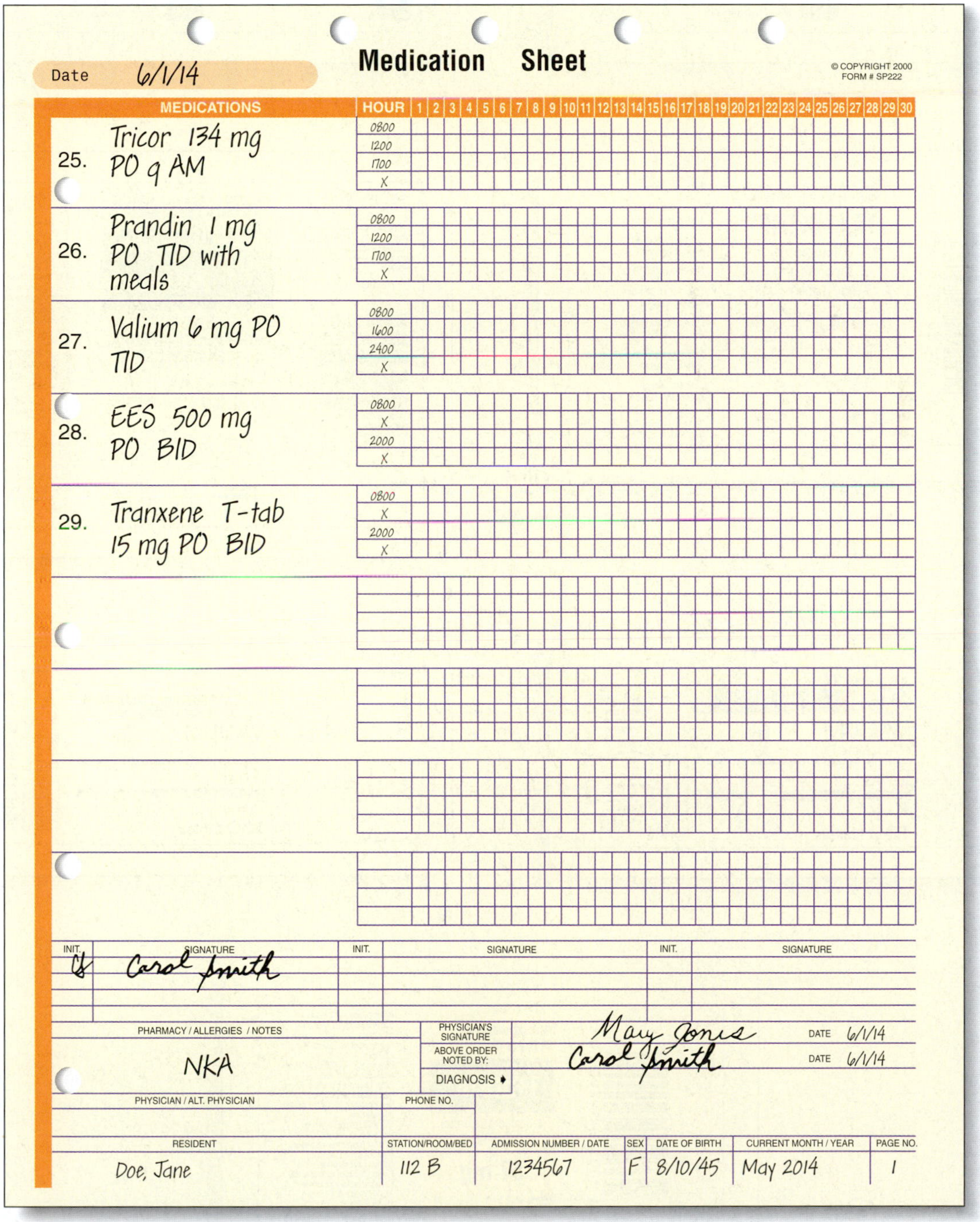

Date 6/1/14	**Medication Sheet**	© COPYRIGHT 2000 FORM # SP222

MEDICATIONS	HOUR	1 2 3 4 5 6 7 8 9 10 11 12 13 14 15 16 17 18 19 20 21 22 23 24 25 26 27 28 29 30
25. Tricor 134 mg PO q AM	0800 / 1200 / 1700 / X	
26. Prandin 1 mg PO TID with meals	0800 / 1200 / 1700 / X	
27. Valium 6 mg PO TID	0800 / 1600 / 2400 / X	
28. EES 500 mg PO BID	0800 / X / 2000 / X	
29. Tranxene T-tab 15 mg PO BID	0800 / X / 2000 / X	

INIT.	SIGNATURE	INIT.	SIGNATURE	INIT.	SIGNATURE
S	Carol Smith				

PHARMACY / ALLERGIES / NOTES	PHYSICIAN'S SIGNATURE	Mary Jones	DATE 6/1/14
NKA	ABOVE ORDER NOTED BY:	Carol Smith	DATE 6/1/14
	DIAGNOSIS ◆		
PHYSICIAN / ALT. PHYSICIAN	PHONE NO.		

RESIDENT	STATION/ROOM/BED	ADMISSION NUMBER / DATE	SEX	DATE OF BIRTH	CURRENT MONTH / YEAR	PAGE NO.
Doe, Jane	112 B	1234567	F	8/10/45	May 2014	1

Figure 13-15   MAR 2

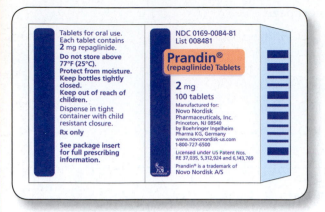

I

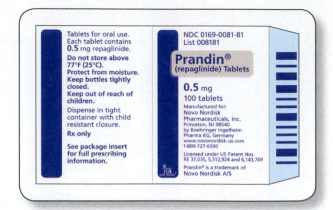

J

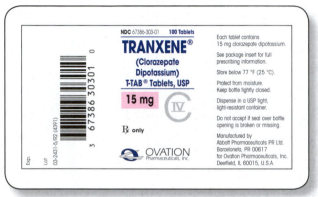

K

E.E.S.® 200 LIQUID

NDC 0074-6306-16
ONE PINT (473 mL)

ERYTHROMYCIN
ETHYLSUCCINATE ORAL
SUSPENSION, USP

Erythromycin activity
200 mg per 5 mL

L

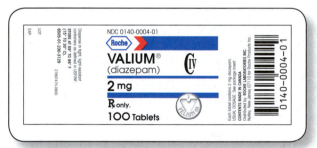

M

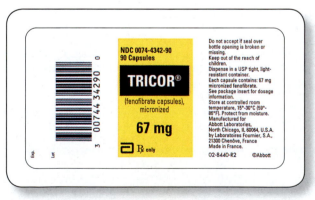

N

TRICOR®

NDC 0074-4342-90
90 Capsules

(fenofibrate capsules),
micronized

67 mg

O

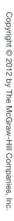

CRITICAL THINKING APPLICATIONS

The following medications are ordered for a patient with a gastrostomy tube who cannot swallow and must receive all medications through the tube.

a. Depakote® ER 250 mg daily

b. Valium® 4 mg qid

c. Vistaril 50 mg PO prn for anxiety

d. Cephalexin 500 mg

On hand: Refer to labels P, Q, R and S. For this exercise Valium® tablets are scored.

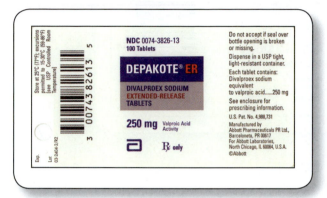

P

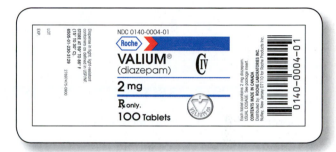

Q

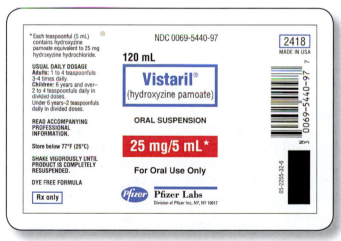

R

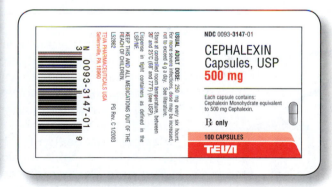

S

1. For each medication, calculate the amount to administer. (LO 13.1a)

2. Are there any medications on the list that cannot be given as ordered? (LO 13.1b)

3. How would you administer these medications? (LO 13.1, 13.1b)

4. What action would you take if you could not give a medication as ordered? (LO 13.1b)

CASE STUDY

Ordered: Biaxin® liquid 187.5 mg PO qid

On hand: Refer to label T.

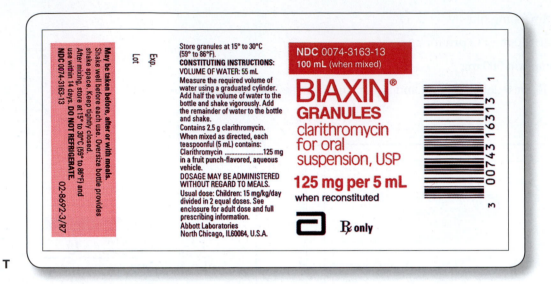

Store granules at 15° to 30°C (59° to 86°F).
CONSTITUTING INSTRUCTIONS:
VOLUME OF WATER: 55 mL
Measure the required volume of water using a graduated cylinder. Add half the volume of water to the bottle and shake vigorously. Add the remainder of water to the bottle and shake.
Contains 2.5 g clarithromycin. When mixed as directed, each teaspoonful (5 mL) contains:
Clarithromycin ....125 mg
in a fruit punch-flavored, aqueous vehicle.
DOSAGE MAY BE ADMINISTERED WITHOUT REGARD TO MEALS.
Usual dose: Children: 15 mg/kg/day divided in 2 equal doses. See enclosure for adult dose and full prescribing information.
Abbott Laboratories
North Chicago, IL60064, U.S.A.

NDC 0074-3163-13
100 mL (when mixed)

BIAXIN®
GRANULES
clarithromycin
for oral
suspension, USP

125 mg per 5 mL
when reconstituted

℞ only

Exp.
Lot

NDC 0074-3163-13
May be taken before, after or with meals. Shake well before each use. Oversize bottle provides shake space. Keep tightly closed. After mixing, store at 15° to 30°C (59° to 86°F) and use within 14 days. **DO NOT REFRIGERATE.**
02-8692-3/R7

3 00743 16313 1

T

1. Describe how you would reconstitute this medication. (LO 13.2b)

2. Calculate the amount to administer. (LO 13.2a)

3. What measuring device would you use to give this dose? (LO 13.2b)

4. Calculate the daily dose. (LO 13.2a)

INTERNET ACTIVITY

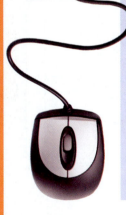

You are working in a physician's office where a patient with diabetes is having difficulty with blood glucose control. The physician discovers that the patient, who has trouble swallowing, has been crushing Glucotrol XL tablets. Because this sustained-release medication should not be crushed, the patient has been receiving too much medication at one time. You realize that this problem could occur with any patient who is taking a sustained-release medication.

Assignment: Search the Internet for patient education materials warning patients about crushing medications.

Suggested key words: medication + crushing; medication + swallowing; pills + swallowing

To check your answers, see the Answer section at the end of the book, which starts on page A-1.

GO TO . . . Open the CD-ROM that accompanies your textbook, and complete a final review of the learning objectives, practice problems, games, slideshow, and other activities presented for this chapter. For a final evaluation, take the chapter test. A score of 95 percent or above indicates mastery of the chapter concepts.

Parenteral Dosages and Other Medication Administration Forms

The best way to escape from a problem is to solve it.

—ALAN SAPORTA

Learning Outcomes

When you have completed Chapter 14, you will be able to:

14.1 Calculate doses of parenteral medication in solution and select a syringe based on the dosage calculation.

14.2 Calculate doses of medications expressed in percent or ratio format.

14.3 Calculate doses of reconstituted parenteral medications.

14.4 Differentiate other medication administration forms and equipment.

KEY TERMS

Absorption rate

Inhalant

Instillations

Metered-dose inhalers (MDIs)

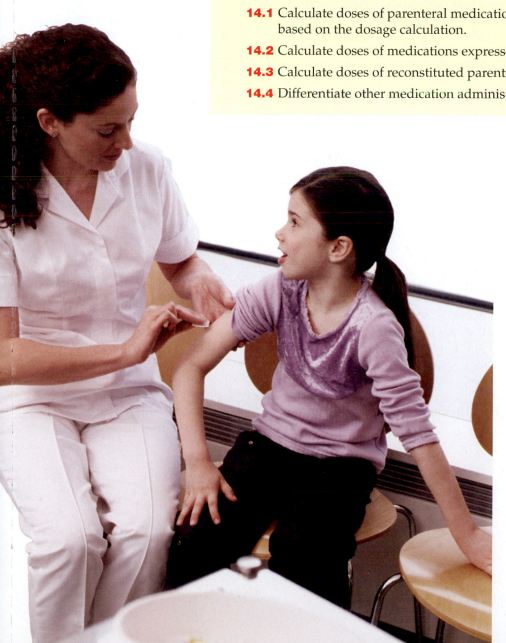

INTRODUCTION

Parenteral medications are *not* taken by mouth, so they bypass the digestive tract. They include medications that are administered by injection and other medications such as inhalants, rectal, and transdermal drugs. Injection routes include intravenous (IV), intramuscular (IM), subcutaneous (subcut), and intradermal (ID). These routes have different **absorption rates**, the rate at which the medication is absorbed and dispersed into the blood stream. Because of this, dosages may vary if the same medication is administered via different routes.

- IV (into a vein)—fastest absorption rate of 30 to 60 seconds
- IM (into a muscle)—absorption rate varies from 10 minutes and longer
- Subcut (under the skin, into fatty tissue)—absorption rate varies 15 minutes and longer
- ID (between layers of skin)—sustained absorption rate because medication is absorbed through the capillaries of skin

This chapter will focus on dosage calculations for parenteral medications with the exception of intravenous and insulin administration, which will be covered in later chapters. So get ready to solve some problems.

14.1 Calculating Parenteral Dosages in Solution

Injections are mixtures that contain the drug dissolved in an appropriate liquid. The dosage or solution strength on an injectable medication's label indicates the amount of drug contained within a volume of solution (see Table 14-1). Dosage strength may be expressed in milligrams per milliliter, as a percent, or as a ratio.

TABLE 14-1 Sample Solution Strengths

LABEL DESCRIPTION	INTERPRETATION
Compazine 5 mg/mL	1 mL contains 5 mg of Compazine
Epogen 3000 units/mL	1 mL contains 3000 units of Epogen
Lidocaine 1%	100 mL contains 1 g of lidocaine
Epinephrine 1:1000	1000 mL contains 1 g of epinephrine

Physicians' orders for injections will usually specify the amount of medication to be administered to the patient. Before the injection can be administered, it is necessary to calculate how many milliliters of the solution contain the desired dose of the medication.

As with oral medications, follow the ABC's of dosage calculation, starting with the dosage ordered, dose on hand, and dosage unit. If the dosage ordered and dose on hand have different units, then you must perform Step A: convert the units of the dosage ordered to the units of the desired dose. Then follow Step B: calculate the amount to administer, using any of the three methods of dosage calculations, that is, proportion, dimensional analysis, or the formula method. Then verify your calculation with Step C: Think! . . . Is it reasonable?

Syringe Sizes

Once you have determined the amount to administer, you must select the appropriate syringe and needle. Rule 14-1 gives you the guidelines to follow for selecting the syringe. See Chapter 8 for a discussion of needles.

RULE 14-1	Select the proper syringe.

1. If the amount of injection to administer is 1 mL or more, round the amount to the tenths and use a standard 3-mL syringe.

2. If the amount of injection to administer is less than 1 mL but greater than or equal to 0.5 mL and calculates evenly to the tenths, use a 1-mL tuberculin syringe or a standard 3-mL syringe.

3. If the amount of injection to administer is less than 1 mL, round to the hundredths and use a 1-mL tuberculin syringe. For amounts less than 0.5 mL use a 0.5-mL tuberculin syringe, if available.

Example 1

The amount to administer is calculated at 2.4 mL. Since this is greater than 1 mL, a standard syringe should be used. See Figure 14-1.

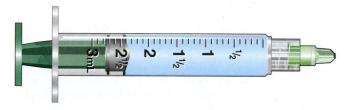

Figure 14-1   Standard syringe with 2.4 mL.

Example 2

The amount to administer is calculated at 0.6 mL. Since this amount is greater than 0.5 mL and calculates evenly to the tenths, either a 1-mL tuberculin syringe or a 3-mL syringe can be used. See Figures 14-2a and 14-2b.

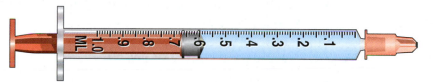

Figure 14-2a   A 1-mL tuberculin syringe with 0.6 mL.

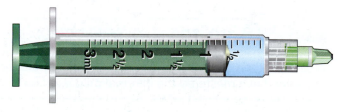

Figure 14-2b   A standard 3-mL syringe with 0.6 mL.

Example 3

The amount to administer is calculated at 0.34 mL. Since this is less than 1 mL, a 1 mL tuberculin syringe or a 0.5-mL tuberculin syringe should be used. See Figure 14-3.

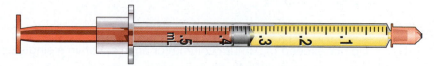

Figure 14-3   A 0.5-mL tuberculin syringe with 0.34 mL.

GO TO . . . Open the CD-ROM that accompanies your textbook, and select Chapter 14, Selecting a Syringe (LO 14.1). Review the animation and example problems, then complete the practice problems. Continue to the next section of the book once you have mastered the information presented.

The amount to administer will not always be in whole milliliters, and it will sometimes be necessary to round your answer.

RULE 14-2	Correctly round the amount of an injection to administer.
	1. Round volumes greater than 1 mL to the nearest tenth because the 3 mL syringe is calibrated in tenths.
	2. Round volumes less than 1 mL to the nearest hundredth because tuberculin syringes are calibrated in hundredths.

Example 1

The amount to administer is calculated at 1.66 mL. Since the volume is greater than 1 mL, you round 1.66 mL to the nearest tenth, which is 1.7 mL.

LEARNING LINK Recall from Chapter 2, Rule 2-4 about rounding decimals.

Example 2

The amount to administer is calculated at 0.532 mL. Since the volume is less than 1 mL, you round 0.532 mL to the nearest hundredth, which is 0.53 mL.

LEARNING LINK Recall from Chapter 2, Rule 2-4 about rounding decimals.

GO TO . . . Open the CD-ROM that accompanies your textbook, and select Chapter 14, Rounding an Injection (14.1). Review the animation and example problems, then complete the practice problems. Continue to the next section of the book once you have mastered the information presented.

Once you determine the proper syringe, you must also decide whether the amount to be administered can be safely injected in a single site. When the amount to administer exceeds the amount that can be safely given in one site, divide the amount into equal (or nearly equal) parts. Then administer them in separate sites.

RULE 14-3	Do not exceed maximum volume for an injection in a single site.
	Intramuscular injections:
	• Adult 3 mL
	• Adult deltoid (arm) 1 mL

- Child 6 to 12 years   2 mL
- Child 0 to 5 years   1 mL
- Premature Infant   0.5 mL

Subcutaneous injections: 1 mL

Dosages larger than these maximum volumes are very rare and should be checked and verified.

Example

The amount to administer to an adult is 4.5 mL. After checking and verifying the amount, you draw up 2 mL into one syringe and 2.5 mL into another. Inject the contents of each syringe into a different site. See Figure 14-4.

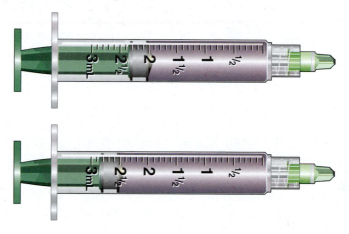

Figure 14-4 Two standard syringes would be used for a dose greater than the maximum volume for an injection such as 4.5 mL.

GO TO . . . Open the CD-ROM that accompanies your textbook, and select Chapter 14, Maximum Volumes for Injections (LO 14.1). Review the animation and example problems, then complete the practice problems. Continue to the next section of the book once you have mastered the information presented.

When calculating the amount to administer for injectable medications, you must determine how many milliliters contain the desired dose of medication and then apply Rules 14-1 to 14-3.

PROPORTION METHOD

EXAMPLE 1

Find the amount to administer and select the proper syringe.

Ordered: Valium® 7.5 mg IM now

On hand: Refer to Figure 14-5 on next page.

Patient: A 175-lb, 45-year-old male

STEP A: CONVERT
The dosage ordered O and the dose on hand H are already expressed in the same units, so the desired dose D is 7.5 mg.

STEP B: CALCULATE

Follow Procedure Checklist 12-1.

1. Fill in the proportion.

$$\frac{H}{Q} = \frac{D}{A} \qquad H : Q = D : A$$

From the label we find that the dosage unit Q is 1 mL and the dose on hand H is 5 mg.

Using Fractions:

$$\frac{5 \text{ mg}}{1 \text{ mL}} = \frac{7.5 \text{ mg}}{A}$$

Using Ratios:

$$5 \text{ mg} : 1 \text{ mL} = 7.5 \text{ mg} : A$$

2. Cancel units.

$$\frac{5 \, \cancel{\text{mg}}}{1 \text{ mL}} = \frac{7.5 \, \cancel{\text{mg}}}{A}$$

$$5 \, \cancel{\text{mg}} : 1 \text{ mL} = 7.5 \, \cancel{\text{mg}} : A$$

3. Cross-multiply and solve

$$5 \times A = 1 \text{ mL} \times 7.5 \qquad\qquad 1 \text{ mL} \times 7.5 = 5 \times A$$

$$A = \frac{1 \text{ mL} \times 7.5}{5} \qquad\qquad \frac{1 \text{ mL} \times 7.5}{5} = A$$

$$A = 1.5 \text{ mL} \qquad\qquad\qquad 1.5 \text{ mL} = A$$

STEP C: THINK! . . . IS IT REASONABLE?

Since 7.5 mg is $1\frac{1}{2}$ times larger than 5 mg, the volume to administer should be $1\frac{1}{2}$ times larger than the volume on hand. 1.5 mL is one and one half times larger than 1 mL, so the answer is reasonable.

The amount to administer is 1.5 mL.

- Referring to Rule 14-1, a standard 3-mL syringe would be used.
- Referring to Rule 14-2, we find that it is not necessary to round in this example.
- Referring to Rule 14-3, the total volume may be given as a single injection.

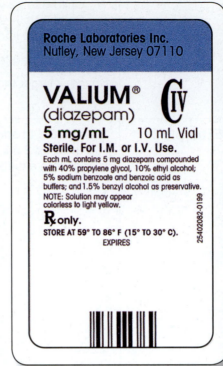

Figure 14-5

EXAMPLE 2 Find the amount to administer and select the proper syringe.

Ordered: Lorazepam 800 mcg IM now

On hand: Refer to Figure 14-6.

Patient: An 85-lb, 12-year-old female

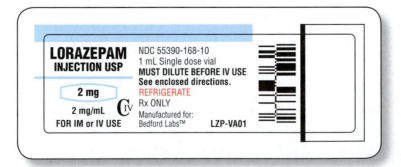

Figure 14-6

STEP A: CONVERT

The dosage ordered O is in micrograms, and the dose on hand H is in milligrams, so the desired dose D, in milligrams, must be calculated.

Follow Procedure Checklist 6-1 using fractions.

1. Fill in the proportion, recalling that 1 mg = 1000 mcg.

$$\frac{1 \text{ mg}}{1000 \text{ mcg}} = \frac{D}{800 \text{ mcg}}$$

2. Cancel units.

$$\frac{1 \text{ mg}}{1000 \text{ \cancel{mcg}}} = \frac{D}{800 \text{ \cancel{mcg}}}$$

3. Cross-multiply and solve for the unknown.

$$1000 \times D = 1 \times 800 \text{ mg}$$

$$D = 0.8 \text{ mg}$$

We now have the necessary pieces of information: D = 0.8 mg, Q = 1 mL, and H = 2 mg.

STEP B: CALCULATE
Follow Procedure Checklist 12-1, using fractions.

1. Fill in the proportion.

$$\frac{2 \text{ mg}}{1 \text{ mL}} = \frac{0.8 \text{ mg}}{A}$$

2. Cancel units.

$$\frac{2 \text{ \cancel{mg}}}{1 \text{ mL}} = \frac{0.8 \text{ \cancel{mg}}}{A}$$

3. Cross-multiply and solve for the unknown.

$$2 \times A = 1 \text{ mL} \times 0.8$$

$$A = 1 \text{ mL} \times \frac{0.8}{2}$$

$$A = 0.4 \text{ mL}$$

STEP C: THINK! . . . IS IT REASONABLE?
Since 1 is half of 2, then A should be half of 0.8. 0.4 is half of 0.8, so the answer is reasonable.

The amount to administer is 0.4 mL.

- Referring to Rule 14-1, a 1-mL or 0.5-mL tuberculin syringe would be used.
- Referring to Rule 14-2, we find that it is not necessary to round in this example.
- Referring to Rule 14-3, the total volume may be given as a single injection.

DIMENSIONAL ANALYSIS

EXAMPLE 1

Find the amount to administer and select the proper syringe.

Ordered: Valium 7.5 mg IM now

On hand: Refer to Figure 14-5 on the previous page.

Patient: A 175-lb, 45-year-old male

STEP A: CONVERT
The dosage ordered O is 7.5 mg. The dose on hand H is 5 mg, and the dosing unit Q is 1 mL. Because the dosage ordered and the dose on hand have the same units, no conversion is needed to find the desired dose D, which is 7.5 mg.

STEP B: CALCULATE

Follow Procedure Checklist 12-2.

1. The unit of measure for the amount to administer will be milliliters.

   A mL =

2. No conversion factor needed.

3. The dosage unit is 1 mL. The dose on hand is 5 mg. This is your first factor.

   $$\frac{1 \text{ mL}}{5 \text{ mg}}$$

4. The dosage ordered is 7.5 mg. Set up the equation.

   $$A \text{ mL} = \frac{1 \text{ mL}}{5 \text{ mg}} \times \frac{7.5 \text{ mg}}{1}$$

5. Cancel units.

   $$A \text{ mL} = \frac{1 \text{ mL}}{5 \text{ \cancel{mg}}} \times \frac{7.5 \text{ \cancel{mg}}}{1}$$

6. Solve the equation.

   $$A \text{ mL} = \frac{1 \text{ mL}}{5} \times \frac{7.5}{1}$$

   $$A = 1.5 \text{ mL}$$

STEP C: THINK! . . . IS IT REASONABLE?

Since 7.5 is $1\frac{1}{2}$ times larger than 5, the volume to be administered should be $1\frac{1}{2}$ times larger than 1. The amount to administer, 1.5, is $1\frac{1}{2}$ times larger than 1, so the answer is reasonable.

The amount to administer is 1.5 mL.

- Referring to Rule 14-1, a standard syringe 3-mL would be used.

- Referring to Rule 14-2, we find that it is not necessary to round in this example.

- Referring to Rule 14-3, the total volume may be given as a single injection.

| **EXAMPLE 2** | Find the amount to administer and select the proper syringe. |

Ordered: Lorazepam 800 mcg IM now

On hand: Refer to Figure 14-6 on page 352.

Patient: An 85-lb, 12-year-old female

STEP A: CONVERT

The unit of measure for the dose on hand is milligrams. The unit of measure for the dose ordered is micrograms. Determine the conversion factor for milligrams to micrograms.

STEP B: CALCULATE

Follow Procedure Checklist 12-2.

1. The unit of measure for the amount to administer will be milliliters.

   A mL =

2. The conversion factor is:

   $$\frac{1 \text{ mg}}{1000 \text{ mcg}}$$

3. The dosage unit is 1 mL. The dose on hand is 2 mg. This is our second factor.

   $$\frac{1 \text{ mg}}{1000 \text{ mcg}} \times \frac{1 \text{ mL}}{2 \text{ mg}}$$

4. The dosage ordered is 800 mcg. Set up the equation.

   $$A \text{ mL} = \frac{1 \text{ mg}}{1000 \text{ mcg}} \times \frac{1 \text{ mL}}{2 \text{ mg}} \times \frac{800 \text{ mcg}}{1}$$

5. Cancel units.

$$A \text{ mL} = \frac{1 \text{ mg}}{1000 \text{ mcg}} \times \frac{1 \text{ mL}}{2 \text{ mg}} \times \frac{800 \text{ mcg}}{1}$$

6. Solve the equation.

$$A \text{ mL} = \frac{1}{1000} \times \frac{1 \text{ mL}}{2} \times \frac{800}{1}$$

$$A = 0.4 \text{ mL}$$

STEP C: THINK! . . . IS IT REASONABLE?

The concentration is 2 mg per 1 mL, so the volume to be administered will be half the dose (in milligrams). 0.4 is half of 0.8 (800 mcg), so it is reasonable.

The amount to administer is 0.4 mL.

- Referring to Rule 14-1, a 1-mL or 0.5-mL tuberculin syringe would be used.
- Referring to Rule 14-2, we find that it is not necessary to round in this example.
- Referring to Rule 14-3, the total volume may be given as a single injection.

FORMULA METHOD

EXAMPLE 1

Find the amount to administer and select the proper syringe.

Ordered: Valium 7.5 mg IM now

On hand: Refer to Figure 14-5 on page 352.

Patient: A 175-lb, 45-year-old male

STEP A: CONVERT
The drug is ordered in milligrams, which is the same unit of measure as that of the dose on hand. No conversion necessary.

STEP B: CALCULATE
Follow Procedure Checklist 12-3.

1. Desired dose $D = 7.5$ mg

Dose on hand $H = 5$ mg

Quantity to be administered $Q = 1$ mL

2. Fill in the formula.

$$\frac{D}{H} \times Q = A$$

$$\frac{7.5 \text{ mg}}{5 \text{ mg}} \times 1 \text{ mL} = A$$

3. Cancel units.

$$\frac{7.5 \text{ mg}}{5 \text{ mg}} \times 1 \text{ mL} = A$$

4. Solve for the unknown.

$$\frac{7.5}{5} \times 1 \text{ mL} = A$$

$$1.5 \text{ mL} = A$$

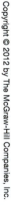

STEP C: THINK! . . . IS IT REASONABLE?

Since the desired dose is $1\frac{1}{2}$ times larger than the dose in 1 mL, the volume to be administered should be $1\frac{1}{2}$ times larger than 1 mL. The amount to administer, 1.5 mL, is one and one half times larger than 1 mL, so it is reasonable.

The amount to administer is 1.5 mL.

- Referring to Rule 14-1, a standard 3-mL syringe would be used.
- Referring to Rule 14-2, we find that it is not necessary to round in this example.
- Referring to Rule 14-3, the total volume may be given as a single injection.

EXAMPLE 2   Find the amount to administer and select the proper syringe.

Ordered: Lorazepam 800 mcg IM now

On hand: Refer to Figure 14-6 on page 352.

Patient: An 85-lb, 12-year-old female

STEP A: CONVERT

The dosage ordered Q is in micrograms, and the dose on hand H is in milligrams, so the desired dose D, in milligrams, must be calculated.

Follow Procedure Checklist 6-1 using fractions.

In this example, Procedure Checklist 6-1 proportion method is used.

1. Fill in the proportion, recalling that 1 mg = 1000 mcg.

$$\frac{1\ \text{mg}}{1000\ \text{mcg}} = \frac{D}{800\ \text{mcg}}$$

2. Cancel units.

$$\frac{1\ \text{mg}}{1000\ \cancel{\text{mcg}}} = \frac{D}{800\ \cancel{\text{mcg}}}$$

3. Cross-multiply and solve for the unknown.

$$1000 \times D = 1 \times 800\ \text{mg}$$
$$D = 0.8\ \text{mg}$$

We now have the necessary pieces of information: $D = 0.8$ mg, $Q = 1$ mL, and $H = 2$ mg.

STEP B: CALCULATE

Follow Procedure Checklist 12-3.

1. Fill in the formula.

$$\frac{0.8\ \text{mg}}{2\ \text{mg}} \times 1\ \text{mL} = A$$

2. Cancel units.

$$\frac{0.8\ \cancel{\text{mg}}}{2\ \cancel{\text{mg}}} \times 1\ \text{mL} = A$$

3. Solve for the unknown.

$$\frac{0.8}{2} \times 1\ \text{mL} = A$$
$$0.4\ \text{mL} = A$$

STEP C: THINK! . . . IS IT REASONABLE?

The concentration is 2 mg per 1 mL, so the volume to administer will be half as large as the desired dose. 0.4 is half as large as 0.8 so it is reasonable.

The amount to administer is 0.4 mL.

- Referring to Rule 14-1, a 1-mL or 0.5-mL tuberculin syringe would be used.
- Referring to Rule 14-2, we find that it is not necessary to round in this example.
- Referring to Rule 14-3, the total volume may be given as a single injection.

Confirming the Physician's Order

A patient in an agitated state is brought to the emergency department. The physician verbally orders 2 mL IM of Vistaril. The healthcare professional draws up 2 mL from a vial labeled 50 mg/mL. She then notices another vial labeled 25 mg/mL.

Think! . . . Is It Reasonable? What should she do? How is the patient's care affected if she does not take action?

REVIEW AND PRACTICE

14.1 Calculating Parenteral Dosages in Solutions

For exercises 1 to 17, find the amount to administer, and then determine the proper syringe and write it in the space provided.

1. Ordered: Thiamine 100 mg IM now

   On hand: Refer to label A.

   Administer: _____   Syringe: _____

```
NDC 63323-013-02        1302

THIAMINE
HYDROCHLORIDE

INJECTION, USP

100 mg/mL

For IM or IV Use          Rx only
2 mL  Multiple Dose Vial
Usual Dosage: See insert.
PROTECT FROM LIGHT.

Abraxis
Pharmaceutical Products
Schaumburg, IL 60173

401818C

LOT/EXP

3   63323-013-02   8
```

A

2. Ordered: Heparin 700 units subcut daily

On hand: Refer to label B.

Administer: _____   Syringe: _____

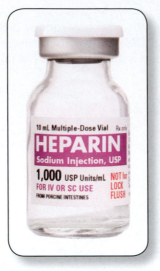

B

3. Ordered: Tigan® 200 mg IM TID

On hand: Refer to label C.

Administer: _____   Syringe: _____

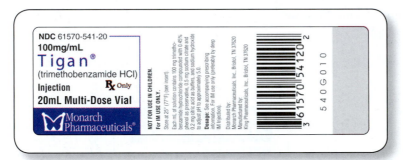

C

4. Ordered: Sandostatin® 200 mcg subcut q12h

On hand: Refer to label D.

Administer: _____   Syringe: _____

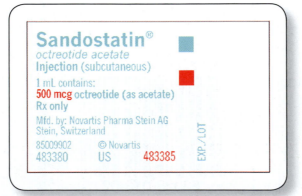

D

5. Ordered: Neupogen® 180 mcg subcut daily

On hand: Refer to label E.

Administer: _____   Syringe: _____

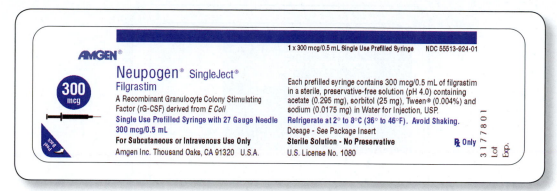

E

6. Ordered: Neupogen® 240 mcg subcut daily

On hand: Refer to label F.

Administer: _____   Syringe: _____

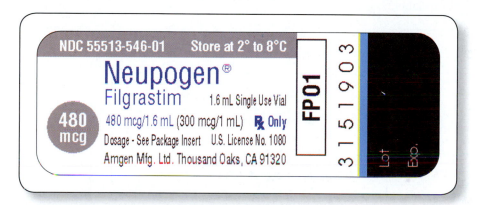

F

7. Ordered: Epogen® 3500 units subcut three times per week

On hand: Refer to label G.

Administer: _____   Syringe: _____

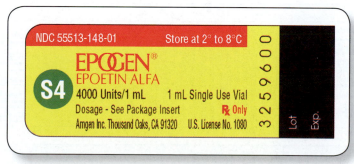

G

8. Ordered: Neulasta® 6 mg subcut now

On hand: Refer to label H.

Administer: _____   Syringe: _____

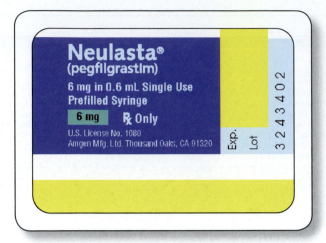

H

9. Ordered: Zemplar™ 3 mcg IM daily

On hand: Refer to label I.

Administer: _____   Syringe: _____

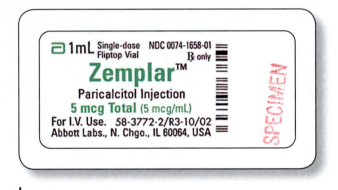

I

10. Ordered: Oxytocin 10 units IM now.

On hand: Refer to label J.

Administer: _____   Syringe: _____

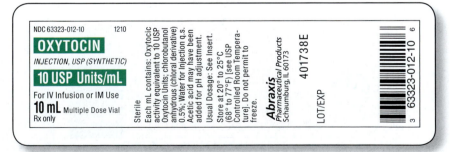

J

11. Ordered: Clindamycin 600 mg IM pre-op

On hand: Refer to label K.

Administer: _____   Syringe: _____

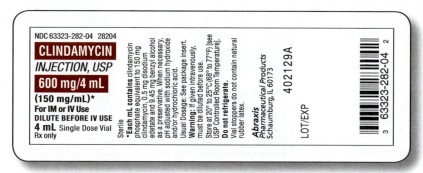

K

12. Ordered: Synagis® 35 mg IM now

On hand: Refer to label L.

Administer: _____   Syringe: _____

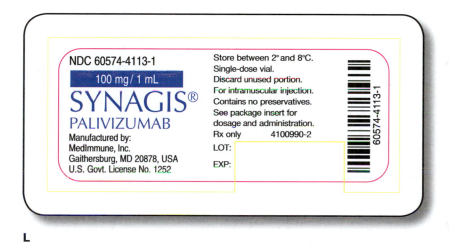

L

13. Ordered: Oxytocin 15 units IM q 12h prn

On hand: Refer to label M.

Administer: _____   Syringe: _____

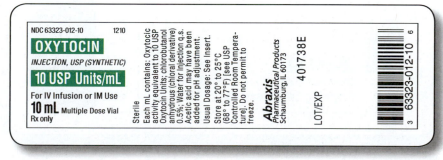

M

14. Ordered: Furosemide 20 mg IM at 0800

On hand: Refer to label N.

Administer: _____   Syringe: _____

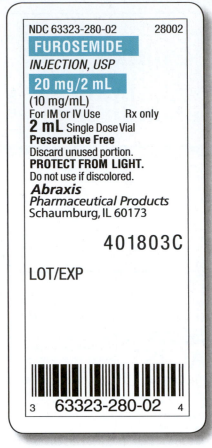

N

15. Ordered: Aranesp® 25 mcg subcut now

On hand: Refer to label O.

Administer: _____   Syringe: _____

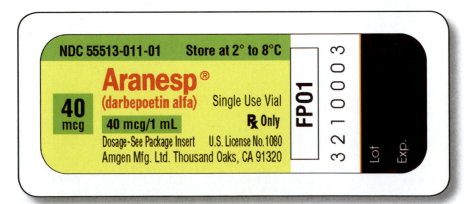

O

16. Ordered: Valium® 10 mg IM stat
On hand: Refer to label P.
Administer: _____   Syringe: _____

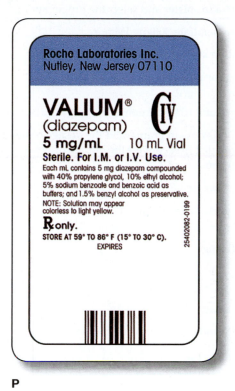

P

To check your answers, see the Answer section at the end of the book, which starts on page A-1.

14.2 Medications Expressed in Percent or Ratio Format

When the dosage strength is expressed as a percent or a ratio, convert it before calculating the amount to administer. For example, to administer 1% lidocaine, rewrite the strength as 1 g (dose on hand) per 100 mL (dosage unit) then calculate. If the labeled strength were 1:2000, rewrite it as 1 g (dose on hand) per 2000 mL (dosage unit). Some drugs, such as heparin, are measured in units and may have their solution strength expressed in ratio format. The ratio indicates the number of units contained in 1 mL. For example, heparin sodium 1:10,000 contains 10,000 units in 1 mL.

RULE 14-4

When a solution strength is expressed as a percent or ratio:

1. Convert the percent or ratio to the dosage strength, such as grams per milliliter, milligrams per milliliter, or units per milliliter.

2. Calculate the amount to administer, then apply Rules 14-1 to 14-3.

PROPORTION METHOD

EXAMPLE 1

Find the amount to administer and select the proper syringe.

Ordered: Magnesium sulfate 300 mg IM now

On hand: Magnesium sulfate 10% solution

Patient: A 75-lb, 8-year-old female

STEP A: CONVERT

The dosage strength of a 10% solution is 10 g (H) per 100 mL (Q).

The dose on hand H is now in grams, and the dosage ordered O is in milligrams. To calculate the desired dose D, we must first convert the dosage ordered—300 mg—to the same unit of measure as that of the dose on hand, grams.

Follow Procedure Checklist 6-1 using fractions.

1. Fill in the proportion, recalling that 1 g = 1000 mg.

$$\frac{1 \text{ g}}{1000 \text{ mg}} = \frac{D}{300 \text{ mg}}$$

2. Cancel units.

$$\frac{1 \text{ g}}{1000 \text{ mg}} = \frac{D}{300 \text{ mg}}$$

3. Cross-multiply and solve for the unknown.

$$1000 \times D = 300 \times 1 \text{ g}$$
$$D = \frac{300 \times 1 \text{ g}}{1000}$$
$$D = 0.3 \text{ g}$$

STEP B: CALCULATE

Follow Procedure Checklist 12-1 using fractions.

1. $D = 0.3$ g, $Q = 100$ mL, and $H = 10$ g. Fill in the proportion.

$$\frac{10 \text{ g}}{100 \text{ mL}} = \frac{0.3 \text{ g}}{A}$$

2. Cancel units.

$$\frac{10 \text{ g}}{100 \text{ mL}} = \frac{0.3 \text{ g}}{A}$$

3. Cross-multiply and solve for the unknown.

$$10 \times A = 100 \text{ mL} \times 0.3$$
$$A = \frac{100 \text{ mL} \times 0.3}{10}$$
$$A = 3 \text{ mL}$$

STEP C: THINK! . . . IS IT REASONABLE?

Since the concentration of the medication is 1 to 10, the volume to be administered should be 10 times larger than the desired dose. 3 is 10 times larger than 0.3 so it is reasonable.
The amount to administer is 3 mL.

- Referring to Rule 14-1, a standard 3-mL syringe would be used.

- Referring to Rule 14-2, we find that it is not necessary to round in this example.

- Referring to Rule 14-3, the dose would need to be divided into two parts because of the age of the patient. Draw 1.5 mL into each of two syringes and administer them into different sites.

| EXAMPLE 2 | Find the amount to administer and select the proper syringe. |

Ordered: Epinephrine 0.2 mg subcut stat

On hand: Vial of epinephrine 1:2000 solution for injection

Patient: A 150-lb, 35-year-old adult

STEP A: CONVERT

The dosage strength of a 1:2000 solution is 1 g (*H*) per 2000 mL (*Q*).

The dose on hand *H* is now in grams, and the dosage ordered *O* is in milligrams. To calculate the desired dose *D*, we must first convert the dosage ordered 0.2 mg to the same unit of measure as that of the dose on hand, grams.

Follow Procedure Checklist 6-1 using fractions.

1. Fill in the proportion, recalling that 1 g = 1000 mg.

$$\frac{1 \text{ g}}{1000 \text{ mg}} = \frac{D}{0.2 \text{ mg}}$$

2. Cancel units.

$$\frac{1 \text{ g}}{1000 \text{ mg}} = \frac{D}{0.2 \text{ mg}}$$

3. Cross-multiply and solve for the unknown.

$$1000 \times D = 0.2 \times 1 \text{ g}$$

$$D = \frac{0.2 \times 1 \text{ g}}{1000}$$

$$D = 0.0002 \text{ g}$$

STEP B: CALCULATE

Follow Procedure Checklist 12-1 using fractions.

1. *D* = 0.0002 g, *Q* = 2000 mL, and *H* = 1 g. Fill in the proportion.

$$\frac{1 \text{ g}}{2000 \text{ mL}} = \frac{0.0002 \text{ g}}{A}$$

2. Cancel units.

$$\frac{1 \text{ g}}{2000 \text{ mL}} = \frac{0.0002 \text{ g}}{A}$$

3. Cross-multiply and solve for the unknown.

$$1 \times A = 2000 \text{ mL} \times 0.0002$$

$$A = \frac{2000 \text{ mL} \times 0.0002}{1}$$

$$A = 0.4 \text{ mL}$$

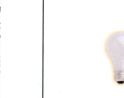

STEP C: THINK! . . . IS IT REASONABLE?

The medication concentration is 1 mg/2 mL. Since 0.4 is twice as much as 0.2 it is reasonable.

The amount to administer is 0.4 mL.

- Referring to Rule 14-1, a 1-mL or 0.5-mL tuberculin syringe would be used.
- Referring to Rule 14-2, we find that it is not necessary to round in this example.
- Referring to Rule 14-3, the dose would not need to be divided into two because the amount is less than 0.5 mL.

| EXAMPLE 3 | Find the amount to administer and select the proper syringe. |

Ordered: Heparin sodium 5,000 units subcut q8h

On hand: Heparin 1:10,000 for injection

Patient: A 145-lb, 60-year-old male

STEP A: CONVERT

The dosage strength of heparin 1:10,000 is 10,000 units (H) per 1 mL (Q).

The dosage ordered O and the dose on hand H are both expressed as units, so no conversion is necessary to find the desired dose, which is 5,000 units.

STEP B: CALCULATE

Follow Procedure Checklist 12-1 using fractions.

1. Fill in the proportion.

$$\frac{10{,}000\text{ units}}{1\text{ mL}} = \frac{5{,}000\text{ units}}{A}$$

2. Cancel units.

$$\frac{10{,}000\ \cancel{\text{units}}}{1\text{ mL}} = \frac{5{,}000\ \cancel{\text{units}}}{A}$$

3. Cross-multiply and solve for the unknown.

$$10{,}000 \times A = 1\text{ mL} \times 5{,}000$$

$$A = 1\text{ mL} \times \frac{5{,}000}{10{,}000}$$

$$A = 0.5\text{ mL}$$

STEP C: THINK! . . . IS IT REASONABLE?

5,000 units is half as much as 10,000 units, so the volume to administer should be half of 1 mL. 0.5 is one-half of 1, so the answer is reasonable.

The amount to administer is 0.5 mL.

- Referring to Rule 14-1, a 1-mL tuberculin syringe would be used.
- Referring to Rule 14-2, we find that it is not necessary to round in this example.
- Referring to Rule 14-3, the total volume may be given as a single injection.

DIMENSIONAL ANALYSIS

| EXAMPLE 1 | Find the amount to administer and select the proper syringe. |

Ordered: Magnesium sulfate 300 mg IM now

On hand: Magnesium sulfate 10% solution

Patient: A 75-lb, 8-year-old female

STEP A: CONVERT

The unit of measure for the dosage ordered is milligrams. The unit of measure for the dose on hand is grams. Recall that 1 g equals 1000 mg. Because we wish to convert to grams (the units of the dose on hand), our first factor must have grams on top. The dosage strength of a 10% solution is 10 g (*H*) per 100 mL (*Q*).

STEP B: CALCULATE

Follow Procedure Checklist 12-2.

1. The unit of measure for the amount to administer will be milliliters.

    A mL =

2. Conversion factor is:

    $$\frac{1 \text{ g}}{1000 \text{ mg}}$$

3. The dosage unit is 100 mL. The dose on hand is 10 g. This is our second factor.

    $$\frac{1 \text{ g}}{1000 \text{ mg}} \times \frac{100 \text{ mL}}{10 \text{ g}}$$

4. The dosage ordered is 300 mg. Place this over 1 and set up the equation.

    $$A \text{ mL} = \frac{1 \text{ g}}{1000 \text{ mg}} \times \frac{100 \text{ mL}}{10 \text{ g}} \times \frac{300 \text{ mg}}{1}$$

5. Cancel units.

    $$A \text{ mL} = \frac{1 \cancel{\text{g}}}{1000 \cancel{\text{mg}}} \times \frac{100 \text{ mL}}{10 \cancel{\text{g}}} \times \frac{300 \cancel{\text{mg}}}{1}$$

6. Solve the equation.

    $$A \text{ mL} = \frac{1}{1000} \times \frac{100 \text{ mL}}{10} \times \frac{300}{1}$$

    $$A = 3 \text{ mL}$$

STEP C: THINK! . . . IS IT REASONABLE?

The medication is in a 1 to 10 solution. 3 is 10 times larger than 0.3, so it is reasonable.

The amount to administer is 3 mL.

- Referring to Rule 14-1, a standard 3-mL syringe would be used.
- Referring to Rule 14-2, we find that it is not necessary to round in this example.
- Referring to Rule 14-3, the dose would need to be divided into two parts because of the age of the patient. Draw 1.5 mL into each of two syringes, and administer them into different sites.

EXAMPLE 2

Find the amount to administer and select the proper syringe.

Ordered: Epinephrine 0.2 mg subcut stat

On hand: Vial of epinephrine 1:2000 solution for injection

Patient: A 150-lb, 35-year-old adult

STEP A: CONVERT

The dosage strength of a 1:2000 solution is 1 g (*H*) per 2000 mL (*Q*).

The dose on hand *H* is now in grams, and the dosage ordered *O* is in milligrams. To calculate the desired dose *D*, we must first change the dosage ordered 0.2 mg to the same unit of measure as that of the dose on hand, grams. Determine the conversion factor.

STEP B: CALCULATE

Follow Procedure Checklist 12-2.

1. The unit of measure for the amount to administer will be milliliters.

    A mL =

2. We wish to convert to grams so our conversion factor must have grams on top.

$$\frac{1 \text{ g}}{1000 \text{ mg}}$$

3. The dosage unit is 2000 mL. The dose on hand is 1 g. This is our next factor.

$$\frac{1 \text{ g}}{1000 \text{ mg}} \times \frac{2000 \text{ mL}}{1 \text{ g}}$$

4. The dosage ordered is 0.2 mg. Place this over 1 and set up the equation.

$$A \text{ mL} = \frac{1 \text{ g}}{1000 \text{ mg}} \times \frac{2000 \text{ mL}}{1 \text{ g}} \times \frac{0.2 \text{ mg}}{1}$$

5. Cancel units.

$$A \text{ mL} = \frac{1 \cancel{\text{g}}}{1000 \cancel{\text{mg}}} \times \frac{2000 \text{ mL}}{1 \cancel{\text{g}}} \times \frac{0.2 \cancel{\text{mg}}}{1}$$

6. Solve the equation.

$$A \text{ mL} = \frac{2000 \text{ mL} \times 0.2 \cancel{\text{mg}}}{1000 \cancel{\text{mg}}}$$

$$A = 0.4 \text{ mL}$$

STEP C: THINK! . . . IS IT REASONABLE?

The medication concentration is 1 mg/2 mL. Since 0.4 is twice as much as 0.2, it is reasonable.

The amount to administer is 0.4 mL.

- Referring to Rule 14-1, a 1-mL or 0.5-mL tuberculin syringe would be used.
- Referring to Rule 14-2, we find that it is not necessary to round in this example.
- Referring to Rule 14-3, the dose would not need to be divided into two because the amount is less than 0.5 mL.

EXAMPLE 3 Find the amount to administer and select the proper syringe.

Ordered: Heparin sodium 5,000 units subcut q8h

On hand: Heparin 1:10,000 for injection

Patient: A 145-lb, 60-year-old male

STEP A: CONVERT

The dosage strength of heparin 1:10,000 is 10,000 units (*H*) per 1 mL (*Q*).

The dosage ordered *O* and the dose on hand *H* are both expressed as units, so no conversion is necessary to find the desired dose, which is 5,000 units.

STEP B: CALCULATE

Follow Procedure Checklist 12-2.

1. The unit of measure for the amount to administer will be milliliters.

$$A \text{ mL} =$$

2. Since the unit of measure for the dosage ordered is the same as that for the dose on hand, this step is unnecessary.

3. The dosage unit is 1 mL. The dose on hand is 10,000 units. This is the first factor.

$$\frac{1 \text{ mL}}{10,000 \text{ units}}$$

4. The dosage ordered is 5,000 units. Set up the equation.

$$A \text{ mL} = \frac{1 \text{ mL}}{10,000 \text{ units}} \times \frac{5,000 \text{ units}}{1}$$

5. Cancel units.

$$A \text{ mL} = \frac{1 \text{ mL}}{10{,}000 \text{ } \cancel{\text{units}}} \times \frac{5{,}000 \text{ } \cancel{\text{units}}}{1}$$

6. Solve the equation.

$$A \text{ mL} = \frac{1 \text{ mL}}{10{,}000} \times \frac{5{,}000}{1}$$

$$A = 0.5 \text{ mL}$$

STEP C: THINK! . . . IS IT REASONABLE?

5,000 units is half as much as 10,000 units, so the volume to administer should be half of 1 mL. 0.5 is one half of 1, so the answer is reasonable.

The amount to administer is 0.5 mL.

- Referring to Rule 14-1, a 1-mL tuberculin syringe would be used.
- Referring to Rule 14-2, we find that it is not necessary to round in this example.
- Referring to Rule 14-3, the total volume may be given as a single injection.

FORMULA METHOD

EXAMPLE 1

Find the amount to administer and select the proper syringe.

Ordered: Magnesium sulfate 300 mg IM now

On hand: Magnesium sulfate 10% solution

Patient: A 75-lb, 8-year-old female

STEP A: CONVERT

The dosage strength of a 10% solution is 10 g (H) per 100 mL (Q).

The dosage ordered O is in milligrams, and the dose on hand H is in grams, so the desired dose D, in grams, must be calculated.

Follow Procedure Checklist 6-1 using fractions.

1. Fill in the proportion, recalling that 1 g = 1000 mg.

$$\frac{1 \text{ g}}{1000 \text{ mg}} = \frac{D}{300 \text{ mg}}$$

2. Cancel units.

$$\frac{1 \text{ g}}{1000 \text{ } \cancel{\text{mg}}} = \frac{D}{300 \text{ } \cancel{\text{mg}}}$$

3. Cross-multiply and solve for the unknown.

$$1000 \times D = 300 \times 1 \text{g}$$

$$D = \frac{300 \times 1 \text{ g}}{1000}$$

$$D = 0.3 \text{ g}$$

STEP B: CALCULATE

Follow Procedure Checklist 12-3.

1. $D = 0.3$ g, $Q = 100$ mL, and $H = 10$ g. Fill in the formula.

$$\frac{0.3 \text{ g}}{10 \text{ g}} \times 100 \text{ mL} = A$$

2. Cancel units.

$$\frac{0.3 \cancel{\text{ g}}}{10 \cancel{\text{ g}}} \times 100 \text{ mL} = A$$

3. Solve for the unknown.

$$\frac{0.3}{10} \times 100 = A$$

$$3 \text{ mL} = A$$

STEP C: THINK! . . . IS IT REASONABLE?

The medication is in a 10 to 1 solution. 3 is 10 times larger than 0.3, so it is reasonable.

The amount to administer is 3 mL.

- Referring to Rule 14-1, a standard 3-mL syringe would be used.
- Referring to Rule 14-2, we find that it is not necessary to round in this example.
- Referring to Rule 14-3, the dose would need to be divided into two parts because of the age of the patient. Draw 1.5 mL into each of two syringes, and administer them into different sites.

EXAMPLE 2

Find the amount to administer and select the proper syringe.
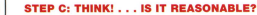

Ordered: Epinephrine 0.2 mg subcut stat

On hand: Vial of epinephrine 1:2000 solution for injection

Patient: A 150-lb, 35-year-old adult

STEP A: CONVERT

The dosage strength of a 1:2000 solution is 1 g (H) per 2000 mL (Q).

The dose on hand H is now in grams, and the dosage ordered O is in milligrams. To calculate the desired dose D, we must first convert the dosage ordered 0.2 mg to the same unit of measure as that of the dose on hand, grams.

Follow Procedure Checklist 6-1 using fractions.

1. Fill in the proportion, recalling that 1 g = 1000 mg.

$$\frac{1 \text{ g}}{1000 \text{ mg}} = \frac{D}{0.2 \text{ mg}}$$

2. Cancel units.

$$\frac{1 \text{ g}}{1000 \cancel{\text{ mg}}} = \frac{D}{0.2 \cancel{\text{ mg}}}$$

3. Cross-multiply and solve for the unknown.

$$1000 \times D = 0.2 \times 1 \text{ g}$$

$$D = \frac{0.2 \times 1 \text{ g}}{1000}$$

$$D = 0.0002 \text{ g}$$

STEP B: CALCULATE

Follow Procedure Checklist 12-3.

1. $D = 0.0002$ g, $Q = 2{,}000$ mL, and $H = 1$ g. Fill in the formula.

$$\frac{0.0002 \text{ g}}{1 \text{ g}} \times 2{,}000 \text{ mL} = A$$

2. Cancel units.

$$\frac{0.0002 \;\cancel{g}}{1 \;\cancel{g}} \times 2{,}000 \text{ mL} = A$$

3. Solve for the unknown.

$$\frac{0.0002}{1} \times 2{,}000 \text{ mL} = A$$

$$0.4 \text{ mL} = A$$

STEP C: THINK! . . . IS IT REASONABLE?

The medication concentration is 1 mg/2 mL. Since 0.4 is twice as much as 0.2, it is reasonable.

The amount to administer is 0.4 mL.

- Referring to Rule 14-1, a 1-mL or 0.5-mL tuberculin syringe would be used.
- Referring to Rule 14-2, we find that it is not necessary to round in this example.
- Referring to Rule 14-3, the dose would not need to be divided into two because the amount is less than 0.5 mL.

EXAMPLE 3 | Find the amount to administer and select the proper syringe.

Ordered: Heparin sodium 5,000 units subcut q8h

On hand: Heparin 1:10,000 for injection

Patient: A 145-lb, 60-year-old male

STEP A: CONVERT

The dosage strength of heparin 1:10,000 is 10,000 units (H) per 1 mL (Q).

The dosage ordered O and the dose on hand H are both expressed as units, so no conversion is necessary to find the desired dose, which is 5,000 units.

STEP B: CALCULATE

Follow Procedure Checklist 12-3.

1. Fill in the formula.

$$\frac{5{,}000 \text{ units}}{10{,}000 \text{ units}} \times 1 \text{ mL} = A$$

2. Cancel units.

$$\frac{5{,}000 \;\cancel{\text{units}}}{10{,}000 \;\cancel{\text{units}}} \times 1 \text{ mL} = A$$

3. Solve for the unknown.

$$\frac{5{,}000 \text{ mL}}{10{,}000} = A$$

$$0.5 \text{ mL} = A$$

STEP C: THINK! . . . IS IT REASONABLE?

5,000 units is half as much as 10,000 units, so the volume to administer should be half of 1 mL. 0.5 is half of 1, so the answer is reasonable.

The amount to administer is 0.5 mL.

- Referring to Rule 14-1, a 1-mL tuberculin syringe would be used.
- Referring to Rule 14-2, we find that it is not necessary to round in this example.
- Referring to Rule 14-3, the total volume may be given as a single injection.

GO TO . . . Open the CD-ROM that accompanies your textbook, and select Chapter 14, Medication Doses as a Percent or Ratio (LO 14.2). Review the animation and example problems, then complete the practice problems. Continue to the next section of the book once you have mastered the information presented.

CRITICAL THINKING ON THE JOB

Confusing the Amount of Solution with the Dosage Unit

A patient is brought to the physician's office with severe vomiting. The physician orders Compazine™ 5 mg IM stat. The healthcare professional obtains a vial labeled 5 mg/mL. The label also lists the total quantity of medication as 5 mL. The healthcare professional misinterprets the solution strength as 5 mg/5 mL and injects a total of 5 mL of Compazine™.

Think ! . . . Is It Reasonable? What mistake was made? How could the healthcare professional have avoided this mistake?

REVIEW AND PRACTICE

14.2 Calculate Medication Doses Expressed in Percent or Ratio Format.

Find the amount to administer for each of the following orders. Then mark the syringe with the correct amount to administer.

1. Ordered: Magnesium sulfate 750 mg stat
   On hand: Magnesium sulfate 20% solution

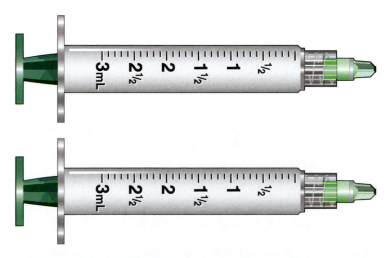

2. Ordered: Lidocaine 200 mg IM stat
   On hand: Lidocaine 10% solution

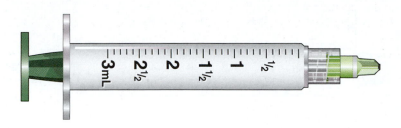

3. Ordered: Epinephrine 0.3 mg subcut stat
   On hand: Epinephrine 1:1000 solution

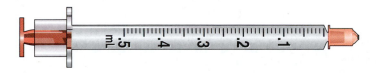

4. Ordered: Adrenalin 0.5 mg subcut stat
   On hand: Adrenalin 1:1000 solution

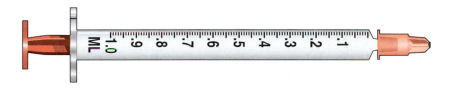

5. Ordered: Prostigmin 0.2 mg IM post-op q6h
   On hand: Prostigmin 1:4000 solution

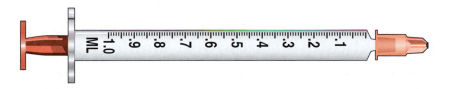

6. Ordered: Prostigmin 0.5 mg IM stat
   On hand: Prostigmin 1:2000 solution

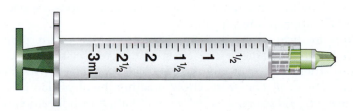

7. Ordered: Heparin sodium 8,000 units subcut q8h

   On hand: Heparin sodium 1:5000 solution

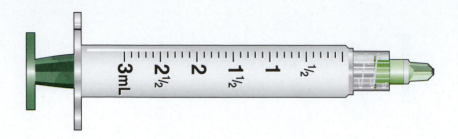

8. Ordered: Heparin sodium 5,000 units subcut q12h × 7 days

   On hand: Heparin sodium 1:10,000 solution

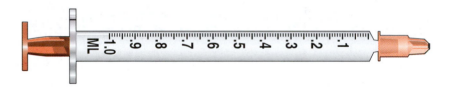

9. Ordered: Lidocaine 25 mg subcut now

   On hand: Lidocaine 5% solution

To check your answers, see the Answer section at the end of the book, which starts on page A-1.

14.3 Reconstituting Parenteral Medications

Medications that lose potency quickly in solution may be supplied in powdered form. When needed, they are reconstituted by dissolving them in an appropriate solvent (or diluent). The drug label, package insert, and PDR provide instructions for reconstituting a medication. Be sure to use the directions specific to the medication you plan to administer.

First, determine what solvent should be used to dilute the medication. Common solvents include sterile water, saline, or a bacteriostatic solution containing a preservative that prevents the growth of microorganisms. Some medications are packaged with a separate container of the appropriate solvent.

Many medications, especially antibiotics, cause severe pain when injected. They may be mixed with lidocaine, a local anesthetic, to reduce this pain. The label or package insert indicates when lidocaine can be used. *Because lidocaine is itself a medication, you need a physician's order to use it.* Therefore, check whether the physician has ordered lidocaine. Be careful to use only lidocaine and *not* a combination of lidocaine and epinephrine in solution, because epinephrine causes vasoconstriction, a tightening of the blood vessels, which delays medication absorption.

The label or package insert lists how much solvent to combine with the medication. Read the directions carefully. Sometimes different amounts of solvent are used, based on whether the medication is for IM or IV use.

RULE 14-5

To reconstitute a powdered medication:

1. Find the directions on the medication label or package insert.

2. Use a sterile syringe and aseptic (germ-free) technique to draw up the correct amount of the appropriate diluent.

3. Inject the diluent into the medication vial.

4. Agitate the mixture by rolling, inverting, or shaking the vial. Check the directions on the label or package insert for which of these methods to use.

5. Make sure that the powdered medication is completely dissolved and that the solution is free of visible particles before you use it.

GO TO . . . Open the CD-ROM that accompanies your textbook, and select Chapter 14, Reconstitute a Powdered Medication (LO 14.3). Review the animation and example problems, then complete the practice problems. Continue to the next section of the book once you have mastered the information presented.

Use the exact amount of solvent indicated in the directions to produce a solution with the correct dosage strength. Powder takes up volume even when dissolved. The volume of the reconstituted medication includes the volume of the solvent and the volume of the powder.

If less than the recommended amount of solvent is used, the powder may not dissolve completely, making the solution unsafe to administer. If too much solvent is used, then the patient will not receive the desired dose. When preparing a suspension, remember that the particles will not dissolve completely. Your goal is to distribute them evenly.

Some vials contain a single dose of medication. Many must be reconstituted immediately before administering them, because they quickly lose potency. Other such medications can be stored for a short time after reconstitution. In some facilities, medications are reconstituted in the pharmacy and delivered ready to use.

RULE 14-6

When you store a medication after reconstituting it:

1. You must record the date, the time of expiration, and your name or initials.

2. For multiple-dose medications, also record the solution strength.

Check the drug label or package insert for the length of time a reconstituted medication may be stored. Storage time may depend on whether the medication is refrigerated.

Example 1	How would you reconstitute and label the following medication?
	Ordered: Glucagon 1 mg IM stat
	On hand: Refer to the labels in Figure 14-7.

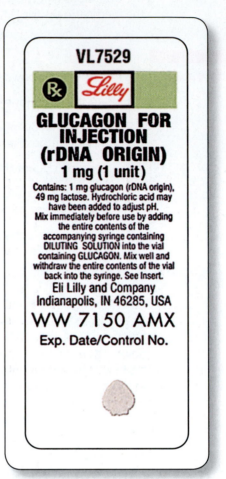

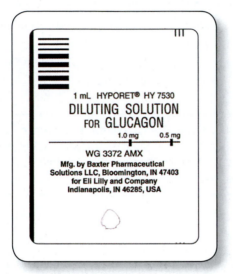

Figure 14-7

A 1-mL vial of diluting solution is provided. Once mixed, the solution must either be used immediately or be discarded. Because the mixed solution will not be stored, you do not need to label the vial.

Example 2	How would you reconstitute and label the following medication? Find the amount to administer.
	Ordered: Zyprexa® 5 mg IM now
	On hand: Refer to the label and portion of package insert shown in Figures 14-8 and 14-9.

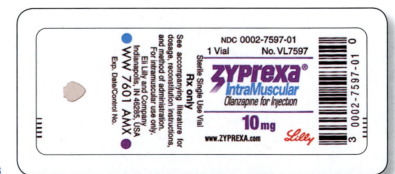

Figure 14-8

ZYPREXA® IntraMuscular (olanzapine for injection) Dosing
ZYPREXA IntraMuscular is approved for the treatment of agitation associated with schizophrenia and bipolar mania.

Dose (mg)	Injection volume (mL)
10.0 mg	Withdraw total contents of vial
7.5 mg	1.5 mL
5.0 mg	1.0 mL
2.5 mg	0.5 mL

10 mg is the recommended dose for agitation associated with bipolar mania and schizophrenia.

Follow the steps below to reconstitute and use ZYPREXA IntraMuscular:

1. Inject 2.1 mL of Sterile Water for Injection into single-packaged vial for up to 10-mg dose.
2. Dissolve contents of vial completely; resulting solution should be clear and yellow.
3. Use solution within 1 hour; discard any unused portion.
4. Refer to table for injection volumes and corresponding doses of ZYPREXA IntraMuscular.
5. Immediately after use, dispose of syringe in approved sharps box.

Figure 14-9   Package insert.

The diluent used to reconstitute this medication is 2.1 mL of sterile water for doses up to 10 mg. Contents must be dissolved completely, and fluid will be clear and yellow. The solution can only be used for 1 h. When it is prepared, you will administer 1 mL to deliver 5 mg of medication.

Example 3

How would you reconstitute and label the following medication? Find the amount to administer.

Ordered: Methylprednisolone 30 mg IM at 0930

On hand: Refer to the label (Figure 14-10) and package insert (Figure 14-11 on next page).

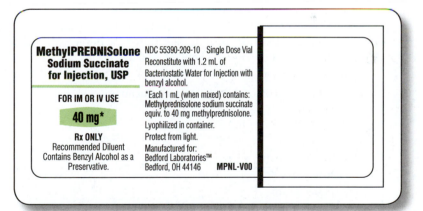

MethylPREDNISolone Sodium Succinate for Injection, USP

FOR IM OR IV USE

40 mg*

Rx ONLY
Recommended Diluent Contains Benzyl Alcohol as a Preservative.

NDC 55390-209-10   Single Dose Vial
Reconstitute with 1.2 mL of Bacteriostatic Water for Injection with benzyl alcohol.

*Each 1 mL (when mixed) contains: Methylprednisolone sodium succinate equiv. to 40 mg methylprednisolone. Lyophilized in container.
Protect from light.
Manufactured for:
Bedford Laboratories™
Bedford, OH 44146   **MPNL-V00**

Figure 14-10

According to the label and package insert the medication should be reconstituted with 1.2 mL bacteriostatic water for injection with benzyl alcohol. Once reconstituted the vial will contain 40 mg/mL.

Methylprednisolone sodium succinate for injection may be administered by intravenous or intramuscular injection or by intravenous infusion, the preferred method for initial emergency use being intravenous injection. To administer by intravenous (or intramuscular) injection, reconstitute the product as follows:

The 40 mg single-dose vial is reconstituted by adding 1.2 mL bacteriostatic water for injection with benzyl alcohol. The 125 mg single-dose vial is reconstituted by adding 2.1 mL bacteriostatic water for injection with benzyl alcohol. The 500 mg single-dose vial is reconstituted by adding 4 mL bacteriostatic water for injection with benzyl alcohol. The 1 gram single-dose vial is reconstituted by adding 7.5 mL bacteriostatic water for injection with benzyl alcohol. The desired dose may be administered intravenously over a period of several minutes.

To prepare solutions for intravenous infusion, first prepare the solution for injection as directed. This solution may then be added to indicated amounts of 5% dextrose in water, isotonic saline solution or 5% dextrose in isotonic saline solution.

Multiple Sclerosis

In treatment of acute exacerbations of multiple sclerosis, daily doses of 200 mg of prednisolone for a week followed by 80 mg every other day for 1 month have been shown to be effective (4 mg of methylprednisolone sodium succinate for injection is equivalent to 5 mg of prednisolone).

STORAGE CONDITIONS

Protect from light.

Store unreconstituted product at 20° to 25°C (68° to 77°F). See USP controlled room temperature.

Store solution at 20° to 25°C (68° to 77°F). See USP controlled room temperature.

Use solution within 48 hours after mixing.

Figure 14-11 Package insert.

According the package insert the resulting solution should be used within 48 hours of mixing. If you mix the medication at 10 a.m. on 6/17/12 and store at room temperature, label the vial Exp. 6/19/12 10 a.m., 40 mg/mL. The medication should also be protected from light before and after reconstitution.

To calculate the amount to administer for Example 3:

PROPORTION METHOD

EXAMPLE

STEP A: CONVERT

The dosage ordered O and the dose on hand H are already expressed in the same units, so the desired dose D is 30 mg. After reconstitution the dosage strength is 40 mg/mL, making the dosage unit Q 1 mL, and the dose on hand H is 40 mg.

STEP B: CALCULATE

Follow Procedure Checklist 12-1 using fractions.

1. Fill in the proportion.

$$\frac{H}{Q} = \frac{D}{A}$$

$$\frac{40 \text{ mg}}{1 \text{ mL}} = \frac{30 \text{ mg}}{A}$$

2. Cancel units.

$$\frac{40 \text{ mg}}{1 \text{ mL}} = \frac{30 \text{ mg}}{A}$$

3. Cross-multiply and solve for the unknown.

$$40 \times A = 1 \text{ mL} \times 30$$

$$A = \frac{1 \text{ mL} \times 30}{40}$$

$$A = 0.75 \text{ mL}$$

STEP C: THINK! . . . IS IT REASONABLE?

Since 30 is $\frac{3}{4}$ of 40, and 0.75 is $\frac{3}{4}$ of 1, it is reasonable.

Using a 1-mL tuberculin syringe, we will administer 0.75 mL.

DIMENSIONAL ANALYSIS

EXAMPLE

STEP A: CONVERT

The dosage ordered O and the dose on hand H are already expressed in the same units, so the desired dose D is 30 mg. After reconstitution the dosage strength is 40 mg/mL, making the dosage unit Q 1 mL, and the dose on hand H is 40 mg.

STEP B: CALCULATE

Follow Procedure Checklist 12-2.

1. The unit of measure for the amount to administer will be milliliters.

A mL =

2. Since the unit of measure for the dosage ordered is the same as that for the dose on hand, this step is unnecessary.

3. The dosage unit is 1 mL. The dose on hand is 40 mg. This is our first factor.

$$\frac{1 \text{ mL}}{40 \text{ mg}}$$

4. The dosage ordered is 30 mg. Place this over one and set up the equation.

$$A \text{ mL} = \frac{1 \text{ mL}}{40 \text{ mg}} \times \frac{30 \text{ mg}}{1}$$

5. Cancel units.

$$A \text{ mL} = \frac{1 \text{ mL}}{40 \text{ \cancel{mg}}} \times \frac{30 \text{ \cancel{mg}}}{1}$$

6. Solve the equation.

$$A \text{ mL} = \frac{1 \text{ mL}}{40} \times \frac{30}{1}$$

$$A = 0.75 \text{ mL}$$

STEP C: THINK! . . . IS IT REASONABLE?

Since 30 is $\frac{3}{4}$ of 40, and 0.75 is $\frac{3}{4}$ of 1, it is reasonable.

Using a 1-mL tuberculin syringe, we will administer 0.75 mL.

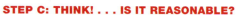

FORMULA METHOD

EXAMPLE

STEP A: CONVERT

The dosage ordered O and the dose on hand H are already expressed in the same units, so the desired dose D is 30 mg. After reconstitution the dosage strength is 40 mg/mL, making the dosage unit Q 1 mL, and the dose on hand H is 40 mg.

STEP B: CALCULATE

Follow Procedure Checklist 12-3.

1. The drug is ordered in milligrams, which is the same unit of measure as that of the dose on hand. Therefore,

Desired dose (D) = 30 mg

Dose on hand (H) = 40 mg

Quantity (Q) = 1 mL

2. Fill in the formula.

$$\frac{D}{H} \times Q = A$$

$$\frac{30 \text{ mg}}{40 \text{ mg}} \times 1 \text{ mL} = A$$

3. Cancel units.

$$\frac{30 \cancel{\text{ mg}}}{40 \cancel{\text{ mg}}} \times 1 \text{ mL} = A$$

4. Solve for the unknown.

$$\frac{30 \text{ mg}}{40} \times 1 \text{ mL} = A$$

$$0.75 \text{ mL} = A$$

STEP C: THINK! . . . IS IT REASONABLE?
Since 30 is $\frac{3}{4}$ of 40, and 0.75 is $\frac{3}{4}$ of 1, it is reasonable.

Using a 1-mL tuberculin syringe, we will administer 0.75 mL.

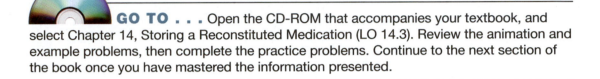 **GO TO . . .** Open the CD-ROM that accompanies your textbook, and select Chapter 14, Storing a Reconstituted Medication (LO 14.3). Review the animation and example problems, then complete the practice problems. Continue to the next section of the book once you have mastered the information presented.

ERROR ALERT!

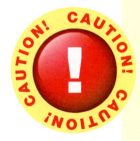

Select the Correct Instructions for the Strength and Route Ordered

The package insert for a 500-mg vial of Maxipime® can be reconstituted for both IM and IV use. Suppose a nurse mistakenly reconstitutes Maxipime® 500 mg IM for 500 mg IV instead. The IV instructions indicate that the nurse should use 5 mL of diluent, producing a solution strength of 100 mg/mL. Calculate the amount to administer.

$$\frac{500 \text{ mg}}{100 \text{ mg}} \times 1 \text{ mL} = A$$

$$\frac{500 \cancel{\text{ mg}}}{100 \cancel{\text{ mg}}} \times 1 \text{ mL} = A = 5 \times 1 \text{ mL} = 5 \text{ mL}$$

The healthcare professional administers two injections of 2.5 mL each. The patient's discomfort increases, and the number of injection sites available for future injections is reduced. Costs increase because more diluent and syringes than necessary are used. The risk of injection complications is doubled. Correctly reconstituted for IM use, 1.3 mL of diluent will be used to produce a solution with a dosage strength of 280 mg/mL. Calculate the amount to administer.

$$\frac{500 \text{ mg}}{280 \text{ mg}} \times 1 \text{ mL} = A$$

$$\frac{500 \cancel{\text{ mg}}}{280 \cancel{\text{ mg}}} \times 1 \text{ mL} = A = \frac{50 \text{ mL}}{28} = 1.785 \text{ rounded to } 1.8 \text{ mL}$$

This amount 1.8 mL is the correct IM dose.

Recording Accurate Information

A healthcare professional receives the following order: Humatrope® 2 mg IM three times a week (see Figure 14-12).

At 0800 on 10/15/12, the healthcare professional prepares the medication to administer later that day. After reading the label (see Figure 14-12), she draws up all the diluent supplied with the medication (see Figure 14-13) and injects it into the vial. According to the drug label, the remaining medication may be refrigerated for 14 days if protected from light. She labels the vial "Exp: 0800 10/29/12. Refrigerate. 5 mg/mL" and signs it with her initials. The vial will not be exposed to light in the refrigerator. Otherwise, the healthcare professional might wrap it in foil or place it inside a paper bag.

Later that day, the healthcare professional calculates the amount to administer, based on the label,

$$\frac{2 \text{ mg}}{5 \text{ mg}} \times 1 \text{ mL} = A$$

$$\frac{2 \cancel{\text{ mg}}}{5 \cancel{\text{ mg}}} \times 1 \text{ mL} = A = \frac{2}{5} \text{ mL} = 0.4 \text{ mL}$$

She uses a 0.5 mL tuberculin syringe to administer the medication.

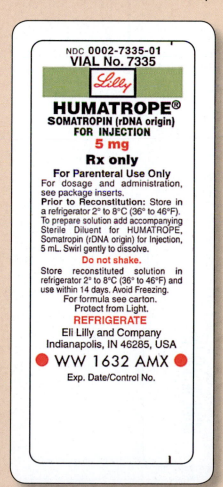

Figure 14-12

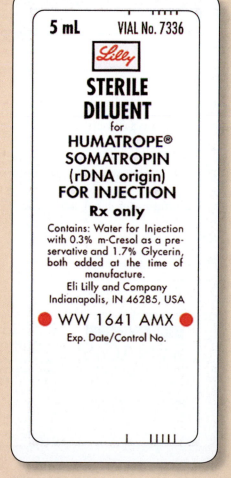

Figure 14-13

(*Continued*)

Think! . . . Is It Reasonable? What mistake did the healthcare professional make? How could she correct her mistake?

REVIEW AND PRACTICE

14.3 Reconstituting Parenteral Medication

For Exercises 1–4, refer to the following label:

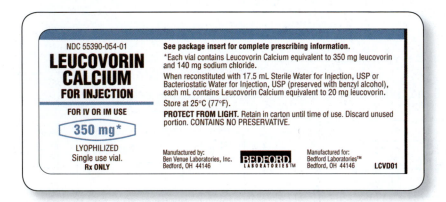

1. How much diluent should you add to the 350-mg vial?

2. What solution strength should you print on the label?

3. What can be used to reconstitute the Leucovorin?

4. If the dose ordered is 15 mg IM, what would be the amount to administer?

For Exercises 5–9, refer to the following order, label, and package insert.

Ordered: Synagis® 75 mg IM q8h.

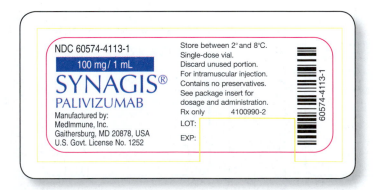

Preparation of Lyophilized Product for Administration:

- To reconstitute, remove the tab portion of the vial cap and clean the rubber stopper with 70% ethanol or equivalent.

- Both the 50 mg and 100 mg vials contain an overfill to allow the withdrawal of 50 mg or 100 mg Synagis®respectively when reconstituted following the directions described below.

- SLOWLY add 0.6 mL of sterile water for injection to the 50 mg vial or add 1.0 mL of sterile water for injection to the 100 mg vial. The vial should be tilted slightly and gently rotated for 30 seconds to avoid foaming. DO NOT SHAKE or VIGOROUSLY AGITATE the vial. This is a critical step to avoid prolonged foaming.

- Reconstituted Synagis® should stand undisturbed at room temperature for a minimum of 20 minutes until the solution clarifies.

- Reconstituted Synagis® should be inspected visually for particulate matter or discoloration prior to administration. The reconstituted solution should appear clear or slightly opalescent (a thin layer of micro-bubbles on the surface is normal and will not affect dosage). DO NOT use if there is particulate matter or if the solution is discolored.

- Reconstituted Synagis® does not contain a preservative and should be administered within 6 hours of reconstitution. Administer immediately after withdrawal from vial. Synagis® is supplied in single-use vials. DO NOT re-enter the vial. Discard any unused portion.

5. What diluent should you use to reconstitute Synagis®?

6. How much diluent should you add to this vial?

7. How many approximate milligrams are in 1 mL?

8. If Synagis is reconstituted at 1000 on January 3, 2013, what should you write on the label?

9. How much solution should you administer?

For Exercises 10–15, refer to the following order, and label information.

Ordered: Gemzar® 100 mg for IV infusion

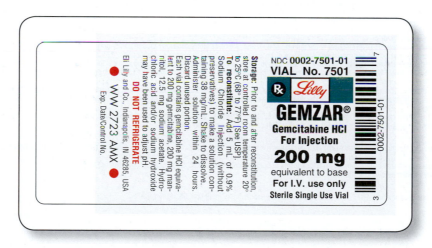

10. What diluent should you use to reconstitute this medication?

11. How much diluent should you add to the vial?

12. What solution strength should you write on the label?

13. If the Gemzar® is reconstituted at 2400 on 6/5/2012 and will be stored at room temperature, what expiration date and time should you write on the label?

14. How should the medication be stored?

15. How much solution would be used to administer 100 mg of medication?

For Exercises 16–19, refer to the following order, label, and package insert.

Ordered: Penicillin G potassium 1 million units IM q2h

READ ACCOMPANYING PROFESSIONAL INFORMATION.

RECOMMENDED STORAGE IN DRY FORM.

Store below 86°F (30°C)

Sterile solution may be kept in refrigerator for one (1) week without significant loss of potency.

CAUTION: Federal law prohibits dispensing without prescription.

6505-00-958-3305

NDC 0049-0520-83

Buffered

Pfizerpen®

(penicillin G potassium)

For Injection

FIVE MILLION UNITS

Pfizer **Roerig**
Division of Pfizer Inc, NY, NY 10017

USUAL DOSAGE
Average single intramuscular injection: 200,000-400,000 units.
Intravenous: Additional information about the use of this product intravenously can be found in the package insert.

mL diluent added	Units per mL of solution
18.2 mL	250,000
8.2 mL	500,000
3.2 mL	1,000,000

Buffered with sodium citrate and citric acid to optimum pH.

PATIENT: _____

ROOM NO.: _____

DATE DILUTED: _____

05-4243-00-3
MADE IN USA

Reconstitution
The following table shows the amount of solvent required for solution of various concentrations:

Approx. Desired Concentration (units/mL)	Approx. Volume (mL) 1,000,000 units	Solvent for Vial of 5,000,000 units	Infusion Only 20,000,000 units
50,000	20.0	–	–
100,000	10.0	–	–
250,000	4.0	18.2	75.0
500,000	1.8	8.2	33.0
750,000	–	4.8	–
1,000,000	–	3.2	11.5

When the required volume of solvent is greater than the capacity of the vial, the penicillin can be dissolved by first injecting only a portion of the solvent into the vial, then withdrawing the resultant solution and combining it with the remainder of the solvent in a larger sterile container.

Buffered Pfizerpen (penicillin G potassium) for Injection is highly water soluble. It may be dissolved in small amounts of Water for Injection, or Sterile Isotonic Sodium Chloride Solution for Parenteral Use. All solutions should be stored in a refrigerator. When refrigerated, penicillin solutions may be stored for seven days without significant loss of potency.

Buffered Pfizerpen for Injection may be given intramuscularly or by continuous intravenous drip for dosages of 500,000, 1,000,000, or 5,000,000 units. It is also suitable for intrapleural, intraarticular, and other local instillations.

THE 20,000,000 UNIT DOSAGE MAY BE ADMINISTERED BY INTRAVENOUS INFUSION ONLY.

(1) Intramuscular Injection: Keep total volume of injection small. The intramuscular route is the preferred route of administration. Solutions containing up to 100,000 units of penicillin per mL of diluent may be used with a minimum of discomfort. Greater concentration of penicillin G per mL is physically possible and may be employed where therapy demands. When large dosages are required, it may be advisable to administer aqueous solutions of penicillin by means of continuous intravenous drip.

(2) Continuous Intravenous Drip: Determine the volume of fluid and rate of its administration required by the patient in a 24 hour period in the usual manner for fluid therapy, and add the appropriate daily dosage of penicillin to this fluid. For example, if an adult patient requires 2 liters of fluid in 24 hours and a daily dosage of 10 million units of penicillin, add 5 million units to 1 liter and adjust the rate of flow so the liter will be infused in 12 hours.

(3) Intrapleural or Other Local Infusion: If fluid is aspirated, give infusion in a volume equal to 1/4 or 1/2 the amount of fluid aspirated, otherwise, prepare as for intramuscular injection.

(4) Intrathecal Use: The intrathecal use of penicillin in meningitis must be highly individualized. It should be employed only with full consideration of the possible irritating effects of penicillin when used by this route. The preferred route of therapy in bacterial meningitides is intravenous, supplemented by intramuscular injection.

Parenteral drug products should be inspected visually for particulate matter and discoloration prior to administration, whenever solution and container permit. Sterile solution may be left in refrigerator for one week without significant loss of potency.

HOW SUPPLIED
Buffered Pfizerpen® (penicillin G potassium) for Injection is available in vials containing respectively 5,000,000 units × 10's (NDC 0049-0520-83) and 20,000,000 units × 1's (NDC 0049-0530-28); buffered with sodium citrate and citric acid to an optimum pH.

Each million units contains approximately 6.8 milligrams of sodium (0.3 mEq) and 65.6 milligrams of potassium (1.68 mEq).
Store the dry powder below 86°F (30°C).

Reference
1. American Heart Association, 1977. Prevention of bacterial endocarditis. Circulation. **56**:139A-143A.

Rx only

©2003 PFIZER INC

16. To make a solution of 500,000 units/mL, how much diluent should you add to the vial?

17. If the medication in the vial is reconstituted with 4.8 mL of diluent, what solution strength should you write on the label?

18. If the penicillin is reconstituted at 1200 on 11/20/13 and will be stored in the refrigerator, what expiration date and time should you write on the label?

19. When reconstituted with 8.2 mL, how much solution should you administer?

For Exercises 20–24, refer to the following label, order, and package insert (on the next page).

Ordered: Rocephin® 750 mg IM q6h
On hand: See label

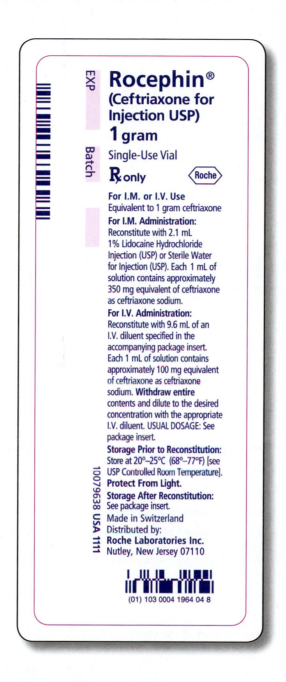

20. What diluent will be used to prepare this medication?

21. How much diluent should you add to one vial?

22. What is the dosage strength of the solution, once reconstituted?

23. If Rocephin® is reconstituted at 1600 on October 4, 2013, and will be stored in the refrigerator, what should you write on the label?

24. How much solution should you administer?

Description:
Caption:

COMPATIBILITY AND STABILITY: Rocephin sterile wder should be stored at room temperature—77°F (25° C)—or below and protected from light. After reconstitution, protection from normal light is not necessary. The color of solutions ranges from light yellow to amber, depending on the length of storage, concentration and diluent used.

Rocephin *intramuscular* solutions remain stable (loss of potency less than 10%) for the following time periods:

Diluent	Concentration mg/ml	Storage	
		Room Temp. (25° C)	Refrigerated (4°C)
Sterile Water for Injection	100	2 days	10 days
	250,350	24 hours	3 days
0.9% Sodium Chloride	100	2 days	10 days
Solution	250,350	24 hours	3 days
5% Dextrose Solution	100	2 days	10 days
	250,350	24 hours	3 days
Bacteriostatic Water +0.9%	100	24 hours	10 days
Benzyl Alcohol	250,350	24 hours	3 days
1% Lidocaine Solution	100	24 hours	10 days
(without epinephrine)	250,350	24 hours	3 days

Rocephin *intravenous* solutions, at concentrations of 10, 20 and 40 mg/ml., remain stable (loss of potency less than 10%) for the following time periods stored in glass or PVC containers:

Diluent	Storage	
	Room Temp. (25°C)	Refrigerated (4°C)
Sterile Water	2 days	10 days
0.9% Sodium Chloride Solution	2 days	10 days
5% Dextrose Solution	2 days	10 days
10% Dextrose Solution	2 days	10 days
5% Dextrose + 0.9% Sodium Chloride Solution*	2 days	Incompatible
5% Dextrose + 0.45% Sodium Chloride Solution	2 days	Incompatible

*Data available for 10 to 40 mg/mL concentration in this diluent in PVC containers only; Excerpt from package insert for Rochephin by Roche.

To check your answers, see the Answer section at the end of the book, which starts on page A-1.

14.4 Other Medication Administration Forms and Equipment

Medications may be given by a variety of routes besides oral and common parenteral routes. These routes are used for intradermal injections, inhalants, and rectal and transdermal medications.

Intradermal Injections

Very small doses of medication can be injected under the first layer of the skin. Although it is parenteral, this route is normally used for diagnostic testing, most often screening for tuberculosis or allergies. When an intradermal (ID) injection is required, the physician usually orders the intended diagnostic test, such as a Mantoux (PPD) test for tuberculosis. You determine the amount of solution to use by checking the vial label or the package insert. If a dose other than the standard diagnostic dose is to be administered, the physician will order the exact amount. No calculation is required. Intradermal injections are usually 0.1 mL or less. A 1-mL tuberculin syringe is always used.

Drops, Sprays, and Mists

Different types of equipment are used to deliver medication to the nose, ears, eyes, and throat in the form of drops, sprays, and mists. Drops, also called **instillations,** deliver medication to the nose, eyes, and ears. Sprays deliver medication to the nose and throat. Drops and sprays are measured according to the dose prescribed and the manufacturer's instructions. Therefore, be sure to use the equipment that accompanies the drug when you administer these medications.

Droppers, similar to those for oral medications, are used to administer drops. Plastic squeeze bottles are used for drops and sprays. Atomizers deliver sprays by using a rubber bulb to propel the spray from a medicine container into the nose.

Another way to administer medication is to use a mist that the patient inhales. Vaporizers, or steam inhalers, use boiling water to create a mist from liquid medication. Nebulizers, often used by patients with asthma, and **metered-dose inhalers (MDIs)** also help deliver medication to the patient.

Inhalants

Inhaled medications, or **inhalants,** are administered either by metered-dose inhaler (MDI), Figure 14-14, or by nebulizer. Metered-dose inhalers provide a measured dose of medication in each puff. The physician orders the number of puffs to be given. No calculation is necessary. MDI must be primed before initial use, or if the MDI has not been used for two weeks. The plastic actuator should be cleaned weekly; the metal canister is not cleaned. See manufacturer's instructions for priming and cleaning methods. There are three common methods for using an MDI inhaler, the closed mouth (Figure 14-14), the open mouth (Figure 14-15), and the closed mouth with a spacer (Figure 14-16). With all methods, shake the MDI, exhale

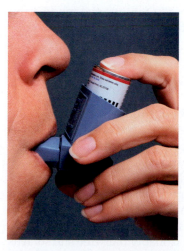

Figure 14-14 An MDI is used to deliver inhalant medications (Closed Mouth Method).

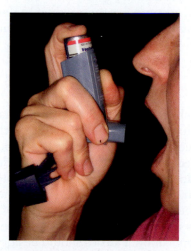

Figure 14-15 MDI Open Mouth Method.

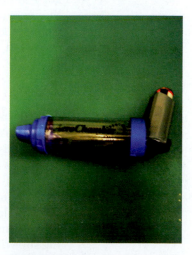

Figure 14-16 Spacer Used for MDI.

fully, inhale slowly while depressing the canister, then hold the inhalation as long as possible, up to 10 seconds. If multiple doses are ordered wait 1 minute between doses, or as manufacturer directs.

Medications given by nebulizer are supplied as liquids which are mixed with sterile saline solution. Single doses premixed with saline are available for most medications. A few are measured in the receptacle of the nebulizer, after which the correct amount of saline is added. Sterile saline is usually provided in 3-mL or 5-mL single-dose ampules.

Inhalant medications in multiple-dose containers are usually packaged with special droppers calibrated for the standard doses. If the dropper is not available or becomes contaminated, a sterile syringe may be used.

The physician usually specifies the solution strength and the amount of inhalant to administer. For example, the order Mucomyst 20% 3 mL via nebulizer QID is a complete order. In some cases, the physician will also order an amount of normal saline to be added to the medication. When calculations are necessary, the same methods proportion, dimensional analysis, and formula—are used for inhalants as are used for parenteral medications.

Vaginal and Rectal Medications

Medications can be administered by the vaginal (pv) or rectal (pr) routes. Liquid vaginal medication is in the form of a douche, and solid vaginal medication is in tablet or suppository form. Liquid rectal medication is in the form of an enema, and solid rectal medication is in suppository form. Generally, suppositories cannot be accurately divided. Therefore, in most cases, only doses that are multiples of the available suppository strength may be administered.

In some cases, according to their manufacturers, suppositories can be safely divided in half. However, they are not scored. Thus, the physician's order should specify that $\frac{1}{2}$ suppository is to be given. For example, if the order reads Tigan® 50 mg p.r. t.i.d., ask the physician to clarify whether $\frac{1}{2}$ of a 100-mg suppository is acceptable. The order should then be rewritten: Tigan® 100 mg supp. Give $\frac{1}{2}$ supp.

Topical Medications

Topical medications, such as gels, creams, ointments, and pastes, are applied directly to the skin. You administer the drug with a glove, tongue blade, or cotton-tipped applicator. Topical medications are usually given for their therapeutic effect in or on the skin. Follow the instructions that accompany the product to determine how to remove the medication from its container and administer it. Avoid letting any of the medication contact your own skin.

Transdermal Systems

Transdermal medication is a form of topical medication absorbed through the skin into the bloodstream. Transdermal medications include patches, ointments, and creams. Patches usually consist of a special membrane that releases liquid medication at a constant rate. The patch has adhesive edges to hold it in place so that the membrane rests against the skin (see Figure 14-17). The dosage rate of a transdermal patch is usually expressed in milligrams or micrograms per hour. Patches cannot be divided. If a dose is larger than the amount provided by a single patch, you can use multiple patches. Before you administer a patch, be certain to remove any patches that are already in place, wipe off any residual medication, and rotate the site with each application. Patches should be applied to a reasonably hair-free site such as abdomen, shoulder, back, or hip. Be careful to avoid placing the patch on skin that is irritated or rubbed, such as under a waistband or bra strap; also avoid skin that is scarred, inflamed, or broken. Date, time, and sign patch when administering. Observe the patient, if febrile, since the rate of absorption may increase.

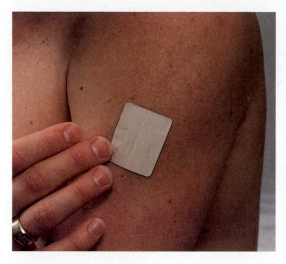

Figure 14-17   Application of a transdermal patch; date, time, and signature will be added to the patch.

FORMULA METHOD

EXAMPLE 1

Find the amount to administer.

Ordered: Deponit® 0.8 mg/hr topically

On hand: Deponit® 0.2 mg/h and 0.4 mg/h patches

STEP A: CONVERT
No conversion needed.

STEP B: CALCULATE

$$\frac{0.8 \text{ mg/h}}{0.4 \text{ mg/h}} \times 1 \text{ patch} = A$$

$$\frac{\overset{2}{\cancel{0.8 \text{ mg/h}}}}{\cancel{0.4 \text{ mg/h}}} \times 1 \text{ patch} = 2 \times 1 \text{ patch} = 2 \text{ patches}$$

STEP C: THINK! . . . IS IT REASONABLE?
Since 0.8 is twice as much as 0.4, and 2 patches are twice as much as 1 patch, it is reasonable.

Administer 2 patches. While you could also administer 4 of the 0.2 mg/h patches, you should use the least amount of dosage units possible to give the ordered dose.

Sometimes the ordered dose can be administered by using a combination of patches. In these cases, use critical thinking skills to determine which combination will work.

EXAMPLE 2

Find the amount to administer.

Ordered: Vivelle® 0.125 mg/day

On hand: Vivelle® in four dosage strengths: 0.0375 mg/day, 0.05 mg/day, 0.075 mg/ day, and 0.1 mg/day

STEP A: CONVERT
No conversion needed.

STEP B: CALCULATE
Start with the patch that has the greatest dosage strength (0.1 mg/day). Because all the patches deliver more than 0.025 mg/day, none will work in combination with this patch. Next, try combinations with the 0.075 mg/day patch.

Administer a combination of one 0.075 mg/day patch and one 0.05 mg/day patch.

STEP C: THINK! . . . IS IT REASONABLE?
0.075 + 0.05 = 0.125 the ordered dose, so it is reasonable.

GO TO . . . Open the CD-ROM that accompanies your textbook, and select Chapter 14, Other Medication Routes (LO 14.4). Review the animation and example problems, then complete the practice problems. Continue to the next section of the book once you have mastered the information presented.

PATIENT EDUCATION

Teach patients to use dosage equipment with the correct calibrations. Stress that attention must be paid to the dosage strength (supply dose), if the patient is administering medications that are prepared in different strengths. Instruct the patient not to divide suppositories (unless directed by the authorized prescriber) or patches. Additionally, transdermal patches should be applied to skin that is free of irritation, does not form skin folds, and does not have a lot of hair. Skin should be free of lotions, or powders, or anything else that might interfere with absorption. Each successive patch must be placed in new site to prevent skin irritation. Discard patches by folding in half, with medicated side together. Place in closed container, to keep away from children and pets.

REVIEW AND PRACTICE

14.4 Other Medication Forms and Equipment

Match the medication forms with their descriptions. Medication forms may be used more than once.

a. Topical
b. Transdermal
c. Drops
d. Sprays
e. Mists
f. Vaginal
g. Rectal

_____ **1.** Can be delivered in the form of a tablet, suppository, or douche.

_____ **2.** Applied directly to the skin.

_____ **3.** Delivered by a nebulizer, vaporizer, or metered-dose inhaler.

_____ 4. Medication from a patch is absorbed through the skin.

_____ 5. Can be delivered in the form of a suppository or an enema.

_____ 6. Must be marked with your initials, date, and time of administration.

_____ 7. Also known as instillations.

_____ 8. An atomizer is used to deliver this medication form.

_____ 9. Are useful when a patient has difficulty or trouble swallowing oral drugs.

_____ 10. Are usually delivered to the nose, eyes, and ears.

For Exercises 11–20, find the amount to administer.

11. Ordered: Acetylcysteine 1 g via nebulizer
    On hand: Acetylcysteine 20% solution 10-mL vial

12. Ordered: Albuterol 2.5 mg via nebulizer
    On hand: Albuterol 5 mg/mL

13. Ordered: Atrovent® 250 mcg via nebulizer
    On hand: Atrovent® 0.02% inhalation solution 500 mcg/2.5-mL vial

14. Ordered: Numorphan 10 mg p.r. PRN
    On hand: Numorphan 5-mg suppositories

15. Ordered: RMS morphine supp 15 mg p.r. PRN
    On hand: RMS 5-mg, 10-mg, and 30-mg suppositories

16. Ordered: Phenergan® 12.5 mg pr PRN
    On hand: Phenergan® 25-mg suppositories

17. Ordered: Testoderm 0.8 mg/day top
    On hand: Testoderm 0.4 mg/day patches

18. Ordered: Catapres® 0.5 mg/day top
    On hand: Catapres® TTS-1 (0.1 mg/day), TTS-2 (0.2 mg/day), TTS-3 (0.3 mg/day)

19. Ordered: Alora® 0.15 mg/day
    On hand: Alora® 0.05 mg/day, 0.075 mg/day, and 0.1 mg/day

20. Ordered: Transderm Nitro 0.3 mg/h top
    On hand: Transderm Nitro 0.1 mg/h, 0.2 mg/h, and 0.6 mg/h patches

To check your answers, see the Answer section at the end of the book, which starts on page A-1.

CHAPTER 14 SUMMARY

LEARNING OUTCOME	KEY POINTS

14.1 Calculate doses of parenteral medication in solution and select syringe based on dose calculation.
Pages 348–363

- Parenteral medication is in solution
- Find the dosage strength
- *Convert* to like units of measurement
- *Calculate* using either proportion method, dimensional analysis, or formula method (see Chapter 12 for discussion of each method)
- *Think! . . . [about your answer, determine] Is It Reasonable?*

Rule 14-1 Select the proper syringe

- If volume to administer is greater than or equal to 1 mL, use a 3-mL syringe
- If volume to administer is less than 1 mL, but greater than or equal to 0.5 mL and calculates evenly to the hundredths, use a 1-mL tuberculin syringe or a 3-mL syringe
- If the volume to administer is less than 0.5 mL, round to the hundredths and use a 1-mL tuberculin syringe. For amounts less than 0.5 mL, use a 0.5-mL tuberculin syringe, if available.

Rule 14-2 Correctly round the amount of an injection to administer

- Round volumes greater than 1 mL to the nearest tenth (3-mL syringe is calibrated in tenths)
- Round volumes less than 1 mL to the nearest hundredth (tuberculin syringe is calibrated in hundredths)

Rule 14-3 Do not exceed maximum volume for an injection in a single site.

- Intramuscular (IM) injections:
  - Adult   3 mL
  - Adult deltoid (arm)   1 mL
  - Child 6–12 years   2 mL
  - Child 0–5 years   1 mL
  - Premature Infant   0.5 mL

LEARNING OUTCOME	KEY POINTS
	▶ Subcutaneous (Subcut) injections: 1 mL
	▶ Volumes greater than above should be divided between two syringes, to meet the above site requirements. *It is rare to administer more than the standard site volume, so verify volume prior to administration.*
14.2 Calculate doses of medications expressed in percent or ratio format. Pages 363–374	*Percent (per 100)* means grams per 100 mL Example: 1% means 1 gram per 100 mL *Ratio* means gram per mL Example 1:2000 means 1 gram per 2000 mL Rule 14-4 *Convert* solution strength to standard format of g/mL, mg/mL, or units/mL . *Calculate* using proportion method, dimensional analysis, or formula method. *Think! . . . Is It Reasonable?* Then apply Rules 14-1 to 14-3.

14.3 Calculate doses of reconstituted parenteral medications. Pages 374–386	● Use the appropriate diluent
	● Use the exact volume of diluents recommended by manufacturer, to render the correct dosage strength
	
	Rule 14-5 To reconstitute a powdered medication
	
	  1. Find directions on label or package insert
	  2. Use sterile syringe and aseptic technique
	  3. Inject diluent into the medication vial
	  4. Mix by rolling, inverting, or shaking the vial
	  5. Completely dissolve powdered medication prior to use

14.4 Differentiate other medication administration forms and equipment. Pages 386–391	Medications may be administered by other routes and require different equipment to administer. Intradermal injections : less than or equal to 0.1 mL; exact volume of specific strength is *ordered* Topical medications, creams, gets, ointments, pastes, patches, administered on top of the skin with glove or applicator (do not let drug get on your skin). Transdermal patch may not be divided. If dose is greater than that of patch, apply multiple patches to achieve desired dose.

LEARNING OUTCOME	KEY POINTS
	Inhalants are administered by metered-dose inhaler (MDI) which has a premeasured dose per puff, or by a nebulizer. Nebulizer medications can be premixed, or the medication may be added to sterile saline in the nebulizer. Medications in multiple-dose containers usually have a calibrated dropper to measure the dose, so no calculation is needed. In the rare instances a calculation is necessary, use the proportion method, dimensional analysis, or formula method.

Vaginal/rectal medications are usually suppositories. Be sure to select the correct dosage strength for administration. Although never scored, some suppositories may be divided per manufacturer's direction. If a suppository is be cut in half, the AP's order will be written indicating medication strength: Give $\frac{1}{2}$ supp. |

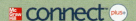
Answer the following questions.

1. What is the correct syringe to select if the amount to be injected is 0.75 mL? (LO 14.1)

2. If the dosage to be administered is 1.75 mL, what syringe would you select and to what amount would the dosage be rounded? (LO 14.1)

3. List the maximum volume for an IM injection for the following patients: an adult, an adult deltoid, a child 6-12 years old. (LO 14.1)

4. If the order for a subcutaneous injection results in an amount of 2.2 mL, what action should be taken before any administration? (LO 14.1)

5. What type of injection is usually less than 0.1 mL? (LO 14.1)

6. What equipment is necessary when the order states to deliver the medication in puffs? (LO 14.4)

7. What is a common drug form for the administration of rectal medications? (LO 14.4)

8. Explain the administration of a transdermal medication. (LO 14.4)

9. List three common diluents used when reconstituting powdered medications? (LO 14.3)

Use the identified drug labels to answer the following questions:

10. Refer to Label A. What is the caution on the label? (LO 14.3)

11. If the order is for 75 mg IM, what amount would be administered? (LO 14.1)

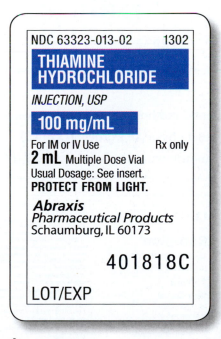

A

12. Refer to Label B. How many units are in each milliliter of this drug? (LO 14.4)

13. If the order is for 800 units subcut, what amount would be administered? (LO 14.1)

14. If the order is for 1000 units, how many times may this vial be used? (LO 14.1)

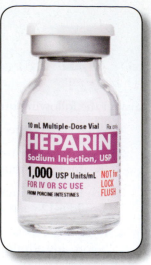

B

15. Refer to Label C. If the order is for 900 mg IM, what amount would be administered? (LO 14.1)

16. What extra preparations would you need to make in order to administer the amount in Question 15? (LO 14.1)

17. Other than IM, what route is acceptable for administration of this drug and what must you do before administration? (LO 14.1)

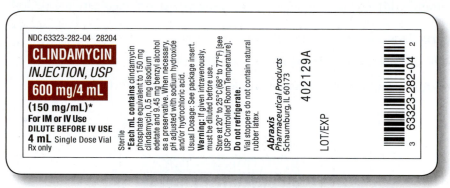

C

18. Refer to Label D. What two diluents, and how much of each, are suggested on the label? (LO 14.3)

19. Which one of the diluents requires a physician's order? (LO 14.3)

20. If the order is 500 mg IM, what amount would be administered? (LO 14.3)

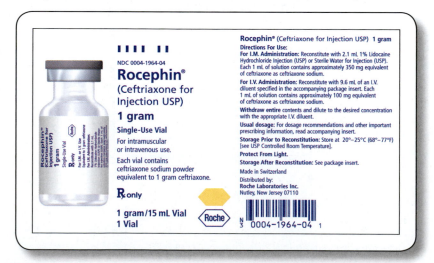

D

CHECK UP

For Exercises 1–10, find the amount to administer, then mark the syringe. (LO 14.1, 14.2)

1. Ordered: INFeD® (iron dextran) 100 mg IM daily
On hand: INFeD® 50 mg/mL

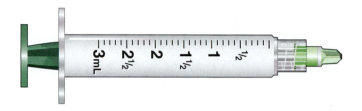

2. Ordered: Haloperidol decanoate 60 mg IM stat
On hand: Haloperidol decanoate 50 mg/mL

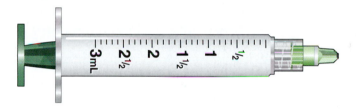

3. Ordered: Loxitane® 30 mg IM bid
On hand: Loxitane® 50 mg/mL

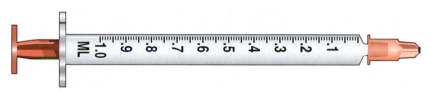

4. Ordered: Epogen® 1400 units subcut three times per week
On hand: Epogen® 2000 units/mL

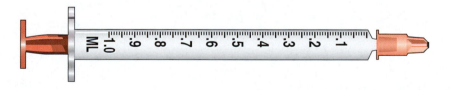

5. Ordered: Lidocaine 300 mg IM stat
   On hand: Lidocaine 20% solution

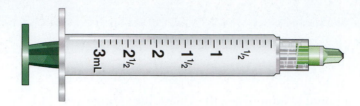

6. Ordered: Magnesium sulfate 250 mg IM daily
   On hand: Magnesium sulfate 10% solution

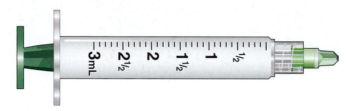

7. Ordered: Levsin® 0.4 mg IM bid
   On hand: Levsin® 0.5 mg/mL

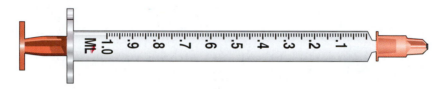

8. Ordered: Robinul® 0.15 mg IM stat
   On hand: Robinul® 0.2 mg/mL

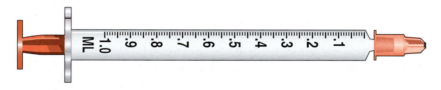

9. Order: Prostigmin 0.75 mg IM q4h
   On hand: Prostigmin 1:1000 solution

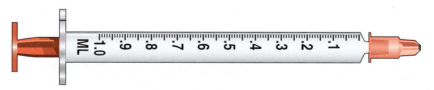

10. Ordered: Epinephrine 0.5 mg subcut stat
   On hand: Epinephrine 1:200 solution

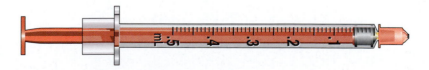

For Exercises 11–21, find the amount to administer, select the proper syringe, and write in the space provided. (LO 14.1, 14.2)

11. Ordered: Adrenalin® 0.2 mg subcut stat
On hand: Adrenalin® 1:2000 solution
Administer: _____ Syringe: _____

12. Ordered: Calciferol 24,000 International Units IM daily
On hand: Calciferol 500,000 International Units/5 mL
Administer: _____ Syringe: _____

13. Ordered: Heparin sodium 7,500 units subcut q8h
On hand: Heparin 1:20,000 solution
Administer: _____ Syringe: _____

14. Ordered: Heparin calcium 7,500 units subcut q8h
On hand: Heparin calcium 5,000 units/0.2 mL
Administer: _____ Syringe: _____

15. Ordered: Thiamine 200 mg IM
On hand: Refer to label A.
Administer: _____ Syringe: _____

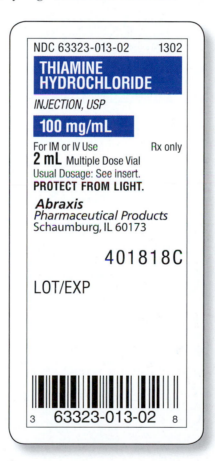

A

16. Ordered: Heparin 400 units subcut daily

On hand: Refer to label B.

Administer: _____ Syringe: _____

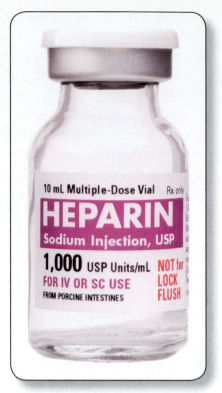

B

17. Ordered: Furosemide 15 mg IM now

On hand: Refer to label C.

Administer: _____ Syringe: _____

NDC 63323-280-02   28002

FUROSEMIDE

INJECTION, USP

20 mg/2 mL

(10 mg/mL)

For IM or IV Use   Rx only

2 mL Single Dose Vial

Preservative Free

Discard unused portion.

PROTECT FROM LIGHT.

Do not use if discolored.

Abraxis
Pharmaceutical Products
Schaumburg, IL 60173

401803C

LOT/EXP

3   63323-280-02   4

C

18. Ordered: Oxytocin 20 units IM q 12h prn

On hand: Refer to label D.

Administer: _____ Syringe: _____

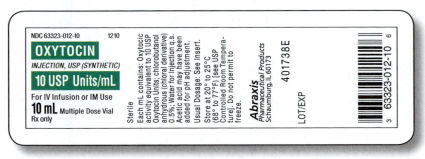

D

19. Ordered: Epogen® 2500 units subcut three times per week

On hand: Refer to label E.

Administer: _____ Syringe: _____

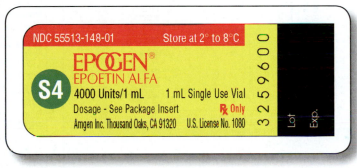

E

20. Ordered: Clindamycin 300 mg IM now

On hand: Refer to label F.

Administer: _____ Syringe: _____

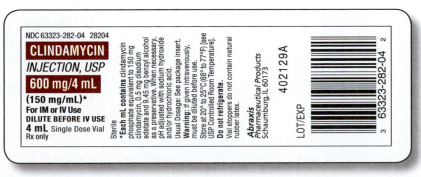

F

21. Ordered: 0.25 mg Sandostatin® subcut daily

On Hand: Refer to label G.

Administer: _____ Syringe: _____

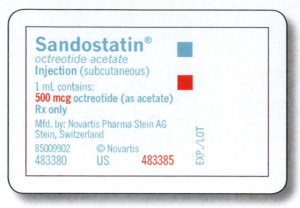

G

22. Explain which vial of medication, label H or I, you would use for the following order. (LO 14.1)

Ordered: Furosemide 40 mg IM

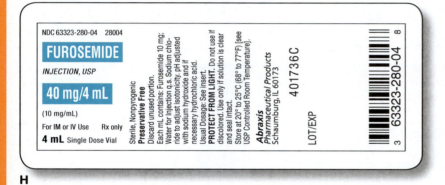

H

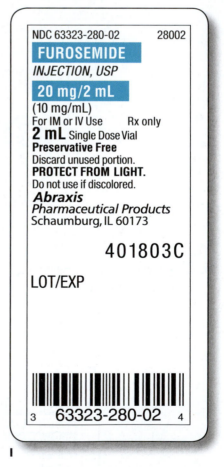

I

For Exercises 23–26, refer to label J and the package insert. (LO 14.3)

23. What diluents may be used to reconstitute Zyprexa® for IM use?

24. How much diluent should be added to the vial?

25. How much would you withdraw for a 5 mg dose?

26. How long will the solution retain its potency at room temperature?

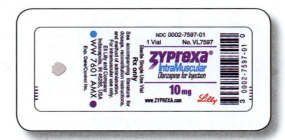

J

ZYPREXA® IntraMuscular (olanzapine for injection) Dosing
ZYPREXA IntraMuscular is approved for the treatment of agitation associated with schizophrenia and bipolar mania.

Dose (mg)	Injection volume (mL)
10.0 mg	Withdraw total contents of vial
7.5 mg	1.5 mL
5.0 mg	1.0 mL
2.5 mg	0.5 mL

10 mg is the recommended dose for agitation associated with bipolar mania and schizophrenia.

Follow the steps below to reconstitute and use ZYPREXA IntraMuscular:

1. Inject 2.1 mL of Sterile Water for Injection into single-packaged vial for up to 10-mg dose.
2. Dissolve contents of vial completely; resulting solution should be clear and yellow.
3. Use solution within 1 hour; discard any unused portion.
4. Refer to table for injection volumes and corresponding doses of ZYPREXA IntraMuscular.
5. Immediately after use, dispose of syringe in approved sharps box.

For Exercises 27–32, find the amount to administer. (LO 14.4)

27. Ordered: Acetylcysteine 800 mg via nebulizer q6h
    On hand: Acetylcysteine 10% solution

28. Ordered: Albuterol 1.25 mg via nebulizer q8h
    On hand: Albuterol 5 mg/mL

29. Ordered: Thorazine® 50 mg q6h pr as needed
    On hand: Thorazine® 25-mg and 100-mg suppositories

30. Ordered: Dilaudid® 6 mg q4h pr as needed
    On hand: Dilaudid® 3-mg suppositories

31. Ordered: Androderm® 5 mg/day top
    On hand: Androderm® 2.5 mg/day patches

32. Ordered: Nitro-Dur® 0.3 mg/h top
    On hand: Nitro-Dur® 0.1 mg/h and 0.2 mg/h patches

CRITICAL THINKING APPLICATIONS

For questions 1–5 on the next page, refer to the following label, order, and package insert. (LO 14.3)

Ordered: PegIntron™ 180 mcg subcut weekly

On hand: Refer to the label A and package insert below.

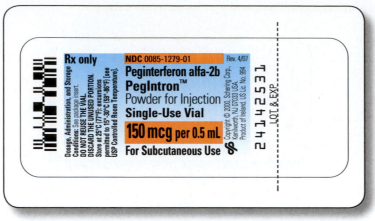

A

Preparation and Administration
PEG-Intron Redipen™
PEG-Intron Redipen™ consists of a dual-chamber glass cartridge with sterile, lyophilized peginterferon alfa-2b in the active chamber and Sterile Water for Injection, USP in the diluent chamber. The PEG-Intron in the glass cartridge should appear as a white to off-white tablet shaped solid that is whole or in pieces, or powder. To reconstitute the lyophilized peginterferon alfa-2b in the Redipen™, hold the Redipen™ upright (dose button down) and press the two halves of the pen together until there is an audible click. Gently invert the pen to mix the solution. DO NOT SHAKE. The reconstituted solution has a concentration of either 50 µg per 0.5 mL, 80 µg per 0.5 mL, 120 µg per 0.5 mL, or 150 µg per 0.5 mL for a single subcutaneous injection. Visually inspect the solution for particulate matter and discoloration prior to administration. The reconstituted solution should be clear and colorless. Do not use if the solution is discolored or cloudy, or if particulates are present.

Keeping the pen upright, attach the supplied needle and select the appropriate PEG-Intron dose by pulling back on the dosing button until the dark bands are visible and turning the button until the dark band is aligned with the correct dose. The prepared PEG-Intron solution is to be injected subcutaneously.

The PEG-Intron Redipen™ is a single use pen and does not contain a preservative. The reconstituted solution should be used immediately and cannot be stored for more than 24 hours at 2°-8°C (see **Storage**). **DO NOT REUSE THE REDIPEN™.** The sterility of any remaining product can no longer be guaranteed. **DISCARD THE UNUSED PORTION.** Pooling of unused portions of some medications has been linked to bacterial contamination and morbidity.

PEG-Intron Vials
Two B-D Safety-Lok™ syringes are provided in the package; one syringe is for the reconstitution steps and one for the patient injection. There is a plastic safety sleeve to be pulled over the needle after use. The syringe locks with an audible click when the green stripe on the safety sleeve covers the red stripe on the needle. Instructions for the preparation and administration of PEG-Intron Powder for Injection are provided below.

Reconstitute the PEG-Intron lyophilized product with only 0.7 mL of 1.25 mL of supplied diluent (Sterile Water for Injection, USP). **The diluent vial is for single use only. The remaining diluent should be discarded.** No other medications should be added to solutions containing PEG-Intron, and PEG-Intron should not be reconstituted with other diluents. Swirl gently to hasten complete dissolution of the powder. The reconstituted solution should be clear and colorless. Visually inspect the solution for particulate matter and discoloration prior to administration. The solution should not be used if discolored or cloudy, or if particulates are present.

The appropriate PEG-Intron dose should be withdrawn and injected subcutaneously. PEG-Intron vials are for single use only and do not contain a preservative. The reconstituted solution should be used immediately and cannot be stored for more than 24 hours at 2°-8°C (see **Storage**). **DO NOT REUSE THE VIAL.** The sterility of any remaining product can no longer be guaranteed. **DISCARD THE UNUSED PORTION.** Pooling of unused portions of some medications has been linked to bacterial contamination and morbidity.

After preparation and administration of the PEG-Intron for injection, it is essential to follow the state and or local procedures for proper disposal of syringes, needles, and the Redipen™. A puncture-resistant container should be used for disposal. Patients should be instructed in how to properly dispose of used syringes, needles, or the Redipen™ and be cautioned against the reuse of these items.

Storage
PEG-Intron Redipen™
PEG-Intron Redipen™ should be stored at 2° to 8°C (36° to 46°F). After reconstitution, the solution should be used immediately, but may be stored up to 24 hours at 2° to 8°C (36° to 46°F). The reconstituted solution contains no preservative, and is clear and colorless. **DO NOT FREEZE.**
PEG-Intron Vials
PEG-Intron should be stored at 25°C (77°F); excursions permitted to 15°-30°C (59°-86°F) [see USP Controlled Room Temperature]. After reconstitution with supplied Diluent the solution should be used immediately, but may be stored up to 24 hours at 2° to 8°C (36° to 46°F). The reconstituted solution contains no preservative, is clear and colorless. **DO NOT FREEZE.**

PegIntron™ package insert

1. How should you prepare this medication?

2. How much diluent is supplied and how much should be used?

3. What should you do with the rest of the diluent?

4. How would this medication most likely be administered?

5. After reconstitution, how should this medication be stored and for how long?

CASE STUDY

For questions 1–4 on the next page, refer to the following label, order, and package insert. (LO 14.2, 14.3)

The physician orders Sandostatin® 75 mcg IM tid.

On hand: See labels a, b, and c.

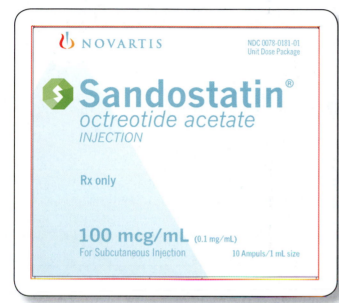

A

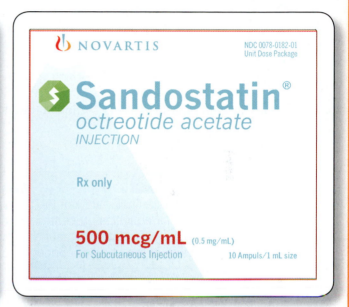

B

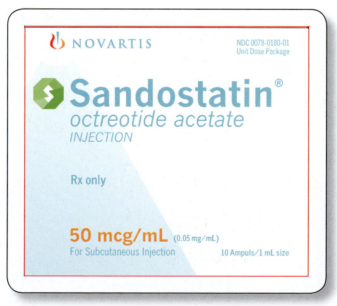

C

1. Describe what actions you should take before administering the medication. If you were going to administer the medication:

2. Which package would you use and why?

3. What would be the amount to administer?

4. What syringe would you use?

INTERNET ACTIVITY

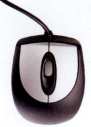

You have a standard 3-g vial of Timentin® on hand and have been ordered to give a 36-year-old patient Timentin® 500 mg IM for a mild urinary tract infection. The package insert is not available, and you are not certain how to reconstitute the medication and calculate the dose. Search the Internet to find a package insert or other reliable source for reconstitution directions. What is the appropriate amount and solution? What is the amount to administer?

To check your answers, see the Answer section at the end of the book, which starts on page A-1.

GO TO . . . Open the CD-ROM that accompanies your textbook, and complete a final review of the learning outcomes, practice problems, games, slideshow, and other activities presented for this chapter. For a final evaluation, take the chapter test and email or print your results for your instructor. A score of 95 percent or above indicates mastery of the chapter concepts.

Intravenous Calculations

One must learn by doing the thing, for though you think you know it, you have no certainty until you try.

—Aristole

Learning Outcomes

When you have completed Chapter 15, you will be able to:

15.1 Identify the components and concentrations of IV solutions.

15.2 Distinguish basic types of IV equipment.

15.3 Calculate IV flow rates for:

  a. Electronic devices in mL/h

  b. Manually controlled devices in gtt/min

  c. IV rate adjustment

15.4 Calculate infusion time and volume.

15.5 Perform calculations for intermittent IV infusions.

KEY TERMS

Central line
Drip chamber
Heparin lock
Hypertonic
Hypotonic
Infiltration
Infusion pumps
Intravenous
Isotonic
KVO or TKO fluids
Maintenance fluids
Patient-controlled
  analgesia (PCA)
Phlebitis
Peripherally inserted
  central catheters (PICC)
Port-A-Cath
Primary line
Rate controllers
Replacement fluids
Saline lock
Secondary line
Syringe pumps
Therapeutic fluids

INTRODUCTION

Intravenous (IV) fluids are solutions, including medications, that are delivered directly into the bloodstream through a vein. Blood, a suspension, is also delivered intravenously. Fluids delivered directly into the bloodstream have a rapid effect, which is necessary during emergencies or other critical care situations when medications are needed. However, the results can be fatal if the wrong medication or dosage is given. Healthcare workers who administer or monitor IV solutions should know the principles discussed in this chapter.

Many IV drugs are available. Each has its own guidelines regarding its use, based on specifications developed by the manufacturers. The guidelines typically outline recommended dosages, infusion rates, compatibility, and patient monitoring. For example, some medications cannot be combined with others, or must be administered over a specific length of time.

Furthermore, most states regulate who may administer IV medications and what training is required. This chapter teaches IV calculations and theory; however, to be proficient, you must obtain the required training and learn by doing.

15.1 IV Solutions

IV solutions fall into four functional categories: **replacement fluids, maintenance fluids, KVO or TKO fluids,** and **therapeutic fluids.** *Replacement fluids* replace electrolytes and fluids lost or depleted due to hemorrhage, vomiting, or diarrhea. Examples include whole blood, nutrient solutions, or fluids administered to treat dehydration. *Maintenance fluids* help patients maintain normal electrolyte and fluid balance. They include IV fluids such as normal saline given during and after surgery. Some IVs provide access to the vascular system for emergency situations. Fluids prescribed at a very slow rate to maintain open venous access are called *KVO (keep vein open) fluids or TKO (to keep open) fluids.* A commonly used *KVO fluid* is 0.9% sodium chloride, also called normal saline (NS). *Therapeutic fluids* deliver medication to the patient.

IV Labels

IV solutions are labeled with the name and exact amount of components in the solution. The label in Figure 15-1 is clearly marked as 5% dextrose and lactated Ringer's injection. Table 15-1 summarizes abbreviations often used for IV solutions.

RULE 15-1	In abbreviations for IV solutions, letters identify the component and numbers identify the concentration.
Example 1	An order for 5% dextrose in lactated Ringer's solution might be abbreviated in any of the following ways: D5LR D_5LR 5%D/LR D5%LR

GO TO . . . Open the CD-ROM that accompanies your textbook, and select Chapter 15, IV Solution Abbreviations (LO 15.1). Review the animation and example problems, then complete the practice problems. Continue to the next section of the book once you have mastered the information presented.

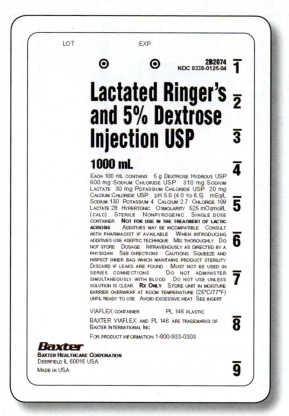

Figure 15-1 1000 mL D5LR label.

TABLE 15-1 Commonly Used Abbreviations	
D10W	10% dextrose in water
D5W	5% dextrose in water
W, H₂O	Water
NS, NSS	Normal saline (0.9% NaCl)
LR	Lactated ringer's
RL	Ringer's lactate
$\frac{1}{2}$ NS, $\frac{1}{2}$ NSS	One-half normal saline solution (0.45% NaCl)
$\frac{1}{3}$ NS, $\frac{1}{3}$ NSS	One-third normal saline solution (0.3% NaCl)
$\frac{1}{4}$ NS, $\frac{1}{4}$ NSS	One-fourth normal saline solution (0.225% NaCl)

IV Concentrations

Solutions may have different concentrations of dextrose (glucose) or saline (sodium chloride, or NaCl). For example, 5% dextrose contains 5 g of dextrose per 100 mL (see Figure 15-2). Normal saline is 0.9% saline; it contains 900 mg, or 0.9 g, of sodium chloride per 100 mL (see Figure 15-3). In turn, 0.45% saline, or $\frac{1}{2}$ NS, has 450 mg of sodium chloride per 100 mL, i.e., one-half the amount of normal saline. Other saline concentrations include 0.3% saline (or $\frac{1}{3}$ NS) and 0.225% saline (or $\frac{1}{4}$ NS).

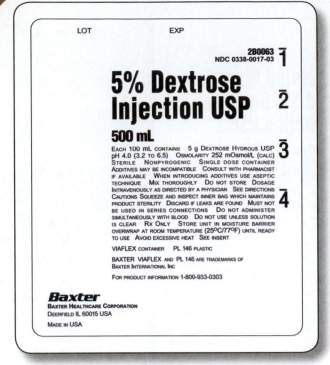

Figure 15-2 500 mL of D5W.

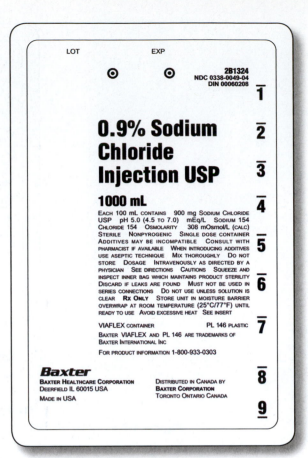

Figure 15-3 1000 mL of NS.

Example 1	How much dextrose is contained in 500 mL D5W? (Refer to Figure 15-2.)
	D5W represents 5% dextrose in water; it has 5 g of dextrose per 100 mL of water. Using the proportion method with fractions (Procedure Checklist 6-1),

$$\frac{5 \text{ g}}{100 \text{ mL}} = \frac{x}{500 \text{ mL}}$$

$$100x = 2500 \text{ g}$$

$$x = 25 \text{ g}$$

So 25 g of dextrose is contained in 500 mL D5W.

Example 2	How much sodium chloride is contained in 1000 mL of NS (Figure 15-3)?

$$\frac{0.9 \text{ g}}{100 \text{ mL}} = \frac{x}{1000 \text{ mL}}$$

$$100x = 900 \text{ g}$$

$$x = 9 \text{ g}$$

So 9 g of sodium chloride is contained in 1000 mL of NS.

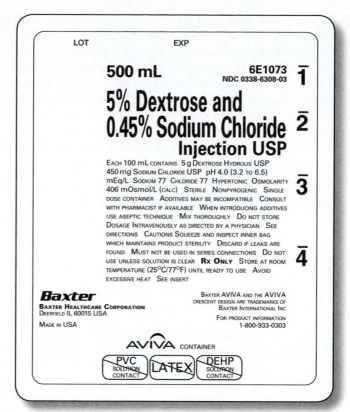

Figure 15-4 D5 1/2 NS.

| Example 3 | How much dextrose and sodium chloride are contained in 1000 mL of D5 $\frac{1}{2}$ NS (Figure 15-4)? |

Dextrose:

$$\frac{5\text{ g}}{100\text{ mL}} = \frac{x}{1000\text{ mL}}$$

$$100x = 5000\text{ g}$$

$$x = 50\text{ g dextrose}$$

Sodium chloride:

$$\frac{0.45\text{ g}}{100\text{ mL}} = \frac{x}{1000\text{ mL}}$$

$$100x = 450\text{ g}$$

$$x = 4.5\text{ g sodium chloride}$$

So there are 50 g of dextrose and 4.5 g sodium chloride in 1000 mL of D5 $\frac{1}{2}$ NS.

Knowledge of a patient's fluid and electrolyte balance is necessary to determine a solution's concentration. Calcium, potassium, chloride, phosphorus, and magnesium are electrolytes that can be added to an IV solution to help correct a fluid or chemical imbalance.

The concentration of these electrolytes determines the osmolarity of the solution. Solutions with approximately the same osmolarity as the fluid within the cell are termed **isotonic.** Solutions with a lower osmolarity than intracellular fluid are termed **hypotonic.** Hypotonic solutions are dilute, which results in fluid moving into the cell. Solutions with a higher osmolarity than intracellular fluid are termed **hypertonic.** Hypertonic solutions are concentrated and cause fluid to shift out of the cell. Authorized prescribers use this knowledge to determine which type of IV fluid to administer. If the patient is dehydrated and there is not enough fluid within the cell, a hypotonic IV fluid is ordered. If the patient has too much fluid in the cell, as in cerebral edema, a hypertonic fluid is ordered. If the patient has a normal fluid balance, but can't take fluids enterally, maintenance IV fluid that is isotonic is ordered. Isotonic IV fluid is also used to replace intravascular fluid if the patient is hypovolemic (does not have enough fluid circulating in the blood vessels).

Examples of isotonic solutions are: lactated Ringer's, Ringer's lactate, normal saline (0.9% NaCl), and D5W. Although D5W has an osmolarity similar to intracellular fluid while it is in the IV bag, the dextrose quickly moves into the cell after administration, leaving a hypotonic solution in the extracellular fluid. For this reason D5W is used as a hypotonic solution. Saline solutions with less NaCl than normal saline (less than 0.9% NaCl) are hypotonic. Examples of these are $\frac{1}{2}$ NS (0.45% NaCl), $\frac{1}{3}$ NS (0.3% NS), and $\frac{1}{4}$ NS (0.225% NaCl). Saline solutions with more NaCl than normal saline (greater than 0.9% NaCl) are hypertonic. Examples of these are 3% NaCl and 5% NaCl.

RULE 15-2	Patients with normal electrolyte levels are likely to receive isotonic solutions. Those with high electrolyte levels will receive hypotonic solutions. Those with low electrolyte levels will receive hypertonic solutions.
Example 1	Patient A is a 35-year-old, healthy female who will have an IV infusion during a diagnostic test. She will require an isotonic solution such as NS, or lactated Ringer's.
Example 2	Patient B is an 8-year-old female who has been vomiting and has had diarrhea for 24 hours and is dehydrated. She may require a hypotonic solution like 0.45% sodium chloride or 0.3% sodium chloride to restore the proper fluid level in her cells and tissues.
Example 3	Patient C is a 50-year-old male with cerebral edema. He may require hypertonic solution such as 3% sodium chloride to help draw fluids from cells and tissues.

GO TO . . . Open the CD-ROM that accompanies your textbook, and select Chapter 15, IV Concentrations (LO 15.1). Review the animation and example problems, then complete the practice problems. Continue to the next section of the book once you have mastered the information presented.

Compatibility

Medications, electrolytes, and nutrients are additives that can be combined with IV solutions. Potassium chloride, vitamins B and C, and antibiotics are common additives. While additives are often prepackaged in the solution, you may need to mix the additive and IV solution yourself. The physician's order will tell you how much additive to administer, the amount and type of basic IV solution to use, and the length of time over which the additive/IV mixture should infuse. For example, an order may call for 20 milliequivalents (mEq) of potassium chloride in 1000 mL of 5% dextrose and normal saline over 8 h, or

1000 mL D5NS c̄ 20 mEq KCl IV over 8 h

RULE 15-3	Before you combine any medications, electrolytes, or nutrients with an IV solution, be sure the components are compatible.

Example	Some incompatible additives may cause the resulting solution to turn cloudy or crystallize, which means it hardens to crystals. If you mix an IV base solution with an additive that is incompatible (see Table 15-2), you may place the patient's health at serious risk. Verify compatibility by checking with a compatibility chart, a drug reference book, the pharmacy, the Internet, or a package insert.

TABLE 15-2 Verifying Compatibility

The following are a few examples of incompatible combinations. Always check the compatibility of IV solutions and additives.

Ampicillin	5% dextrose in water
Cefotaxime sodium	Sodium bicarbonate
Diazepam	Potassium chloride
Dopamine HCl	Sodium bicarbonate
Penicillin	Heparin
Penicillin	Vitamin B complex
Sodium bicarbonate	Lactated Ringer's
Tetracycline HCl	Calcium chloride

GO TO . . . Open the CD-ROM that accompanies your textbook, and select Chapter 15, Compatibility (LO 15.1). Review the animation and example problems, then complete the practice problems. Continue to the next section of the book once you have mastered the information presented.

REVIEW AND PRACTICE

15.1 IV Solutions

For Exercises 1–5, calculate the number of grams of NaCL and/or dextrose in each of the following IV solutions.

1. 1000 mL $D_{10}W$ _____ g dextrose

2. 500 mL D5 $\frac{1}{2}$ NS _____ g dextrose _____ g NaCl

3. 250 mL D_5NS _____ g dextrose _____ g NaCl

4. 1000 mL D_5LR _____ g dextrose

5. 500 mL $D_5 \frac{1}{4}$ NS _____ g dextrose _____ g NaCl

To check your answers, see Answer section at the end of the book, which starts on page A-1.

Checking Compatibility

A patient in respiratory distress with congestive heart failure is started on D5/0.45% NaCl. The next day she is diagnosed with an upper respiratory infection. The physician orders 500 mg ampicillin IVPB q6h.

The healthcare professional begins to administer the ampicillin. She notices that the solution in the tubing has become cloudy.

Think! . . . Is It Reasonable? Why would the solution in the tubing be cloudy? What should the healthcare professional do?

15.2 IV Equipment

IV equipment is available in several forms. Most are electronic or have electronic components, while some are still manual.

The Primary Line

The typical IV setup consists of a bag or bottle of IV solution and tubing. IV bags come in different sizes, often containing 500 or 1000 mL of solution. You should mark them at regular time intervals to record the amount of solution that is being infused. Your facility will have specific guidelines for you to follow.

The tubing, which is the **primary line,** usually includes a **drip chamber,** clamp, and injection ports (see Figure 15-5). The drip chamber is a transparent enclosure through which the drops of IV fluid can be counted in order to estimate the rate of infusion. The drip chamber attaches to the IV bag. To measure the flow rate, squeeze and release the drip chamber until it is half filled with IV solution. Fluid in the chamber makes it easy to count the drops that

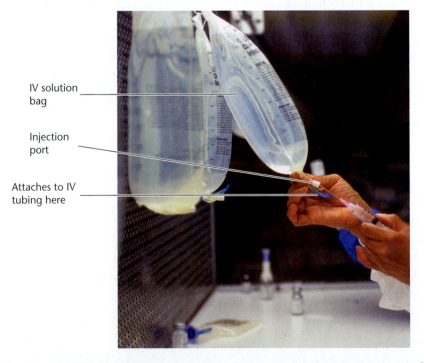

IV solution bag

Injection port

Attaches to IV tubing here

Figure 15-5 A bag of IV fluid may have medication added through the injection port before administration.

fall into it from the bag. Use a roller clamp (Figure 15-6) or a screw clamp to set or adjust the flow rate of the IV solution. A slide clamp shuts off the IV solution flow completely without disturbing the flow rate setting at the roller or screw clamp. Injection ports allow you to inject medications or compatible fluids into the primary line or to attach a second IV line. IV bags may have ports for additives injected directly into the solution.

Tubing is available in two sizes: macrodrip or microdrip. Macrodrip tubing (see Figure 15-7) allows larger drops to form before falling into the drip chamber. It is used for infusions of 80 mL/h or more and is always used for operating room infusions. Microdrip tubing allows smaller drops to enter the drip chamber. It is used for flow rates of less than 80 mL/h and is often used for KVO infusions. Microdrip tubing is especially useful for pediatric and critical care IVs, when very small volumes are used and accuracy is extremely important. Accidental increases in volume can be fatal in these situations.

Secondary Lines (Piggyback)

A **secondary line,** also known as a piggyback or IVPB, is an IV setup that attaches to a primary line. It can be used to infuse medication or other compatible fluids on an intermittent basis, such as q6h. Although shorter than primary tubing, secondary tubing has the same basic components. IVPB bags are usually smaller, often holding 50, 100, or 150 mL of fluid. (See Figure 15-8.) Some medications require a larger amount of fluid as a diluent, such as 250 mL.

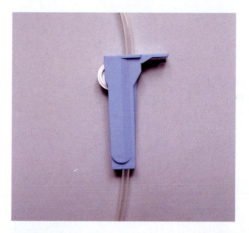

Figure 15-6   Roller clamp.

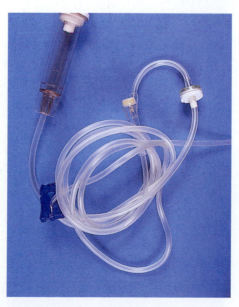

Figure 15-7   IV tubing.

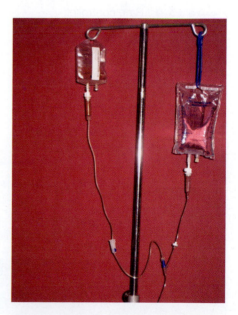

Figure 15-8   Secondary IV solution piggybacked to primary IV solution.

Monitoring IV Equipment

IVs may be monitored manually. The bag is hung 36 inches (in.) above the patient's heart to allow gravity to draw the fluid through the tubing and into the vascular system. Whoever administers and monitors the IV adjusts the flow rate, using roller or screw clamps. Manually delivered IV fluids are usually adjusted in drops per minute (gtt/min).

Electronic devices—rate controllers, infusion pumps, syringe pumps, and *patient-controlled analgesia* (PCA) devices—can be used to regulate the flow of IV infusions. These devices often use tubing specific to the equipment. Some types of tubing may be used only with specific pumps (see Figures 15-9, 15-10, 15-11, 15-12).

Rate controllers rely on gravity to infuse the solution, but no clamp is used to adjust the flow rate. Tubing is threaded through the controller, where a pincher maintains a preset flow rate. The controller is attached to a sensor that measures the drops or volume of solution that is delivered. An alarm sounds when the preset flow rate cannot be maintained.

Infusion pumps apply pressure sufficient to deliver a set volume of liquid every minute into the vein. They can introduce liquid into a central vein, where pressure is much higher than in peripheral veins. The desired flow rate is set on an infusion pump, either in milliliters per hour or by dosage. The unit does not rely on gravity, but forces the IV solution through

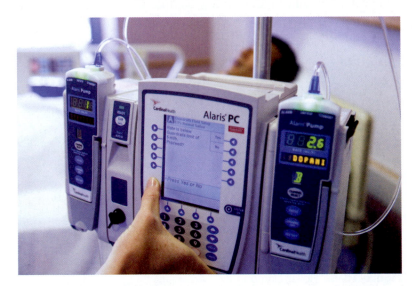

Figure 15-9   Rate controller.

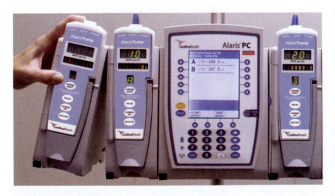

Figure 15-10   Infusion pump.

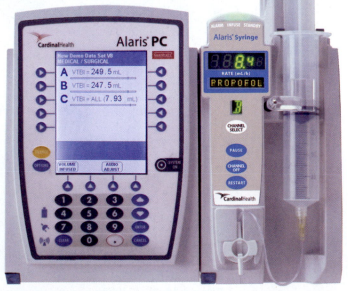

Figure 15-11   Syringe pump.

the tubing. A sensor detects when the IV bag is empty or the flow is too rapid by sounding an alarm. An alarm also sounds if the flow rate cannot be maintained or if the bag is empty. A rate that is too slow may indicate too much resistance in the vein, suggesting blockage, a kink in the tubing, or that the IV catheter has come out of the vein. In some cases, the equipment will continue to pump the IV fluid, even though the catheter is out of the vein. Thus, when you use an infusion pump, you must monitor the patient's infusion site regularly for signs of infiltration (such as swelling, coolness, or discomfort).

Syringe pumps allow you to insert a syringe in the pump unit (see Figure 15-11). The syringe can deliver medication or fluids that cannot be combined with other medications or solutions. Syringe pumps are useful for pediatric medications as well as for medications that must be administered at a precisely controlled rate. Syringe pumps are often used in cases when a medication must be administered over half an hour or less; they are also used for longer time periods as well.

Patient-controlled analgesia (PCA) devices are used by patients in pain, including pain from cancer or surgery (see Figure 15-12). PCA pumps allow patients to control their own medication within limits preset according to the order of the authorized prescriber. By pressing a button on a hand-held device, a patient administers medication. The PCA device helps monitor the effectiveness of the pain relief prescription, recording the number of times the patient uses the device.

Volume control sets such as Buretrol, Soluset, and Volutrol are used with manual IV setups and electronic rate controllers to improve accuracy, especially for small volumes of medication or fluid (see Figure 15-13). They are calibrated in 1-mL increments, with a total volume capacity ranging from 100 to 150 mL. Medication is injected through an injection port into a burette—a chamber that holds a smaller controlled amount of fluid. An exact amount of IV fluid is added as a diluent to the burette chamber, where it is mixed. The fluid is delivered to the patient in microdrips. Burettes are often used in critical care or pediatric IVs because of their accuracy.

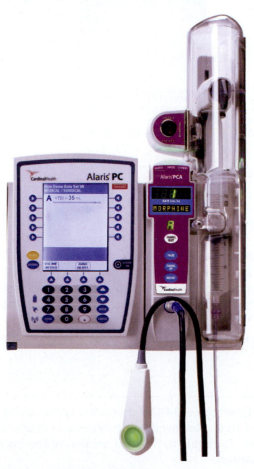

Figure 15-12 PCA pump.

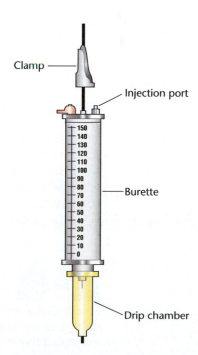

Figure 15-13 Volume control set.

Peripheral and Central IV Therapy

Peripheral IV therapy accesses the circulatory system through a peripheral vein. Sites are usually located in the hand, forearm, foot, and leg. Because peripheral veins can be difficult to locate in small or premature infants, a peripheral IV line may be set up using a vein in the scalp.

Central IV therapy provides direct access to major veins. See Figure 15-14. A **central line** is used when the patient needs large amounts of fluids, a rapid infusion of medication, infusion of highly concentrated solutions, or long-term IV therapy. Central lines can be inserted using a catheter through the chest wall (see Figure 15-15) or by threading a catheter through a peripheral vein. In newborn infants, a central line can be inserted into the umbilical vein or artery. These procedures are usually performed by a physician. A **peripherally inserted central catheter (PICC)** is inserted in arm veins and threaded into a central vein, often by specially trained nurses. A **Port-A-Cath** is used to deliver medication to a central vein. It is surgically placed under the skin and accessed through the skin to administer IV medication on an intermittent basis.

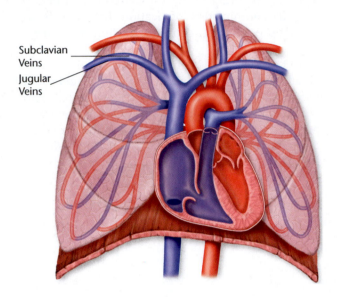

Subclavian
Veins
Jugular
Veins

Figure 15-14 A central venous line is usually inserted into the internal jugular or subclavian veins.

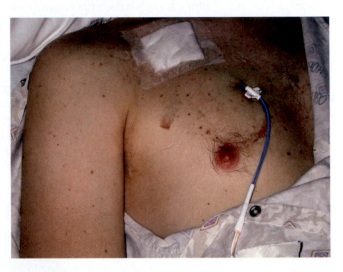

Figure 15-15 Central venous line inserted through the chest wall.

RULE 15-4	Never flush a sluggish IV with a syringe.
Example	If you flush or irrigate an IV catheter that is clogged, you may be pushing a clot into the circulatory system. This clot, known as an *embolism,* can travel through the bloodstream and block a blood vessel. An obstruction or blockage of any blood vessel in the body is dangerous. An obstruction of a blood vessel in a vital organ such as the heart or lungs can be fatal.

GO TO . . . Open the CD-ROM that accompanies your textbook, and select Chapter 15, IV Flush (LO 15.2). Review the animation and example problems, then complete the practice problems. Continue to the next section of the book once you have mastered the information presented.

Pain or swelling near an IV site may indicate an infiltration or phlebitis. An **infiltration** occurs when the needle or catheter is dislodged from the vein or penetrates the vein. Fluid is then infused into the surrounding tissue (see Figure 15-16). Signs of infiltration include swelling, discomfort, and coolness at the infiltration site, as well as a sizable decrease in flow rate. The table in Figure 15-16 lists the manifestations associated with varying grades of IV infiltration. **Phlebitis** is an inflammation of the vein. It can develop when the vein is irritated by IV additives, by movement of the needle or catheter, or during long-term IV therapy. In most cases of phlebitis, patients will complain of pain at or near the site. Other signs include heat, redness, and swelling of the injection site. In the case of either infiltration or phlebitis, stop the IV infusion and restart it in another limb. In the case of phlebitis, also notify the patient's physician.

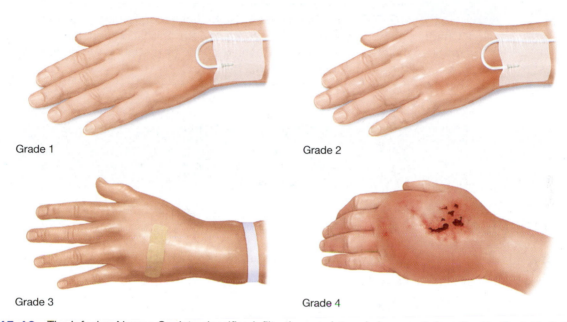

Grade 1

Grade 2

Grade 3

Grade 4

Figure 15-16   The Infusion Nurses Society classifies infiltration as pictured above and described in the table below.

INS Infiltration Scale	
GRADE	CLINICAL CRITERIA
0	No symptoms
1	Skin blanched Edema < 1 in. around site Cool to touch With or without pain
2	Skin blanched Edema < 6 in. around site Cool to touch With or without pain
3	Skin blanched and translucent Gross edema > 6 in. around site Cool to touch Mild to moderate pain Possible numbness

(Continued)

GRADE	CLINICAL CRITERIA
4	Skin blanched and translucent Skin tight, leaking Skin discolored, bruised, swollen Gross edema > 6 in. around site Deep pitting tissue edema Circulatory impairment Moderate to severe pain Infiltration of any amount of blood product, irritant, or vesicant

GO TO . . . Open the CD-ROM that accompanies your textbook, and select Chapter 15, IV Equipment (LO 15.2). Review the animation and example problems, then complete the practice problems. Continue to the next section of the book once you have mastered the information presented.

REVIEW AND PRACTICE

15.2 IV Equipment

For Exercises 1–8, identify the IV equipment that you would use in each instance.

1. Add a dose of medication to an existing line.

2. Adjust the flow rate of an IV solution.

3. Stop the IV flow without disturbing the flow rate.

4. Introduce IV fluid into a central vein.

5. Set up tubing to infuse D5W at the rate of 40 mL/h.

6. Allow patient to self-administer medication for pain.

7. Administer a small amount of fluid over 15 minutes.

8. Administer an exact amount of IV fluid added as a diluent that is mixed and delivered in microdrips to a pediatric patient.

Provide a brief response to each of the following questions.

9. When would central IV therapy be used?

10. What do you look for when you monitor an IV?

11. How might you recognize infiltration?

12. What are three possible causes of phlebitis?

13. How high should the IV bag be hung?

14. What four electronic devices can be used to regulate the flow of IV infusions?

15. When is an injection port used?

To check your answers, see the Answer section at the end of the book, which starts on page A-1.

15.3 Calculating Flow Rates

An order for IV fluids indicates the *amount of an IV fluid* to be administered and the *length of time* over which it is to be given. Before you can administer the IV, you must calculate a *flow rate* for the intravenous solution from these two values. For most electronic devices that regulate the flow of IV solutions, the flow rate will be expressed in milliliters per hour (mL/h).

RULE 15-5

To calculate flow rates in milliliters per hour, identify the following:

- *V* (volume) is expressed in milliliters.

- *T* (time) must be expressed in hours. (Convert the units when necessary by using the proportion method or dimensional analysis.)

- *F* (flow rate) will be rounded to the nearest whole number.

Use the formula method with $F = \frac{V}{T}$ or dimensional analysis to determine the flow rate in milliliters per hour.

FORMULA METHOD

EXAMPLE 1

Find the flow rate.

Ordered: 500 mg ampicillin in 100 mL NS to infuse over 30 minutes

In this case the volume is expressed in milliliters, and $V = 100$ mL.

STEP A: CONVERT

Since time is expressed in minutes, you must first convert 30 minutes (min) to hours to find *T*. In this example Procedure Checklist 6-1, the proportion method is used.

$$\frac{1\,h}{60\,min} = \frac{x}{30\,min}$$

$$\frac{1\,h}{60\,\cancel{min}} = \frac{x}{30\,\cancel{min}}$$

$$60 \times x = 1\,h \times 30$$

$$x = \frac{1\,h \times 30}{60}$$

$$x = 0.5\,h$$

STEP B: CALCULATE

We now have the information needed in the proper units.

$$V = 100\,mL \quad \text{and} \quad T = 0.5\,h$$

Using the formula $F = \frac{V}{T}$, we find that

$$F = \frac{100\,mL}{0.5\,h}$$

$$F = \frac{200\,mL}{h}$$

STEP C: THINK! . . . IS IT REASONABLE?

If 100 mL infuses in $\frac{1}{2}$ hour then 200 mL would infuse in 1 hour.

Find the flow rate.

Ordered: 500 mL D5 1/2 NS over 3 h

STEP A: CONVERT
No conversion needed.

STEP B: CALCULATE
In this case the units are already expressed in milliliters and hours; $V = 500$ mL and $T = 3$ h. Using the formula $F = \frac{V}{T}$, we have

$$F = \frac{500 \text{ mL}}{3 \text{ h}}$$

$$F = 166.7 \text{ mL/h}$$

$$F = 167 \text{ mL/h} \qquad \text{rounded to nearest whole number}$$

STEP C: THINK! . . . IS IT REASONABLE?
If 500 mL is divided by 3 hours it equals 167 mL/h

DIMENSIONAL ANALYSIS

EXAMPLE 1

Find the flow rate.

Ordered: 500 mg ampicillin in 100 mL NS to infuse over 30 min

STEP A: CONVERT
Since the time is expressed in minutes and the flow rate is mL/h, you must determine the conversion factor for minutes to hours.

$$\frac{60 \text{ min}}{1 \text{ h}}$$

STEP B: CALCULATE

1. Determine the units of measure for the answer (F), and place it as the unknown on one side of the equation.

   F mL/h =

2. Write the first conversion factor for hours to minutes as determined in Step A, with minutes in the numerator.

   $$\frac{60 \text{ min}}{1 \text{ h}}$$

3. Write a second factor with the number of milliliters to be administered on top (V) and the length of time to be administered (T) on the bottom. Set up the equation.

   $$F \text{ mL/h} = \frac{60 \text{ min}}{1 \text{ h}} \times \frac{100 \text{ mL}}{30 \text{ min}}$$

4. Cancel units on the right side of the equation. The remaining unit of measure on the right side of the equation should match the unknown unit of measure on the left side of the equation.

   $$F \text{ mL/h} = \frac{60 \text{ \cancel{min}}}{1 \text{ h}} \times \frac{100 \text{ mL}}{30 \text{ \cancel{min}}}$$

5. Solve the equation.

   $$F \text{ mL/h} = \frac{60 \times 100}{30}$$

   $$F = 200 \text{ mL/h}$$

STEP C: THINK! . . . IS IT REASONABLE?
If 100 mL infuses in 1/2 hour then 200 mL would infuse in 1 hour.

Find the flow rate.

Ordered: 500 mL D5 1/2 NS over 3 h

STEP A: CONVERT

No conversion needed.

STEP B: CALCULATE

1. Determine the units of measure for the answer (*F*) and place it as the unknown on one side of the equation.

   F mL/h =

2. On the right side of the equation, write a factor with the number of milliliters to be administered on top (*V*) and the length of time to be administered (*T*) on the bottom.

   $$F \text{ mL/h} = \frac{500 \text{ mL}}{3 \text{ h}}$$

3. Since the units of measure on the left side of the equation match the units of measure on the right side of the equation, no additional conversion factors are necessary. Solve the equation.

   $$F \text{ mL/h} = \frac{500 \text{ mL}}{3 \text{ h}}$$

   $$F = 166.7 \text{ mL/h}$$

   $$F = 167 \text{ mL/h, rounded to nearest whole number}$$

STEP C: THINK! . . . IS IT REASONABLE?

If 500 mL is divided by 3 hours it equals 167 mL/h

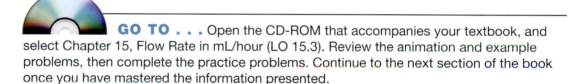

GO TO . . . Open the CD-ROM that accompanies your textbook, and select Chapter 15, Flow Rate in mL/hour (LO 15.3). Review the animation and example problems, then complete the practice problems. Continue to the next section of the book once you have mastered the information presented.

For a manually regulated IV, the flow rate needs to be calculated as the number of drops per minute (gtt/min). Before this can be calculated, you must first know how many drops are in a milliliter. IV tubing packages are labeled with a drop factor, which tells you how many drops of IV solution are equal to 1 mL when using that tubing (Figures 15-17 and 15-18). *Macrodrip* tubing has larger drops and one of three typical drop factors: 10 gtt/mL, 15 gtt/mL, or 20 gtt/mL. *Microdrip* tubing has a drop factor of 60 gtt/mL. See Figure 15-19.

In most circumstances you will determine the flow rate in milliliters per hour and then need to determine the flow rate in drops per minute. For example, you may be using an electronic device to monitor the flow rate of an IV. These devices are usually set at a flow rate of milliliters per hour. If an electronic device needs to be checked manually, then you will need

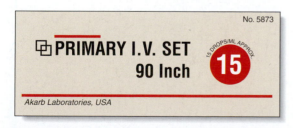

Figure 15-17 15 gtt/mL calibrated macrodrip tubing.

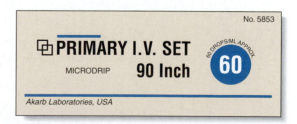

Figure 15-18 60 gtt/mL calibrated microdrip tubing.

CHAPTER 15 Intravenous Calculations **423**

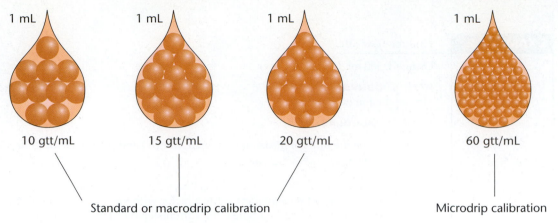

10 gtt/mL   15 gtt/mL   20 gtt/mL   60 gtt/mL

Standard or macrodrip calibration   Microdrip calibration

Figure 15-19 Macrodrip and microdrip calibration.

to convert the flow rate of milliliters per hour to drops per minute to count the drops delivered to a patient in a minute. Once you know the desired flow rate in drops per minute and the IV is not attached to an electronic device, you adjust the roller or screw clamp so that the drops fall at the desired rate.

RULE 15-6

To determine the flow rate *f* in drops per minute:

Change the flow rate in milliliters per hour (*F*) to drops per minute (*f*), using the formula

$$f = \frac{F \times C}{60}$$

where *F* = flow rate, mL/h
  C = calibration factor of tubing, gtt/mL
  60 = number of minutes in 1 h

Round your answer to the nearest whole number.

Note: You can also use the dimensional analysis method for calculating the flow rate, adding the gtt factor of your tubing to the equation used for determining the flow rate F in mL/h.

FORMULA METHOD

EXAMPLE 1

Find the flow rate in drops per minute that is equal to 75 mL/h when you are using 20 gtt/mL macrodrip tubing.

CALCULATE

  F = 75 mL/h

  C = 20 gtt/mL

Substituting into the formula gives

$$f = \frac{F \times C}{60 \text{ min/h}}$$

$$f = \frac{75 \text{ mL/h} \times 20 \text{ gtt/mL}}{60 \text{ min/h}}$$

Cancel units.

$$f = \frac{75 \; \cancel{mL}/\cancel{h} \times 20 \; gtt/\cancel{mL}}{60 \; min/\cancel{h}}$$

Solve the equation.

$$f = 25 \; gtt/min$$

Find the flow rate in drops per minute that is equal to 35 mL/h when you are using 60 gtt/mL microdrip tubing.

CALCULATE

$$F = 35 \; mL/h$$

$$C = 60 \; gtt/mL$$

Substituting into the formula gives

$$f = \frac{F \times C}{60}$$

$$f = \frac{35 \; mL/h \times 60 \; gtt/mL}{60 \; min/h}$$

Cancel the units.

$$f = \frac{35 \; \cancel{mL}/\cancel{h} \times 60 \; gtt/\cancel{mL}}{60 \; min/\cancel{h}}$$

$$f = 35 \; gtt/min$$

Note: The value of the flow rate is the same in drops per minute or milliliters per hour when 60 gtt/mL microdrip tubing is used. In other words, for microdrop tubing, $F = f$.

DIMENSIONAL ANALYSIS

Find the flow rate in drops per minute that is equal to 75 mL/h when you are using 20 gtt/mL macrodrip tubing.

CALCULATE

1. Determine the unit of measure for the answer (f) and place it as the unknown on one side of the equation.

$$f \; gtt/min =$$

2. Determine the first factor. The number of milliliters to be administered on top (V) and the length of time to be administered (T) on the bottom.

$$\frac{75 \; mL}{1 \; h}$$

3. Multiply by a second factor to convert the hours to minutes, placing hours in the numerator.

$$75 \; mL/h \times \frac{1 \; h}{60 \; min}$$

4. Multiply by the drop factor of the tubing being used. This is the third factor. Set up the equation.

$$f \; gtt/min = \frac{75 \; mL}{1 \; h} \times \frac{1 \; h}{60 \; min} \times \frac{20 \; gtt}{1 \; mL}$$

5. Cancel units on the right side of the equation. The remaining unit of measure on the right side of the equation should match the unknown unit of measure on the left side of the equation.

$$f \text{ gtt/min} = \frac{75 \text{ mL}}{1 \text{ h}} \times \frac{1 \text{ h}}{60 \text{ min}} \times \frac{20 \text{ gtt}}{1 \text{ mL}}$$

6. Solve the equation.

$$f = \frac{75 \times 20 \text{ gtt}}{60 \text{ min}}$$

$$f = 25 \text{ gtt/min}$$

EXAMPLE 2 Find the flow rate in drops per minute that is equal to 35 mL/h when you are using 60 gtt/mL microdrip tubing.

CALCULATE

1. Determine the unit of measure for the answer (f) and place it as the unknown on the left side of the equation.

$$f \text{ gtt/min} =$$

2. Determine the first factor. The number of milliliters to be administered on top (V) and the length of time to be administered (T) on the bottom.

$$\frac{35 \text{ mL}}{h}$$

3. Multiply by a second factor to convert the hours to minutes; place hours in the numerator.

$$35 \text{ mL/h} \times \frac{1 \text{ h}}{60 \text{ min}}$$

4. Multiply by the drop factor of the tubing being used. Set up the equation.

$$f \text{ gtt/min} = \frac{35 \text{ mL}}{1 \text{ h}} \times \frac{1 \text{ h}}{60 \text{ min}} \times \frac{60 \text{ gtt}}{1 \text{ mL}}$$

5. Cancel units on the right side of the equation. The remaining unit of measure on the right side of the equation should match the unknown unit of measure on the left side of the equation.

$$f \text{ gtt/min} = \frac{35 \text{ mL}}{1 \text{ h}} \times \frac{1 \text{ h}}{60 \text{ min}} \times \frac{60 \text{ gtt}}{1 \text{ mL}}$$

6. Solve the equation.

$$f \text{ gtt/min} = 35 \times \frac{1}{60 \text{ min}} \times \frac{60 \text{ gtt}}{1}$$

$$f = 35 \text{ gtt/min}$$

Note: The value of the flow rate is the same in drops per minute or milliliters per hour when 60 gtt/mL microdrip tubing is used. In other words, for microdrip tubing, $F = f$.

GO TO . . . Open the CD-ROM that accompanies your textbook, and select Chapter 15, Flow Rate in gtt/min (LO 15.3). Review the animation and example problems, then complete the practice problems. Continue to the next section of the book once you have mastered the information presented.

Adjusting Flow Rates

Counting drops and timing are not always precise. What you calibrated as 25 drops per minute may actually be 25.4 drops per minute. Therefore, adjustments to flow rates sometimes need to be made. You should check at least once every hour that the IV is infusing to see if it is behind or ahead of schedule. The policy at the facility where you are employed will dictate whether you may adjust the IV flow rate or whether you should notify the physician. Always check this policy before you adjust a flow rate.

RULE 15-7	To adjust the flow rate: • Recalculate the infusion, using the volume remaining in the IV and the time remaining in the order. • Check the guidelines at your facility before you adjust the flow rate.
Example 1	Original order: 1500 mL NS over 12 h The IV was infused at an original rate of 42 gtt/min using 20 gtt/mL macrodrip tubing. After 3 h, 1200 mL remains in the bag. **CALCULATE** $V = 1200$ mL (volume remaining) $T = 12$ h original $- 3$ h elapsed $= 9$ h remaining $C = 20$ gtt/mL Using the formula $f = C \times \frac{V}{T}$, we must first convert 9 h to minutes. Using the proportion method with ratios, we find $60 \text{ min} : 1 \text{ h} = T : 9 \text{ h}$ $60 \text{ min} : 1 \cancel{h} = T : 9 \cancel{h}$ $T \times 1 = 60 \text{ min} \times 9$ $T = 540$ min Insert the appropriate numbers into the formula. $f = 20 \text{ gtt/mL} \times \dfrac{1200 \text{ mL}}{540 \text{ min}}$ Cancel units. $f = 20 \text{ gtt/}\cancel{mL} \times \dfrac{1200 \ \cancel{mL}}{540 \text{ min}}$ Solve for the unknown. $f = 20 \text{ gtt} \times \dfrac{1200}{540 \text{ min}}$ $f = 44.4$ gtt/min Round to the nearest whole number. $f = 44$ gtt/min = adjusted flow rate *Note:* IV rate adjustment can be determined in mL/h by dividing remaining hours into remaining volume. For this example: 1200 mL/9 h = 133.33 or 133 mL/h.

Example 2

Original order: 1500 mL NS over 12 h

Using 15 gtt/mL macrodrip tubing, the IV should have infused at 31 gtt/min. After 4 h, 1100 mL remains in the bag.

CALCULATE

V = 1100 mL (volume remaining)

T = 12 h − 4 h = 8 h remaining

C = 15 gtt/mL

Using the formula $f = C \times \frac{V}{T}$, we must first convert 8 h to minutes. Using the proportion method with fractions, we have

$$\frac{1 \cancel{h}}{60 \text{ min}} = \frac{8 \cancel{h}}{x}$$

$1 \times x$ min $= 60 \times 8$

x min $= 480$

Insert the appropriate numbers into the formula.

$$f = 15 \text{ gtt/mL} \times \frac{1100 \text{ mL}}{480 \text{ min}}$$

Cancel units.

$$f = 15 \text{ gtt/m}\cancel{L} \times \frac{1100 \text{ m}\cancel{L}}{480 \text{ min}}$$

Solve for the unknown.

$$f = 15 \text{ gtt} \times \frac{1100}{480 \text{ min}}$$

f = 34.4 gtt/min

Round to the nearest whole number.

f = 34 gtt/min = adjusted flow rate

Note: Adjusted flow rate in mL/h: 1100 mL/8 h = 137.5 or 138 mL/h.

GO TO . . . Open the CD-ROM that accompanies your textbook, and select Chapter 15, Adjusting the Flow Rate (LO 15.3). Review the animation and example problems, then complete the practice problems. Continue to the next section of the book once you have mastered the information presented.

CRITICAL THINKING ON THE JOB

Adjusting the Flow Rate

Earlier in the day, Pat set up an IV based on the following physician's order: 750 mL D5NS to infuse over 8 h. Pat calculated that the patient should receive 94 mL of fluid per hour, with a flow rate of 16 gtt/min using 10 gtt/mL tubing.

After 4 h (one-half the time ordered for the infusion), Pat observed that 450 mL remained in the IV bag. Only one-half of the fluid, or 375 mL, should have remained in the bag. The patient had received 75 mL less fluid than expected. Pat decided to reset the flow rate for the next hour so that the patient would receive the original 94 mL/h plus the 75 mL that should have already been administered, for a total of 169 mL. After the next hour, Pat planned to reset the IV to the original flow rate of 16 gtt/min. Pat calculated the new flow rate as

$$\frac{10 \text{ gtt}}{1 \text{ mL}} \times \frac{169 \text{ mL}}{1 \text{ h}} \times \frac{1 \text{ h}}{60 \text{ min}} =$$

$$\frac{28.17 \text{ gtt}}{1 \text{ min}} = 28 \text{ gtt/min}$$

Thus, Pat adjusted the flow rate to 28 gtt/min.

 Think! . . . Is It Reasonable? What mistake did Pat make? What should Pat have done to avoid the mistake?

REVIEW AND PRACTICE

15.3 Calculating Flow Rates

For Exercises 1–4, find the flow rate in milliliters per hour.

1. Ordered: 1000 mL LR over 6 h

2. Ordered: 300 mL NS over 2 h

3. Ordered: 3000 mL 1/2 NS q24h

4. Ordered: 40 mEq KCl in 100 mL NS over 45 min

For Exercises 5–10, calculate the flow rate for IVs using electronic devices.

5. Ordered: 1500 mL RL over 12 h, using an infusion pump

6. Ordered: 1000 mL NS over 12 h, using an infusion pump

7. Ordered: 750 mL NS over 8 h, using an electronic controller set in milliliters per hour

8. Ordered: 20 mEq KCl in 50 mL NS over 30 min, using an electronic rate controller set in milliliters per hour

9. Ordered: 1800 mL 1/2 NS per day by infusion pump

10. Ordered: 250 mL D5W over 3 h by infusion pump

For Exercises 11–16, calculate the flow rate for manually regulated IVs.

11. Ordered: 1000 mL NS over 24 h, tubing is 20 gtt/mL

12. Ordered: 400 mL RL over 8 h, tubing is 10 gtt/mL

13. Ordered: 1500 mL 0.45% S over 12 h, tubing is 15 gtt/mL

14. Ordered: 250 mL D5W over 3 h, tubing is 10 gtt/mL

15. Ordered: 40 mEq KCl in 100 mL NS over 40 min, tubing is 20 gtt/mL

16. Ordered: 500 mL NS over 8 h, tubing is 15 gtt/mL

For Exercises 17–20, look at the drop factor (gtt/mL) on labels A–D to calculate flow rates.

17. Ordered: 3000 mL NS over 24 h, refer to label A.

18. Ordered: 50 mL penicillin IV over 1 h, refer to label B.

19. Ordered: 750 mL 5%D NS over 5 h, refer to label C.

20. Ordered: 100 mL gentamicin over 30 min, refer to label D.

For Exercises 21 and 22, calculate the flow rate in drops per minute.

21. Ordered: 1000 mL D5W over 9 h, using an electronic controller set in drops per minute, tubing calibration is 15 gtt/mL

22. Ordered: 750 mL RL over 8 h by electronic rate controller set in drops per minute, tubing calibration is 15 gtt/mL

For Exercises 23–25, calculate the original flow rate. Then determine if an adjustment is necessary and calculate the adjusted flow rate.

23. Ordered: 375 mL RL over 3 h (10 gtt/mL tubing) After 1 h, 175 mL has infused.

24. Ordered: 1000 mL NS over 8 h (20 gtt/mL tubing) With 5 h remaining, 550 mL of NS remains in the IV bag.

25. Ordered: 500 mL D5W over 4 h (15 gtt/mL tubing) After 2 h, 200 mL has infused.

For Exercises 26 to 30, you must manually check the IV infusion rate. Calculate the rate in drops per minute.

26. Rate controller set at 200 mL/h, tubing 10 gtt/mL

27. Infusion pump set at 125 mL/h, tubing 15 gtt/mL

28. Electronic pump set at 150 mL/h, tubing 15 gtt/mL

29. Pediatric infusion set at 75 mL/h, tubing 60 gtt/mL

30. Rate controller set at 100 mL/h, tubing 10 gtt/mL

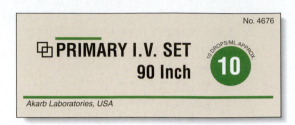

No. 4676

⊞ PRIMARY I.V. SET
90 Inch
10 DROPS/ML APPROX
10

Akarb Laboratories, USA

A

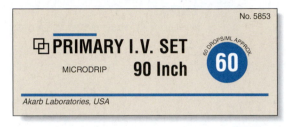

No. 5853

⊞ PRIMARY I.V. SET
MICRODRIP   **90 Inch**
60 DROPS/ML APPROX
60

Akarb Laboratories, USA

B

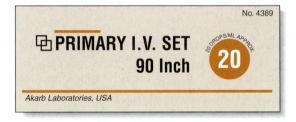

No. 4389

⊞ PRIMARY I.V. SET
90 Inch
20 DROPS/ML APPROX
20

Akarb Laboratories, USA

C

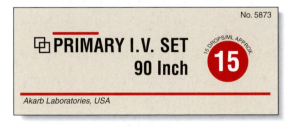

No. 5873

⊞ PRIMARY I.V. SET
90 Inch
15 DROPS/ML APPROX
15

Akarb Laboratories, USA

D

To check your answers, see the Answer section at the end of the book, which starts on page A-1.

15.4 Infusion Time and Volume

An order may call for a certain amount of fluid to infuse at a specific rate, without specifying the duration. In this case you will need to calculate the duration or amount of time the IV will take to infuse, so that you can monitor the IV properly. In other cases, you may know the duration and the flow rate, and you will need to calculate the fluid volume.

Calculating Infusion Time

In the previous section, you calculated the rate of infusion when given the volume and time. Sometimes the infusion rate and volume are given in the order, and you will need to calculate the duration or amount of time the infusion will take to be administered.

RULE 15-8	To calculate infusion time in hours *T*, identify: • *V* (volume) expressed in milliliters. • *F* (flow rate) expressed in milliliters per hour. • Fractional hours expressed in minutes by multiplying by 60. Use the formula $T = \frac{V}{F}$ or dimensional analysis to find *T*, the infusion time in hours.

FORMULA METHOD

EXAMPLE 1

Find the total time to infuse.

Ordered: 1000 mL NS to infuse at a rate of 75 mL/h

CALCULATE

The volume $V = 1000$ mL. The flow rate F is expressed in milliliters per hour, $F = 75$

Substitute the values into the formula $T = \frac{V}{F}$.

$$T = \frac{1000 \text{ mL}}{75 \text{ mL/h}}$$

Cancel the units.

$$T = \frac{1000 \text{ mL}}{75 \text{ mL/h}}$$

$$T = 13.33 \text{ h} = \text{total time to infuse 1000 mL}$$

Note that 0.33 h does not represent 33 minutes. Because there is 60 min in 1 h, you must multiply the fractional hours by 60 to convert it to minutes.

$$0.33 \text{ h} \times 60 \text{ min/h} = 20 \text{ min}$$

The total time to infuse the solution is 13 h 20 min.

EXAMPLE 2

Find the total time to infuse.

Ordered: 750 mL LR to infuse at a rate of 125 mL/h started at 11 p.m.

CALCULATE

The volume $V = 750$ mL. The flow rate F is expressed in milliliters per hour, $F = 125$ mL/h.

Substitute the values into the formula $T = \frac{V}{F}$.

$$T = \frac{750 \text{ mL}}{125 \text{ mL/h}}$$

$$T = 6 \text{ h} = \text{total time to infuse 750 mL}$$

DIMENSIONAL ANALYSIS

EXAMPLE 1

Find the total time to infuse.

Ordered: 1000 mL NS to infuse at a rate of 75 mL/h

CALCULATE

1. Determine the unit of measure for the answer T, and place it as the unknown on the left side of the equation.

   $T\,h =$

2. The first factor is the number of milliliters to be administered on over 1. The second factor is the inverted flow rate. The flow rate is inverted in order to solve for hours (h). Set up the equation.

   $T\,h = \dfrac{1000\text{ mL}}{1} \times \dfrac{1\text{ h}}{75\text{ mL}}$

3. Cancel units on the right side of the equation. The remaining unit of measure on the right side of the equation should match the unknown unit of measure on the left side of the equation.

   $T\,h = \dfrac{1000\text{ m\cancel{L}}}{1} \times \dfrac{1\text{ h}}{75\text{ m\cancel{L}}}$

4. Solve the equation.

   $T\,h = \dfrac{1000\text{ h}}{75}$

   $T = 13.33\text{ h} =$ total time to infuse 1000 mL

Note that 0.33 h does not represent 33 min. Because there is 60 min in 1 h, you must multiply the fractional hours by 60 to convert it to minutes.

   $0.33\text{ h} \times 60\text{ min/h} = 20\text{ min}$

The total time to infuse the solution is 13 h 20 min.

EXAMPLE 2

Find the total time to infuse.

Ordered: 750 mL LR to infuse at a rate of 125 mL/h, started at 11 p.m.

CALCULATE

1. Determine the unit of measure for the answer T, and place it as the unknown on the left side of the equation.

   $T\,h =$

2. The first factor is the number of milliliters to be administered on top V over 1. The second factor is the inverted flow in order to solve for hours.

   $T\,h = \dfrac{750\text{ mL}}{1} \times \dfrac{1\text{ h}}{125\text{ mL}}$

3. Cancel units on the right side of the equation. The remaining unit of measure on the right side of the equation should match the unknown unit of measure on the left side of the equation.

   $T\,h = \dfrac{750\text{ m\cancel{L}}}{1} \times \dfrac{1\text{ h}}{125\text{ m\cancel{L}}}$

4. Solve the equation.

   $T\,h = \dfrac{750\text{ h}}{125}$

   $T = 6\text{ h} =$ total time to infuse 750 mL

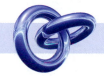 **GO TO . . .** Open the CD-ROM that accompanies your textbook, and select Chapter 15, Infusion Time in Hours (LO 15.4). Review the animation and example problems, then complete the practice problems. Continue to the next section of the book once you have mastered the information presented.

In some cases, you will need to determine the time an infusion will be complete.

RULE 15-9	To calculate the time when an infusion will be completed, you must first know the time the infusion started in military time and the total time in hours and minutes to infuse the solution ordered. Since each day is only 24 hours long, when the sum is greater than 2400 (midnight), you must start a new day by subtracting 2400. This will determine the time of completion, which will be the next calendar day.
Example 1	Determine when the following infusion will be completed.
	Ordered: 1000 mL NS to infuse at a rate of 75 mL/h
	You start the infusion at 7 a.m. on 6/06/12 First determine the start time in military or international time: 7 a.m. = 0700

Learning Link Recall from Chapter 7, Rule 7-2 using the 24-h clock.

Next, calculate the infusion time, $T = \frac{V}{F}$

$$T = \frac{1000 \text{ mL}}{75 \text{ mL/h}}$$

$T = 13.33$ h or 13 h 20 min

Now, add the total amount of time (in hours and minutes) writing the hours followed by minutes. Since the infusion time is 13 h 20 min, add 1320.

0700	time started in military or international time
+1320	total amount of time in hours and minutes
2020	

The infusion will be completed at 2020, which is 8:20 p.m.

Example 2	Determine when the infusion will be completed.
	Ordered: 750 mL LR to infuse at a rate of 125 mL/h, started at 11 p.m. on 8/04/12
	Next, calculate the infusion time, $T = \frac{V}{F}$

$$T = \frac{750 \text{ mL}}{125 \text{ mL/h}}$$

$T = 6$ h

Copyright © 2012 by The McGraw-Hill Companies, Inc.

First determine the start time in military or international time: 11 p.m. = 2300 Add the total amount of time to infuse, which was determined as 6 h, 00 minutes, therefore add 600 to the starting time.

$$
\begin{array}{rl}
2300 & \text{time started in military or international time} \\
+\ 600 & \text{total amount of time of infusion in hours and minutes} \\
\hline
2900 & \text{sum is greater than 2400} \\
-2400 & \text{subtract 2400} \\
\hline
500 &
\end{array}
$$

The infusion will be complete at 0500, or 5:00 a.m., on 8/05/12.

GO TO . . . Open the CD-ROM that accompanies your textbook, and select Chapter 15, Calculating an IV Completion (LO 15.4). Review the animation and example problems, then complete the practice problems. Continue to the next section of the book once you have mastered the information presented.

Calculating Infusion Volume

When infusion rate and infusion time are given in the order, the volume infused over a given period of time can be calculated so that you can monitor the IV properly.

RULE 15-10

To calculate infusion volume:

Use the formula $V = T \times F$ or dimensional analysis to find the infusion volume V in milliliters, where:

- T (time) must be expressed in hours.

- F (flow rate) must be expressed in milliliters per hour.

FORMULA METHOD

EXAMPLE 1 Find the total volume infused in 5 h if the infusion rate is 35 mL/h.

CALCULATE

$T = 5\ \text{h}$

$F = 35\ \text{mL/h}$

Substitute the values into the formula $V = T \times F$.

$V = 5\ \text{h} \times 35\ \text{mL/h}$

$V = 175\ \text{mL} = $ volume that will infuse over 5 h

EXAMPLE 2

Find the total volume infused in 12 h if the infusion rate is 200 mL/h.

CALCULATE

Substitute the values into the formula.

$$V = 12 \text{ h} \times 200 \text{ mL/h}$$

$$V = 2400 \text{ mL} = \text{volume that will infuse over 12 h}$$

DIMENSIONAL ANALYSIS

EXAMPLE 1

Find the total volume infused in 5 h if the infusion rate is 35 mL/h.

CALCULATE

1. Determine the unit of measure for the answer V, and place it as the unknown on the left side of the equation.

   V mL =

2. The first factor is the length of time of the infusion over 1.

   $$\frac{5 \text{ h}}{1}$$

3. Multiply by the first factor by the flow rate. Set up the equation.

   $$V \text{ mL} = \frac{5 \text{ h}}{1} \times \frac{35 \text{ mL}}{1 \text{ h}}$$

4. Cancel units on the right side of the equation. The remaining unit of measure on the right side of the equation should match the unknown unit of measure on the left side of the equation.

   $$V \text{ mL} = \frac{5 \cancel{\text{h}}}{1} \times \frac{35 \text{ mL}}{\cancel{\text{h}}}$$

5. Solve the equation.

   $$V \text{ mL} = 175 \text{ mL to be infused in 5 h}$$

EXAMPLE 2

Find the total volume infused in 12 h if the infusion rate is 200 mL/h.

CALCULATE

1. Determine the unit of measure for the answer (V), and place it as the unknown on the left side of the equation.

   V mL =

2. The first factor is the length of time of the infusion over 1.

   $$\frac{12 \text{ h}}{1}$$

3. Multiply by the first factor by the flow rate.

   $$V \text{ mL} = \frac{12 \text{ h}}{1} \times \frac{200 \text{ mL}}{\text{h}}$$

4. Cancel units on the right side of the equation. The remaining unit of measure on the right side of the equation should match the unknown unit of measure on the left side of the equation.

   $$V \text{ mL} = \frac{12 \cancel{\text{h}}}{1} \times \frac{200 \text{ mL}}{\cancel{\text{h}}}$$

5. Solve the equation.

   $$V \text{ mL} = 2400 \text{ mL to be infused in 12 h}$$

GO TO . . . Open the CD-ROM that accompanies your textbook, and select Chapter 15, Infusion Volume (LO 15.4). Review the animation and example problems, then complete the practice problems. Continue to the next section of the book once you have mastered the information presented.

REVIEW AND PRACTICE

15.4 Infusion Time and Volume

For Exercises 1–5, find the total time to infuse.

1. Ordered: 1000 mL NS at 83 mL/h using an infusion pump

2. Ordered: 500 mL LR at 125 mL/h using microdrip tubing

3. Ordered: 750 mL 1/2 NS at 31 mL/h

4. Ordered: 1000 mL NS at 200 mL/h

5. Ordered 250 mL D5W at 100 mL/h using an infusion pump

For Exercises 6–10, find when the infusion will be completed.

6. Ordered: 1500 mL D5W with 30 mEq KCl/L at a rate of 75 mL/h. You start the infusion at noon.

7. Ordered: 2000 mL NS via infusion pump at 100 mL/h. You start the infusion at 3:30 p.m.

8. Ordered: 750 mL RL at 50 mL/h. You start the IV at 1000

9. Ordered: 250 mL via a microdrip set at 40 mL/h. You start the infusion at 9:45 p.m.

10. Ordered: 500 mL $\frac{1}{2}$ NS at 75 mL/h. The infusion started at 1615.

For Exercises 11–14, find the total volume to administer.

11. 75 mL/h 1/2 NS for 2 h 30 min using a rate controller

12. D5RL set at 100 mL/h for 8 h

13. D5W at 125 mL/h for 12 h using an infusion pump

14. An antibiotic solution infused over 2 h at 75 mL/h

To check your answers, see the Answer section at the end of the book, which starts on page A-1.

15.5 Intermittent IV Infusions

IV medications are sometimes delivered on an intermittent basis. Intermittent medications can be delivered through an IV secondary line or a saline or heparin lock. Intermittent IV infusions are usually delivered through an IV secondary line when the patient is receiving continuous IV therapy. Intermittent IV infusions or IV push medications can also be delivered through a saline or heparin lock when the patient does not require continuous or replacement fluids.

Secondary Lines (Piggyback)

As stated in Section 15.2, a secondary line is used to infuse medications through an intravenous piggyback (IVPB) system. IVPB medications are typically infused via mini-bags of 50, 100, 150, 200, or 250 mL of fluid. (See Figure 15-20.)

Intermittent Peripheral Infusion Devices

You can administer medication to a patient on a regular, though not continuous, schedule by using an *intermittent peripheral infusion device.* These devices are more commonly known as **heparin locks** or **saline locks.** To create a lock, attach an infusion port to an already inserted IV catheter. This port allows you to inject medication directly into the vein by using a syringe or to infuse medication intermittently. (See Figure 15-21.) Physicians' orders will list IV push or bolus for medication that is injected into an IV line or through a saline or heparin lock.

Fluids do not flow continuously through the IV needle or catheter when a lock is used. To prevent blockage of the line, the device must be flushed 2 or 3 times a day or after administering medication. A saline lock is flushed or irrigated with saline. A heparin lock is flushed or irrigated with heparin, an anticoagulant that retards clot formation. The policy of the facility and the device will dictate the amount and concentration of solution to use. Saline or heparin fills the infusion port and IV catheter, preventing blood from entering and becoming trapped. If blood were trapped, a clot would form, blocking the catheter.

Preparing and Calculating Intermittent Infusions

Frequently intermittent medications are already reconstituted and prepared for administration by piggyback or through a heparin or saline lock. The flow rate for prepared medications is calculated in the same manner as regular IV infusions. The amount of fluid may be less (see Figure 15-21) and the amount of time to infuse may be less than an hour, so to calculate the flow rate you will need to change the number of minutes into hours (see Example 1 for Rule 15-5).

In some cases, you will be required to reconstitute and prepare a medication for IV infusion or calculate the amount to administer for an IV push medication.

When intermittent IV infusions are given through a saline or heparin lock, the lock should be irrigated or flushed before and/or after administration. If you meet resistance when flushing a saline or heparin lock, stop the procedure immediately so that you do not force a clot into the bloodstream.

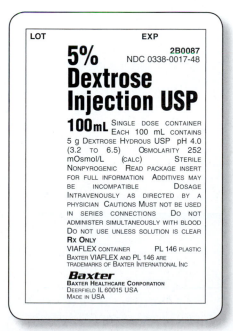

Figure 15-20 A 100 mL bag of IV fluid like this one may be used to mix and administer intermittent IV infusions.

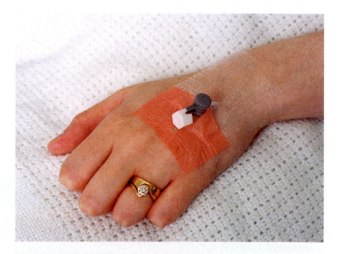

Figure 15-21 Intermittent peripheral infusion device— also called saline lock or heparin lock.

RULE 15-11	When you prepare medication for an intermittent IV infusion:
	• Reconstitute the medication, using the label and package insert.
	• Calculate the amount to administer and the flow rate.
Example	Ordered: Eloxatin® 75 mg in 250 mL D5W IV piggyback over 90 min
	On hand: Eloxatin® (oxaliplatin injection) 5 mg/mL injection 100 mg single-use vial
	According to the package insert, Eloxatin® should be reconstituted with 20 mL of water for injection or 5% dextrose for injection. The dosage strength of the medication will be 100 mg/20 mL. First, calculate the amount of medication to administer using the proportion method, dimensional analysis, or the formula method.

PROPORTION METHOD

EXAMPLE

STEP A: CONVERT
Since the ordered dose and dose on hand are both in milligrams, there is no conversion needed.

STEP B: CALCULATE
Since the dosage ordered is 75 mg, you will calculate the amount to administer using the following information:

D (desired dose) = 75 mg H (dose on hand) = 100 mg Q (dosage unit) = 20 mL

Follow Procedure Checklist 12-1.

1. Fill in the proportion using fractions.

$$\frac{H}{Q} = \frac{D}{A}$$

$$\frac{100 \text{ mg}}{20 \text{ mL}} = \frac{75 \text{ mg}}{A}$$

2. Cancel units.

$$\frac{100 \text{ mg}}{20 \text{ mL}} = \frac{75 \text{ mg}}{A}$$

3. Cross-multiply and solve for the unknown.

$$100 \times A = 20 \text{ mL} \times 75$$

$$A = 20 \text{ mL} \times \frac{75}{100}$$

$$A = 15 \text{ mL}$$

STEP C: THINK . . . IS IT REASONABLE?
Since the ordered dose is $\frac{3}{4}$ of the supply dose, the ordered volume, 15 mL, is reasonable as it is $\frac{3}{4}$ of the supply volume (dosage unit).

DIMENSIONAL ANALYSIS

EXAMPLE

STEP A: CONVERT
Since the ordered dose and dose on hand are both in milligrams, there is no conversion needed.

STEP B: CALCULATE

Since the dosage ordered is 75 mg, you will calculate the amount to administer using the following information:

D (desired dose) = 75 mg H (dose on hand) = 100 mg Q (dosage unit) = 20 mL

Follow Procedure Checklist 12-2.

1. The unit of measure for the amount to administer will be milliliters.

   A mL =

2. Since the unit of measurement for the dosage ordered is the same as that for the dose on hand, this step is unnecessary.

3. The dosage unit is 20 mL. The dose on hand is 100 mg. This is the first factor.

   $$\frac{20 \text{ mL}}{100 \text{ mg}}$$

4. The dosage ordered is 75 mg.

   $$A \text{ mL} = \frac{20 \text{ mL}}{100 \text{ mg}} \times \frac{75 \text{ mg}}{1}$$

5. Cancel units.

   $$A \text{ mL} = \frac{20 \text{ mL}}{100 \text{ m\cancel{g}}} \times \frac{75 \text{ m\cancel{g}}}{1}$$

6. Solve the equation.

   $$A \text{ mL} = \frac{20 \text{ mL}}{100} \times \frac{75}{1}$$

   $$A = 15 \text{ mL}$$

STEP C: THINK . . . IS IT REASONABLE?

Since the ordered dose is $\frac{3}{4}$ of the supply dose, the ordered volume, 15 mL, is reasonable as it is $\frac{3}{4}$ of the supply volume (dosage unit).

FORMULA METHOD

EXAMPLE

STEP A: CONVERT

Since the ordered dose and dose on hand are both in milligrams, there is no conversion needed.

STEP B: CALCULATE

Since the dosage ordered is 75 mg, you will calculate the amount to administer using the following information:

D (desired dose) = 75 mg H (dose on hand) = 100 mg Q (dosage unit) = 20 mL

Follow Procedure Checklist 12-3.

1. The drug is ordered in milligrams, which is the same unit of measure as that for the dose on hand. No conversion is necessary.

2. Fill in the formula.

   $$\frac{D}{H} \times Q = A$$

   $$\frac{75 \text{ mg}}{100 \text{ mg}} \times 20 \text{ mL} = A$$

3. Cancel units.

   $$\frac{75 \text{ m\cancel{g}}}{100 \text{ m\cancel{g}}} \times 20 \text{ mL} = A$$

4. Solve for the unknown.

   $$\frac{75}{100} \times 20 \text{ mL} = A$$

   $$15 \text{ mL} = A$$

Once you have determined the amount of medication to administer you will need to calculate the flow rate.

From the package insert, you determine the reconstituted solutions must be further diluted with an infusion solution of 250 to 500 mL of 5% dextrose injection, USP. The order reads to use 250 mL of D5W; so using a sterile needle and proper aseptic technique, you withdraw 15 mL of the diluted medication and inject it into the 250-mL bag of D5W. Now you have a solution of 75 mg of Eloxatin® in 250 D5W, which you must deliver over 90 min. Add 15 mL medication plus 250 mL of D5W for a total volume of 265 mL. Calculate the flow rate in milliliters per hour, using Rule 15-5.

Note: Check your facility policy. In some cases, 15 mL of IV solution is withdrawn from the IV bag before adding the 15 mL of medication. This will allow the calculation to be based on the original volume of IV fluid, 250 mL.

In this case the volume is expressed in milliliters, and we will use the volume $V = 265$ mL.

DIMENSIONAL ANALYSIS

EXAMPLE

CONVERT
Since time is expressed in minutes, you must first convert 90 min to hours to find T. (In this example we will use the proportion method to convert.)

$$\frac{1\ h}{60\ min} = \frac{x}{90\ min}$$

$$\frac{1\ h}{60\ \cancel{min}} = \frac{x}{90\ \cancel{min}}$$

$$60 \times x = 1\ h \times 90$$

$$x = \frac{1\ h \times 90}{60}$$

$$x = 1.5\ h$$

CALCULATE
We now have the information needed in the proper units.

$$V = 265\ mL \qquad \text{and} \qquad T = 1.5\ h$$

Using the formula $F = \frac{V}{T}$, we find that

$$F = \frac{265\ mL}{1.5\ h}$$

$$F = 177\ mL/h$$

You would set the infusion pump to 177 mL/h.

If an infusion pump is not used, you will need to calculate the drops per minute. For this example we will use standard tubing that is 15 gtt/mL. Always check the drop factor on the tubing packaging.

CALCULATE
Follow Rule 15-6. In this example we will use dimensional analysis to calculate the flow rate in gtt/min (f).

1. Determine the units of measure for the answer (f) and place it as the unknown on one side of the equation.

   f gtt/min =

2. The first factor is the number of mL to be administered on top (V) and the length of time to be administered (T) on the bottom.

   $$\frac{177\ mL}{h}$$

3. Multiply by a second factor to convert the hours to minutes to placing hour in the numerator.

$$\frac{177 \text{ mL}}{\text{h}} \times \frac{1 \text{ h}}{60 \text{ min}}$$

4. Multiply by the drop factor of the tubing being used.

$$f \text{ gtt/min} = \frac{177 \text{ mL}}{\text{h}} \times \frac{1 \text{ h}}{60 \text{ min}} \times \frac{15 \text{ gtt}}{1 \text{ mL}}$$

5. Cancel units on the right side of the equation. The remaining unit of measure on the right side of the equation should match the unknown unit of measure on the left side of the equation.

$$f \text{ gtt/min} = \frac{177 \cancel{\text{ mL}}}{\cancel{\text{h}}} \times \frac{1 \cancel{\text{h}}}{60 \text{ min}} \times \frac{15 \text{ gtt}}{1 \cancel{\text{ mL}}}$$

6. Solve the equation.

$$f = \frac{177 \times 15 \text{ gtt}}{60 \text{ min}}$$

$$f = 44 \text{ gtt/min}$$

GO TO . . . Open the CD-ROM that accompanies your textbook, and select Chapter 15, Intermittent IV Infusion (LO 15.5). Review the animation and example problems, then complete the practice problems. Continue to the next section of the book once you have mastered the information presented.

PATIENT EDUCATION

Instruct patients who are sent home with a saline or heparin lock to care for the device and administer their medications. Teach them about infiltration and phlebitis, and to contact their physician immediately should signs of either problem arise.

1. Avoid getting the injection site wet when bathing or washing hands.
2. Collect all necessary supplies before irrigating the lock or administering medication.
3. Irrigate the device at least twice a day to prevent clotting around the needle or catheter. Develop a schedule.
4. Clean the injection port with an antiseptic swab before injecting the irrigant or prescribed medication.
5. Before administering medication, flush a heparin lock with 1 to 10 mL NS to clear any residual heparin.
6. Attach syringe to the lock, and pull the plunger back. Watch for blood in the chamber to confirm access to the vein. This step must be followed for every injection with the device.
7. After injecting the saline, withdraw the syringe. Inject the medication according to the physician's instructions.
8. After withdrawing the syringe, flush any residual medication from the device.
9. If heparin is used as an irrigant, inject it according to the physician's instructions. Then withdraw the syringe.
10. After completing the injections, swab the port with an antiseptic wipe.

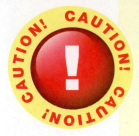

ERROR ALERT!

Select the Correct Strength of Heparin for an Intermittent IV Flush

A heparin flush is a diluted solution of heparin administered to maintain patency of an intravenous line. The concentration of a heparin flush is 10 units/mL or 100 units/mL. Heparin to be administered for therapeutic purposes is available in 1,000 units/ mL (see Figure 15-24, Label A, below), 5,000 units/mL and 10,000 units/mL. If the medication technician administered 1 mL of the 10,000:1 solution instead of the 100:1 solution, the patient would receive 100 times the dose ordered! Serious, sometimes fatal, errors have occurred as a result of administering the wrong concentration of heparin.

REVIEW AND PRACTICE

15.5 Intermittent IV Infusions

For Exercises 1 to 4, refer to labels A and B.

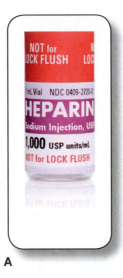

A

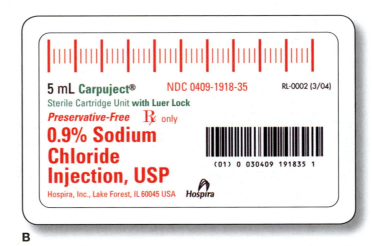

B

Figure 15-24 Heparin injection solution and saline lock flush.

1. Which would be used to flush a saline lock?

2. Which would be used to flush a heparin lock?

3. Standing order reads 3 mL saline lock flush q8h. Calculate the amount to administer.

4. Standing order reads Heparin 5,000 units IV q12h. Calculate the amount to administer.

For Exercises 5–10, determine the amount to administer and calculate the flow rate in milliliters per hour and drops per minute.
Ordered: Gemzar® 150 mg in 500 mL NS over 2 h
On hand: Refer to IV tubing packaging C, label D, and package insert E (Figure 15-25).

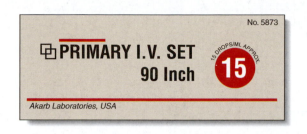

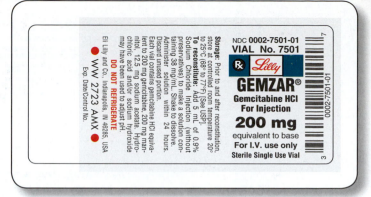

C

D

Gemzar® may be administered on an outpatient basis.

Instructions for Use/Handling—The recommended diluent for reconstitution of Gemzar® is 0.9% Sodium Chloride Injection without preservatives. Due to solubility considerations, the maximum concentration for Gemzar® upon reconstitution is 40 mg/mL. Reconstitution at concentrations greater than 40 mg/mL may result in incomplete dissolution, and should be avoided.

To reconstitute, add 5 mL of 0.9% Sodium Chloride Injection to the 200-mg vial or 25 mL of 0.9% Sodium Chloride Injection to the 1-g vial. Shake to dissolve. These dilutions each yield a gemcitabine concentration of 38 mg/mL which includes accounting for the displacement volume of the lyophilized powder (0.26 mL for the 200-mg vial or 1.3 mL for the 1-g vial). The total volume upon reconstitution will be 5.26 mL or 26.3 mL, respectively. Complete withdrawal of the vial contents will provide 200 mg or 1 g of gemcitabine, respectively. The appropriate amount of drug may be administered as prepared or further diluted with 0.9% Sodium Chloride Injection to concentrations as low as 0.1 mg/mL.

Reconstituted Gemzar® is a clear, colorless to light straw-colored solution. After reconstitution with 0.9% Sodium Chloride Injection, the pH of the resulting solution lies in the range of 2.7 to 3.3. The solution should be inspected visually for particulate matter and discoloration, prior to administration, whenever solution or container permit. If particulate matter or discoloration is found, do not administer.

When prepared as directed, Gemzar® solutions are stable for 24 hours at controlled room temperature 20° to 25°C (68° to 77°F) [*See* USP]. Discard unused portion. Solutions of reconstituted Gemzar® should not be refrigerated, as crystallization may occur.

The compatibility of Gemzar® with other drugs has not been studied. No incompatibilities have been observed with infusion bottles or polyvinyl chloride bags and administration sets.

E

Figure 15-25   IV tubing packaging, Gemzar® label, and package insert.

5. Amount to administer: _____

6. Flow rate in milliliters per hour: _____

7. Flow rate in drops per minute: _____

Ordered: Doxycycline 75 mg IVPB in 100 mL of D5W over 1 hour

On hand: Refer to label F, package insert G, and IV tubing packaging H (Figure 15-26 on the next page).

8. Amount to administer: _____

9. Flow rate in milliliters per hour: _____

10. Flow rate in drops per minute: _____

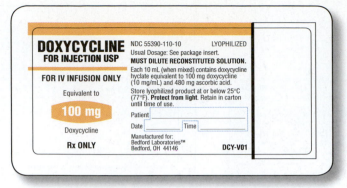

F

Preparation of Solution: To prepare a solution containing 10 mg/mL, the contents of the vial should be reconstituted with 10 mL of Sterile Water for Injection, or any of the ten intravenous infusion solutions listed below. Each 100 mg of doxycycline (i.e., withdraw entire solution from the 100 mg vial) is further diluted with 100 to 1000 mL of the intravenous solutions listed below:

1. 0.9% Sodium Chloride Injection
2. 5% Dextrose Injection
3. Ringer's Injection
4. Invert Sugar, 10% in Water
5. Lactated Ringer's Injection
6. Dextrose 5% in Lactated Ringer's
7. Normosol-M® in D5-W (Abbott)
8. Normosol-R® in D5-W (Abbott)
9. Plasma-Lyte® 56 in 5% Dextrose (Travenol)
10. Plasma-Lyte® 148 in 5% Dextrose (Travenol)

This will result in desired concentrations of 0.1 to 1 mg/mL. Concentrations lower than 0.1 mg/mL or higher than 1 mg/mL are not recommended.

G

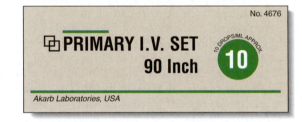

H

Figure 15-26 Doxycycline label, package insert, and IV tubing package.

Excerpt from Doxycycline Package Insert found at www.bedfordlabs.com

To check your answers, see the Answer section at the end of the book, which starts on page A-1.

CHAPTER 15 SUMMARY

Copyright © 2012 by The McGraw-Hill Companies, Inc.

LEARNING OUTCOME	KEY POINTS
15.1 Identify components and concentrations of IV solutions. Pages 408–414	D = Dextrose; W = Water D5W = Dextrose 5% in Water Percent = grams/100 mL, therefore 1000 mL D5W contains 50 g Dextrose calculated: $1 \text{ g}/100 \text{ mL} = x/1000 \text{ mL}$ NS = Normal saline (0.9% NaCl, i.e. 0.9 g/100 mL) $\frac{1}{2}$ NS = 0.45% NS (0.45 g/100 mL)

LEARNING OUTCOME	KEY POINTS
	$\frac{1}{4}$ NS = 0.225% NS (0.225 g/100 mL) LR or RL = Lactated Ringers or Ringer's lactate IV solutions are ordered for: Replacement fluids—replace fluids and electrolytes lost due to hemorrhage, illness, surgery Maintenance fluids—maintain normal fluid and electrolyte balance KVO fluids—fluids delivered at a very slow rate to keep vein open Therapeutic fluids—deliver medication
15.2 Distinguish basic types of IV equipment. Pages 414–420	Primary line—Larger IV bag (e.g., 500 mL or 1000 mL) connected to long tubing with a drip chamber (to count drops), roller clamp (to adjust the flow rate), and injection ports (to inject medications, fluids, or attach a secondary line) Secondary line—Smaller IV Bag (e.g. 250 mL) or mini-bag (e.g., 50 mL, 100 mL) connected to shorter tubing with similar tubing components as primary line; aka IVPB or intravenous piggyback because it is hung higher than the primary line in order to infuse or piggyback an intermittent infusion into the primary line Rate controller—sensor applied to the drip chamber to measure drops or volume that is delivered Infusion pump—device that delivers a set volume per minute or per hour; equipped with alarm to indicate tubing blockage or empty bag Syringe pump—infusion device to which a syringe is attached for delivery of intravenous medications PCA device—pump in which the patient presses a button to deliver pain medication (patient-controlled analgesia) within preset limits per order of authorized prescriber Volume control sets—a burette chamber (calibrated in 1 mL increments) with an injection port to which up to 150 mL fluid and medications can be added Peripheral line—IV access through a peripheral vein Central line—IV access through a large major vessel, such as the jugular vein or femoral vein PICC line—peripherally inserted (central catheter) line threaded into a central vein Port-a-Cath—device implanted under the skin connected to a central vein used for long-term intermittent medication administration
15.3 Calculate IV flow rates. Pages 421–430	mL/h (F) Calculate 250 mL over 2 hours in mL/h: **Formula method:** Flow rate $(F) = \dfrac{\text{Volume (mL)}}{\text{Time (hours)}};\ \dfrac{250\text{ mL}}{2\text{ h}} = 125\text{ mL/h}$ Calculate 100 mL over 45 minutes in mL/h: **Formula method:** convert 45 min to 0.75 h using the proportion method $\left(\dfrac{60\text{ min}}{1\text{ h}} = \dfrac{45\text{ min}}{x}\right)$, then apply the formula $F = \dfrac{V}{T}$. $F = \dfrac{100\text{ mL}}{0.75\text{ h}} = 133.33$ or 133 mL/h **Dimensional Analysis:** $\dfrac{F\text{ mL}}{\cancel{h}} = \dfrac{100\text{ mL}}{45\ \cancel{\text{min}}} \times \dfrac{60\ \cancel{\text{min}}}{1\ \cancel{h}};$ cancel units: $\dfrac{100}{3} \times \dfrac{4}{1} = \dfrac{400}{3} = 133.33$ or 133 mL/h

Copyright © 2012 by The McGraw-Hill Companies, Inc.

LEARNING OUTCOME	KEY POINTS
	gtt/min (f): Calculate 125 mL/h using a drop factor (calibration) of 15 gtt/mL **Formula method:** $f\,(\text{gtt/min}) = \dfrac{F\,(\text{mL/h}) \times C}{60\,\text{min/h}};$ $f = \dfrac{(125\,\text{mL/h} \times 15\,\text{gtt/mL})}{60\,\text{min/h}};$ cancel units: $f = \dfrac{125}{4} = 31.25$ or 31 gtt/min **Dimensional Analysis:** $f\,\text{gtt/min} = F \times 1\,\text{h}/60\,\text{min} \times C$ or $\dfrac{125\,\text{mL}}{1\,\text{h}} \times \dfrac{1\,\text{h}}{60\,\text{min}} \times \dfrac{15\,\text{gtt}}{1\,\text{mL}};$ $f = \dfrac{125}{4} = 31.25$ or 31 gtt/min IV Rate Adjustment $= \dfrac{\text{Volume left}}{\text{Time left}}$
15.4 Calculate infusion time and volume. Pages 430–436	Time: ▶ **Formula Method:** Time $= \dfrac{\text{Volume (mL)}}{F\,(\text{mL/h})};$ convert fractional hours to minutes by multiplying by 60 Calculate time to infuse 500 mL at 60 mL/h: $T = \dfrac{500\,\text{mL}}{60\,\text{mL/h}} = 8.33$ h or 8 h, 20 min (0.33 h × 60 min/h = 20 min) ▶ **Dimensional Analysis:** $T\,\text{h} = \dfrac{500\,\text{mL}}{1\,\text{h}} \times \dfrac{1\,\text{h}}{60\,\text{mL}}$ $= \dfrac{500}{60} = 8.33$ h or 8 h, 20 min Volume: ▶ **Formula Method:** $V = T \times F$ Calculate the volume infused in 2 hours 30 minutes for IV running at 150 mL/h $V = 2.5\,\text{h} \times 150\,\text{mL/h} = 375\,\text{mL}$ ▶ **Dimensional Analysis:** $V\,\text{mL} = \dfrac{2.5\,\text{h}}{1} \times \dfrac{150\,\text{mL}}{\text{h}} = 375\,\text{mL/h}$

15.5 Perform calculations for intermittent IV infusions.
Pages 436–444
	Saline lock—a port through which a medication can be injected directly into the vein or to which an intermittent infusion can be attached; flushed intermittently with saline to maintain patency
	Heparin lock—similar to a saline lock except it is flushed intermittently with low-dose heparin to maintain patency
	Calculations:
	1. Use formula method, proportion method or dimensional analysis (from Parenteral Dosages Chapter) to determine amount to administer after medication is reconstituted.
	2. Use formula method or dimensional analysis to calculate flow rate:
	  a. First convert minutes to hours, if necessary, then apply Formula:
	    • To calculate mL/h: $F = V/T$
	    • To calculate gtt/min: $f = \dfrac{F \times C}{60\,\text{min/h}}$
	  b. Dimensional Analysis:
	    • To calculate mL/h: $F = \dfrac{\text{mL}}{1\,\text{min}} \times \dfrac{60\,\text{min}}{1\,\text{h}}$
	    • To calculate gtt/min: $f = \dfrac{\text{mL}}{1\,\text{h}} \times \dfrac{1\,\text{h}}{60\,\text{min}} \times \dfrac{C\,\text{gtt}}{1\,\text{min}}$

HOMEWORK ASSIGNMENT

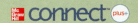

Answer the following questions.

1. List the four functional categories of IV solutions. (LO 15.1)

2. In the IV label abbreviation D5W, which component identifies the concentration level? (LO 15.1)

3. Define the terms isotonic, hypertonic, and hypotonic. (LO 15.1)

4. Before combining any medication with an IV solution, what must be verified first? (LO 15.1)

5. List three parts of a primary IV line. (LO 15.2)

6. List four types of electronic infusion devices. (LO 15.2)

7. Under what circumstances would a patient most likely need central line IV therapy? (LO 15.2)

8. What is the drop factor for microdrip tubing? (LO 15.2)

9. How is the flow rate measured when an infusion pump is used? (LO 15.2)

10. Name and explain two types of intermittent IV infusion methods. (LO 15.2)

11. If the order is 1000 mL to infuse over 12 hours (10 gtt/mL tubing), calculate the flow rate. (LO 15.3)

12. If the order is 50 mL to infuse over 90 minutes (microdrip tubing), calculate the flow rate. (LO 15.3)

13. If the order is 500 mL to infuse at 150 mL/hour (10 gtt/mL tubing), how long will it take to infuse? (LO 15.3)

14. If an IV is infusing at 20 gtt/minute with a drop factor (calibration) of 20 gtt/mL and the volume of the IV bag is 500 mL, how many hours will it take to infuse? (LO 15.4)

15. An IV of 500 mL is begun at 11 a.m. and the flow rate is 15 gtt/minute (10 gtt/mL tubing). At what time will the infusion be complete? (LO 15.4)

16. If the order is 250 mL over 3 hours, what mL/hour setting will you use on an infusion pump? (LO 15.4)

17. If the order is 150 mL over 30 minutes, how many mL/hour will you set on the infusion pump? (LO 15.4)

18. What is the total volume to be infused for an IV infusing at 80 mL/hours for 6 hours? (LO 15.4)

19. At the end of 4 hours, what is the total volume infused for an IV infusing at 20 drops per minute (10 gtt/mL tubing)? (LO 15.4)

20. If the order is 500 mL over 4 hours (10 gtt/mL tubing), after one hour there should be how much remaining in the bag? (LO 15.4)

CHECK UP

For Exercises 1–7, match the term to its description. Write the answer in the space provided. (LO 15.1, 15.2)

_____	**1.** Roller clamp	**a.**	type of solution that causes fluid to move out of the cell
_____	**2.** KVO fluids	**b.**	type of fluid given to a patient who is dehydrated
_____	**3.** Hypertonic	**c.**	the patient is in charge of delivering his or her own pain medications
_____	**4.** Phlebitis	**d.**	provide access to the vascular system for emergency situations
_____	**5.** PCA	**e.**	redness, swelling, and pain at an IV site
_____	**6.** Infusion pump	**f.**	applies pressure to administer an IV fluid
_____	**7.** Hypotonic	**g.**	used to control the rate of an IV infusion

For Exercises 8–13, calculate the flow rate for orders to be administered by an infusion pump. (LO 15.3)

8. 3000 mL D5W IV q24h

9. 500 mL LR IV q8h

10. 1200 mL 1/2 NS IV q12h

11. 250 mL NS IV q4h

12. 1 g Claforan in 100 mL D5W IV over 90 min

13. 500 mg ampicillin in 50 mL D5W IV over 30 min

For Exercises 14–19, find the flow rate for the orders, rounded to the nearest drop/min. (LO 15.3)

14. 2200 mL IV RL q24h (15 gtt/mL tubing)

15. 300 mL IV NS q8h (10 gtt/mL tubing)

16. 1000 mL IV D5W q6h (15 gtt/mL tubing)

17. 1800 mL IV D5/$\frac{1}{2}$ NS q12h (20 gtt/mL tubing)

18. 1500 mL IV $\frac{1}{3}$ NS q8h (10 gtt/mL tubing)

19. 300 mL D5LR IV q6h (microdrip tubing)

For Exercises 20–22, calculate the original flow rate. Then determine if an adjustment is necessary and calculate the adjusted flow rate. Determine if the rate can be adjusted safely. (LO 15.3)

20. Ordered: 1000 mL RL over 8 h (15 gtt/mL tubing)
After 2 h, 125 mL has infused.

21. Ordered: 2500 mL NS over 24 h (10 gtt/mL tubing)
After 3 h, 200 mL has infused.

22. Ordered 500 mL $\frac{1}{2}$ NS over 8 h (60 gtt/mL tubing)
After 2 h, 450 mL is remaining in the IV bag.

For Exercises 23–26, find the total time to infuse. (LO 15.4)

23. Ordered: 1000 mL D5/0.45% NS at 125 mL/h via infusion pump

24. Ordered: 800 mL $\frac{1}{4}$ NS at 50 mL/h via rate controller

25. Ordered: 600 mL LR IV at 25 mL/h

26. Ordered: 1200 mL D5/NS IV at 70 mL/h

For Exercises 27–30, find when the infusion will be completed. (LO 15.4)

27. 800 mL via infusion pump at 90 mL/h, starting at 0820

28. 1000 mL at 125 mL/h, starting at 1 p.m.

29. 500 mL at 175 mL/h, starting at 2230

30. 750 mL at 35 mL/h, starting at 4 p.m.

For Exercises 31–34, find the total volume to administer. (LO 15.4)

31. $\frac{1}{4}$ NS at 125 mL/h over 5 h 30 min via infusion pump

32. RL at 25 mL/h over 12 h

33. NS at 125 mL/h over 7 h 30 min

34. D5W at 80 mL/h over 8 h 20 min

CRITICAL THINKING APPLICATION

The physician has ordered an adult patient with pneumonia to have clindamycin 500 mg IV q8h. On hand: See clindamycin label A and package insert B on next page. (LO 15.5)

1. How would you prepare the medication?

2. Calculate the amount to administer.

3. Is this the correct dose for treatment of pneumonia? Why or why not?

4. What fluid should not be used as a diluent for children?

5. The medication cannot be administered immediately because the patient is having a diagnostic test. What should you do?

6. Calculate the flow rate of the infusion.

A

CLINDAMYCIN PHOSPHATE INJECTION USP

Usual adult and adolescent dose

Antibacterial
Intramuscular or intravenous, 300 to 600 mg (base) every six to eight hours; or 900 mg every eight hours.[13]

[Babesiosis (treatment)][1]
Intravenous, 300 to 600 mg clindamycin (base) four times a day with concurrent oral administration of 650 mg of quinine, three or four times a day for seven to ten days.[49] [50]

[Pneumonia, *Pneumocystis carinii* (treatment)][1]
Intravenous, 2400 to 2700 mg (base) per day in divided doses in combination with 15 to 30 mg of primaquine daily.[35] [36] [53]

[Toxoplasmosis, central nervous system (CNS) (treatment)][1]
Intravenous, 1200 to 4800 mg (base) per day in divided doses in combination with 50 to 100 mg of pyrimethamine daily.[31] [32] [33] [34] [52] [55] [56]

Usual adult prescribing limits
Up to 2.7 grams (base) daily.

Note: Doses up to 4.8 grams daily have been used. However, some medical experts recommend a maximum dose of 2.7 grams daily.

Preparation of dosage form:
To prepare initial dilution for intravenous use, each dose must be diluted as follows (it must not be administered undiluted as a bolus):

Dose (mg)	Diluent (mL)	Duration of administration (min)
300	50	10
600	100	20
900	100	30

Caution: Products containing benzyl alcohol are not recommended for use in neonates. A fatal toxic syndrome consisting of metabolic acidosis, CNS depression, respiratory problems, renal failure, hypotension, and possibly seizures and intracranial hemorrhages has been associated with this use.

Stability:
Clindamycin phosphate retains its potency for 24 hours at room temperature in intravenous infusions containing sodium chloride, dextrose, potassium, vitamin B complex, cephalothin, kanamycin, gentamicin, penicillin, or carbenicillin.[13]

Incompatibilities:
Clindamycin phosphate is physically incompatible with ampicillin, phenytoin sodium, barbiturates, aminophylline, calcium gluconate, and magnesium sulfate.[13]

*Excerpt from package insert for Clindamycin made by Abraxis

B

CASE STUDY

A patient has a PCA pump with morphine sulfate 50 mg in 500 mL D5W. Hospital policy requires you to document the dose of morphine administered during your shift. When you came on duty, the pump showed that 227 mL had infused. At the end of your shift the pump shows that 272 mL has infused. How much morphine did the patient receive during your shift? (LO 15.3)

INTERNET ACTIVITY

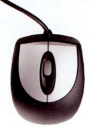

You are applying for a new job that will require you to work with IV fluids exclusively. To prepare for the position, you want to learn more about the types of fluids and when and how they are used. Additionally you would like to become familiar with IV equipment made by various companies. Research the Internet and learn more about fluids and IV equipment. You may want to make yourself a chart or table with pictures to use as a reference tool.

To check you answers, see the Answer section at the end of the book, which starts on page A-1.

GO TO . . . Open the CD-ROM that accompanies your textbook, and complete a final review of the learning outcomes, practice problems, games, slideshow, and activities presented for this chapter. For a final evaluation, take the chapter test and email or print your results for your instructor. A score of 95 percent or above indicates mastery of the chapter concepts.

UNIT FOUR ASSESSMENT

For questions 1–5 answer the following questions pertaining to enteral medication administration equipment.

1. 30 milliliters (mL) equals how many cubic centimeters (cc)?

2. The best equipment for administering 2.5 mL of fluid, enterally is a:
   a. medicine cup   b. hypodermic syringe   c. tablespoon   d. oral syringe

3. At which part of the meniscus is liquid measured in a measuring cup?

4. An order calls for 2 teaspoons of a liquid oral medication. The only available medicine cup is calibrated in mL. How many mL will you pour into the medicine cup?

5. If a medicine is a thick liquid, which may not flow through a dropper, what device might be a good choice for administering this liquid to a child?

For questions 6–10 answer the following questions pertaining to parenteral medication administration equipment.

6. What would be the best syringe to administer 0.25 mL of fluid IM?

7. What would be the best syringe to administer 1.5 mL of fluid IM?

8. What would be the best syringe to administer 8 mL of fluid IV?

9. What would be the best syringe to administer 50 units of U-100 insulin?

10. What would be the best syringe to administer 0.1 mL of fluid ID?

Calculate one dose of the following medication orders.

11. Ordered: levothyroxine 75 mcg PO daily
    On hand: levothyroxine 0.15 mg tablets
    Administer: _____ tablet(s)

12. Ordered: cefadroxil 1 g PO q6h
    On hand: cefadroxil 500 mg tablets
    Administer: _____ tablet(s)

13. Ordered: cefprozil 1 g PO daily
    On hand: cefprozil 250 mg/5 mL
    Administer: _____ tsp

14. Ordered: potassium chloride 60 mEq PO daily
    On hand: potassium chloride 20 mEq/15 mL
    Administer: _____ oz

15. Ordered: azithromycin 0.5 g PO daily
    On hand: azithromycin 200 mg/5 mL
    Administer: _____ mL

16. Determine the concentration of dextrose and/or sodium chloride in each of the following intravenous solutions:
    a. D5NS   b. D10W   c. D5 $\frac{1}{2}$ NS   d. D5 $\frac{1}{4}$ NS

17. Match the IV equipment to the most appropriate description:
    a. Primary line _____   i. The calibration is 60 gtt/mL.
    b. Central line _____   ii. This device is surgically implanted under the skin.
    c. Secondary line _____   iii. This tubing has injection ports for additional lines.
    d. Port-a-Cath _____   iv. This device can be peripherally inserted and provides direct access to major veins.
    e. Microdrip tubing _____   v. Intravenous piggyback (IVPB) medications are given through this device.

18. Calculate the following IV flow rates:
    a. Ordered: 3000 mL D5NS over 24 h using an infusion pump
       Rate: _____ mL/h
    b. Ordered: 50 mL D5W over 45 min using an infusion pump
       Rate: _____ mL/h
    c. Ordered: 1000 mL NS over 10 h; tubing is 15 gtt/mL
       Rate: _____ gtt/min
    d. Ordered: 80 mg tobramycin in 100 mL D5W over 20 min
       Rate: _____ mL/h
    e. Ordered: 1000 mL D5 ½ NS to run at 85 mL/h; tubing is 10 gtt/mL
       Rate: _____ gtt/min

19. Calculate the IV infusion time or volume as indicated:
    a. Ordered: 1000 mL NS at 125 mL/h started at 1500
       At what time will the IV finish? _____
    b. Ordered: D5W at 50 mL/h started at 0730 and finished at 1230
       What volume infused? _____
    c. Ordered: 1000 mL D5 $\frac{1}{2}$ NS at 100 mL/h started at 2145
       At what time will the IV finish? _____
    d. Ordered: $\frac{1}{2}$ NS at 80 mL/h infused for 3 h 45 min
       What volume infused? _____

20. Determine the IV flow rate for the following intermittent infusion orders:
    a. Ordered: ampicillin 125 mg in 50 mL D5W to be administered over 20 min
       Rate: _____ mL/h
    b. Ordered: cefazolin 1 g in 100 mL NS to be administered over 40 min
       Rate: _____ mL/h
    c. Ordered: gentamicin 35 mg in 25 mL D5W to be administered over 15 min; tubing is 60 gtt/mL
       Rate: _____ gtt/min
    d. Ordered: oxacillin sodium 500 mg in 50 mL NS to be administered over 10 min
       Rate: _____ mL/h

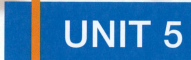

UNIT 5

Calculations Used in Specialty Areas

16

CHAPTER

Preparation of Noninjectable Solutions

Everything should be made as simple as possible, but not one bit simpler.

—ALBERT EINSTEIN

Learning Outcomes

When you have completed Chapter 16, you will be able to:

16.1 Write a recipe for preparing a percent solution or solid.

16.2 Calculate the amount of solute and solvent needed to prepare a desired strength for:

a. Topical solutions/irrigants

b. Enteral feedings

KEY TERMS

Diluent
qsad
Solute
Solution
Solvent
Universal solvent

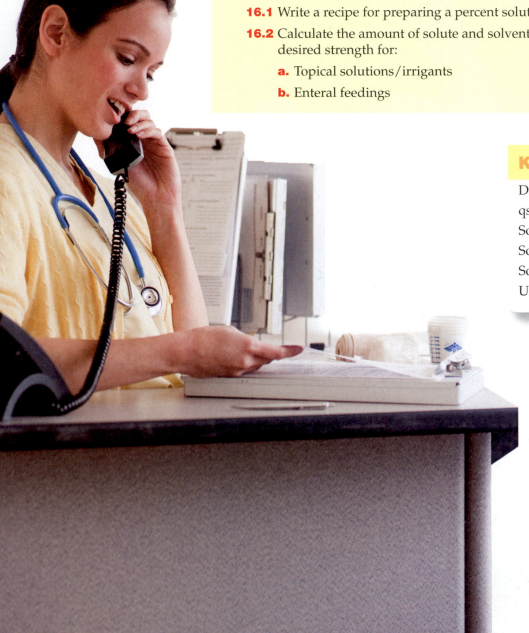

INTRODUCTION

Sometimes it is necessary to prepare nutritional formulas from a powder or to dilute nutritional formulas or irrigating solutions to make a weaker solution. Since it is often the responsibility of the nurse or other healthcare professionals to reconstitute non-injectable solutions, this chapter will review concepts and calculations related to nutritional formulas and topical irrigants.

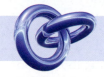

LEARNING LINK Recall from Chapter 14 that reconstitution is the process of mixing and diluting solutions.

16.1 Preparation of Solutions

Solutions are liquid mixtures containing two or more different chemicals. The liquid that is used to dissolve the other chemicals is called the **solvent,** while the chemicals dissolved in the solvent are called **solutes.** The most commonly used solvent is water, which is sometimes referred to as the **universal solvent.** Another name for solvent is **diluent,** which is a substance used to dilute. An example of a solution is normal saline, which contains 0.9 g of sodium chloride (table salt) in every 100 mL of solution. In this example, sodium chloride is the solute, and water is used as the solvent (diluent).

The manufacturer prepares most of the solutions used in healthcare. Some common examples are injections, eye drops, and cough syrups. It is occasionally necessary to prepare a solution from a powder or to dilute a solution that is more concentrated than what is needed. To do this, you will need to know how concentrations of solutions are expressed.

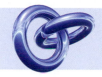

LEARNING LINK Recall from Chapter 15 that percent on a solution label means the number of grams per 100 mL, for example dextrose 5% IV solution contains 5 grams of dextrose per 100 mL of IV solution.

Percent Concentration

One of the most common ways of expressing the concentration is as a percent. Remember that *percent* means *per hundred.* When a concentration is expressed as a percent, it tells you how much of the solute is found in every 100 mL of the solution. When the solute is a solid or semisolid, the percent concentration tells you how many grams of the solute are contained in every 100 mL of the solution.

RULE 16-1	For fluid mixtures prepared with a dry medication, the percent strength represents the number of grams of the medication contained in 100 mL of the mixture.
	For fluid mixtures prepared with a liquid medication, the percent strength represents the number of milliliters of medication contained in 100 mL of the mixture.
Example 1	Determine the amount of hydrocortisone powder in 300 mL of 2% hydrocortisone lotion.
	Each percent represents 1 gram (g) of hydrocortisone per 100 mL of lotion. A 2% hydrocortisone lotion will contain 2 g of hydrocortisone powder in every 100 mL.
	Therefore, 300 mL of the lotion will contain 3 times as much, or 6 g, of hydrocortisone powder.
Example 2	Determine the amount of lidocaine in a 2% lidocaine solution.
	A 2% lidocaine solution contains 2 g of lidocaine in every 100 mL of solution. In other words, 100 mL of 2% lidocaine solution = 2 g lidocaine mixed with enough solvent to make a total of 100 mL.

Example 3	Determine the amount of isopropyl alcohol in 100 mL of a 70% isopropyl alcohol solution. The percent strength is 70. A 70% isopropyl alcohol solution has 70 mL of isopropyl alcohol in every 100 mL of solution. In this case, 100 mL of 70% isopropyl alcohol = 70 mL isopropyl alcohol mixed with enough solvent to make a total of 100 mL.

GO TO . . . Open the CD-ROM that accompanies your textbook, and select Chapter 16, Percent Concentration for Solutions (LO 16.1). Review the animation and example problems, then complete the practice problems. Continue to the next section of the book once you have mastered the information presented

When the solute is a solid and the solvent is a solid, the percent concentration tells you how many grams of the solute are contained in 100 g of the product.

RULE 16-2	For solid or semisolid mixtures prepared with a dry medication, the percent strength represents the number of grams of the medication contained in 100 g of the mixture.
	For solid or semisolid mixtures prepared with a liquid medication, the percent strength represents the number of milliliters of medication contained in 100 g of the mixture.
Example 1	Determine the amount of hydrocortisone in 2% hydrocortisone ointment.
	Every 100 g of ointment will contain 2 g of hydrocortisone. If the preparation were being compounded in the pharmacy, 2 g of hydrocortisone would be incorporated in 98 g of petroleum jelly.
Example 2	Determine the amount of hydrocortisone powder in 50 g of a 1% hydrocortisone ointment.
	Each percent represents 1 g of hydrocortisone per 100 g of ointment. A 1% hydrocortisone ointment will contain 1 g of hydrocortisone powder in every 100 g.
	Therefore, 50 g of the ointment will contain $\frac{1}{2}$ as much, or 0.5 g of hydrocortisone powder.

GO TO . . . Open the CD-ROM that accompanies your textbook, and select Chapter 16, Percent Concentration for Solids (LO 16.1). Review the animation and example problems, then complete the practice problems. Continue to the next section of the book once you have mastered the information presented

Preparing Percent Solutions and Solids

Note that in the above examples we stated that the solution contained *enough solvent to make a total of 100 mL*. In Rule 16.1, Example 2 , the 2% lidocaine solution, you may think that you would need 100 mL of solvent. This, however, would not take into account the volume occupied by the lidocaine. To prepare a solution, you would first measure the solute and then add a *sufficient quantity of solvent to bring the total to the desired volume.*

RULE 16-3	When preparing a solution, first measure the solute, then add a sufficient quantity of solvent to bring the total to the desired volume.
Example 1	A "recipe" for preparing 100 mL of 2% lidocaine solution would look like this:

2% Lidocaine Solution

Lidocaine	2 g
Water	qsad 100 mL

(The abbreviation **qsad or QSAD** is taken from a Latin phrase meaning "a sufficient quantity to adjust the dimensions to . . . .") In this case, you are adding enough water to make the final volume 100 mL. When you are preparing a liquid solution, the diluents should be added up to the desired volume.

In this example you were asked how to prepare 100 mL of the solutions, and no calculations were needed. For a percent solution prepared from a solid solute, the percent strength is equal to the number of grams of solute contained in 100 mL of the solution.

Example 2	Write a recipe for preparing 100 g of 10% zinc oxide from zinc oxide powder and petroleum jelly.

10% Zinc Oxide

Zinc oxide	10 g
Petroleum jelly	90 g

In this example a solid (zinc oxide) is being added to another solid (an ointment base). Once you determine the number of grams for the solute, you must subtract from the total number of grams to create the recipe to compound this ointment. You do not use the expression *qsad* when preparing solid mixtures.

To this point, you have been shown how to make 100 mL of solution. You can calculate a different quantity of solution by applying the proportion method or dimensional analysis. The steps for each of these methods were introduced in chapter 6 through Procedure Checklists 6-1 and 6-2. For the following examples we will use these procedure checklists and the ABC steps of dosage calculations to calculate quantities for a percent solid or solution.

PROPORTION METHOD

Calculating Quantities for a Percent Solution or Solid by Proportion Method using Procedure Checklist 6-1

1. Write a conversion factor (ratio or fraction) with the units needed in the answer in the numerator (before the colon) and the units you are converting from in the denominator (after the colon).

2. Write a factor (ratio or fraction) with the unknown, x, in the numerator and the number that you need to convert in the denominator.

3. Set up the two ratios (fractions) as a proportion.

4. Cancel units.

5. Cross-multiply, then solve for the unknown value.

EXAMPLE   Write out a recipe for preparing 250 mL of 0.9% sodium chloride.

STEP A: CONVERT

This step is not applicable.

STEP B: CALCULATE

Follow the Procedure Checklist 6-1 using fractions.

1. The percent concentration tells us that 100 mL solution contains 0.9 g NaCl. We need to calculate how many grams of NaCl are needed to prepare 250 mL of solution. Since we are calculating grams, our conversion factor first ratio will be written.

$$\frac{0.9\ g}{100\ mL}$$

2. The other ratio for our proportion has the unknown, x, for a numerator and 250 mL solution as the denominator:

$$\frac{x}{250\ mL}$$

3. Setting up the two ratios as a proportion gives us the following equation:

$$\frac{x}{250\ mL} = \frac{0.9\ g}{100\ mL}$$

4. Cancel units:

$$\frac{x}{250\ \cancel{mL}} = \frac{0.9\ g}{100\ \cancel{mL}}$$

5. Cross-multiply to solve for the unknown:

$$100x = 0.9 \times \frac{250}{100}$$

$$x = 2.25\ g\ NaCl$$

STEP C: THINK! . . . IS IT REASONABLE?

Since there is 0.9 g of NaCl in 100 mL, there should be more than 2 times that amount in 250 mL, so, yes, 2.25 g is a reasonable answer.

DIMENSIONAL ANALYSIS METHOD

Calculating Quantities for a Percent Solution or Solid by the Dimensional Analysis Method using Procedure Checklist 16-2

1. Write the unknown, x, alone on one side of an equation.

2. On the other side of the equation, write a conversion factor with the units of measure for the answer in the numerator and the units you are converting from in the denominator.

3. Multiply the conversion factor by the number that is being converted over 1

4. Cancel units.

5. Solve the equation.

EXAMPLE   Write out a recipe for preparing 250 mL of 0.9% sodium chloride.

STEP A: CONVERT

This step is not applicable.

Copyright © 2012 by The McGraw-Hill Companies, Inc.

STEP B: CALCULATE

Follow the Procedure Checklist 6-2.

1. $x\text{ g} =$

2. The percent concentration tells us that 100 mL solution contains 0.9 g NaCl. We need to calculate how many grams of NaCl are needed to prepare 250 mL of solution. Since we are calculating grams, our conversion factor will be written.

$$\frac{0.9\text{g}}{100\text{ mL}}$$

3. Setting up the two ratios as a proportion gives us the following equation:

$$x\text{ g} = \frac{0.9\text{ g}}{100\text{ mL}} \times \frac{250\text{ mL}}{1}$$

4. Cancel units:

$$x\text{ g} = \frac{0.9\text{ g}}{100\text{ m\cancel{L}}} \times \frac{250\text{ m\cancel{L}}}{1}$$

5. Cross-multiply to solve for the unknown:

$$x\text{ g} = 2.25\text{ g NaCl}$$

STEP C: THINK! . . . IS IT REASONABLE?

Regardless of the method used, we find that 2.25 g of NaCl is needed to prepare 250 mL of a 0.9% solution. Our "recipe" looks like this:

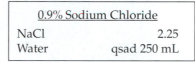

0.9% Sodium Chloride	
NaCl	2.25
Water	qsad 250 mL

REVIEW AND PRACTICE

16.1 Preparation of Solutions and Solids

For Exercises 1 to 5, write a recipe for creating a percent solution or solid.

1. Write a recipe for preparing 500 mL of 0.9% sodium chloride.

2. Write a recipe for preparing 50 mL of a 2% lidocaine solution.

3. Write a recipe for preparing 100 g of a 3% hydrocortisone ointment from hydrocortisone powder and petroleum jelly.

4. Write a recipe for preparing 250 mL of a $\frac{1}{2}$ NS solution.

5. Write a recipe for preparing 75 g of a 20% zinc oxide ointment from zinc oxide powder and petroleum jelly.

To check your answers, see the Answer section at the end of the book, which starts on page A-1.

16.2 Preparing a Dilution from a Concentrate

In the preceding section you were asked to calculate how to prepare a solution using a solid solute or a percent solution. Sometimes, however, you need to prepare a solution by mixing a solution that is more concentrated than needed with one that is less concentrated than needed. The less concentrated solution often is the solvent (solution that dilutes) while the

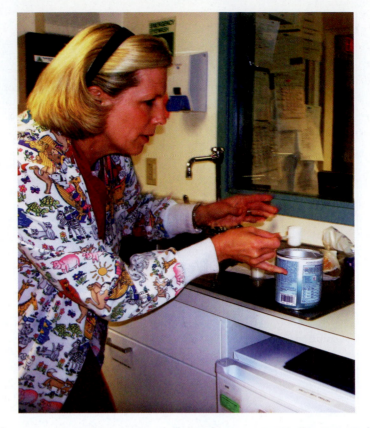

Figure 16-1 A nurse may need to prepare a dilution from a concentrate or a powder when mixing nutritional or infant formulas.

more concentrated solution is the solute. For example, you may need a $\frac{3}{4}$ strength nutritional formula, in which case you would dilute the formula with water. (See Figure 16-1.) Nurses or other health professionals may need to dilute stock solutions, such as hydrogen peroxide (H_2O_2), with a less concentrated liquid such as normal saline, to be used as a topical solution or irrigant. To prepare a dilution from a concentrated solution, you must know what quantity of concentrate (solute) must be added to what quantity of diluent (solvent), to generate a volume of dilution at a prescribed concentration. See Rule 16-4 for preparing dilutions from a concentrate. Use the formula method shown or you can use alligation to calculate how to prepare solutions. The formula method is shown here. If you prefer to use the alligation method, it can be found in Appendix A.

RULE 16-4

Preparing Dilutions from a Concentrate
1. To prepare a dilution from a concentrate, determine:
   The volume of solution needed = V
   - The concentration of solution needed = C
   - The amount of solute = St
   - The amount of solvent = Sv

2. To determine the amount of solute, multiple the volume times the concentration:
   $C \times V = St$

3. To determine the amount of solvent, subtract the solute from the total volume:
   $V - St = Sv$

FORMULA METHOD

EXAMPLE 1

1 ounce of $\frac{1}{4}$ strength hydrogen peroxide, diluted with normal saline, is prescribed for wound care to be administered three times per day. Determine the recipe to create a two-day supply of this wound irrigant.

STEP A: CONVERT

Convert the volume (V) from ounces to mL. 6 ounces will be needed for a two-day supply (1 ounce three times per day × 2 days = 6 oz), convert 6 ounces to mL:

$$\frac{1\ oz}{30\ mL} = \frac{6\ oz}{x}$$

$$x = 180\ mL$$

STEP B: CALCULATE

1. Determine the components of the formula.

   $V = 180\ mL \qquad C = \frac{1}{4}$

2. Fill in the formula $C \times V = St$ to determine the solute.

   $\frac{1}{4} \times 180\ mL = 45\ mL$ (solute/hydrogen peroxide)

3. Fill in the formula $V - St = Sv$ to determine the solvent.

   $180\ mL - 45\ mL = 135\ mL$ (solvent/normal saline)

$\frac{1}{4}$ Strength Hydrogen Peroxide—180 mL	
H_2O_2	45 mL
NS	135 mL

STEP C: THINK ! . . . IS IT REASONABLE?

Since 45 is one-fourth of the total volume of solution (180 mL) and 135 + 45 = 180 mL, then this answer is reasonable.

EXAMPLE 2

Administer 2 oz of $\frac{3}{4}$ strength Pulmocare® every 2 hours via feeding tube. Determine the recipe to create a one-day supply of this nutritional supplement. NOTE: When no solvent is given, the universal solvent, water, is used as the diluent.

STEP A: CONVERT

Convert the volume (V) from ounces to mL. 24 oz will be needed for a one-day supply (2 oz × 12 intervals [there are twelve 2-hour intervals in 24 hours] = 24 ounces), convert 24 ounces to mL.

$$\frac{1\ oz}{30\ mL} = \frac{24\ oz}{x}$$

$$x = 720\ mL$$

STEP B: CALCULATE

1. Determine the components of the formula.

   $V = 720\ mL \qquad C = \frac{3}{4}$

2. Fill in the formula $C \times V = St$ to determine the solute.

   $\frac{3}{4} \times 720 = 540\ mL$ (solute/Pulmocare®)

3. Fill in the formula $V - St = Sv$ to determine the solvent.

   $720\ mL - 540\ mL = 180\ mL$ (solvent/water)

$\frac{3}{4}$ Strength Pulmocare®—720 mL	
Pulmocare®	540 mL
H_2O	180 mL

PATIENT EDUCATION

Sometimes the caloric content of infant formulas requires adjustment based on the infant's caloric requirements. Parents should be provided with the following information regarding mixing infant formulas

1. Most infant formulas have 20 calories in each ounce. To grow, some babies may need to get more calories in less volume.

2. Before you mix infant formula, wash your hands with soap and water. Also, wash the top of the formula can before opening to prevent germs from getting into the formula. Use clean measuring utensils and containers.

3. Let the cold tap water run for 2 minutes before mixing with the formula to reduce the amount of lead that may be in the water. Well water may contain bacteria and should not be used to make infant formula.

4. When using liquid concentrate:
   a. Check the formula label. It should read "concentrate," not "ready-to-use."
   b. Shake the can before opening.
   c. Follow the recipe provided by the authorized prescriber.
   d. Pour the formula concentrate from the can into another container.
   e. Measure the desired amount of water in a clear liquid measuring cup.
   f. Add to the concentrate and mix well.

5. When using powdered formula:
   a. Follow the recipe provided by the authorized prescriber.
   b. Using a clear liquid measuring cup, measure the desired amount of water.
   c. Set the measuring cup on a flat surface, and check the level of the liquid at eye level.
   d. Add unpacked, level measures of formula powder to the water.
   e. Use only the scoop provided in the formula can or measuring cups intended for dry ingredients.
   f. Mix or shake well until all lumps are gone.

6. Storage Information:
   a. Store prepared formula in a covered container in the refrigerator.
   b. Throw away any unused prepared formula after 48 hours.
   c. Throw away any unused formula powder one month after opening the can.

7. Feeding Instructions:
   a. Shake the formula well.
   b. Warm it by running warm tap water over the bottler or setting the bottle in a pan of warm water.
   c. Do not use a microwave because it heats unevenly, causing "hot spots" that could burn the baby's mouth.
   d. After warming, shake the bottle again.
   e. Always test the temperature of the formula before feeding.
   f. Discard any formula left in the bottle after a feeding.

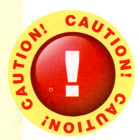

ERROR ALERT!

Label All Patient Tubing

Enteral Nutrition (EN), aka "tube feeding," is the administration of food directly into the gastrointestinal tract (GI) through a tube placed in the nose, the stomach, or the small intestines. Patients receiving tube feedings are unable to feed themselves and are typically critically ill. Such patients usually have other types of tubes such as IVs, oxygen, or drainage tubes. An infant in Madrid, Spain, died when formula was given to him through an IV catheter. This error is tragic and can be prevented by tagging all patient tubing with identification labels.

GO TO . . . Open the CD-ROM that accompanies your textbook, and select Chapter 16, Preparing Dilutions from a Concentrate (LO 16.2). Review the animation and example problems, then complete the practice problems. Continue to the next section of the book once you have mastered the information presented.

CRITICAL THINKING ON THE JOB

Order: Give 90 mL $\frac{1}{2}$ Strength Sustacal® Now

The nurse prepares the order with 30 mL of Sustacal® + 60 mL of water.

Think ! . . . Is It Reasonable? How will this error impact the patient? How should the formula have been prepared?

16.2 Preparing a Dilution from a Concentrate

For Exercises 1 to 5, write a recipe for a wound irrigation solution, using NS as the diluent (solvent). The recipe volume should reflect the total supply indicated

1. Clean sacral wound with 4 ounces of $\frac{1}{2}$ strength acetic acid q6h × 2 days.

2. Perform pin care with 2 ounces of $\frac{1}{3}$ strength hydrogen peroxide q4h × 3 days.

3. Irrigate foot wound with 0.24 L of $\frac{1}{4}$ strength sodium hypochlorite solution daily × 1 week.

4. Cleanse abdominal wound with 2 ounces of $\frac{3}{4}$ strength hydrogen peroxide t.i.d. × 1 week.

5. Use 60 mL of $\frac{2}{3}$ strength povidine-iodine solution q2h × 24 hours to clean open wound prior to surgery.

For Exercises 6–10, write a recipe for the total supply of each nutritional supplement.

6. Three–day supply of 90 mL $\frac{1}{4}$ strength Enfamil® to be given q4h.

7. Two-day supply of 4 oz of $\frac{3}{4}$ strength Boost® to be given q3h.

8. One week supply of 2 oz of $\frac{1}{3}$ strength Ensure® to be administered q6h.

9. Daily supply of 1 oz per hour of $\frac{2}{3}$ strength Sustacal®.

10. 48-hour supply of 60 mL of $\frac{1}{2}$ strength Similac® to be administered q2h.

To check your answers, see the Answer section at the end of the book, which starts on page A-1.

CHAPTER 16 SUMMARY

LEARNING OUTCOME	KEY POINTS
16.1 Write a recipe for preparing a percent solutions or solid. Pages 457–461	Solution—liquid mixture containing both solute and solvent

Solute—chemical that is dissolved or diluted

Solvent—liquid used to dilute or dissolve (aka diluent)

Universal solvent—water

Percent concentration for solutions

- ▸ With a liquid solute, percent concentration is number of mL per 100 mL, e.g. 70% isopropyl alcohol = 70 mL/100 mL.

- ▸ With a solid solute, percent concentration is the number of grams per 100 mL, e.g. 2% lidocaine solution = 2 g lidocaine/100 mL solution

Percent concentration for solids—when the solute and solvent are both solids, percent concentration is the number of grams per 100 g, e.g., 2% hydrocortisone cream = 2 g hydrocortisone powder/100 g ointment

qsad = quantity sufficient to adjust the dimensions to a particular volume

To prepare a percent solution—add enough solvent to the solute to make 100 mL solution, e.g., to prepare a 0.9% NaCl solution, add enough solution to 0.9 g of NaCl to make 100 mL.

To prepare a percent solution, for solutions other than 100 mL—calculate the proportionate number of grams of solute and solvent, using

The Proportion Method: For example, to prepare 250 mL of 0.9% NaCl, set up the proportion:

$$\frac{0.9 \text{ g}}{100 \text{ mL}} = \frac{x}{250 \text{ mL}}$$

$$x = 2.25 \text{ g}$$

Add enough solution to 2.25 g NaCl to make 250 mL.

The Dimensional Analysis Method:

$$x = \frac{0.9 \text{ g}}{100 \text{ mL}} \times \frac{250 \text{ mL}}{1}$$

$$x = \frac{0.9 \text{ g}}{100 \text{ mL}} \times \frac{250 \text{ mL}}{1}$$

$$x = 2.25 \text{ g NaCl}$$

To prepare a percent solid mixture—determine the number of grams of solute and subtract it from the total mixture to determine the solvent or ointment base, e.g., 10% zinc oxide (10 g/100 g) = 10 g of zinc oxide powder in 90 g of petroleum jelly.

LEARNING OUTCOME	KEY POINTS

16.2 Calculate the amount of solute and solvent needed to prepare a desired strength for:
a. Enteral feedings
b. Topical solutions/irrigants.
Pages 461–465

Preparing a Dilution from a Concentrate

1. Identify the following information in the problem (following rule 16-4).

   a. The volume of solution needed = V

   b. The concentration of the solution needed = C

   c. The amount of solute = St

   d. The amount of solvent = Sv

2. Plug the values into the following formula: $C \times V = St$

3. Determine the amount of solvent by subtracting the solute from the total volume: $V - St = Sv$

For example, create a two-day supply of 1 ounce of $\frac{1}{4}$ strength hydrogen peroxide, diluted with normal saline, for wound care t.i.d.

Step A: Convert Convert ounces to mL: 1 oz three times per

day $\times$ 2 days = $\dfrac{6 \text{ oz}}{\text{day}}$

$$\frac{1 \text{ oz}}{30 \text{ mL}} = \frac{6 \text{ oz}}{x}; \qquad x = 180 \text{ mL}$$

Step B: Calculate

Calculate: $C \times V = St;$ $\qquad \dfrac{1}{4} \times 180 \text{ mL} = 45 \text{ mL}$

$V - St = Sv;$ $\qquad 180 \text{ mL} - 45 \text{ mL} = 135 \text{ mL}$

Recipe: 45 mL solute (peroxide) + 135 mL solvent (NS) = 180 mL

Step C: Think! . . . Is it Reasonable? Since 45 is one-fourth of 180 mL, the recipe makes sense.

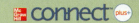
Answer the following questions.

1. A liquid solution labeled 10% hydrogen peroxide would have how many mL of hydrogen peroxide in each 100 mL of solution? (LO 16.1)

2. Write a recipe for 100 g of a 5% hydrocortisone cream using hydrocortisone powder and petroleum jelly. (LO 16.1)

3. Write a recipe for 500 mL of $\frac{1}{4}$ NS solution. (LO 16.1)

4. Write a recipe for 150 mL of 2% lidocaine solution. (LO 16.1)

5. Write a recipe for 250 mL Dextrose 5% in water. (LO 16.1)

For Exercises 6–10, define the terms. (LO 16.1)

6. Solute

7. Solvent

8. Solution

9. Universal solvent

10. qsad

For Exercises 11–15, identify the solute and solvent in each solution. (LO 16.1)

11. 1000 mL D10W

12. 500 mL 0.45% sodium chloride (sodium chloride in water)

13. 12 oz $\frac{1}{2}$ strength Sustacal®

14. 10 mL 2% lidocaine solution (lidocaine in water)

15. 4 oz $\frac{1}{4}$ strength Enfamil®

For Exercises 16–20, calculate the total volume and amount of solute and solvent for each order. Use NS for the solvent for wound irrigation, water for the solvent for nutritional formulas. (LO 16.2)

16. Cleanse wound with 90 mL $\frac{2}{3}$ strength povidine-iodine solution q3h × 48 hours, prior to surgery.

17. Prepare a daily supply of $\frac{1}{4}$ strength Enfamil® 45 mL q2h.

18. Irrigate wound with 2.5 oz of $\frac{1}{2}$ strength hydrogen peroxide q.i.d. × 3 days.

19. 0.1 L of $\frac{3}{4}$ strength Ensure® q.i.d. × 2 days

20. Three-day supply of $\frac{2}{3}$ strength Isomil®, 4 oz q4h

CHECK UP

For Exercises 1–5, match the terms, a–e, with the definition, 1–5. (LO 16.1)

_____ 1. The most commonly used solvent

_____ 2. Also known as diluent

_____ 3. Chemical that is diluted

_____ 4. Liquid mixture containing two or more chemicals

_____ 5. Sufficient quantity to produce a desired volume

a. solution

b. qsad

c. universal solvent

d. solute

e. solvent

For Exercises 6–10, identify the solute (St) and solvent (Sv) in each order. (LO 16.1)

6. 500 mL D5W (dextrose 5% in water)

7. 100 mL NS (0.9% sodium chloride in water)

8. 10% zinc oxide ointment (zinc powder in petroleum jelly)

9. 1% lidocaine solution (lidocaine in water)

10. 1 L of $\frac{1}{4}$ strength Ensure® for tube feedings

For Exercises 11–15, write a recipe for each. (LO 16.1)

11. 500 mL D10W (dextrose 10% in water)

12. 100 mL $\frac{1}{2}$ NS (0.45% sodium chloride)

13. 200 g of 20% zinc oxide ointment (zinc powder in petroleum jelly)

14. 50 mL of a 1% lidocaine solution

15. 100 g of a 2% hydrocortisone ointment (hydrocortisone powder in petroleum jelly)

For Exercises 16–20, calculate the solute and solvent for each order. Dilute wound irrigants with normal saline (NS) and nutritional formulas with water. (LO 16.2)

16. Use 2 oz $\frac{1}{2}$ strength hydrogen peroxide q6h for skeletal pin care × 5 days.

17. Give 4 oz $\frac{1}{4}$ strength Enfamil® q4h × 48 hours.

18. Give 0.5 L of $\frac{3}{4}$ strength Pulmocare® b.i.d. × 3 days

19. Cleanse wound with 30 mL $\frac{1}{3}$ strength povidine-iodine solution daily × 1 week

20. Give 12 oz $\frac{2}{3}$ strength Sustacal® a.c. today.

CRITICAL THINKING APPLICATIONS

The patient care technician is making up $\frac{3}{4}$ strength formula for several patients on the unit. (LO 16.2)

1. If 8 oz cans of full strength formula are available, how many cans will be needed to create 64 ounces of $\frac{3}{4}$ strength formula?

2. How many cups of water will be added to the formula?

CASE STUDY

A 130-pound patient in a comatose state, unable to take foods orally, has a nasogastric tube inserted for feedings. Half-strength Ensure® at 50 mL/hour is ordered for the first 24 hours, and then advanced to 75 mL/h × 2 days. On day 4, the formula is advanced to full strength Ensure, continued at 75 mL/h × 2 days. On day 6, the full strength formula is increased to 100 mL/h and maintained at that rate. (LO 16.2)

1. If the formula contains 1 calorie per mL, how many calories did the patient receive after one week?

2. After the first week, what was the average daily caloric intake for this patient?

3. If the patient's caloric requirement is 40 cal/kg/day, was the patient's caloric requirement met after one week with this feeding order?

4. Will the patient's caloric requirement be met during week 2?

INTERNET ACTIVITY

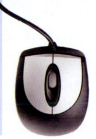

Research the formulas and determine which type of patient would benefit from each.
1. Pulmocare®
2. Jevity®
3. Glucerna®
4. Sustacal®

To check your answers, see the Answer section at the end of the book, which starts on page A-1.

GO TO . . . Open the CD-ROM that accompanies your textbook, and complete a final review of the learning outcomes, practice problems, games, slide show and other activities presented for this chapter. For a final evaluation, take the chapter test and email or print your results for your instructor. A score of 95 percent or above indicates mastery of the chapter concepts.

17

CHAPTER

Calculations for Special Populations

*Perfection consists not in doing extraordinary things,
but in doing ordinary things extraordinarily well.*

—ANGELIQUE ARNAULD

Learning Outcomes

When you have completed Chapter 17, you will be able to:

17.1 Identify factors that impact drug dosing in special populations.

17.2 Calculate safe dosages based on body weight.

17.3 Determine safe doses based on ideal weight vs. actual weight.

17.4 Calculate dosages based on body surface area (BSA).

17.5 Calculate Daily Maintenance Fluid Needs (DMFN).

KEY TERMS

Absorption
Biotransformation
Body surface area
Daily maintenance fluid needs
Distribution
Elimination
Geriatric
Nomogram
Pediatric
Pharmacokinetics
Polypharmacy

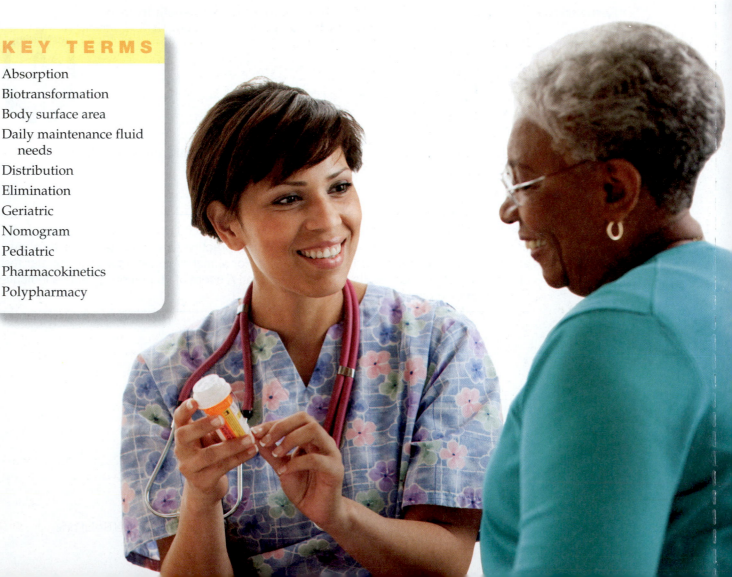

INTRODUCTION

There are two special populations that require extra consideration when you are calculating medication dosages. These are pediatric (children) and geriatric (mature adult) patients. Generally speaking; **pediatric** patients are under the age of 18, and **geriatric** patients are 65 and over. See Figures 17-1 and 17-2. The risk of harm to these populations is far greater because of how they break down and absorb medications. You must clarify all confusing drug orders, calculate with absolute accuracy, verifying that the dose is safe, and seek assistance from your supervisor if you have concerns. No matter how rushed you may feel, you may not take shortcuts with medication calculations for patients from special populations, but rather you must calculate their dosages extraordinarily well!

17.1 Factors that Impact Dosing and Medication Administration

For most drugs, there is a normal recommended dose standardized for an average adult weighing approximately 150 pounds. This standardized dose of a medication is based on a number of assumptions about the patient's body and age. It is assumed that the body systems are fully developed and functioning at a certain level. While these assumptions hold true for most patients, there are many situations in which the dose needs to be adjusted. If the liver or kidneys are not functioning normally, for example, the dose of many drugs needs to be decreased. If the digestive system is not functioning normally, the dose of oral medications may need to be adjusted. These changes in dosage are necessary because the drug is affecting each patient's body differently.

Pharmacokinetics—How Drugs Are Used by the Body

Pharmacokinetics is the study of what happens to a drug after it is administered to a patient. There are four processes that affect a drug after it is administered: *absorption, distribution, biotransformation* (metabolism), and *elimination*. Pharmacokinetics is the study of these four processes, which you can remember using the acronym ADME. Understanding the processes allows adjustments to be made for patients whose body systems are not fully developed or are not functioning at a certain level.

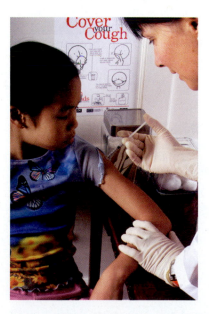

Figure 17-1 Pediatric patients, less than 18 years, require extra attention to detail when performing calculations.

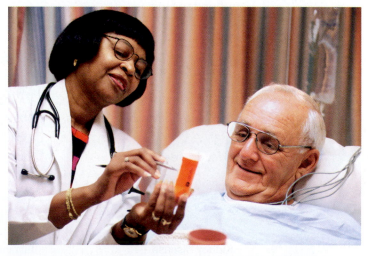

Figure 17-2 Dosage calculation for geriatric patients, those 65 years and older, require extraordinary accuracy.

Absorption is the process that moves a drug from the site where it is given into the bloodstream. Intravenous medications bypass the absorption process because they are administered directly into the bloodstream. Oral medications are absorbed through the digestive system, while topical medications are absorbed through the skin.

Distribution is the process that moves a drug from the bloodstream into other body tissues and fluids. The blood and each of these other areas are called *compartments.* Some compartments include blood, fat, cerebrospinal fluid, and the target site. The *target site* is the site where the drug produces its desired effect. The compartments that a drug will go to are different for different drugs, and depend on the chemical nature of the drug.

Biotransformation (metabolism) is the process that chemically changes the drug in the body. These changes, which occur primarily in the liver, help to protect the body from foreign chemicals, including drugs.

Elimination is the process in which the drug leaves the body. The main way of eliminating most drugs is through the urine, although the drug can also be eliminated in the air that we exhale, sweat, feces, breast milk, or any other body secretion.

The dose of a drug may need to be adjusted if one of these four processes is not functioning within certain limits. Certain conditions affect these four processes, thus affecting the dose. Some examples are found in Table 17-1. A dose adjustment is made based upon the nature and severity of the patient's condition. Thus, the dose ordered might be lower or higher than normal in some circumstances, yet still be the proper dose for the patient. These dosing considerations for various conditions are normally included in the package insert and are considered when the order for the medication is written. You are not expected to make the dosage adjustments; however, understanding these processes will make you *aware* of the many factors that need to be taken into consideration when determining the appropriate dose for an individual.

The function of many body systems changes over the life of a person. In newborns, some systems are not yet fully developed. This is especially true for premature infants. In geriatric patients, those 65 and over, the function of some body systems begins to deteriorate. Skin and veins become more fragile. The functions of the digestive and urinary systems may be affected. Table 17-2 describes examples of age-related factors that can affect dosing. This chapter will show you several methods that are used for calculating dosages for pediatric and geriatric patients.

There are other things to consider when working with special populations. Pediatric and geriatric patients will have a parent or caretaker who will administer or assist them with medications. These individuals will need education. You may be called upon to teach the patients or the caregivers about the medications they will be taking. Table 17-3 provides a list of what each patient or caregiver should know about medications. Geriatric patients may require extra consideration based upon their level of awareness and understanding.

TABLE 17-1 Conditions That May Impact Dosing

CONDITION	PROCESS AFFECTED	EFFECT ON DOSING
Stomach or intestinal disorders	Absorption	Dose of oral medications may need to be changed.
Liver disorders	Biotransformation	The dose of some drugs needs to be decreased.
Obesity	Distribution	Dose of drugs distributed to fat may need to be increased.
Kidney disease	Elimination	Dose of drugs eliminated in urine may need to be changed.

TABLE 17-2 Age-Related Factors That May Impact Dosing

AGE GROUP	CONDITION	PROCESS AFFECTED	EFFECT ON DOSING
Pediatric	pH of stomach is lower	Absorption	Dose of oral medications may need to be changed.
	Thinner skin	Absorption	Dose of topical medications may need to be decreased.
	Liver still developing	Biotransformation	Dose of some drugs needs to be decreased.
	Less circulation to muscles	Absorption	Dose of IM medications may need to be increased.
Geriatric	Thinner skin	Absorption	Dose of topical medications may need to be decreased.
	Decreased liver function	Biotransformation	Dose of some drugs needs to be decreased.
	Decreased kidney function	Elimination	Dose of drugs eliminated in the urine may need to be decreased.
	Poor circulation	Absorption and distribution	Dose of some drugs needs to be adjusted.
	Decreased HCl in stomach (pH is lower)	Absorption	Dose of oral acidic drugs needs to be adjusted

TABLE 17-3 What Patients and Caregivers Should Know about Medications

Name of the medication

Purpose of taking the medication

How to store the medication

How long the patient will need to take the medication

How and when to take the medication

How to know if the medication is effective

Required follow-up (lab tests, doctor appointments)

Possible side effects and what to do about them

Interactions with other drugs and foods

Symptoms to report to the doctor

What to do if a dose is missed

Keeping a list of all medications

When the medication expires

Pediatric Patients

Physiological differences between children and adults make children more susceptible to the effects and adverse reactions of medications. Not only the difference in body size and composition but also the immaturity of organ systems contribute to increased risks associated with pediatric medication administration. As seen in Table 17-2, because children have an increased metabolism and a higher percentage of water per kilogram of body weight, the pharmacokinetic processes—absorption, distribution, biotransformation (metabolism), and excretion are different in children than adults. Appropriate drug dosages in children are typically calculated based on body weight or body surface area (BSA). Rules for calculating drug dosages based on body weight and body surface area will be explored later in this chapter.

Geriatric Patients

When you work with geriatric patients, show them respect. Encourage them, if they are able, to participate in planning their schedule. Listen to their concerns. Recommend that they use the same pharmacy to fill all prescriptions. Encourage them to have one doctor as their primary physician to monitor and approve all medications. Remind them to keep a list of all their medications including vitamins, herbals, and alternative medications. They should take the list or medication bottles when they see their primary physician and all their specialists.

In some cases, geriatric patients may have decreased manual dexterity that can interfere with their ability to inject medications, administer eye drops, or even open bottles. Patients may need to specifically ask their pharmacist for bottle caps that are not childproof. Patients with difficulty swallowing will need information about which medications may be crushed and mixed with applesauce or pudding. In addition, they need information about which medications may *not* be broken or crushed.

Many patients cannot read small print. Medications may need labels that can easily be read and will clearly describe the purpose of each medication. Do not assume patients can distinguish between colors of tablets; white and yellow may be confused, as may blue and green, or orange and pink. Make a chart for the patient with the medications, time, and description to prevent errors.

PATIENT EDUCATION

Family members or others who care for special population patients at home must understand and follow directions when they administer drugs. Talk to parents or caretakers about the following:

1. Explain how much medication to administer at one time, how often during the day, and for how many days. Give parents or caretakers this information in writing. Have them repeat this information, especially if their English or literacy skills are limited.

2. Discuss expected side effects. Provide a telephone number or resource for them to call in case of unexpected or serious side effects. Explain how to reach a Poison Control Center.

3. No one should ever be given someone else's medication. Patients may react differently to medications than expected.

4. Over-the-counter, herbal, and alternative remedies should never be given to a child under age 2 without first speaking to a healthcare provider.

5. Parents or caregivers must check dosage information on over-the-counter medications. The amount to administer changes with age and weight. Some medications may *not* be administered to children below a certain age (often 2) without first checking with a physician.

6. Demonstrate how to measure doses accurately. Calibrated equipment should be used. Droppers are not automatically interchangeable between medications.

7. The full course of prescription medications such as antibiotics must be administered, even if the patient appears to be well or resists taking the medication.

8. Never refer to medication as candy or physically force a patient to take a medication.

9. Replace childproof caps properly and keep medications out of reach of children or patients with mental confusion.

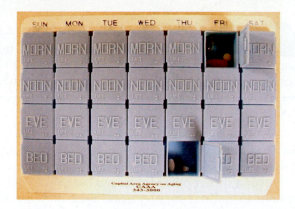

Figure 17-3 A medication container like this one would be very useful for a patient taking multiple daily medications.

Geriatric patients often have some form of hearing loss. They may even try to hide their hearing loss from you. Have patients repeat to you the information that you give them. They may also have short-term memory loss. Determine if they need written directions and explanations. Help them work with memory tools, such as medication calendars that tell them which medications to take each day. Pharmacies often sell weekly dispensers that have a container for each day of the week; patients or family members can prepare in advance the medications for the week (see Figure 17-3).

Instruct patients who regularly take prescription medications not to take over-the-counter or herbal medications without first checking with their physician. They should not take more of any medication than is indicated by the label. They should avoid any medications that have expired (show them how to read the expiration date). They should never borrow medications, especially prescription ones, from anyone else.

CREATININE CLEARANCE Liver and kidney functions are often reduced in geriatric patients. Decreased liver function results in slower metabolism of certain drugs, delaying or prolonging the desired effect of the medication. It can also lead to a higher level of drug in the blood system, producing more intense results.

Decreased kidney function, along with decreased cardiac output, slows the excretion of medications from the body. Slower excretion (resulting from decreased kidney function) and a reduced metabolism (resulting from decreased liver function) combine their effects. Medication accumulates in the body, causing increased side effects or even toxicity. Many chronic diseases common in the elderly can damage the kidneys. These diseases include hypertension, diabetes, and congestive heart failure. Also, some commonly used drugs, such as Lasix® and aminoglycoside antibiotics, can further impair kidney function. Geriatric patients who have these diseases or are prescribed these medications must be monitored especially closely for their kidney functions.

Many package inserts discuss safe dosage levels based on creatinine clearance. Creatinine is a byproduct found in the blood as a result of muscle metabolism. Creatinine clearance (CL_{CR}) is an indicator of the rate at which the kidneys filter the blood. Creatinine clearance often decreases with age because the elderly tend to have lower muscle mass, thus producing less creatinine in the blood. The filtration rate of creatinine by their kidneys is often slower. For many, this decrease is a normal part of the aging process. The creatinine clearance level of an elderly patient is often lower than the level of an average younger adult. For example, creatinine clearance is measured in mL/min and normal values usually drop by 6 mL/min for every 10 years past the age of 20. If a patient has decreased kidney function, then the amount of creatinine excreted through the urine will decrease. At the same time, the amount of creatinine in the blood (or serum creatinine level) may increase.

The creatinine clearance level is calculated by using information that comes from an analysis of blood and urine samples. You may not know this information for every patient. The authorized prescriber will usually factor in a patient's creatinine clearance when preparing a drug order. If you have any questions about administering a medication when creatinine clearance is a factor, speak with your supervisor or authorized prescriber.

GO TO . . . Open the CD-ROM that accompanies your textbook, and select Chapter 17, Factors that Impact Drug Dosing (LO 17.1). Complete the practice problems. Continue to the next section of the book once you have mastered the rule presented.

POLYPHARMACY Many geriatric patients take several medications. They often have more than one physician and one or more specialists who treat very specific diseases and ailments. **Polypharmacy** refers to the practice of taking many medications at a time. Many patients take over a dozen prescription medications each year and numerous over-the-counter medications or natural supplements. They may use medications that were initially prescribed years earlier and are past their expiration date. They may borrow medications. Because of financial pressures, they may also look for ways to limit physician costs by using older medications instead of visiting the physician. They may also order medications by mail or through the internet, without having direct contact with the pharmacist. In addition, some medications may be prescribed without consideration of their interaction with other medications the patient is already taking.

Each additional medication a patient takes increases the likelihood of a drug interaction. These interactions can interfere with the effectiveness of one or more medications. They can also cause serious or even fatal side effects. Adverse drug reactions can be caused by a variety of factors. These include advanced age, small body size, multiple illnesses (including chronic problems), multiple medications, living alone (patients with failing memories or mental capacities), and malnutrition. Elderly patients often take more than one medication to treat the same problem. Sometimes they have neglected to inform a new physician about medications prescribed by other physicians. Sometimes multiple medications are needed to bring a problem under control. The patient may then continue to take all the medications, even though only one or two are still needed. This overuse is especially common with patients being treated for high blood pressure, constipation, or behavioral problems that occur with dementia. Healthcare providers should periodically review with their elderly patients the list of medications the patients are taking. They should look especially for medications that are no longer needed as well as for multiple medications being used to treat the same condition. Certain medications should be avoided by patients with specific diseases. Table 17-4 provides a list of some of these medications.

TABLE 17-4 Drugs to Be Avoided in Specific Diseases

These drugs are likely to cause significant adverse effects in elderly patients with the diseases noted.

SEVERE RISK	DRUGS	LESS SEVERE RISK	DRUGS
Benign prostatic hypertrophy	Antihistamines, anti-Parkinson's drugs, GI antispasmodics, antidepressants	Benign prostatic hypertrophy	Narcotics
Cardiac dysrhythmia	Tricyclic antidepressants	Constipation	Antihistamines, anti-Parkinson's drugs, GI antispasmodics, antidepressants
Clotting disorders	Antiplatelet drugs, ASA (aspirin)	Diabetes mellitus	Steroids, beta blockers
COPD	Hypnotics, sedatives, beta blockers	GI diseases	Aspirin, potassium supplements
GI diseases	NSAIDs, ASA (aspirin)	Insomnia	Decongestants, bronchodilators, some antidepressants
Seizures	Metoclopramide (Reglan)	Seizures	Antipsychotics

To identify cases of polypharmacy and reduce the risk of drug interactions, ask elderly patients about:

1. All medications they take that are prescribed by either their primary physician or specialists.

2. Any over-the-counter medications they take, including vitamins, laxatives, and allergy medications.

3. Any social drugs that they use, including alcohol, tobacco, and marijuana.

4. Medications that they borrow from family and friends.

5. Herbal and home remedies that they use, including natural supplements such as ginseng, gingko biloba, and St. John's Wort.

6. Bringing all the medications they take to be checked. This includes prescriptions, over-the-counter drugs, vitamins, minerals, and herbals.

GO TO . . . Open the CD-ROM that accompanies your textbook, and select Chapter 17, Polypharmacy and Drug Interactions (LO 17.1). Review the animation and example problems, then complete the practice problems. Continue to the next section of the book once you have mastered the rule presented.

REVIEW AND PRACTICE

17.1 Factors that Impact Dosing and Medication Administration

For Exercises 1–10, match the terms with the definition.

1. Process that moves a drug into the bloodstream   **a.** biotransformation

2. Chemical changing of a drug in the body   **b.** pharmacokinetics

3. Process in which a drug is removed from the body   **c.** distribution

4. Movement of a drug from the bloodstream to body tissues and fluids   **d.** elimination

5. What happens to a drug after it is administered   **e.** absorption

6. The rate at which the kidneys filter the blood   **f.** geriatric

7. Practice of taking many medications at one time   **g.** drug interaction

8. Patients under the age of 18   **h.** polypharmacy

9. Alteration of the effect of a drug due to another drug   **i.** creatinine clearance

10. Patients over the age of 65   **j.** pediatric

For Exercises 11–15, identify the special population with a G (geriatric) or P (pediatric) that may be impacted by the age-related factor.

11. Decreased liver function _____

12. Poor circulation _____

13. Lower stomach pH _____

14. Decreased circulation to the muscles _____

15. Thinner skin _____

To check your answers, see the Answer section at the end of the book, which begins on page A-1.

17.2 Dosages Based on Body Weight

Many medication orders, especially pediatric and geriatric orders, are based on body weight. This is especially common for small children. An order based on body weight will often state an amount of medication per weight of the patient per unit of time. For example, the order may read 8 mg/kg/day PO q6h. This order says that, over the course of the day, the patient is to be administered 8 mg of medication for every kilogram that he or she weighs. It also says that the total daily dosage is to be divided into 4 doses given at 6-hour intervals. You will calculate the amount to administer from the information on the drug order, the patient's weight, and the dose on hand.

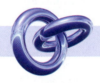

LEARNING LINK   Recall from Chapter 5, Table 5-4 that 1 kg = 2.2 lb.

RULE 17-2 | Calculating Dosage Based on Body Weight

Note: Body weight may require rounding to the whole number, tenths, or hundredths in accordance with the policy of the institution.

Step A: Convert
Convert the patient's weight to kilograms. For accuracy, when converting to kilograms round to the nearest tenth.

Step B: Calculate
Calculate the desired dose *D* by multiplying the dose ordered by the weight in kilograms, such as

$$\frac{mg}{kg} \times kg = \text{desired dose} \qquad or \qquad \frac{mcg}{kg} \times kg = \text{desired dose}$$

Step C: Think! . . . Is It Reasonable?
Confirm whether the desired dose is safe by checking the label, package insert, or product literature. If it is unsafe, consult the authorized prescriber.

After calculating the dosage based on body weight, calculate the amount to administer, using the proportion method, dimensional analysis, or formula method.

PROPORTION METHOD

EXAMPLE 1

Calculate the amount to administer to a 3-year-old who weighs 34 lbs.

Ordered: Hyoscyamine sulfate 5 mcg/kg subcut 1 h preanesthesia

On hand: Hyoscyamine sulfate 0.5 mg/mL

STEP A: CONVERT
Convert the patient's weight to kilograms.

$$\frac{1 \text{ kg}}{2.2 \text{ lb}} = \frac{x}{34 \text{ lb}} \qquad \text{or} \qquad 1 \text{ kg} : 2.2 \text{ lb} = x : 34 \text{ lb}$$

$$2.2 \times x = 34 \times 1 \text{ kg}$$

$$x = \frac{34 \text{ kg}}{2.2}$$

$$x = 15.5 \text{ kg} = \text{patient's weight in kilograms}$$

STEP B: CALCULATE
Calculate the desired dose.

$$\frac{5 \text{ mcg}}{\text{kg}} \times 15.5 \text{ kg} = 77.5 \text{ mcg rounded to } 78 \text{ mcg}$$

STEP C: THINK! . . . IS IT REASONABLE?
Confirm that the desired dose is safe.

Checking the PDR, you find that 5 mcg/kg is the recommended dosage for pediatric patients over 2 years of age.

Calculate the amount to administer.

STEP A: CONVERT
Convert ordered dose 78 mcg to mg, the same unit of measurement as dose on hand, by using the proportion method (Procedure Checklist 6-1).

$$\frac{1 \text{ mg}}{1000 \text{ mcg}} = \frac{x}{78 \text{ mcg}}$$

$$1000 \times x = 78 \times 1 \text{ mg}$$

$$x = \frac{78 \text{ mg}}{1000}$$

$$x = 0.078 \text{ mg}$$

STEP B: CALCULATE
Follow Procedure Checklist 12-1.

$$\frac{H}{Q} = \frac{D}{A} \qquad \text{or} \qquad H : Q = D : A$$

$$\frac{0.5 \text{ mg}}{1 \text{ mL}} = \frac{0.078 \text{ mg}}{A}$$

$$\frac{0.5 \text{ mg}}{1 \text{ mL}} = \frac{0.078 \text{ mg}}{A}$$

$$0.5 \times A = 0.078 \times 1 \text{ mL}$$

$$0.5A = 0.078 \text{ mL}$$

$$A = 0.16 \text{ mL}$$

STEP C: THINK! . . . IS IT REASONABLE?
. . . Since the ordered dose, 0.078 mg, is a lot less than the dose on hand, 0.5 mg, the amount administered should be a lot less than the volume on hand, 1 mL, so 0.16 mL is a reasonable answer!

EXAMPLE 1

Calculate the amount to administer to a 3-year-old who weighs 34 lbs.

Ordered: Hyoscyamine sulfate 5 mcg/kg subcut 1 h preanesthesia

On hand: Hyoscyamine sulfate 0.5 mg/mL

STEP A: CONVERT
Convert the patient's weight to kilograms.

$$x = \frac{1\ kg}{2.2\ \cancel{lb}} \times 34\ \cancel{lb}$$

$$x = 15.5\ kg$$

STEP B: CALCULATE
Calculate the desired dose.

$$\frac{5\ mcg}{\cancel{kg}} \times 15.5\ \cancel{kg} = 77.5\ mcg\ \text{rounded to } 78\ mcg$$

STEP C: THINK! . . . IS IT REASONABLE?
Confirm that the desired dose is safe.

Checking the PDR, you find that 5 mcg/kg is the recommended dose for pediatric patients over 2 years of age.

Calculate the amount to administer.

STEP A: CONVERT
Determine the conversion factor. This will be the first factor in the equation.

The unit of measure for the dosage ordered is mcg. The unit of measure for the dose on hand is mg. Use the conversion factor 1 mg = 1000 mcg. Since we will be converting the dosage ordered to mg, place mg in the numerator. This is the first factor.

$$\frac{1\ mg}{1000\ mcg}$$

STEP B: CALCULATE
Follow Procedure Checklist 12-2.

$$A\ mL = \text{conversion factor} \times \frac{Q}{H} \times \frac{D}{1}$$

The dosage unit is 1 mL; the dose on hand is 0.5 mg. This is the second factor.

$$\frac{1\ mg}{1000\ mcg} \times \frac{1\ mL}{0.5\ mg}$$

The desired dose is 0.078 mg. Place this over one and set up your equation.

$$A\ mL = \frac{1\ \cancel{mg}}{1000\ \cancel{mcg}} \times \frac{1\ mL}{0.5\ \cancel{mg}} \times \frac{78\ \cancel{mcg}}{1}$$

$$A = \frac{78\ mL}{1000} \times 0.5$$

$$A = 0.156\ mL$$

Since the volume of the injection is less than 1 mL, we round to hundredth (two decimals).

$$A = 0.16\ mL$$

STEP C: THINK! . . . IS IT REASONABLE?
. . . Since the ordered dose, 0.078 mg is a lot less than the dose on hand, 0.5 mg, the amount administered should be a lot less than the volume on hand, 1 mL, so 0.16 mL is a reasonable answer!

FORMULA METHOD

EXAMPLE 1

Calculate the amount to administer to a 3-year-old who weighs 34 lb.

Ordered: Hyoscyamine sulfate 5 mcg/kg subcut 1 h preanesthesia

On hand: Hyoscyamine sulfate 0.5 mg/mL

STEP A: CONVERT
Convert the patient's weight to kilograms.

$$x \text{ kg} = \frac{1 \text{ kg}}{2.2 \text{ lb}} \times 34 \text{ lb}$$

$$x = 15.5 \text{ kg}$$

STEP B: CALCULATE
Calculate the desired dose.

$$\frac{5 \text{ mcg}}{\text{kg}} \times 15.5 \text{ kg} = 77.5 \text{ mcg rounded to } 78 \text{ mcg}$$

STEP C: THINK! . . . IS IT REASONABLE?
Confirm that the desired dose is safe. Checking the PDR, you find that 5 mcg/kg is the recommended dose for pediatric patients over 2 years of age.

Calculate the amount to administer.

STEP A: CONVERT
Because the unit of measure for the dose on hand is milligrams, the desired dose must also be expressed in milligrams. Convert the desired dose to mg using Procedure Checklist 6-1.

$$\frac{1 \text{ mg}}{1000 \text{ mcg}} = \frac{x}{78 \text{ mcg}}$$

$$1000 \times x = 78 \times 1 \text{ mg}$$

$$x = \frac{78 \text{ mg}}{1000}$$

$$x = 0.078 \text{ mg}$$

STEP B: CALCULATE
Calculate the amount to administer, using Procedure Checklist 12-3.

$$\frac{D}{H} \times Q = A$$

$$D = 0.078 \text{ mg}$$

$$H = 0.5 \text{ mg}$$

$$Q = 1 \text{ mL}$$

1. Fill in the formula.

$$\frac{0.178 \text{ mg}}{0.5 \text{ mg}} \times 1 \text{ mL} = A$$

2. Cancel units.

$$\frac{0.178 \text{ mg}}{0.5 \text{ mg}} \times 1 \text{ mL} = A$$

3. Solve for the unknown.

$$\frac{0.178}{0.5} \times 1 \text{ mL} = A$$

$$A = 0.156 \text{ mL}$$

4. Since the volume of the injection is less than 1 mL, we round to hundredth (two decimals).

$$A = 0.16 \text{ mL}$$

STEP C: THINK! . . . IS IT REASONABLE?
. . . Since the ordered dose, 0.078 mg is a lot less than the dose on hand, 0.5 mg, the amount administered should be a lot less than the volume on hand, 1 mL, so 0.16 mL is a reasonable answer!

For Example 2 below, refer to the following information to find the amount to administer to a 6 year old patient who weighs 49 lb. and midzolam 0.025 mg/kg IV now is ordered.

According to the package insert at right, pediatric patients from 6 to 12 may have 0.025 to 0.05 mg/kg; up to 0.4 mg/kg not to exceed 10 mg. The dosage ordered corresponds to the low end of the range and is a safe order.

Reading the label below, you determine that Midazolam has a dosage strength of 2 mg/2 mL. We now know that

D (desired dose) = 0.5575 mg

H (dose on hand) = 2 mg

Q (dosage unit) = 2 mL

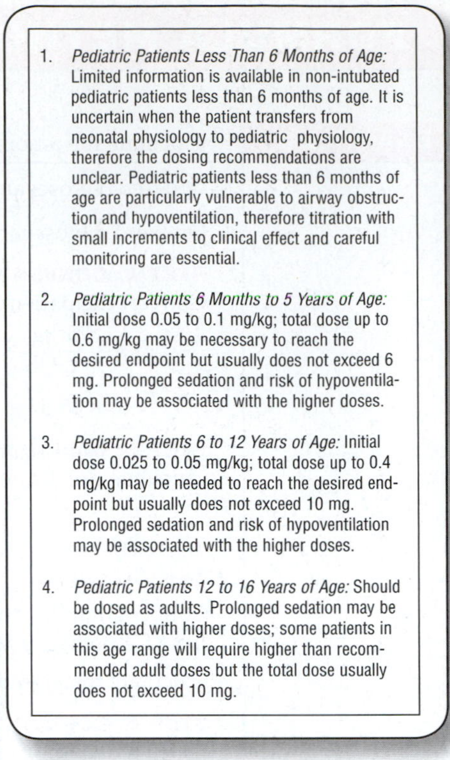

1. *Pediatric Patients Less Than 6 Months of Age:* Limited information is available in non-intubated pediatric patients less than 6 months of age. It is uncertain when the patient transfers from neonatal physiology to pediatric physiology, therefore the dosing recommendations are unclear. Pediatric patients less than 6 months of age are particularly vulnerable to airway obstruction and hypoventilation, therefore titration with small increments to clinical effect and careful monitoring are essential.

2. *Pediatric Patients 6 Months to 5 Years of Age:* Initial dose 0.05 to 0.1 mg/kg; total dose up to 0.6 mg/kg may be necessary to reach the desired endpoint but usually does not exceed 6 mg. Prolonged sedation and risk of hypoventilation may be associated with the higher doses.

3. *Pediatric Patients 6 to 12 Years of Age:* Initial dose 0.025 to 0.05 mg/kg; total dose up to 0.4 mg/kg may be needed to reach the desired endpoint but usually does not exceed 10 mg. Prolonged sedation and risk of hypoventilation may be associated with the higher doses.

4. *Pediatric Patients 12 to 16 Years of Age:* Should be dosed as adults. Prolonged sedation may be associated with higher doses; some patients in this age range will require higher than recommended adult doses but the total dose usually does not exceed 10 mg.

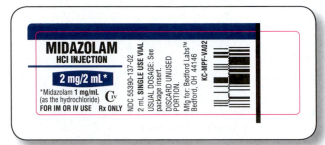

Figure 17-4a Midazolam label.

Figure 17-4b Midazolam package insert.

PROPORTION METHOD

EXAMPLE 2

Find the amount to administer. The patient is 6 years old and weighs 49 lb.

Ordered: Midazolam 0.025 mg/kg IV now.

Refer to Figure 17-4a and 17-4b.

STEP A: CONVERT
Since the ordered dose, 0.5575 mg, and the dose on hand, 2 mg, are both in mg, no conversion is necessary.

STEP B: CALCULATE
Follow Procedure Checklist 12-1.

1. Fill in the proportion.

$$\frac{H}{Q} = \frac{D}{A} \qquad \text{or} \qquad H : Q = D : A$$

$$\frac{2 \text{ mg}}{2 \text{ mL}} = \frac{0.5575 \text{ mg}}{A}$$

2. Cancel units.

$$\frac{2 \text{ mg}}{2 \text{ mL}} = \frac{0.5575 \text{ mg}}{A}$$

3. Cross-multiply and solve for the unknown.

$$2 \times A = 2 \text{ mL} \times 0.5575$$

$$A = 2 \text{ mL} \times \frac{0.5575}{2}$$

$$A = 0.5575 \text{ mL or } 0.56 \text{ mL rounded to the nearest hundredth.}$$

DIMENSIONAL ANALYSIS METHOD

EXAMPLE 2

Find the amount to administer. The patient is 6 years old and weighs 49 lb.

Ordered: Midazolam 0.025 mg/kg IV now.

Refer to Figure 17-4a and 17-4b.

STEP A: CONVERT

Since the ordered dose, 0.5 mg, and the dose on hand, 2 mg, are both in mg, no conversion factor is needed.

STEP B: CALCULATE

Follow Procedure Checklist 12-2.

$$A \text{ mL} = \text{conversion factor} \times \frac{Q}{H} \times \frac{D}{1}$$

1. The amount to administer (A) will be in milliliters.

   A mL =

2. No conversion factor is needed.

3. The dosage unit (Q) is 2 mL; the dose on hand (H) is 2 mg.

   $\dfrac{2 \text{ mL}}{2 \text{ mg}}$ This is the first factor.

4. The desired dose (D) is 0.5575 mg. Place this over one and set up the equation.

   $$A \text{ mL} = \frac{2 \text{ mL}}{2 \text{ mg}} \times \frac{0.5575 \text{ mg}}{1}$$

   $$A = 2 \text{ mL} \times \frac{0.5575}{2}$$

   $A = 0.5575$ mL or 0.56 mL rounded to the nearest hundredth.

STEP C: THINK! . . . IS IT REASONABLE?

. . . Since the ordered dose (0.5575 mg) is about one-fourth of the dose on hand (2 mg), the amount to administer should be approximately one-fourth of the dosage unit (2 mL), so 0.56 mL is a reasonable answer!

FORMULA METHOD

EXAMPLE 2

Find the amount to administer. The patient is a 6-year-old child who weighs 49 lb.

Ordered: Midazolam 0.025 mg/kg IV now

Available: Refer to the label and package insert in Figures 17-4a and 17-4b.

STEP A: CONVERT

1. Convert the child's weight from pounds to kilograms.

   1 kg : 2.2 lb = x kg : 49 lb

   2.2 lb × x kg = 1 kg × 49 lb

   x = 22.3 kg

STEP B: CALCULATE

Find the daily desired dose.

$$\frac{0.025 \text{ mg}}{1 \text{ kg}} \times 22.3 \text{ kg} = \frac{0.025 \text{ mg}}{1 \text{ kg}} \times 22.3 \text{ kg} = 0.5575 \text{ mg}$$

STEP C: THINK! . . . IS IT REASONABLE?

Confirm the desired dose is safe.

STEP A: CONVERT

This step is not applicable since the ordered dose, 0.5575 mg, and the dose on hand, 2 mg, are both in the same unit of measurement, mg.

STEP B: CALCULATE

Follow Procedure Checklist 12-3.

$$\frac{D}{H} \times Q = A$$

1. We know that

   D = 0.5575 mg

   H = 2 mg

   Q = 2 mL

2. Fill in the formula.

   $$\frac{0.5575 \text{ mg}}{2 \text{ mg}} \times 2 \text{ mL} = A$$

3. Cancel units.

   $$\frac{0.5575 \text{ mg}}{2 \text{ mg}} \times 2 \text{ mL} = A$$

4. Solve for the unknown.

   $$\frac{0.5575}{2} \times 2 \text{ mL} = A$$

   A = 0.5575 mL or 0.56 mL rounded to the nearest hundredth.

STEP C: THINK! . . . IS IT REASONABLE?

Since the ordered dose (0.5 mg) is about one-fourth of the dose on hand (2 mg), the amount to administer (0.56 mL) should be approximately one-fourth of the dosage unit (2 mL). Since this is the case, the answer makes sense and is reasonable!

GO TO . . . Open the CD-ROM that accompanies your textbook, and select Chapter 17, Dosages Based on Body Weight (LO 17.2). Review the animation and example problems, then complete the practice problems. Continue to the next section of the book once you have mastered the rule presented.

The total volume of a pediatric injection is limited based on the size and the age of the child. (See Chapter 14, Table 14-3). The length and gauge of the needle used will also vary with the age and size of the patient as well as the location. Smaller muscles need smaller needles. The depth of an injection may also vary for geriatric patients due to their reduced muscle size. You must be aware of all these factors when administering injections to special populations. Additional details regarding these injection techniques are outside the scope of this book. Please review injection techniques before you administer any injection.

Ensuring Safe Dosages

Drug orders may be written in several ways. If you measure or administer the medication, you have the responsibility to check whether the dose is the standard recommended dose. The recommended dose is sometimes written as a range, with a minimum and a maximum recommended dose. In this case, you will need to determine if the dose ordered is not less than the minimum or greater than the maximum recommended dose.

RULE 17-3	Ensuring Safe Dosages
	When you are working with special populations, always check the package insert, drug label, or product literature to ensure the safety of the dose to be administered.

Example 1

Determine whether the following order is safe. If safe, calculate the amount to administer.

Patient: Child who weighs 14.5 kg

Ordered: Erythromycin 125 mg PO q4h

On hand: Refer to the label in Figure 17-5.

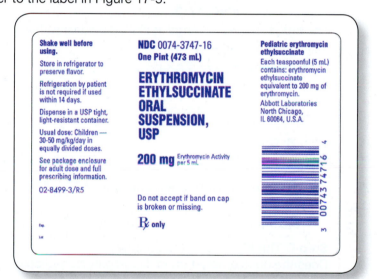

Figure 17-5

Step A: Convert
Since the dose on hand and ordered dose are both mg, no conversion is needed.

Step B: Calculate

Calculate the recommended dose range: mg/kg/day × kg

$$\text{Minimum recommended dosage} = \frac{30 \text{ mg}}{\text{kg}} \times 14.5 \text{ kg} = 435 \text{ mg/day}$$

$$\text{Maximum recommended dosage} = \frac{50 \text{ mg}}{\text{kg}} \times 14.5 \text{ kg} = 725 \text{ mg/day}$$

$$\text{Dosage ordered} = \frac{125 \text{ mg}}{\text{dose}} \times \frac{6 \text{ doses}}{\text{day}} = 750 \text{ mg/day}$$

Step C: Think! . . . Is It Reasonable?
Does the dose ordered fall in the recommended dose range?

The dosage ordered does not fall within the recommended dosage range. You should contact the authorized prescriber.

Example 2

Determine whether the following order is safe. If it is safe, calculate the amount to administer.

Patient: 1-year-old child who weighs 27 lb

Ordered: Amoxil® oral suspension drops 120 mg po q8h

On hand: Refer to the label in Figure 17-6.

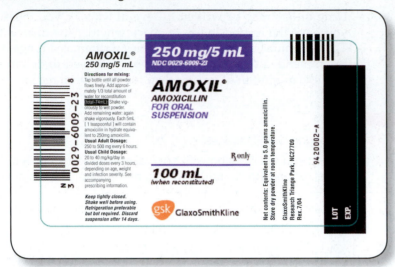

Figure 17-6

The drug label lists a range of child dosages, with a minimum of 20 mg/kg/day and a maximum of 40 mg/kg/day.

Step A: Convert
Convert lb to kg

$$27 \text{ lb} \times \frac{1 \text{ kg}}{2.2 \text{ lb}} = 12.3 \text{ kg}$$

Step B: Calculate
Calculate the recommended dose range: mg/kg/day x kg

$$\text{Minimum recommended dosage} = \frac{20 \text{ mg}}{\text{kg}} \times 12.3 \text{ kg} = 246 \text{ mg/day}$$

$$\text{Maximum recommended dosage} = \frac{40 \text{ mg}}{\text{kg}} \times 12.3 \text{ kg} = 492 \text{ mg/day}$$

Step C Think! . . . Is It Reasonable?
Does the dose ordered fall in the recommended dose range?

$$\text{Dosage ordered} = \frac{120 \text{ mg}}{\text{dose}} \times \frac{3 \text{ doses}}{\text{day}} = 360 \text{ mg/day}$$

The dosage ordered is within the recommended dosage range. Calculate the amount to administer.

$$D = 120 \text{ mg} \qquad H = 250 \text{ mg} \qquad Q = 5 \text{ mL}$$

PROPORTION METHOD

EXAMPLE 2

Calculate the amount to administer.

Ordered: Amoxil® oral suspension drops 120 mg po q8h

On hand: Refer to the label in Figure 17-6.

STEP A: CONVERT
This step is not applicable, since the ordered dose, 120 mg, and the dose on hand, 100 mg, are the same unit of measurement, mg.

STEP B: CALCULATE

Follow Procedure Checklist 12-1.

1. Fill in the proportion.

$$\frac{H}{Q} = \frac{D}{A} \qquad \text{or} \qquad H : Q = D : A$$

$$\frac{250 \text{ mg}}{5 \text{ mL}} = \frac{120 \text{ mg}}{A}$$

2. Cancel units.

$$\frac{250 \text{ \cancel{mg}}}{5 \text{ mL}} = \frac{120 \text{ \cancel{mg}}}{A}$$

3. Cross-multiply and solve for the unknown.

$$250 \times A = 5 \text{ mL} \times 120$$

$$A = 5 \text{ mL} \times \frac{120}{250}$$

$$A = 2.4 \text{ mL}$$

STEP C: THINK! . . . IS IT REASONABLE?

Since the ordered dose 120 mg is less than the dose on hand, 250 mg, then the ordered volume should be less than the supply volume, 5 mL, so an answer of 2.4 mL is a reasonable answer!

DIMENSIONAL ANALYSIS

EXAMPLE 2

Calculate the amount to administer.

Ordered: Amoxil® oral suspension drops 120 mg po q8h

On hand: Refer to the label in Figure 17-6.

STEP A: CONVERT
There is no conversion factor.

STEP B: CALCULATE
Follow Procedure Checklist 12-2.

$$A \text{ mL} = \text{conversion factor} \times \frac{Q}{H} \times \frac{D}{1}$$

1. The unit of measure will be milliliters.

$$A \text{ mL} =$$

2. No conversion factor is needed.

3. The dosage unit is 5 mL; the dose on hand is 250 mg.

$$\frac{5 \text{ mL}}{250 \text{ mg}}$$

4. The desired dose is 120 mg. Place this over 1 and set up the equation.

$$A \text{ mL} = \frac{5 \text{ mL}}{250 \text{ \cancel{mg}}} \times \frac{120 \text{ \cancel{mg}}}{1}$$

$$A = 5 \text{ mL} \times \frac{120}{250}$$

$$A = 2.4 \text{ mL}$$

STEP C: THINK! . . . IS IT REASONABLE?

Since the ordered dose 120 mg is less than the dose on hand, 250 mg, then the ordered volume should be less than the supply volume, 5 mL, so an answer of 2.4 mL is a reasonable answer!

EXAMPLE 2

Calculate the amount to administer.

Ordered: Amoxil® oral suspension drops 120 mg po q8h

On hand: Refer to the label in Figure 17-6.

STEP A: CONVERT
This step is not applicable, since mg is ordered and mg is available.

STEP B: CALCULATE
Follow Procedure Checklist 12-3.

1. We know that

   $D = 120$ mg

   $H = 250$ mg

   $Q = 5$ mL

2. Fill in the formula.

   $$\frac{120 \text{ mg}}{250 \text{ mg}} \times 5 \text{ mL} = A$$

3. Cancel units.

   $$\frac{120 \text{ m\cancel{g}}}{250 \text{ m\cancel{g}}} \times 5 \text{ mL} = A$$

4. Solve for the unknown.

   $$\frac{120}{250} \times 5 \text{ mL} = A$$

   $$A = 2.4 \text{ mL}$$

STEP C: THINK! . . . IS IT REASONABLE?
Since the ordered dose 120 mg is less than the dose on hand, 250 mg, then the ordered volume should be less than the supply volume, 5 mL, so an answer of 2.4 mL is a reasonable answer!

GO TO . . . Open the CD-ROM that accompanies your textbook, and select Chapter 17, Ensuring Safe Dosages Based Upon Weight (LO 17.2). Review the animation and example problems, then complete the practice problems. Continue to the next section of the book once you have mastered the information presented.

ERROR ALERT!

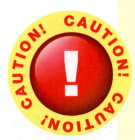

Converting Ounces Carefully

When infants are weighed in pounds and ounces, you will need to convert the weight to kilograms to perform safe dose calculations. Before converting pounds to kilograms, convert ounces to pounds. Remember 16 oz = 1 lb. An ounce is not one-tenth of a pound. A baby whose weight is 8 lb 6 oz does not weigh 8.6 lb. Convert 6 oz to pounds, using the conversion factor of $\frac{1 \text{ lb}}{16 \text{ oz}}$.

Here, 6 oz $\times \frac{1 \text{ lb}}{16 \text{ oz}}$ = 0.375 lb. Thus, 8 lb 6 oz = 8.375 lb.

17.2 Dosages Based on Body Weight

For Exercises 1–10, convert the following weights to kilograms. Rounding to the nearest ten.

1. 66 lb   **2.** 77 lb   **3.** 54 lb   **4.** 37 lb

5. 152 lb   **6.** 202 lb   **7.** 16 lb 4 oz   **8.** 11 lb 10 oz

9. 9 lb 14 oz   **10.** 14 lb 5 oz

For Exercises 11–22, determine if the order is safe. If it is, then determine the amount to administer.

11. The patient is a 3-day-old newborn who weighs 6 lb 5 oz.

Ordered: Nebcin® 5 mg IM q12h

On hand: Nebcin® multidose vial, 20 mg/2 mL. According to the package insert, a premature or full-term neonate up to 1 week of age may be administered up to 4 mg/kg/day in 2 equal doses every 12 h.

12. The patient is a 4-year-old child who weighs 32 lb.

Ordered: Proventil® 1 tsp syrup po tid

On hand: Proventil® Syrup, 2 mg/5 mL. According to the package insert, for children 2 to 6 years of age, dosing should be initiated at 0.1 mg/kg of body weight 3 times a day.

13. The patient is a 3-year old child who weighs 32 lb and has a severe infection.

Ordered: Amoxicillin 750 mg PO q8h

On hand: Refer to label A. According to the package label, the dosing regimen for children is 20 to 40 mg/kg/day q8h.

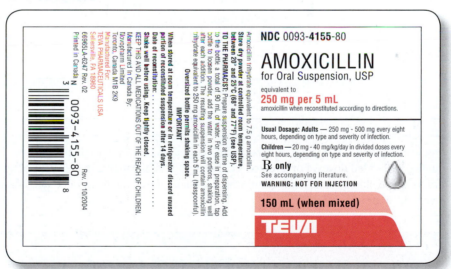

A

14. The patient is a 7-year-old child who weighs 52 lb.

Ordered: Ranitidine 30 mg IV q8h

On hand: Refer to labels B and C.

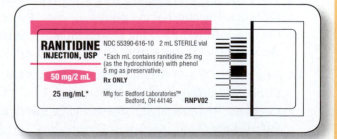

B

C

15. The patient is an 8-year-old child who weighs 55 lb and is being treated for streptococcal pharnygitis.

    Ordered: Cephalexin Susp. 200 mg PO q6h

    On hand: See label D and package insert information E below.

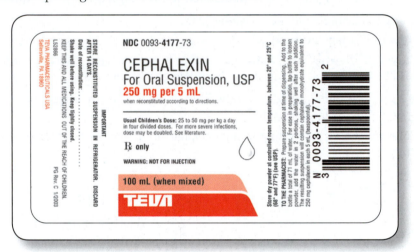

D

Pediatric Patients The usual recommended daily dosage for pediatric patients is 25 to 50 mg/kg in divided doses. For streptococcal pharyngitis in patients over 1 year of age and for skin and skin structure infections, the total daily dose may be divided and administered every 12 hours.

E

16. The patient is a 44-lb child who is $5\frac{1}{2}$ years old.

    Ordered: Tolectin 100 mg po qid

    On hand: Tolectin 200-mg scored tablets. The package insert indicates that for children 2 years and older, the usual dose ranges from 15 to 30 mg/kg/day.

17. The patient is a 44-lb child who is $5\frac{1}{2}$ years old.

    Ordered: Midazolam 1.5 mg IV

    On hand: Refer to label F. The package insert indicates that for children the usual dose ranges from 0.05–0.4 mg/kg.

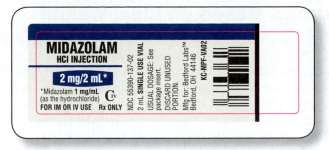

F

18. The same patient from Exercise 17 is given the following order: Midazolam 1 mg IM now.

On hand: Refer to label F. The package insert indicates that for children the usual dose ranges from 0.05–0.4 mg/kg.

19. The patient is a 4-month-old child who weighs 12 lb.

Ordered: Erythromycin suspension 65 mg po q12h

On hand: Erythromycin oral suspension 100 mg/2.5 mL. According to the package insert, the following are usual dosages for children over 3 months of age: For mild to moderate ear, nose, throat infections, either 25 mg/kg/day in divided doses every 12 h, or 20 mg/kg/day in divided doses every 8 h.

20. The patient is a 1-year-old child who weighs 18 lb.

Ordered: Erythromycin suspension 160 mg po q8h.

On hand: Refer to label G.

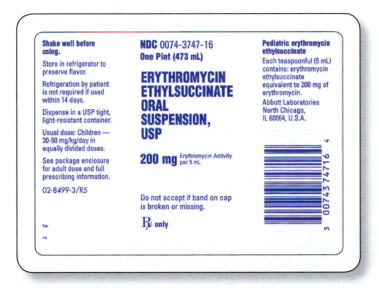

G

21. The patient weighs 47 lb.

Ordered: Antibiotic 3 mcg/kg/day IM divided in 2 equal doses

On hand: Antibiotic in 50 mcg/mL vials

22. The patient weighs 27 kg.

Ordered: Muscle relaxant 10 mg/kg/day IM daily

On hand: Muscle relaxant in 50 mg/mL suspension

To check your answers, see the Answer section at the end of the book, which begins on page A-1.

17.3 Dosages Based on Ideal Weight

A geriatric patient's body generally has a decreased proportion of lean body mass and water, along with an increased proportion of body fat. These proportions alter the distribution of drugs. Some water-soluble drugs, such as aminoglycosides (antibiotics) and digitalis preparations (cardiac medications), are strongly bound to lean tissues. Because the elderly have less lean tissue, more of these water-soluble drugs remain in the circulating blood. Higher levels can lead to toxicity. Thus, serum drug levels (the level of drug dissolved in the blood) must be monitored. Fat-soluble drugs are distributed to body fat. Because the elderly have a larger proportion of body fat, these drugs are distributed to more tissues. The drugs do not remain in the body fat, but are slowly released back into circulation. Thus, fat-soluble drugs have a longer duration of action, resulting in residual effects such as drowsiness. For medications strongly bound to lean tissues (water-soluble), the dose for an overweight patient should be based on the *ideal body weight*. For patients whose weight is below ideal, the *actual* weight should be used. For medications strongly bound to body fat (fatsoluble), the dose is based on the *actual* weight.

RULE 17-4	Determining Safe Dosages Based on Ideal Weight
	Check the package insert or product literature. Double check the order to determine if it is a safe dose based upon renal function and the ideal or actual body weight of the patient. If the dose is safe, calculate the amount to administer.
Example	A 78-year-old male, 5 ft 4 in. tall, and weighing 180 lb, is given the following order. He has normal renal function and is being treated for a serious, but not life-threatening, infection.
	Ordered: Garamycin® 70 mg IM q8h
	On hand: Garamycin® Injectable, 40 mg/mL. According to the package insert, for patients with normal renal function, the usual dosage for serious infections is 1 mg/kg q8h. The dosage for obese patients should be based on lean body mass. For a 5 ft 4 in. patient, the ideal weight range is 122 to 157 lb. Because 122 lb = 55 kg and 157 lb = 71 kg, after rounding, the safe dose for this patient is from 55 to 71 mg q8h. The dosage ordered, 70 mg, falls within that range and is safe. The amount to administer per dose is $$\frac{70 \text{ mg}}{40 \text{ mg}} \times 1 \text{ mL} = 1.75 \text{ mL rounded to } 1.8 \text{ mL}$$

GO TO . . . Open the CD-ROM that accompanies your textbook, and select Chapter 17, Ensuring Safe Dosage Based upon Ideal Weight (LO 17.3). Review the animation and example problems, then complete the practice problems. Continue to the next section of the book once you have mastered the information presented.

CRITICAL THINKING ON THE JOB

Consulting the Authorized Prescriber

While transcribing orders for Mrs. Bekins, who is 83 years old and weighs 118 lb, Karen notes that one of Mrs. Bekins' diagnoses is chronic renal failure. Mrs. Bekins has been given the following drug order: Tazidime 1 g IV q8h for pneumonia. Karen knows that safe doses of antibiotics are often lower for patients with kidney disease than usual prescribed doses. From the package insert, she knows the recommended maintenance dose for Tazidime should be adjusted based on CL_{CR}. According to a table in the insert, for creatinine clearance levels of 31 to 50 mL/min, the recommended dosage is 1 g q12h; for levels of 16 to 30 mL/min, the dosage is 1 g q24h; for levels 6 to 15 mL/min, the dosage is 500 mg q24h; and for levels < 5 mL/min, the dosage is 500 mg q48h. Karen is able to determine that the patient's creatinine clearance level is 9.5 mL/min. This value is between 6 and 15 mL/min. Therefore, the safe dose of Tazidime for the patient is 500 mg q24h. This amount is considerably less than the one indicated by the drug order.

 Think! . . . Is It Reasonable? What should Karen do? By using critical thinking skills, what patient problem was avoided?

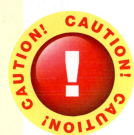

ERROR ALERT!

For Medications That Are Strongly Bound to Lean Body Tissue, Calculate an Overweight Patient's Dose on Ideal Body Weight, Not Actual Weight

Suppose a 75-year-old female, 5 ft 1 in. tall, 190 lb with a CL_{CR} of 30 mL/min is prescribed an initial daily dose of 0.25 mg of Lanoxin® injection. According to the package insert, the level of Lanoxin® is based on the patient's creatinine clearance and lean body weight, not actual body weight. The patient's safe dose is 125 mcg/day (0.125 mg/day), one-half the amount prescribed. By getting too much medication, the patient could suffer digoxin toxicity. The physician who initially ordered the Lanoxin® makes the first error. Still, the healthcare professional who administers the Lanoxin® should check the safety of the amount and verify the order with the authorized prescriber before administration.

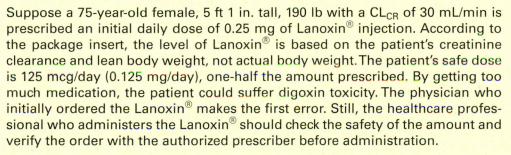

REVIEW AND PRACTICE

17.3 Dosages Based on Ideal Weight

For Exercises 1–4, determine if the dosage ordered is safe.

1. The patient: 92-year-old female, 5 ft 6 in. tall, 130 lb, and CL_{CR} of 61 mL/min. Patient is in ideal weight range.

   Ordered: Amikacin 375 mg IM q12h

   According to the package insert, patients with normal renal function may be administered 7.5 mg/kg q12h or 5 mg/kg q8h. This patient has normal renal function.

2. The patient: 76-year-old female, 5 ft 2 in. tall, 126 lb, and CL_{CR} of 50 mL/min. Patient is in ideal weight range.

   Ordered: Tazidime 1 g IV q12h

   According to the package insert, for creatinine clearance levels of 31 to 50 mL/min, the recommended dosage is 1 g q12h; for levels of 16 to 30 mL/min, the dosage is 1 g q24h; for levels of 6 to 15 mL/min, the dosage is 500 mg q24h; and for levels less than 5 mL/min, the dosage is 500 mg q48h.

3. The patient: 68-year-old male, 5 ft 7 in. tall, 188 lb, CL_{CR} of 60 mL/min, and impaired renal function. Ideal weight should be 172 lb.

   Ordered: Vancocin® HCl 150 mg IV q6h

   According to the package insert, the daily dosage for patients with normal renal function is 2 g divided into doses q6h or q12h. The daily dosage for patients with impaired renal function is 1545 mg/24 h for creatinine clearance of 100 mL/min; 1390 mg/24 h for 90 mL/min; 1235 mg/24 h for 80 mL/min; 1080 mg/24 h for 70 mL/min; 925 mg/24 h for 60 mL/min; 770 mg/24 h for 50 mL/min; 620 mg/24 h for 40 mL/min; 425 mg/24 h for 30 mL/min; 310 mg/24 h for 20 mL/min; and 155 mg/24 h for 10 mL/min.

4. The patient: 79-year-old female, 5 ft tall, 110 lb, CL_{CR} of 90 mL/min, and normal renal function. Patient is within ideal weight range.

   Ordered: Vancocin® HCl 0.5 g IV q6h

   See Exercise 3 above for information about the recommended daily dosage.

For Exercises 5 and 6, determine if the dosage ordered is safe. Then find the amount to administer.

5. The patient: 75-year-old female, 5 ft 3 in. tall, 198 lb, CL_{CR} of 56 mL/min, diagnosed with hypertension and renal impairment. Ideal weight should be 152 lb.

   Ordered: Vasotec® 2.5 mg po daily

   On hand: Vasotec® 5-mg scored tablets

   According to the package insert, the usual dose for patients with normal renal function (over 80 mL/min creatinine clearance) is 5 mg/day; for mild impairment (over 30 and up to 80 mL/min), 5 mg/day; for moderate to severe impairment (30 or less mL/min), 2.5 mg/day.

6. The patient: 81-year-old male, 5 ft tall, 138 lb, CL_{CR} of 63 mL/min, and renal impairment. Patient is within ideal weight range.

   Ordered: Ticarcillin 2 g IV q4h

   On hand: Ticar 1-g vial, 200 mg/mL when reconstituted

   According to the package insert, the usual dose, after the initial loading dose, for patients with infections complicated by renal insufficiency, is 3 g q4h with creatinine clearance over 60 mL/min; 2 g q4h for 30 to 60 mL/min; 2 g q8h for 10 to 30 mL/min; 2 g q12h for less than 10 mL/min; other amounts for patients with complications.

To check your answers, see the Answer section at the end of the book, which begins on page A-1.

17.4 Dosages Based on Body Surface Area (BSA)

Some medications are prescribed based on a patient's body weight. Others factor in both weight and height to determine a patient's **body surface area,** or BSA. Many pediatric medications use a patient's BSA to determine the daily dosage. BSA is also important for burn victims and for patients undergoing chemotherapy, radiation treatments, and open heart surgery. BSA calculations are used to provide more accurate dosage calculations specific to the patient's size and severity of the illness.

Calculating a Patient's BSA

A patient's BSA is stated in square meters (m^2) You can calculate the BSA by using one of the two formulas listed in Rule 17-5. Your calculator should have a program or button that will help you find a square root ($\sqrt{}$) You can also use a special chart called a *nomogram*. **Nomograms** provide an estimate of BSA and are easier to use. Nomograms are available for children and adults. See Figures 17-7 and 17-8 on the next page.

RULE 17-5	Calculating the Body Surface Area Using a Formula To determine a patient's BSA (body surface area): **1.** If you know the height in centimeters and weight in kilograms, calculate $$BSA = \sqrt{\frac{\text{height (cm)} \times \text{weight (kg)}}{3600}} \; m^2$$ **2.** If you know the height in inches and weight in pounds, calculate $$BSA = \sqrt{\frac{\text{height (in)} \times \text{weight (lb)}}{3131}} \; m^2$$ *Note: When using a formula to calculate BSA, if the result is less than one, round to the nearest hundredth. When the result is greater than one, round to the nearest tenth.*
Example 1	Find the body surface area for a child who is 85 cm tall and weighs 13.9 kg. Use the first of the formulas from Rule 17-5. $$BSA = \sqrt{\frac{85 \times 13.9}{3600}} \; m^2 = \sqrt{\frac{1181.5}{3600}} \; m^2 = 0.572 \; m^2 = 0.57 \; m^2$$
Example 2	Find the body surface area for a baby who is 24 in. tall and who weighs 12 lb × oz. Use the second of the formulas from Rule 17-5. First, convert the pounds and ounces to pounds. 12 lb 3 oz = 12.2 lb $$BSA = \sqrt{\frac{24 \times 12.2}{3131}} \; m^2 = \sqrt{\frac{292.8}{3131}} \; m^2 = 0.305 \; m^2 = 0.31 \; m^2$$
Example 3	Find the body surface area for an adult who is 5 ft 6 in. tall and who weighs 168 lb. First, convert the height to inches. Since 1 ft equals 12 in., multiply the number of feet by 12 and then add the inches. 5 × 12 = 60 60 + 6 = 66 in. $$BSA = \sqrt{\frac{66 \times 168}{3131}} \; m^2 = \sqrt{\frac{11,088}{3131}} \; m^2 = 1.88 \; m^2 = 1.9 \; m^2$$

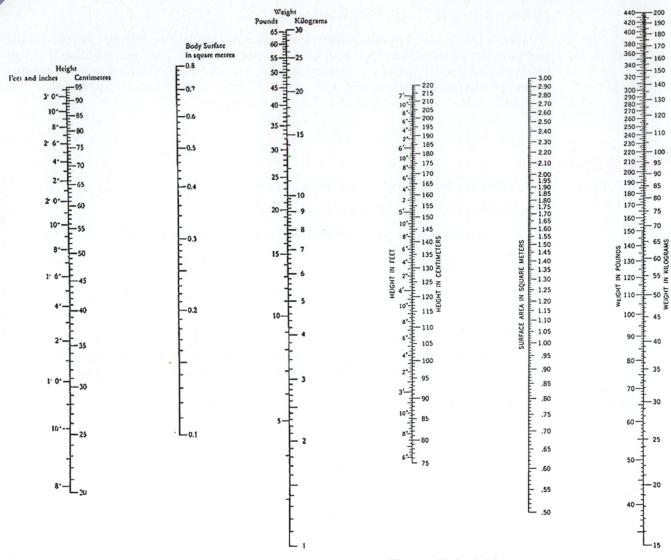

Figure 17-7   Child's nomogram.

Figure 17-8   Adult's nomogram.

GO TO . . . Open the CD-ROM that accompanies your textbook, and select Chapter 17, Calculating BSA-Formula (LO 17.3). Review the animation and example problems, then complete the practice problems. Continue to the next section of the book once you have mastered the information presented.

RULE 17-6	**Calculating the Body Surface Area by Using a Nomogram**
	Using a straightedge (such as a ruler or piece of paper), align the straightedge so that it intersects at the height and weight. Doing so will create an intersection in the BSA scale. *Note: Read the calibrations carefully, the spaces and lines vary based upon where you intersect the line.*
Example 1	Find the body surface area for a child who is 95 cm tall and weighs 13.9 kg, using the child's nomogram (Figure 17-9). $BSA = 0.60 \text{ m}^2$

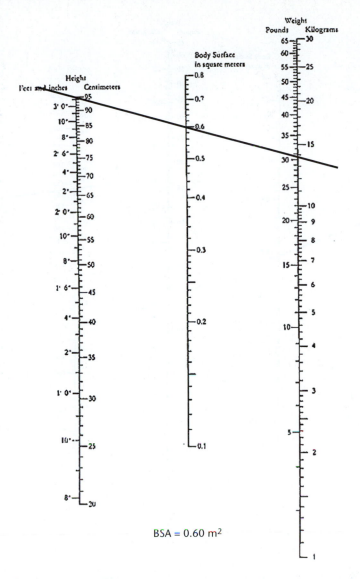

Height
Feet and inches   Centimeters

Body Surface
in square meters

Weight
Pounds   Kilograms

BSA = 0.60 m²

Figure 17-9 Child nomogram for Example 1.

Example 2	Find the body surface area for a baby who is 24 in. tall and weighs 12 lb 3 oz, using the child's nomogram (Figure 17-10). $\qquad$ BSA = 0.29 m²
Example 3	Find the body surface area for an adult who is 5 ft 6 in. tall and who weighs 168 lb, using the adult nomogram (Figure 17-11). $\qquad$ BSA = 1.9 m²

GO TO . . . Open the CD-ROM that accompanies your textbook, and select Chapter 17, Calculate BSA-Nomogram (LO 17.3). Review the animation and example problems, then complete the practice problems. Continue to the next section of the book once you have mastered the information presented.

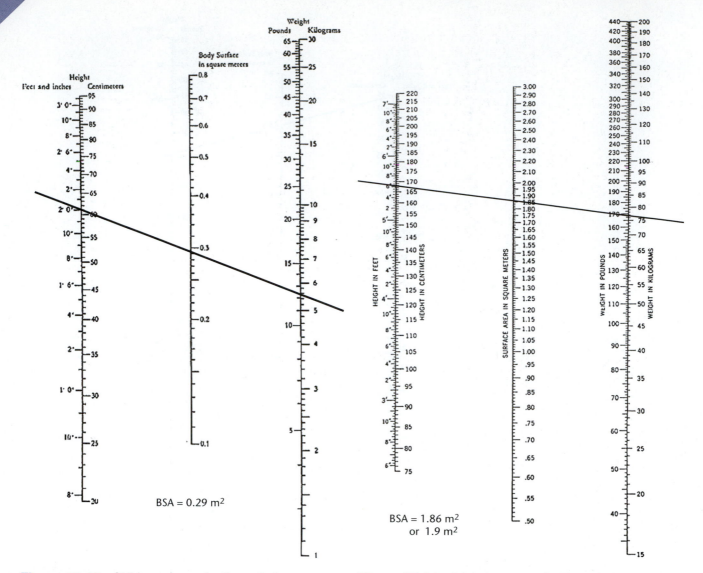

BSA = 0.29 m²

BSA = 1.86 m²
or 1.9 m²

Figure 17-10   Child nomogram for Example 2.

Figure 17-11   Adult nomogram for Example 3.

RULE 17-7	Calculating Dosage Based on BSA
	Step A: Convert Convert the height and weight into BSA m².
	Step B: Calculate Calculate the desired dose: mg/m² × m² (or mcg/m² × m² or units/m² × m² . . . .)
	Step C: Think! . . . Is It Reasonable? Confirm whether the desired dose is safe. If it is unsafe, consult the physician who wrote the order.
	If the dose is safe, calculate the amount to administer, using the proportion method, dimensional analysis, or the formula method.
Example 1	Ordered: CeeNU® (first dose) 140 mg now for a patient whose height is 38 in. and weight is 47 lb. According to the package insert, the first recommended dose of CeeNU® is a single oral dose providing 130 mg/m².
	Step A: Convert Convert the height and weight into BSA m².

Because the recommended dose is per square meter (m^2), you need to find the patient's BSA. You know the patient's height and weight in inches and pounds. Use the second formula in Rule 17-5 or a nomogram.

$$BSA = \sqrt{\frac{\text{height (in.)} \times \text{weight (lb)}}{3131}}\ m^2$$

$$BSA = \sqrt{\frac{38 \times 47}{3131}}\ m^2 = \sqrt{\frac{1786}{3131}}\ m^2 = 0.76\ m^2$$

Step B: Calculate
Calculate the desired dose.

$$\frac{130\ mg}{m^2} \times 0.76\ m^2 = 98.8\ mg$$

Step C: Think! . . . Is It Reasonable?
CeeNU® is available in 100-mg, 40-mg, and 10-mg capsules. The dose ordered, 140 mg, is above the first recommended dose of 98.8 mg. Consult the authorized prescriber who wrote the order.

No calculation is necessary at this time.

Example 2

Ordered: CeeNU® (first dose) 150 mg now for a patient who is 99 cm tall and weighs 50 kg. According to the package insert, the first recommended dose of CeeNU® is a single oral dose providing 130 mg/m^2.

Step A: Convert
Convert the height and weight into BSA m^2.

Use the first formula in Rule 17-5.

$$BSA = \sqrt{\frac{99 \times 50}{3600}}\ m^2 = \sqrt{\frac{4950}{3600}}\ m^2 = 1.2\ m^2.$$

Step B: Calculate
Calculate the desired dose.

$$\frac{130\ mg}{m^2} \times 1.2\ m^2 = 156\ mg$$

Step C: Think! . . . Is It Reasonable?
The dose ordered is safe since the dose or 150 mg is less than the calculated desired dose 156 mg.

Calculate the amount to administer. CeeNU® is available in 100-mg, 40-mg, and 10-mg capsules. Thinking critically and realizing the capsules cannot be divided you must provide the dose to the nearest whole number. This would be 150 mg. You determine to administer 1 capsule of each strength, 100 mg + 40 mg + 10 mg.

REVIEW AND PRACTICE

17.4 Dosages Based on Body Surface Area (BSA)

For Exercises 1–8, use the appropriate formula to calculate the BSA for patients with the following heights and weights.

1. 88 cm and 13.2 kg
2. 58 cm and 21 kg
3. 38 cm and 6 kg
4. 48 cm and 10 kg

5. 52 in and 64 lb
6. 43 in and 35 lb
7. 22 in and 18 lb
8. 26 in and 21 lb

For Exercises 9–12, calculate the recommended dosage in the appropriate unit.

9. The child's BSA is 0.82 m². The recommended dosage is 175 mcg/m².

10. The child's BSA is 0.65 m². The recommended dosage is 0.4 mg/m².

11. The child's height is 62 cm and weight is 5 kg. The recommended dosage is 50 mcg/m².

12. The child's height is 41 in. and weight is 63 lb. The recommended dosage is 0.2 mg/m².

For Exercises 13–16, calculate the amount to administer.

13. The patient is 42 in. tall and weighs 71 lb.
Ordered: Chemotherapy medication 6 mg/m²/day IV q12h
On hand: Chemotherapy medication 200 mcg/mL for IV use.

14. The patient is 86 cm tall and weighs 12 kg.
Ordered: Antibiotic 25 mg/m²/day IM q6h
On hand: Antibiotic 2 mg/mL for IM use.

15. The patient is 34 cm tall and weighs 5 kg.
Ordered: Cerubidine® 25 mg/m² IV weekly
On hand: Cerubidine® for injection. When reconstituted, each milliliter contains 5 mg of drug. The recommended pediatric dosage is 25 mg/m² IV the first day every week.

16. The patient, who is over 1 year old, is 42 in. tall and weighs 45 lb.
Ordered: Oncaspar® 2500 International Units/m² IM every 14 days
On hand: Oncaspar® 5 mL/vial, 750 International Units/mL. The recommended pediatric dosage is 2500 International Units/m² for children whose BSA is greater than or equal to 0.6 m² and 82.5 IU/kg for children whose BSA is less than 0.6 m².

For exercises 17–18, determine if the order is safe. If so, calculate the amount to administer.

17. The patient is 125 cm tall and weighs 45 kg.
Ordered: Gemzar® 800 mg IV weekly.
On hand: Refer to label A. The usual dose is 1000 mg/m² over 30-min IV.

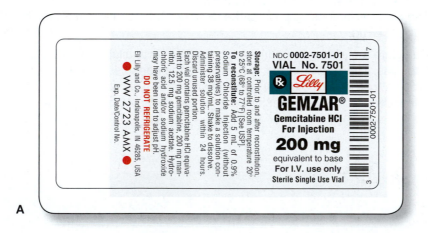

A

18. The patient is 63 in. tall and weighs 125 lb.

Ordered: Cisplatin 125 mg IV every four weeks

On hand: Refer to label B. The usual dose is 75 to 100 mg/m².

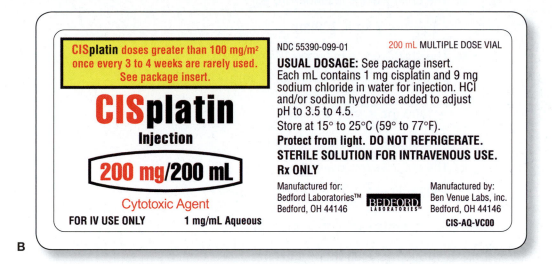

B

To check your answers, see the Answer section at the end of the book, which begins on page A-1.

17.5 Daily Maintenance Fluid Needs (DMFN)

Children's bodies contain a higher percentage of water than adults' bodies. Children, as well as critically ill patients, are at greater risk for fluid overload, dehydration, or electrolyte imbalances. Therefore, you must monitor not only the amount of medication but also the amount of fluid the patient receives. Fluids may be calculated based on body weight, body surface area (BSA), metabolism, or age.

Daily maintenance fluid needs (DMFN) represent the fluid a patient needs over 24 h. It combines maintenance fluids (both orally and parenterally), medications, diluent for medications, and fluids used to flush the injection port. The amount of maintenance fluid required varies according to weight, with the smallest children requiring 100 mL/kg/day. DMFN does not include fluids needed to replace those lost to vomiting, diarrhea, or fever. These are called *replacement fluids* and are based on each patient's condition.

RULE 17-8

To calculate daily maintenance fluid needs (DMFN) based on weight:

1. If the patient weighs up to 10 kg, find

$$\frac{100 \text{ mL}}{1 \text{ kg}} \times \text{kg} = \text{DMFN mL}$$

2. If the patient weighs 10 to 20 kg, find

$$1000 \text{ mL} + \left[\frac{50 \text{ mL}}{1 \text{ kg}} \times (\text{kg} - 10)\right] = \text{DMFN mL}$$

3. If the patient weighs over 20 kg, find

$$1500 \text{ mL} + \left[\frac{20 \text{ mL}}{1 \text{ kg}} \times (\text{kg} - 20)\right] = \text{DMFN mL}$$

Example 1

Find the DMFN for a patient who weighs

    a. 7 kg   **b.** 16 kg   **c.** 24 kg

    a. The child weighs less than 10 kg.

$$\frac{100 \text{ mL}}{1 \text{ kg}} \times 7 \text{ kg} = 700 \text{ mL}$$

    b. The child weighs between 10 and 20 kg.

$$1000 \text{ mL} + \left[\frac{50 \text{ mL}}{1 \text{ kg}} \times (16 \text{ kg} - 10) \right]$$

$$= 1000 \text{ mL} + \left[\frac{50 \text{ mL}}{1} \times 6 \right]$$

$$= 1000 \text{ mL} + 300 \text{ mL} = 1300 \text{ mL}$$

    c. The child weighs over 20 kg.

$$1500 \text{ mL} + \left[\frac{20 \text{ mL}}{1 \text{ kg}} \times (24 \text{ kg} - 20) \right]$$

$$= 1500 \text{ mL} + \left[\frac{20 \text{ mL}}{1} \times 4 \right]$$

$$= 1500 \text{ mL} + 80 \text{ mL} = 1580 \text{ mL}$$

Example 2

What is the flow rate using microdrip tubing for DMFN for a child who weighs 14 kg? Find the DMFN. The patient weighs between 10 and 20 kg.

$$1000 \text{ mL} + \left[\frac{50 \text{ mL}}{1 \text{ kg}} \times (14 \text{ kg} - 10) \right]$$

$$= 1000 \text{ mL} + \left[\frac{50 \text{ mL}}{1} \times 4 \right]$$

$$= 1000 \text{ mL} + 200 \text{ mL} = 1200 \text{ mL}$$

LEARNING LINK   Recall from Chapter 15, that microdrip tubing has a drop factor of 60 gtt/mL.

Next, find the microdrip tubing flow rate for 1200 mL/day.

$$\frac{1200 \text{ mL}}{1 \text{ day}} \times \frac{1 \text{ day}}{24 \text{ h}} \times \frac{1 \text{ h}}{60 \text{ min}} \times \frac{60 \text{ gtt}}{1 \text{ mL}}$$

$$= \frac{1200 \times 60 \text{ gtt}}{24 \times 60 \text{ min}} = \frac{50 \text{ gtt}}{1 \text{ min}}$$

LEARNING LINK   The flow rate is 50 gtt/min. Recall from Chapter 15 that for microdrip tubing, $\frac{\text{mL}}{\text{h}} = \frac{\text{gtt}}{\text{min}}$. In this example, the patient should receive

$$\frac{1200 \text{ mL}}{24 \text{ h}} = \frac{50 \text{ mL}}{1 \text{ h}} = \frac{50 \text{ gtt}}{1 \text{ min}}$$

Example 3

Find the DMFN for a patient who weighs 154 lb. What would be the IV flow rate F mL/h? First convert 154 lb to kilograms.

$$154 \text{ lb} \times \frac{1 \text{ kg}}{2.2 \text{ lb}} = 70 \text{ kg}$$

The patient weighs over 20 kg.

$$1500 + \left[\frac{20 \text{ mL}}{1 \text{ kg}} \times (70 \text{ kg} - 20) \right] = \text{DMFN mL}$$

$$2500 \text{ mL} = \text{DMFN}$$

$$\frac{2500 \text{ mL}}{24 \text{ h}} = \frac{104.1 \text{ mL}}{1 \text{ h}} = 104 \text{ mL/h}$$

rounded to nearest whole number

If this patient took 1300 mL of fluids by mouth, what would be the flow rate for the IV in milliliters per hour?

$$2500 - 1300 = 1200 \text{ mL IV fluids needed in 24 h}$$

$$\frac{1200 \text{ mL}}{24 \text{ h}} = \frac{50 \text{ mL}}{1 \text{ h}} = 50 \text{ mL/h}$$

RULE 17-9 | For pediatric and critically ill patients, the amount of solution in the IV tubing must be considered when you determine infusion times and volumes.

Five feet of standard IV tubing contains about 10 mL of solution. If this tubing is used along with a volume control chamber, a child will not begin receiving medication until the 10 mL of solution already in the tubing has infused. Low-volume (small-diameter) tubing contains only 0.3 mL of solution per 5 ft and effectively eliminates this problem. Additionally most medical facilities will use electronic flow regulators or infusion pumps to ensure accuracy of medications delivered.

GO TO . . . Open the CD-ROM that accompanies your textbook, and select Chapter 17, Daily Maintenance Fluid Needs (DMFN) (LO 17.5). Review the animation and example problems, then complete the practice problems. Continue to the next section of the book once you have mastered the information presented.

REVIEW AND PRACTICE

17.5 Daily Maintenance Fluid Needs

For Exercises 1–5, calculate the daily maintenance fluid needs, based on the following weights.

1. 8 kg   **2.** 33 kg   **3.** 37 lb   **4.** 58 lb   **5.** 121 lb

In Exercises 6–10, find the microdrip tubing flow rate for DMFN for patients, based on the following weights.

6. 21 kg   **7.** 15 kg   **8.** 17 lb   **9.** 41 lb   **10.** 165 lb

For Exercises 11 and 12, determine the recommended IV flow rate.

11. A patient who weighs 180 lb had an oral intake of 1000 mL. What should be the flow rate of his IV per hour to maintain his fluids?

12. A patient weighs 31 kg and has an oral intake of 200 mL. What would be the flow rate of his IV per hour to maintain fluids?

To check your answers, see the Answer–section at the end of the book, which begins on page A-1.

LEARNING OUTCOME	KEY POINTS

17.1 Identify factors that impact drug dosing in special populations. Pages 473–480	1. Pharmacokinetics—the study of how drugs are used by the body.
	
	  a. Absorption—movement of drug into the bloodstream
	
	  b. Distribution—movement of drug from bloodstream into body fluids/tissues
	
	  c. Biotransformation—chemical changing of a drug in the body (liver)
	
	  d. Elimination—excretion of a drug via exhalation or body secretions (urine, sweat, feces, breast milk)
	
	2. Age-Related Variables
	
	  a. Pediatric (age <18)—increased metabolism, less stomach acid, thinner skin, immature liver, decreased circulation to muscles
	
	  b. Geriatric—(age > 65)
	
	    i. Creatinine Clearance (CL_{CR})—an indicator of the rate at which kidneys excrete waste, CL_{CR} decreases with age
	
	    ii. Polypharmacy—the practice of taking multiple medications at the same time; polypharmacy leads to drug interactions.

17.2 Calculate safe dosages based on body weight. Pages 480–493	Three Step Method:
	
	Step A: Convert weight to kg
	
	Step B: Calculate the desired dose: mg/kg $\times$ kg (or mcg/kg $\times$ kg or Units/kg $\times$ kg . . .)
	
	Step C: Think! . . . Is It Reasonable? Confirm the desired dose is safe.
	
	Example: Tobramycin 50 mg IV q8h is ordered for a 44 lb child. The safe dose range is 2–2.5 mg/kg q8h. Is the ordered dose safe?
	
	Step A: Convert
	    44 lb $\times$ 1 kg/2.2 lb = 20 kg
	
	Step B: Calculate
	    2 mg/kg $\times$ 20 kg = 40 mg;
	    2.5 mg/kg $\times$ 20 kg = 50 mg
	
	Step C: Think . . . Is It Reasonable? Since the safe range is 40 to 50 mg q8h and the ordered dose is 50 mg q8h, the ordered dose is safe/reasonable.

LEARNING OUTCOME	KEY POINTS
17.3 Determine safe doses based on ideal weight vs. actual weight. Pages 493–496	When distribution of drugs is altered due to a change in lean body mass, safe doses should be calculated based on ideal body weight instead of actual body weight. Example: Gentamicin 75 mg IV q8h is ordered for a 5 ft, 6 in, 200 lb male for treatment of infection. The usual dose is 1 mg/kg/day. The dose for obese patients with normal renal function should be based on ideal body weight. The ideal weight for a 5 ft, 6 in. male is 136 to 164 lb **Step A: Convert** $\qquad$ 136 lb × 1 kg/2.2 lb/kg = 61.8; $\qquad$ 164 lb × 1 kg/2.2.lb/kg = 74.5 kg **Step B: Calculate** $\qquad$ 1 mg/kg × 61.8 kg = 61.8 mg; $\qquad$ 1 mg/kg × 74.5 kg = 74.5 mg **Step C: Think . . . Is It Reasonable?** Since the ordered dose 75 mg, falls in the range of 62 to 75 mg, the order is safe/reasonable.
17.4 Calculate safe dosages based on body surface area (BSA). Pages 496–502	Body surface area incorporates both the height and weight of the patient and can be determined in one of two ways: 1. Using a formula: $\quad$ a. $\text{BSA in m}^2 = \sqrt{\dfrac{(\text{ht (cm)} \times \text{wt (kg)})}{3600}}$ $\quad$ b. $\text{BSA in m}^2 = \sqrt{\dfrac{(\text{ht (in)} \times \text{wt (lb)})}{3131}}$ 2. Using a nomogram and aligning the height and weight with a straightedge and locating the BSA in the center Safe dose calculations using BSA are used for medications that require very precise amounts. Calculating safe doses based on BSA is a three-step process: **Step A: Convert** height and weight into BSA (m^2) **Step B: Calculate** the desired dose $\text{mg/m}^2 \times \text{m}^2$ $\qquad$ (or $\text{mcg/m}^2 \times \text{m}^2 \dots$) **Step C: Think . . . Is It Reasonable?** Confirm the desired dose is safe. Example: 1000 mg of calcium EDTA is ordered for a 6 ft, 3 in. patient who weighs 185 lb. The safe dose calcium EDTA is 500 mg/m^2. Is the dose ordered safe?

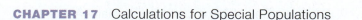

LEARNING OUTCOME	KEY POINTS

17.5 Calculate Daily Maintenance Fluid Needs (DMFN). Pages 503–505	**Step A: Convert**
	
	▸ ft to in. to cm: 6 ft, 3 in. = 75 inches; 75 in. × 2.5 cm/in. = 187.5 cm
	
	▸ lb to kg: 185 lb divided by 2.2 lb/kg = 84.1 kg
	
	▸ height and weight to BSA in m²:
	
	   • $\sqrt{\dfrac{(30\text{ cm} \times 84.1\text{ kg})}{3600}} = 2.1\text{ m}^2$ or
	
	   • $\sqrt{\dfrac{(75\text{ in.} \times 185\text{ lb})}{3131}} = 2.1\text{ m}^2$
	
	Step B: Calculate
	
	    $500\text{ mg/m}^2 \times 2.1\text{ m}^2 = 1050\text{ mg}$
	
	Step C: Think . . . Is It Reasonable? Since the dose ordered (1000 mg) is close to and does not exceed the safe dose (1050 mg), the order is reasonable.
	
	Calculation of DMFN is based on weight in kilograms:
	
	▸ Up to 10 kg: 100 mL/kg
	
	▸ 10–20 kg: 1000 mL + (50 mL/kg × [kg − 10])
	
	▸ Over 20 kg: 1500 mL + (20 mL/kg × [kg − 20])
	
	Example 1: Patient weighs 7.3 kg; 100 mL/kg × 7.3 kg = 730 mL/day
	
	Example 2: Patient weighs 12 kg; 1000 mL + (50 mL/kg × [2]) = 1100 mL/day
	
	Example 3: Patient weighs 24 kg; 1500 mL + (20 mL/kg × [4]) = 1580 mL/day

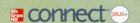
Answer the following questions.

1. List and explain the four processes in the body that affect a drug after it is administered. (LO 17.1)

2. Name two special populations of patients who require extra consideration when calculating medication dosages. (LO 17.1)

3. List four age-related factors that may affect the dosage of a medication for a pediatric patient. (LO 17.1)

4. List four age-related factors that may affect the dosage of a medication for a geriatric patient. (LO 17.1)

5. Explain the impact of creatinine clearance on drug dosages. (LO 17.1)

6. Explain the term "recommended dosage range." (LO 17.2)

7. Body surface area (BSA) uses what two body measurements to provide a more accurate dosage? (LO 17.4)

8. Explain the difference between daily maintenance fluids and replacement fluids. (LO 17.5)

9. What type of medication is strongly bound to lean tissue? (LO 17.1)

10. When would the dose of a medication be calculated on ideal body weight rather than actual weight? (LO 17.3)

11. Explain why a medication dosage may be altered based on the patient's result of a creatine clearance test. (LO 17.3)

12. Define the term polypharmacy and explain how it would increase the risk of drug interactions in a geriatric patient. (LO 17.1)

For Exercises 13–18, use the identified drug labels and package insert information to answer the following questions: (LO 17.2)

13. What is the safe initial dosage range of Depakene® for a 4-year-old child weighing 41.8 pounds? See label A and package insert information.

14. If 850 mg of Depakene® is ordered, what amount would you administer? See label A and package insert information.

Depakene® package insert information:

> PO (children) initial dose of
> 15–45 mg/kg/day

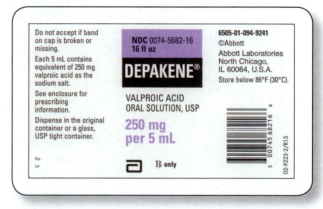

Label A

15. Calculate the correct dosage of Kytril® and amount to administer for a 7-year-old child weighing 61.6 pounds. See label B and package insert information.

Kytril® package insert information:

> IV (adults & children 2–16 yr.) 10 mcg/kg within 30 min. prior to chemotherapy

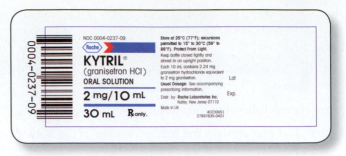

Label B

16. Calculate the safe IM dosage range of clindamycin for a 3-week-old infant weighing 6 pounds 12 ounces. See label C and package insert information.

17. Calculate the safe IM dosage range of clindamycin for a 3-year-old weighing 33 pounds. See label C and package insert information.

Clindamycin package insert information:

> IM, IV (infants <1 month) 3.75–5 mg/kg every 6 hours
> IM, IV (children >1 month) 5–13.3 mg/kg every 8 hours

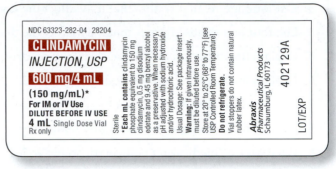

Label C

18. Calculate the safe dosage range of gammagard liquid for a 66-year-old woman weighing 110 pounds. See label D and package insert information. (LO 17.2)

19. If the order for gammagard is 15 g, what amount would you administer? See label D and package insert information. (LO 17.2)

Gammagard Liquid package insert information:

> Monthly doses of approximately 300–600 mg/kg infused at 3 to 4 week intervals are commonly used.

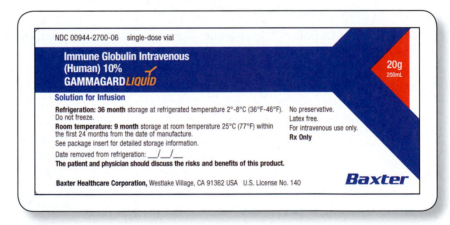

Label D

20. Using the blank nomogram, label E and the package insert information, calculate the correct dosage of Camptosar® for a 5 ft 8 in. tall, 70-year-old man weighing 170 pounds. (LO 17.4)

NOMOGRAM

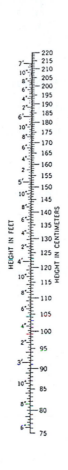
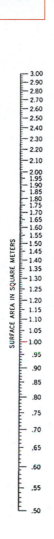
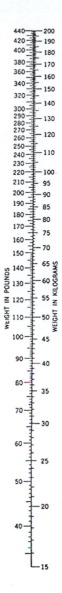

Camptosar® package insert information

CAMPTOSAR® 180 mg/m² as 90-minute infusion

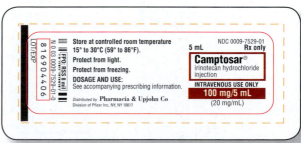

Label E

CHECK UP

In Exercises 1–4, convert the following weights to kilograms. (LO 17.2)

1. 49 lb   **2.** 61 lb   **3.** 6 lb 9 oz   **4.** 12 lb 13 oz

In Exercises 5–8, calculate the BSA for patients with the following heights and weights. (LO 17.4)

5. 105 cm and 19 kg   **6.** 74 cm and 12.1 kg   **7.** 41 in. and 33 lb   **8.** 30 in. and 23 lb

In Exercises 9–15, determine if the order is safe. If it is, then determine the amount to administer.

9. The child weighs 30 lb. (LO 17.2)

Ordered: Depakene® syrup 100 mg po q12h

On hand: Depakene® syrup 250 mg/5 mL. According to the package insert, the initial daily dose for pediatric patients is 15 mg/kg/day.

10. The patient is a 4-year-old child who weighs 16 kg. (LO 17.2)

Ordered: Ventolin syrup 1.6 mg po tid

On hand: Ventolin syrup 2 mg/5 mL. According to the package insert, for children from 2 to 6 years of age, dosing should be initiated at 0.1 mg/kg of body weight 3 times a day. This starting dosage should not exceed 2 mg 3 times a day.

11. The patient is 72 cm tall and weighs 16 kg. (LO 17.4)

Ordered: Oncaspar® 1300 IU IM every 14 days

On hand: Oncaspar® 5 mL/vial, 750 International Units/mL. The recommended pediatric dosage is 2500 International Units/m^2 for children whose BSA is greater than or equal to 0.6 m^2 and 82.5 International Units/kg for children whose BSA is less than 0.6 m^2.

12. The child weighs 31 kg. (LO 17.2)

Ordered: Biaxin® susp 225 mg po q12h × 10

On hand: Refer to label A. According to the package insert, the usual recommended daily dosage for children is 15 mg/kg/day for 10 days.

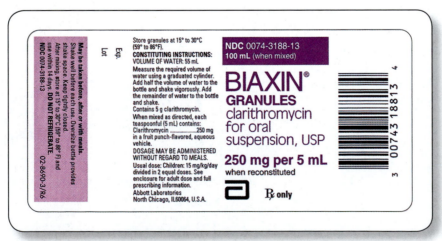

A

13. The child weighs 66 lb. (LO 17.2)

Ordered: Oxcarbazepine 150 mg po BID

On hand: Refer to label B. According to the package insert. Treatment should be initiated at a daily <u>dose</u> of 8–10 mg/kg generally not to exceed 600 mg/day, given in a BID regimen. The <u>target</u> maintenance <u>dose</u> of Trileptal® should be achieved over 2 weeks and is dependent upon <u>patient</u> weight, according to the following chart:

20–29 kg	900 mg/day
29.1–39 kg	1200 mg/day
39 kg	1800 mg/day

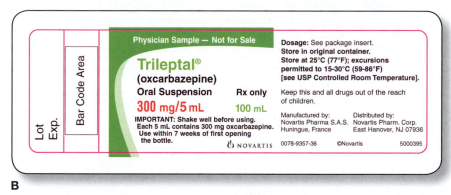

B

14. The patient is a 58-lb child with severe infection. (LO 17.2)

Ordered: Erythromycin 650 mg PO tid.

On hand: Refer to label C. According to the package insert, in mild to moderate infections the usual dosage of erythromycin ethylsuccinate for children is 30 to 50 mg/kg/day in equally divided doses every 6 hours. For more severe infections this dosage may be doubled. If twice-a-day dosage is desired, one-half of the total daily dose may be given every 12 hours. Doses may also be given three times daily by administering one-third of the total daily dose every 8 hours.

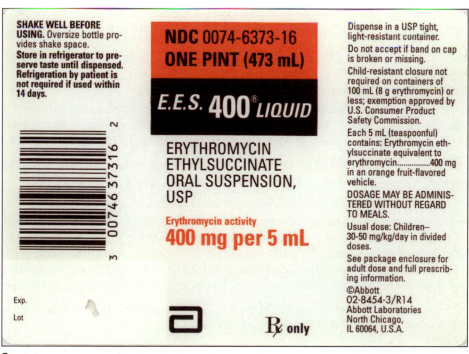

C

15. The patient is a 25-kg child receiving myelosuppressive chemotherapy. (LO 17.2)

Ordered: Neupogen® 125 mcg IVPB over 30 min

On hand: Refer to label D. According to the package insert, for patients receiving myelosuppressive chemotherapy, the recommended daily starting dose is 5 mcg/kg/day, administered as a single daily injection by subcut bolus injection, by short IV infusion (15 to 30 min), or by continuous <u>subcut</u> or continuous IV infusion.

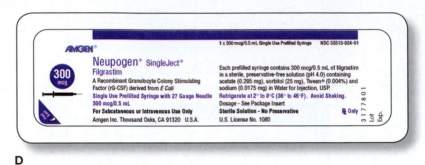

D

In Exercises 16–18, calculate the daily maintenance fluid needs, based on the following weights. Then find the flow rate in milliliters per hour (*F*) for the DMFN. (LO 17.5)

16. 24 kg

17. 39 lb

18. 110 lb (The patient has taken 800 mL fluid orally.)

19. Define creatinine clearance and describe its impact on pharmacokinetics. (LO 17.1)

For Exercises 20–25, determine if the dosage ordered is safe. If the order is safe, then find the amount to administer. Assume that the patients have impaired renal functions. (LO 17.3)

20. The patient: 85-year-old male, 6 ft 1 in. tall, 210 lb, CL_{CR} of 64 mL/min. Ideal weight should be 195 lb.

Ordered: Cartrol 2.5 mg po q24h

On hand: Cartrol 2.5 mg/tablet

According to the package insert, the usual dosage interval for 2.5 mg is as follows: for patients with creatinine clearance above 60 mL/min, 24 h; for 20 to 60 mL/min, 48 h; and for less than 20 mL/min, 72 h.

21. The patient: 68-year-old female, 5 ft 5 in. tall, 166 lb, CL_{CR} of 60 mL/min. Ideal weight should be 162 lb.

Ordered: Capastat 600 mg IM qd

On hand: Capastat sulfate, diluted to 300 mg/mL

According to the package insert, the estimated daily dosage required to maintain a steady level of drug is 1.29 mg/kg for creatinine clearance of 0 mL/min; 2.43 mg/kg for 10 mL/min; 3.58 mg/kg for 20 mL/ min; 4.72 mg/kg for 30 mL/min; 5.87 mg/kg for 40 mL/min; 7.01 mg/kg for 50 mL/min; and 8.16 mg/kg for 60 mL/min.

22. The patient: 82-year-old female, 4 ft 10 in. tall, 102 lb, CL_{CR} of 26 mL/min. Patient is within ideal weight range.

Ordered: Acyclovir sodium (Zovirax®) 450 mg IV q12h infused over 1 h

On hand: Zovirax® for injection, 50 mg/mL when reconstituted

According to the package insert, the recommended dose for this diagnosis for patients with normal renal function is 10 mg/kg q8h. The dose is adjusted as follows for patients with impaired renal function: for creatinine clearance over 50 mL/min, 100 percent of the recommended dose every 8 h; from 25 to 50 mL/min, 100 percent of the recommended dose every 12 h; from 10 to 25 mL/min, 100 percent of the recommended dose every 24 h; for 0 to 10 mL/min, 50 percent of the recommended dose every 24 h.

23. The patient: 73-year-old male, 5 ft 8 in. tall, 154 lb, CL_{CR} of 49 mL/min, diagnosed with a complicated urinary tract infection. Patient is within ideal weight range.

Ordered: Fortaz® 1 g IV q12h

On hand: Fortaz® for injection, reconstituted at 10 mg/mL

According to the package insert, the usual recommended dosage for patients with complicated urinary tract infections is 500 mg to 1 g given q8–12h. For patients with renal insufficiency, the following maintenance dosages are recommended (however, if the usual dosage is less, administer the lower amount): for creatinine clearance of 31 to 50 mL/min, 1 g q12h; for 16 to 30 mL/min, 1 g q24h; for 6 to 15 mL/min, 500 mg q24h; for less than 5 mL/min, 500 mg q48h.

24. The patient: 79-year-old male, 5 ft 9 in. tall, 149 lb, CL_{CR} of 55 mL/min. The patient does not have a life-threatening infection. Patient is within ideal weight range.

    Ordered: Mandol 2 g IV q6h

    On hand: Mandol reconstituted to 1 g/10 mL

    According to the package insert, for patients with renal impairment and less severe infections, the following maintenance dosages are recommended: for creatinine clearance of over 80 mL/min, 1 to 2 g q6h; for 50 to 80 mL/min, 0.75 to 1.5 g q6h; for 25 to 50 mL/min, 0.75 to 1.5 g q8h; for 10 to 25 mL/min, 0.5 to 1 g q8h; for 2 to 10 mL/min, 0.5 to 0.75 g q12h; for less than 2 mL/min, 0.25 to 0.5 g q12h.

25. The patient: 92-year-old female, 5 ft 1 in. tall, 112 lb, CL_{CR} of 32 mL/min. Patient is within ideal weight range.

    Ordered: Timentin® 2 g IV q4h

    On hand: Timentin® reconstituted to 20 mg/mL

    According to the package insert, for patients with renal impairment, the following maintenance dosages are recommended: for creatinine clearance over 60 mL/min, 3.1 g q4h; for 30 to 60 mL/min, 2 g q4h; for 10 to 30 mL/min, 2 g q8h; for less than 10 mL/min, 2 g q12h. For patients with more advanced impairments, lower dosages are recommended.

CRITICAL THINKING APPLICATIONS

You are preparing medication for two patients. Patient A has nosocomial pneumonia and a creatinine clearance of 37 mL/min. He has been ordered Zosyn® 4.5 gram q6h IV. Patient B has pelvic inflammatory disease and a normal creatinine clearance. She has been ordered 3.375 gram IV q6h. You have the following Zosyn® medication vials (see labels E, F, and G) and package insert information.

1. Are the dosages for Patient A and B safe?

2. If safe, what medication will you use and how will you prepare the medication?

3. If not safe, what action should you take?

4. According to the package insert, you further dilute each medication with 150 mL of sterile water for injection. To infuse the medication over 30 minutes, what would the IV flow rate be in mL per hour for administration of the medication to Patient B?

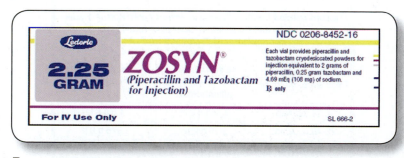

E

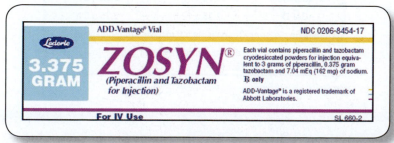

F

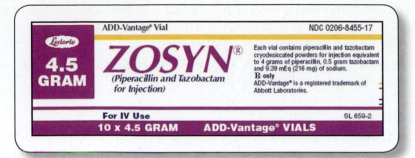

G

Directions for Reconstitution and Dilution for Use
Intravenous Administration

For conventional vials, reconstitute Zosyn® per gram of piperacillin with 5 mL of a compatible reconstitution diluent from the list provided below.

2.25 g, 3.375 g, and 4.5 g Zosyn® should be reconstituted with 10 mL, 15 mL, and 20 mL, respectively. Swirl until dissolved.

Pharmacy vials should be used immediately after reconstitution. Discard any unused portion after 24 hours if stored at room temperature [20°C to 25°C (68°F to 77°F)], or after 48 hours if stored at refrigerated temperature [2°C to 8°C (36°F to 46°F)].

Compatible Reconstitution Diluents

0.9% sodium chloride for injection
Sterile water for injection
Dextrose %
Bacteriostatic saline/parabens
Bacteriostatic water/parabens
Bacteriostatic saline/benzyl alcohol
Bacteriostatic water/benzyl alcohol
Reconstituted Zosyn® solution should be further diluted (recommended volume per dose of 50 mL to 150 mL) in a compatible intravenous diluent solution listed below. Administer by infusion over a period of at least 30 minutes. During the infusion it is desirable to discontinue the primary infusion solution.

Recommended Dosing of Zosyn in Patients with Normal Renal Function and Renal Insufficiency (As total grams piperacillin/tazobactam)		
Renal Function (Creatinine Clearance, mL/min)	**All Indications (except nosocomial pneumonia)**	**Nosocomial Pneumonia**
> 40 mL/min	3.375 q 6 h	4.5 q 6 h
20-40 mL/min*	2.25 q 6 h	3.375 q 6 h
< 20 mL/min*	2.25 q 8 h	2.25 q 6 h
Hemodialysis**	2.25 q 12 h	2.25 q 8 h
CAPD	2.25 q 12 h	2.25 q 8 h
*Creatinine clearance for patients not receiving hemodialysis		
** 0.75 g should be administered following each hemodialysis session on hemodialysis days		

CASE STUDY

You are working in a pediatric ICU where your patient is a 3-year-old boy who has a staphylococcal skin infection in the area surrounding his incision. His attending physician has prescribed the following treatment. You know from his chart that he weighs 40 lb. (LO 17.2)

Ordered: Rocephin® 600 mg IV over 30 min bid

On hand: Refer to label H. According to the package insert, for pediatric patients with skin infections, the recommended total daily dose is 50 to 75 mg/kg/day given once a day (or in equally divided doses twice a day). The total daily dose should not exceed 2 g. The Rocephin® is reconstituted to a dosage strength of 40 mg/mL.

1. What is the recommended range of doses for this patient?

2. Calculate the flow rate for the infusion pump used to deliver this order.

3. Is this order a safe dose for your patient? If it is not a safe dose, what steps should you take?

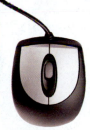

ROCHE LABORATORIES INC.
Nutley, New Jersey 07110

2 grams Single Use Vial
ROCEPHIN®
(ceftriaxone sodium)
For I.M. or I.V. Use
equivalent to 2 grams ceftriaxone
Rx only.

For I.M. Administration: Reconstitute with 4.2 mL 1% Lidocaine Hydrochloride Injection (USP) or Sterile Water for Injection (USP). Each 1 mL of solution contains approximately 350 mg equivalent of ceftriaxone.
For I.V. Administration: Reconstitute with 19.2 mL of an I.V. diluent specified in the accompanying package insert. Each 1 mL of solution contains approximately 100 mg equivalent of ceftriaxone. Withdraw entire contents and dilute to the desired concentration with the appropriate I.V. diluent.
USUAL DOSAGE: See package insert.
Storage Prior to Reconstitution: Store powder at room temperature 77° F (25° C) or below.
Protect From Light.
Storage After Reconstitution: See package insert.

LOT   EXP.

26008278-0698

H

INTERNET ACTIVITY

When you are calculating dosage for special populations, you need to know the patient's actual weight. In some circumstances, it is also important to know the ideal weight for a patient based upon the patient's height. Various charts are available to determine if a patient is of ideal weight. Search the Internet and find a current and reliable height-to-weight ratio chart. Keep this chart handy when you are calculating for special populations.

To check your answers, see the Answer–section at the end of the book, which starts on page A-1.

GO TO . . . Open the CD-ROM that accompanies your textbook, and make a final review of the rules, practice problems, and activities presented for this chapter. For a final evaluation, take the chapter test. A score of 95 percent or above indicates mastery of the chapter concepts.

18 CHAPTER

High-Alert Medications

When on the brink of complete discouragement, success is discerning that the line between failure and success is so fine that often a single extra effort is all that is needed to bring victory out of defeat.

—ELBERT GREEN HUBBARD

Learning Outcomes

When you have completed Chapter 18, you will be able to:

18.1 Differentiate important information needed for administration of insulin

18.1a Identify information on insulin labels

18.1b Read calibrations on insulin syringes

18.1c Explain the procedure for combining insulin

18.2 Identify information on heparin labels

18.3 Calculate subcutaneous dosages of heparin

18.4 Calculate intravenous dosages of heparin

18.4a Calculate weight-based bolus dosages

18.4b Calculate weight-based intravenous rates

KEY TERMS

Anticoagulant
Bolus
Duration
Heparin
Heparin protocol
High-alert medication
Insulin
Loading dose
Onset
Peak
U-100
U-500

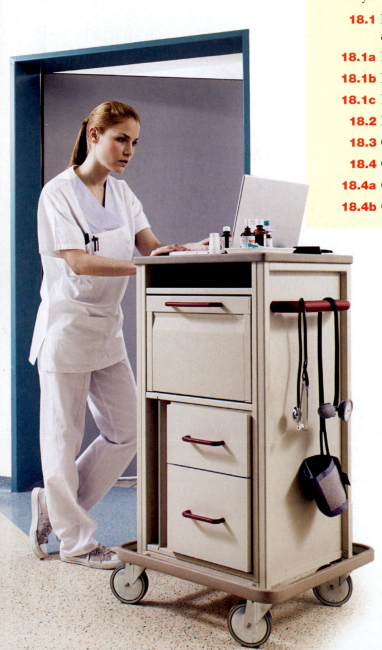

INTRODUCTION

Any calculation error may result in patient harm; however some medications that are routinely administered, termed **high-alert medications,** have a higher risk of devastating harm or death, if the dosage is miscalculated. Additionally, these medications are ones in which healthcare providers do make calculation errors. Because of this, special attention should be used when performing dosage calculation for high-alert medications. A separate nurse should calculate the dosage independently, to verify the dosage, before administering the medication, or changing the rate of IV administration. In other words the dosage calculation is always double-checked by another nurse. Heparin and insulin, both high-alert medications, are discussed in this chapter. There are other high-alert medications identified by the Institute for Safe Medication Practice (ISMP). Be sure to follow your agency's policy and procedure for administering any high-alert medication.

18.1 Insulin Administration

Insulin is a pancreatic hormone that stimulates glucose metabolism. People who have low or no insulin production may have insulin-dependent diabetes. They often need routine subcutaneous injections of insulin to keep their glucose (blood sugar) from rising to levels that could be life-threatening. These regular injections must be rotated to various sites of the body to prevent scarring of the tissue at a single injection site. Sometimes regular insulin is administered as a continuous IV infusion to move glucose into the cells when the blood sugar is at life-threatening high levels.

Types of Insulin

Many types of injectable insulin exist. The oldest types are beef insulin and pork insulin, extracted from the pancreas of a cow or a pig. In the United States, animal-based insulin has been replaced by human insulin, including those types produced by using genetically engineered bacteria. A synthetic form, insulin lispro, is also available. Some types of insulin are clear, while other types of insulin are suspensions, causing them to be cloudy.

Timing of Action

Insulins are classified by the timing of their action (see Table 18-1). Mealtime insulin has a quick onset and a short duration. It is administered to quickly lower an elevated blood sugar, or in anticipation of carbohydrates that are about to be consumed. Rapid-acting mealtime insulin should be administered within 15 minutes of the meal, or with the "first bite" so that it is available as the carbohydrates enter the bloodstream. Basal insulins have a slower onset, but a longer duration. They are administered to meet the patient's basal metabolic requirements for insulin or basic insulin needs. Individuals with Type I diabetes usually require both mealtime and basal insulin doses; for convenience some mealtime and basal insulins come premixed in the same container.

As mentioned above, insulin must be given at a specific time relative to food intake. Therefore, before you administer insulin, you must know the onset, peak, and duration of action of each type. The **onset** is the time when the insulin begins to lower the glucose level. The **peak** is the time at which the insulin's effect is strongest. Both onset and peak are measured from the time the insulin is administered. The **duration** is the length of time the effect of the insulin lasts. It is measured from the time of onset.

For example, a dose of regular insulin administered at 0700 will begin to take effect after 30 min, at 0730 (the onset). Its peak will be 2.5 to 5 hours after it is administered, between 0930 and 1200. Its effect will last until 1530 (the duration), about 8 hours after the onset. Table 18-1 summarizes the action times of many types of insulin, including mixed insulins which are described later.

TABLE 18-1 Timing of Insulin Action

TYPES OF INSULIN*	ONSET	PEAK	DURATION
Mealtime insulin			
Rapid-acting: starts acting quickly, but doesn't last as long as others	15–20 minutes	1–3 hours	3–5 hours
Insulin Aspart *Novolog;* Insulin Glulisine *Apidra;* Insulin lispro *Humalog*			
Shorter-acting: starts more slowly, but works longer than rapid-acting	30 minutes	1–3 hours	6–8 hours
Regular Insulin *Humulin R, Novolin R, Velosulin BR;*			
Basal insulin			
Intermediate-acting: (insulin zinc suspension *Novolin L,* Isophane insulin (NPH) *Humulin N, Novolin N*	2–4 hours	4–8 hours	18–26 hours
Longer-acting: (Insulin Glargine *Lantus, Lantus SoloStar;* Insulin Detemir *Levemir*	4–8 hours (insulin glargine 70–90 minutes)	10–30 hours (insulin glargine does not have a significant peak)	24 to greater than 30 hours
Mixed insulin			
Contains both mealtime *and* basal insulins *Note: Insulin Glargine is NOT mixed with other insulins.*			

*This chart identifies different types of insulin, but is not a complete list.

Insulin Labels

Like other drug labels, insulin labels identify the manufacturer, the brand name, storage information, and the expiration date (Figures 18-1 and 18-2). The concentration is usually listed twice, as the traditional dosage strength (e.g., 100 units/mL) and as the concentration. In most cases, the concentration is **U-100,** meaning that 100 units of insulin is contained in 1 mL of solution. Occasionally, the concentration is **U-500,** with 500 units/mL. Insulin labels also list the type (e.g., R or Regular) and the origin.

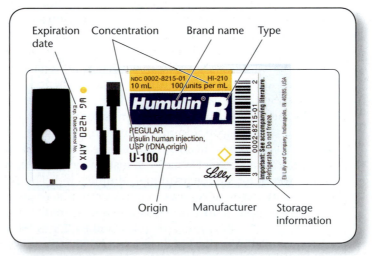

Figure 18-1 Short acting Humulin® R.

Copyright © 2012 by The McGraw-Hill Companies, Inc.

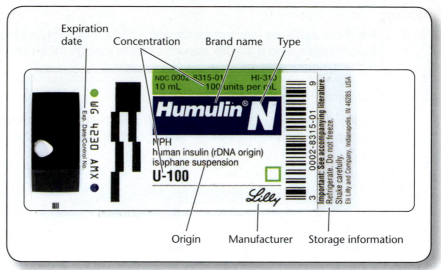

Figure 18-2 Intermediate acting Humulin® N.

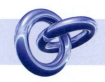

GO TO . . . Open the CD-ROM that accompanies your textbook, and select Chapter 18, Insulin Labels. (LO 18.1a) Review the animation and example problems, then complete the practice problems. Continue to the next section of the book once you have mastered the information presented.

Insulin Syringes

Insulin is administered with special insulin syringes marked in units. Pictures in this chapter do not include safety syringes or needles, so that visualization of key points will not be obstructed. Figure 8-9 in Chapter 8 is an example of three different insulin syringes with needle protection.

LEARNING LINK Recall from Chapter 8, Rule 8-4, that insulin syringes should be used only for administration of insulin.

A standard U-100 insulin syringe holds 100 units or 1 mL of solution (see Figures 18-3 and 18-4). These syringes are calibrated for every 2 units, though some are marked for each unit. Insulin administration is different from the administration of most other injectable medications because the syringe measures units of insulin rather than a volume of solution.

Smaller U-100 insulin syringes, holding up to 50 units (0.5 mL of solution) or 30 units (0.3 mL), are calibrated for each unit (see Figures 18-5 and 18-6). Their larger numbers and expanded calibration scales ensure accuracy with low insulin doses.

RULE 18-1	For more accurate measurements use a 50-unit capacity syringe for insulin doses of less than 50 units, and a 30-unit capacity insulin syringe for insulin doses less than 30 units if these syringes are available.

Example 1

Ordered: Novolin® N 66 units

Because this order is for more than 50 units, use a 100-unit insulin syringe. Find the mark for 66 units and fill the syringe to that calibration (Figure 18-3).

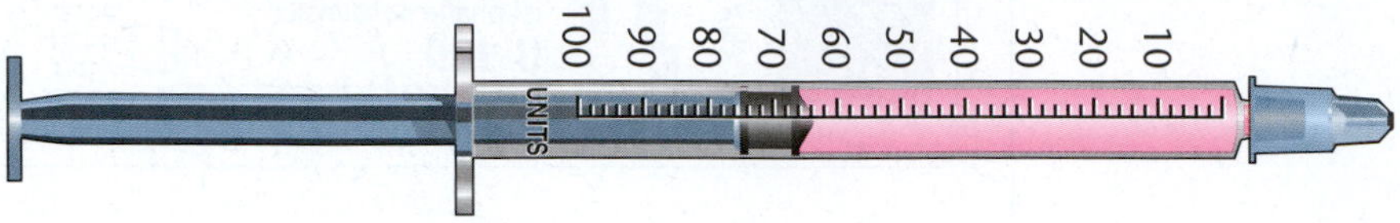

Figure 18-3 100-unit insulin syringe.

Example 2

Ordered: Humulin® R 55 units

Because this order is for more than 50 units, you will need a U-100 syringe. Your best choice would be a syringe calibrated for each unit (Figure 18-4). If you use a syringe calibrated for every 2 units, then fill it to the imaginary line between 54 and 56 units.

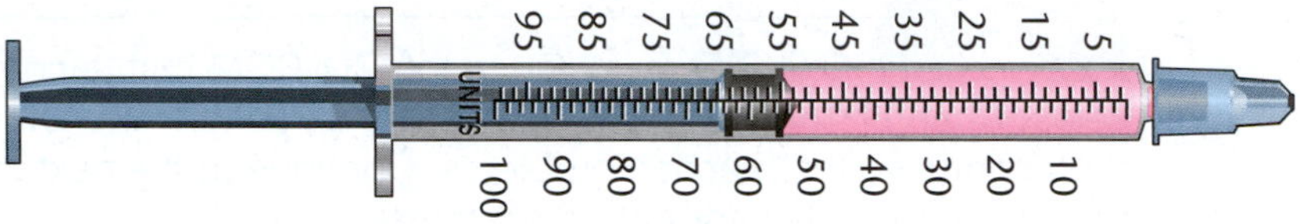

Figure 18-4 100-unit insulin syringe.

Example 3

Ordered: Humulin® R 35 units

Because this order is for less than 50 units, you may use a smaller syringe in which each unit is calibrated (Figure 18-5).

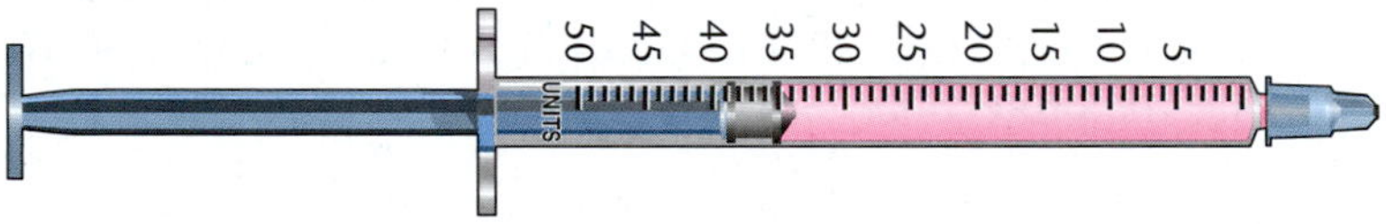

Figure 18-5 50-unit insulin syringe.

Example 4

Ordered: Novolin® R 8 units

Because this order is for less than 30 units, you may use either a 30-unit or 50-unit insulin syringe in which each unit is calibrated (Figure 18-6).

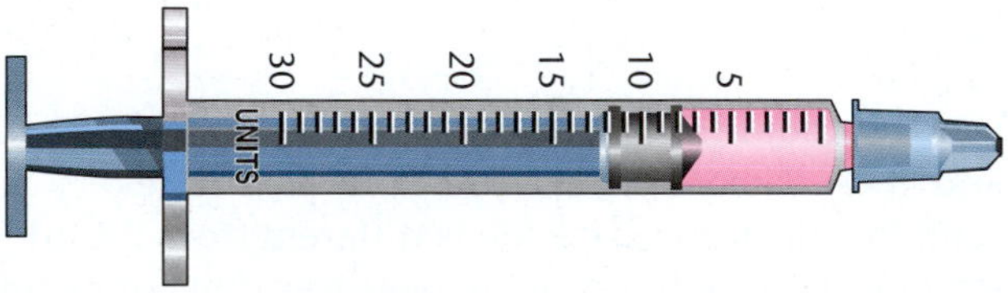

Figure 18-6 30-unit insulin syringe.

GO TO . . . Open the CD-ROM that accompanies your textbook, and select Chapter 18, Small Dose Insulin Syringes (LO 18.1b). Review the animation and example problems, then complete the practice problems. Continue to the next section of the book once you have mastered the information presented.

U-500 insulin is used for patients who are insulin resistant and require high dosages of insulin to maintain a normal blood sugar. It is rarely used and the label includes a warning (See Figure 18-7). U-100 insulin is the insulin that is commonly used. Always check how many units are in 1 mL, since accidentally substituting U-500 insulin for U-100 insulin could result in a fatal overdose. On the occasion that U-500 is ordered or an insulin dose is over 100 units, a tuberculin or standard syringe will be necessary.

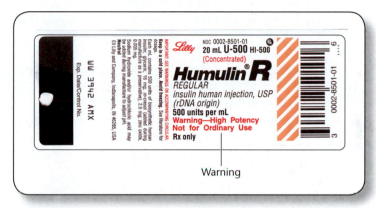

Figure 18-7 U-500 insulin is rarely used. Notice the warning on the label. Check all insulin labels carefully before administering.

RULE 18-2	If the order is for U-500 insulin (which contains 500 units in each milliliter), use a 1-mL tuberculin syringe. Calculate the amount to administer in milliliters.
Example	Ordered: Humulin® R U-500 insulin 80 units

$$\frac{80 \text{ units}}{500 \text{ units}} \times 1 \text{ mL} = A$$

$$\frac{\overset{4}{\cancel{80 \text{ units}}}}{\underset{25}{\cancel{500 \text{ units}}}} \times 1 \text{ mL} = 4 \times \frac{1}{25} \text{ mL} = \frac{4}{25} \text{ mL} = 0.16 \text{ mL}$$

Administer 0.16 mL drawn up in a tuberculin syringe (see Figure 18-8).

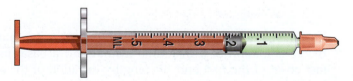

Figure 18-8 0.5 mL tuberculin syringe.

Measuring a Single Insulin Dose

Give the following information to patients:

1. Always wash your hands before handling insulin and syringes.

2. If you are using a basal or mixed insulin, roll the vial between your palms to mix the insulin, until all the insulin looks cloudy (Lantus insulin is not a suspension, so it will remain clear and does not need to be rolled).

3. Cleanse the rubber stopper of the vial with an alcohol wipe, using a circular motion. Start at the center of the circle and work outward.

4. Draw up an amount of air equal to your insulin dose in the syringe. Pull back the plunger until the leading ring is aligned with the correct marking on the syringe (Figure 18-9a).

5. Inject the air into the insulin vial; this will make it easier to withdraw the insulin later, without introducing mealtime insulin into the basal insulin vial. (Figure 18-9b).

6. Keeping the needle inserted through the stopper, turn the vial upside down. Make sure the bevel of the needle is in the insulin. Draw up your ordered dose of insulin (Figure 18-9c).

7. Avoid touching the needle during the procedure.

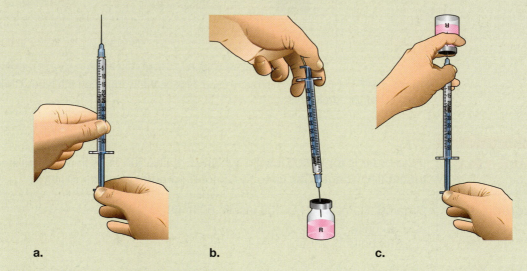

a. b. c.

Figure 18-9 Measuring insulin. **a.** Draw up air. **b.** Inject air into insulin. **c.** Draw up dose of insulin. *Syringes drawings for demonstration purposes only. All syringes should have a safe-needle device.*

Insulin Combinations

In some cases, the physician will prescribe two types of insulin for a patient. For example, the combination of a mealtime insulin and a basal insulin provides the patient with the fast onset of the first and the lengthy duration of the second. The two types of insulin can be .of insulin may be combined by the drug manufacturer. For example, Novolin® 70/30 is 70 percent intermediate-acting NPH insulin and 30 percent shorter-acting regular insulin (Figure 18-11). Humalog® 50/50 has 50 percent intermediate-acting lispro protamine insulin and 50 percent rapid-acting lispro insulin (Figure 18-12) Humalog Mix 75/25 has the same types of insulin only in a different combination (Figure 18-10). In some cases, you will need to prepare the insulin combination yourself.

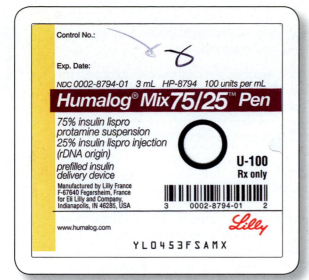

Figure 18-10 Insulin is sometimes self-administered with a pen device. A new needle must be attached for each dose. Manufacturers directions should be followed carefully to ensure air is displaced and the entire dose is administered. Patients should not share insulin pens.

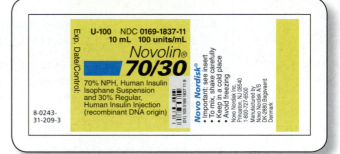

Figure 18-11 This insulin has 70% NPH and 30% R.

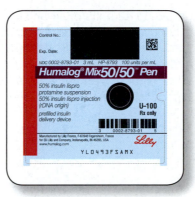

Figure 18-12 This insulin has 50% of two types of insulin.

RULE 18-3	When you are preparing a combined insulin dose, always draw up the mealtime insulin first. *Remember:* The insulin that will act first is drawn up first. Another way to remember Rule 18-3 is to draw up the clear insulin (mealtime) before the cloudy insulin (intermediate-acting). Keep in mind you must first make sure the types of insulin can be mixed. For example, Lantus is longer acting, clear, and cannot be mixed.
Example	Ordered: Novolin® R 20 units, Humulin® N 15 units subcut now Novolin® R is shorter-acting. Humulin® N is intermediate-acting. The shorter-acting insulin (Novolin® R) will be drawn into the syringe first.

RULE 18-4	To prepare a combined insulin dose (note: not all insulin can be combined): **1.** Calculate the total dose of insulin. Dose of mealtime insulin + dose of basal insulin = total dose insulin **2.** Draw up an amount of air equal to the dose of basal insulin. Inject it into the basal insulin vial but do not draw up the dose. Withdraw the needle from this vial. **3.** Draw up an amount of air equal to the dose of mealtime insulin. Inject it into the mealtime insulin vial. **4.** Without withdrawing the needle from the stopper, invert the vial. Draw up the dose of mealtime insulin.

Example

Ordered: Humulin® N 42 units and Humulin® R 10 units subcut daily

First calculate the total dose of insulin:

10 units of Humulin® R + 42 units Humulin® N = 52 units total

Next draw up 42 units of air and inject it into the vial of Humulin® N. Withdraw the needle from Humulin® N without drawing up the dose. Then draw up 10 units of air and inject it into the vial of Humulin® R. Without withdrawing the needle, invert the vial of Humulin® R and draw up 10 units of insulin (Figure 18-13a). Finally, insert the needle into the vial of Humulin® N and invert the vial. Withdraw 42 units of Humulin® N, until the leading ring of the syringe is at the calibration of 52 units, the total dose (Figure 18-13b).

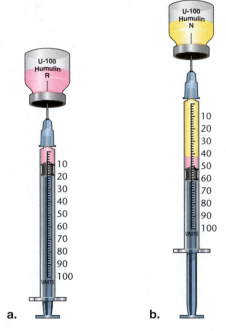

Figure 18-13 **a.** Draw up the mealtime (clear) insulin first. **b.** Be careful when drawing up the basal insulin (cloudy). *Syringes drawings for demonstration purposes only. All syringes should have a safe-needle device.*

GO TO . . . Open the CD-ROM that accompanies your textbook, and select Chapter 18, Drawing Combined Insulin (18.1c). Review the animations and example problems, then complete the practice problems. Continue to the next section of the book once you have mastered the information presented.

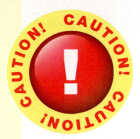

When Two Types of Insulins Are Combined, Measure the Correct Amount of Each

An order reads Novolin® N 37 units and Novolin® R 5 units subcut stat. Suppose you draw up 37 units from the Novolin® R vial and 5 units from the Novolin® N vial. Although the patient receives 42 units of insulin, he receives a much larger dose of regular (shorter-acting) insulin than was ordered—37 units rather than 5 units. The insulin metabolizes the patient's glucose too quickly; he becomes hypoglycemic and loses consciousness; this could lead to brain damage and death. Fortunately, the hypoglycemia is noted in time so glucagon and 50% dextrose are administered, and the patient recovers. This error can be avoided if you carefully check the order against the labels 3 times.

CRITICAL THINKING ON THE JOB

Timing is Essential

The authorized prescriber ordered a routine dose of NPH insulin 15 units at 0730 and a prn dose of regular insulin 4 units at 0730, if the patient's blood sugar is greater than 140. The patient's 0730 blood sugar is 141.

Think! . . . Is It Reasonable?

1. What type or types of insulin should be administered?
2. What is the total dose of insulin to be administered?
3. What syringe should be used to administer the insulin?
4. What might happen if you gave the insulin at 0730 and the breakfast tray was delayed until 0930? What could you do to prevent this from happening?

REVIEW AND PRACTICE

18.1 Insulin Administration

For Exercises 1–14, refer to labels A–G. Select the label corresponding to each order. Then mark the desired amount of insulin on the syringe.

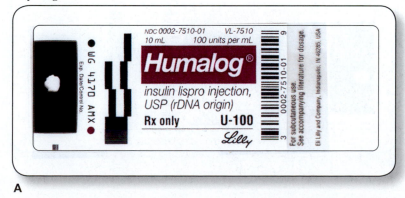

A

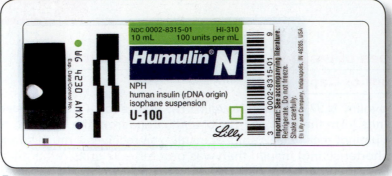

B

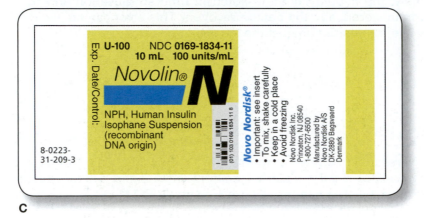

C

NDC 0169-1833-11
10 mL   100 units/mL
U-100

Novolin® **R**

Regular, Human Insulin Injection (recombinant DNA origin) USP

Novo Nordisk®
• Important: see insert
• Keep in a cold place
• Avoid freezing

Novo Nordisk Inc.
Princeton, NJ 08540
1-800-727-6500
Manufactured by
Novo Nordisk A/S
DK-2880 Bagsvaerd
Denmark

Exp. Date/Control:

8-0203-31-209-3

(01) 103 0169 1833 11 1

D

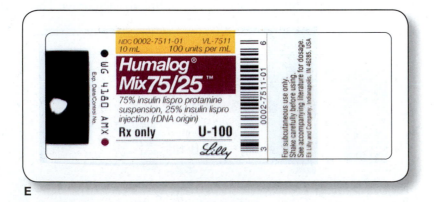

E

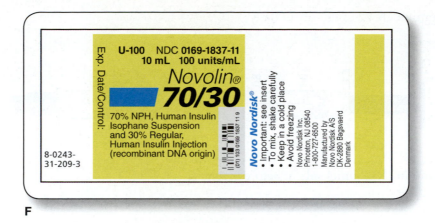

F

G

1. Ordered: Novolin® R 12 units subcut before breakfast

   Select vial: _____

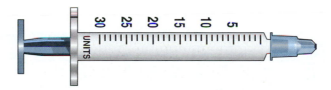

2. Ordered: Humalog® 5 units subcut 15 min before lunch

   Select vial: _____

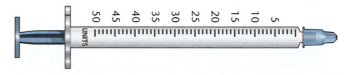

3. Ordered: Novolin® N 35 units subcut daily

   Select vial: _____

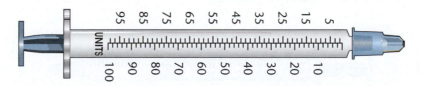

4. Ordered: Humulin® N 72 units subcut daily

Select vial: _____

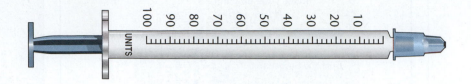

5. Ordered: Humulin® R 42 units subcut before breakfast

Select vial: _____

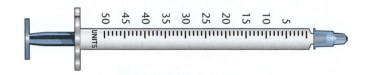

6. Ordered: Humalog® 75/25 17 units subcut before breakfast

Select vial: _____

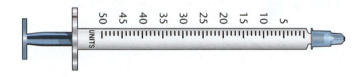

7. Ordered: Novolin® 70/30 53 units subcut before dinner

Select vial: _____

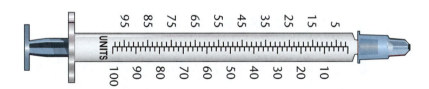

8. Ordered: Novolin® 70/30 R 26 units subcut before breakfast

Select vial: _____

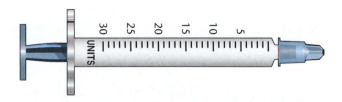

9. Ordered: Humulin® N 44 units subcut before dinner

Select vial: _____

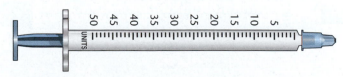

10. Ordered: Humalog® 15 units subcut before breakfast

Select vial: _____

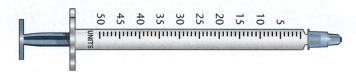

11. Ordered: Novolin® N 64 units subcut daily

Select vial: _____

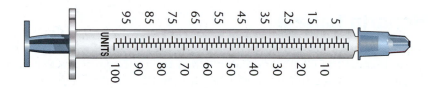

12. Ordered: Humulin® R 36 units subcut before dinner

Select vial: _____

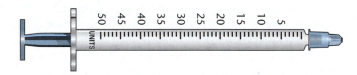

13. Ordered: Humalog® 75/25 7 units subcut stat

Select vial: _____

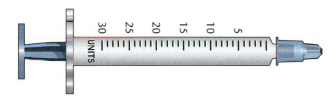

14. Ordered: Novolin® R 14 units subcut before breakfast

Select vial: _____

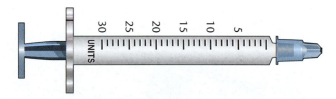

For Exercises 15 and 16, first mark on the syringe the dose of shorter-acting insulin ordered. Then mark where the leading ring will be after you draw up the intermediate-acting insulin into the same syringe.

15. Novolin® N 65 units and Novolin® R 12 units subcut qam

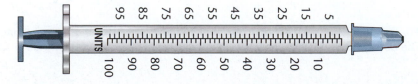

16. Humulin® N 53 units and Humulin® R 4 units subcut qam

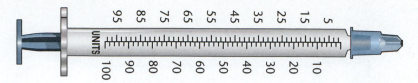

To check your answers, see the Answer section at the end of the book, which starts on page A-1.

To check your answers, see the Answer section at the end of the book, which starts on page A-1.

18.2 Heparin Labels

Heparin is an anticoagulant medication that decreases the patient's ability to form clots. It is administered in USP units. Patients that receive heparin are at risk of bleeding or hemorrhage. As discussed in Chapter 15, heparin may be used as an irrigant to keep the blood from clotting in a heparin lock. For this purpose it is packaged in prefilled syringes, cartridges or vials of 10 to 100 units (see Figure 18-14). Heparin may also be administered intermittently subcutaneously (subcut) or IV in larger dosages. When multiple injections of heparin are administered subcut, the sites of the injection should be rotated to prevent bruising. Heparin is never administered IM because of the risk of hematoma. Bleeding is a great concern for patients receiving heparin, so the dosage calculations must be accurate..

Even after the identification of heparin as a high-alert medication and the publicity that surrounds heparin dosage errors, heparin dosage errors continue to occur. Some errors have stemmed from mixing up the concentration of the vials, for example, a vial of 10,000 units of heparin/mL was used instead of 10 units/mL. Heparin doses should be written with commas between thousands and hundreds to help prevent this error, for example write 1,000 units not 1000 units. When administering heparin, it is critically important that you read the information on the drug label and question anything that is unfamiliar. (See Figures 18-15 to 18-20)

When administered as a continuous IV infusion to prevent a CVA (cerebrovascular accident) or MI (myocardial infarction), or to prevent further clot formation in a patient with a DVT (deep vein thrombosis) or PE (pulmonary embolism), the heparin infusion rate may be ordered as units per hour (units/h) or individualized by weight as units per kilogram per hour (units/kg/h). Initially, a **bolus** dose (volume administered rapidly, in this case, IV push) is administered to attain a therapeutic blood level. This is followed by a continuous IV infusion.

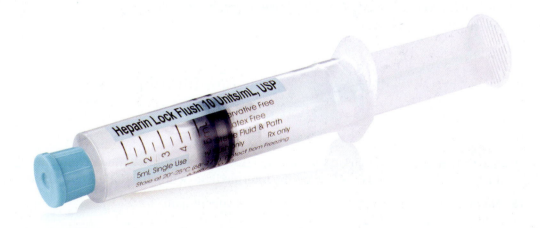

Figure 18-14 Heparin lock flush solution may be available in prefilled syringes such as this one. The dosage strength is 10 units/mL and the amount of flush in the syringe is 5 mL.

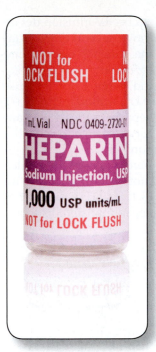

Figure 18-15 Heparin sodium 1,000 USP units/mL in 1 mL bottle.

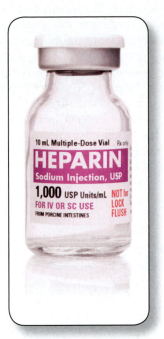

Figure 18-16 Heparin sodium 1,000 USP units/mL in 10 mL bottle.

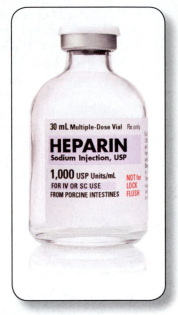

Figure 18-17 Heparin sodium 1,000 USP units/mL in 30 mL bottle.

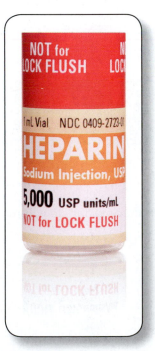

Figure 18-18 Heparin sodium 5,000 USP units/mL in 1 mL bottle.

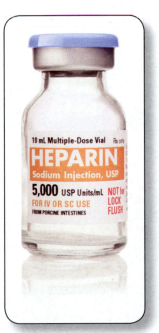

Figure 18-19 Heparin sodium 5,000 USP units/mL in 10 mL bottle.

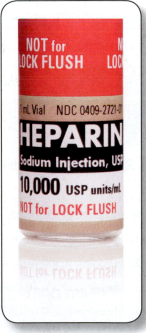

Figure 18-20 Heparin sodium 10,000 USP units/mL in 1 mL bottle.

To maintain a constant rate, heparin is always administered by an electric IV infusion device. Dosage rates are adjusted according to lab results, which may be drawn several times a day. The nurse must carefully recalculate the heparin dosage to meet the patient's new requirements. *Remember a second nurse must calculate the dosage independently, to ensure accuracy.*

The practitioner chooses which dosage strength of heparin, and volume bottle to use, based on the ordered dose. Heparin dosage strength ranges from 10 USP units/mL to 20,000 USP units/mL, so extreme caution should be used when selecting heparin bottles. For example, if the ordered dose is heparin 5,000 units subcut, the most appropriate concentration and volume would be 5,000 USP units/mL in a 1-mL bottle (see Figure 18-18). This is appropriate because the desired dose is 1 mL, which is easily drawn up, there is no wasted medication, and it is an acceptable volume to administer subcut. It would not be appropriate to use heparin sodium 1,000 USP units/mL in a 1-mL bottle (see Figure 18-15), since it would take 5 bottles to achieve the dose, and the volume of 5 mL is too large to be administered subcut.

 LEARNING LINK   Recall from Chapter 14, Rule 14-3, that 1 mL is the maximum volume for an adult subcutaneous injection.

RULE 18-5   Check the dosage strength on the label to ensure the correct amount of heparin is used in your dosage calculation

GO TO . . . Open the CD-ROM that accompanies your textbook, and select Chapter 18, Heparin Concentrations (LO 18.2). Review the animation and example problems, then complete the practice problems. Continue to the next section of the book once you have mastered the rule presented.

REVIEW AND PRACTICE

18.2 Heparin Labels

For exercises 1–10 use the medication labels in Figures 18-14 through 18-20 to identify the appropriate volume bottle and dosage strength for the intended purpose.

1. Heparin 5,000 units IV bolus   _____

2. Heparin 7,500 units subcut   _____

3. Heparin flush 10 units IV push   _____

4. Heparin 8,000 units IV bolus   _____

5. Heparin 2,500 units subcut   _____

6. Heparin 1,000 units in NS 500 mL   _____

7. Heparin 10,000 units subcut   _____

8. Heparin 2,000 units IV bolus   _____

9. Heparin 750 units IV bolus _____

10. Heparin 2,500 units IV bolus _____

To check your answers, see the answer section at the end of the book, which starts on page A-1.

18.3 Calculating Subcutaneous Heparin Dosages

You have learned, in Chapter 12, how to calculate dosages. Use the proportion method, dimensional analysis, or the formula method to calculate the volume of heparin to be administered. *Remember to use the abc's of dosage calculation to ensure your answer is correct.*

PROPORTION METHOD

EXAMPLE

Find the amount (A) of subcut heparin to administer.

Ordered: heparin 2,500 units subcut

On hand: heparin 5,000 USP units/mL

STEP A: CONVERT
Since the dosage ordered is units, and the dose on hand is units, no conversion is necessary.

STEP B: CALCULATE
Follow Procedure Checklist 12-1.

1. Fill in the proportion

$$\frac{H}{Q} = \frac{D}{A}$$

$$\frac{5{,}000 \text{ units}}{1 \text{ mL}} = \frac{2{,}500 \text{ units}}{A}$$

2. Cancel units leaving mL for the answer.

$$\frac{5{,}000 \text{ units}}{1 \text{ mL}} = \frac{2{,}500 \text{ units}}{A}$$

3. Cross-multiply and solve for the answer.

$$5{,}000 \times A = 2{,}500 \times 1 \text{ mL}$$

$$A = \frac{2{,}500}{5{,}000} \times 1 \text{ mL}$$

$$A = \frac{1}{2} \text{ mL}$$

$$A = 0.5 \text{ mL}$$

STEP C: THINK! . . . IS IT REASONABLE?
Since 2,500 units is half as much as 5,000 units, it stands to reason that the amount to give would be half of 1 mL, so the answer is reasonable.

DIMENSIONAL ANALYSIS

EXAMPLE

Find the amount subcut heparin to administer.

Ordered: heparin 2,500 units subcut

On hand: heparin 5,000 ISP units/mL

STEP A: CONVERT

The dose ordered is measured in units and the dosage strength is also measured in units. No conversion factor is needed.

STEP B: CALCULATE

Follow Procedure Checklist 12-2.

1. The unit of measure for the amount to administer will be milliliters.

A mL =

2. No conversion factor is necessary.

3. The dosage unit is 1 mL. The dose on hand is 5,000 units. This is our first factor.

$$\frac{1 \text{ mL}}{5{,}000 \text{ units}}$$

4. The dosage ordered is 2,500 units. Place this over 1 and set up the equation.

$$A \text{ mL} = \frac{1 \text{ mL}}{5{,}000 \text{ units}} \times \frac{2{,}500 \text{ units}}{1}$$

5. Cancel units.

$$A \text{ mL} = \frac{1 \text{ mL}}{5{,}000 \text{ \sout{units}}} \times \frac{2{,}500 \text{ \sout{units}}}{1}$$

6. Solve the equation.

$$A \text{ mL} = \frac{2{,}500 \text{ mL}}{5{,}000}$$

$$A = \frac{1}{2} \text{ mL}$$

$$A = 0.5 \text{ mL}$$

STEP C: THINK! . . . IS IT REASONABLE?

Since 2,500 units is half as much as 5,000 units, it stands to reason that the amount to give would be half of 1 mL, so the answer is reasonable.

FORMULA METHOD

EXAMPLE

Find the amount (A) of subcut heparin to administer.

Ordered (D): heparin 2,500 units subcut

On hand (H/Q): heparin 5,000 units/mL

STEP A: CONVERT

The drug is ordered in units, which is the same unit of measure as that of the dose on hand. No conversion necessary.

STEP B: CALCULATE

$D = 2{,}500$ units, $Q = 1$ mL, and $H = 5{,}000$ units.

Follow Procedure Checklist 12-3

1. Fill in the formula.

$$\frac{2{,}500 \text{ units}}{5{,}000 \text{ units}} \times 1 \text{ mL} = A$$

2. Cancel units.

$$\frac{2{,}500 \text{ \sout{units}}}{5{,}000 \text{ \sout{units}}} \times 1 \text{ mL} = A$$

3. Solve for the unknown.

$$\frac{1}{2} \times 1 \text{ mL} = A$$

$$\frac{1}{2} \text{ mL} = A$$

The amount to administer is 0.5 mL.

STEP C: THINK! . . . IS IT REASONABLE?
Since 2,500 units is half as much as 5,000 units, it stands to reason that the amount to give would be half of 1 mL, so the answer is reasonable.

GO TO . . . Open the CD-ROM that accompanies your textbook, and select Chapter 18, Calculating Subcutaneous Heparin Dosages (LO 18.3). Review the animation and example problems, then complete the practice problems. Continue to the next section of the book once you have mastered the rule presented.

REVIEW AND PRACTICE

18.3 Calculating Subcutaneous Heparin Doses

For Exercises 1–5, using any one of the above methods, calculate the volume of heparin to be administered.

1. Ordered: Heparin 5,000 units subcut
   On hand: 5,000 USP units/1 mL

2. Ordered: Heparin 7,500 units subcut
   On hand: 10,000 USP units/1 mL

3. Ordered: Heparin 5,000 units subcut
   On hand: Heparin 10,000 USP units/1 mL

4. Ordered: Heparin 8,000 units subcut
   On hand: Heparin 20,000 USP units/1 mL

5. Ordered: Heparin 2,500 units subcut
   On hand: Heparin 5,000 USP units/1 mL

To check your answers, see the Answer section at the end of the book, which starts on page A-1.

18.4 Intravenous Heparin Dosages

You have learned to calculate how many milliliters of solution were needed to administer a dose of heparin. Calculating the flow rate is very similar. Before, the desired dose D represented only a quantity of units. Here, the desired dose D represents a flow rate, a quantity of units per time period.

To determine the rate at which to administer a solution containing heparin with an electronic device that measures the infusion in milliliters per hour, find A, where:

D = rate of desired dose (units/h)

Q = dosage unit (units)

H = dose on hand (mL)

A = amount to administer (mL/h)

Use the proportion method, dimensional analysis, or formula method.

PROPORTION METHOD

EXAMPLE

Find the hourly rate at which to administer IV heparin.

Ordered: 1,000 units/h IV heparin using an infusion pump

On hand: 25,000 units heparin in 500 mL of D5W

STEP A: CONVERT
The dosage ordered and the dose on hand have the same units; no conversion is necessary.

STEP B: CALCULATE
The dosage ordered D is 1,000 units/h. The dose on hand H is 25,000 units, and the dosage unit Q is 500 mL.

Follow Procedure Checklist 12-1.

1. Fill in the proportion.

$$\frac{25{,}000 \text{ units}}{500 \text{ mL}} = \frac{1{,}000 \text{ units/h}}{A}$$

2. Cancel units, leaving mL/h for the answer.

$$\frac{25{,}000 \text{ units}}{500 \text{ mL}} = \frac{1{,}000 \text{ units/h}}{A}.$$

3. Cross-multiply and solve for the answer.

$$25{,}000 \times A = 500 \text{ mL} \times 1{,}000/h$$

$$25{,}000 \times A = 500{,}000 \text{ mL/h}$$

$$A = \frac{500{,}000 \text{ mL/h}}{25{,}000}$$

$$A = 20 \text{ mL/h}$$

STEP C: THINK! . . . IS IT REASONABLE?
Since the dosage strength of a 25,000 units/500 mL solution is 50 units/1 mL, and 50 × 20 is 1,000, it is reasonable.

DIMENSIONAL ANALYSIS

EXAMPLE

Find the hourly rate at which to administer IV heparin.

Ordered: 1,000 units/h IV heparin using an infusion pump

On hand: 25,000 units heparin in 500 mL of D5W

STEP A: CONVERT
No conversion factor necessary.

STEP B: CALCULATE
Follow Procedure Checklist 12-2.

1. The unit of measure will be milliliters per hour.

   A mL/h =

2. The dosage unit is 500 mL; the dose on hand is 25,000 units. This is your first factor.

   $$\frac{500 \text{ mL}}{25,000 \text{ units}}$$

3. The desired dose is 1,000 units/h. Set up the equation.

   $$A \text{ mL/h} = \frac{500 \text{ mL}}{25,000 \text{ units}} \times \frac{1,000 \text{ units}}{1 \text{ h}}$$

   $$A \text{ mL/h} = \frac{500 \text{ mL}}{25,000 \text{ units}} \times \frac{1,000 \text{ units}}{1 \text{ h}}$$

   $$A = 20 \text{ mL/h}$$

STEP C: THINK! . . . IS IT REASONABLE?
Since the dosage strength of a 25,000 unit/500 mL solution is 50 units/1 mL, and 50 × 20 is 1,000, it is reasonable.

To ensure the maximum and/or safe dose is not exceeded, you will need to determine the hourly dose of a heparin infusion.

RULE 18-7

To calculate the hourly dose of heparin (desired dose *D*). Determine the following:

   H = dose on hand or total amount to administer

   Q = dosage unit for total amount

   A = amount to administer or flow rate of infusion

Calculate, using the proportion method, dimensional analysis, or formula method.

PROPORTION METHOD

EXAMPLE

What is the hourly dose?

Ordered: 30,000 units of IV heparin in 500 mL of D5W to infuse at 25 mL/h

   H = 30,000 units (dose on hand or total amount to administer)

   Q = 500 mL (dosage unit for total amount)

$A = 25$ mL/h (amount to administer or flow rate of infusion)

$D =$ desired hourly dose

STEP A: CONVERT

Since the dosage unit is mL and the amount to administer is in mL, no conversion is necessary.

STEP B: CALCULATE

Follow Procedure Checklist 12-1.

1. Fill in the proportion.

$$\frac{H}{Q} = \frac{D}{A} \quad \text{or} \quad \frac{\text{dose on hand}}{\text{dosage unit}} = \frac{\text{desired dose}}{\text{amount to administer}}$$

Thinking critically, we realize we already know the amount to administer A or flow rate of the infusion and we need to determine the hourly dose D or desired dose.

$$\frac{30{,}000 \text{ units}}{500 \text{ mL}} = \frac{D}{25 \text{ mL/h}}$$

2. Cancel units.

$$\frac{30{,}000 \text{ units}}{500 \text{ m\cancel{L}}} = \frac{D}{25 \text{ m\cancel{L}/h}}$$

3. Cross-multiply and solve for the unknown.

$$500 \times D = 30{,}000 \text{ units} \times 25/h$$

$$D = \frac{30{,}000 \text{ units}}{500} \times 25/h$$

$$D = \frac{30{,}0\cancel{0}0 \text{ units}}{50\cancel{0}} \times 25/h$$

$$D = 1500 \text{ units/h}$$

STEP C: THINK! . . . IS IT REASONABLE?

Since a dosage strength of 30,000 unit/500 mL provides 60 units/1 mL, and 60 × 25 = 1500, it is reasonable.

DIMENSIONAL ANALYSIS

EXAMPLE

What is the hourly dose?

Ordered: 30,000 units of IV heparin in 500 mL of D5W to infuse at 25 mL/h

$H = 30{,}000$ units (dose on hand or total amount to administer)

$Q = 500$ mL (dosage unit for total amount)

$A = 25$ mL/h (amount to administer or flow rate of infusion)

$D =$ desired hourly dose

STEP A: CONVERT

The dosage unit and the amount to administer are both mL, so no conversion factor is necessary.

STEP B: CALCULATE

Follow Procedure Checklist 12-2.

1. The hourly rate for the unknown D will be in units per hour. Place this on the left side of the equation.

D units/h =

2. The dose on hand is 30,000 units. The dosage unit is 500 mL. This is your first factor.

$$\frac{30{,}000 \text{ units}}{500 \text{ mL}}$$

3. The flow rate of the infusion is 25 mL/h. Use this as your second factor. Set up the equations.

$$D \text{ units/h} = \frac{30{,}000 \text{ units}}{500 \text{ mL}} \times \frac{25 \text{ mL}}{1 \text{ h}}$$

4. Cancel units. The remaining units on the right side of the equation must match those on the left side of the equation.

$$D \text{ units/h} = \frac{30{,}000 \text{ units}}{500 \text{ mL}} \times \frac{25 \text{ mL}}{1 \text{ h}}$$

5. Solve the equation.

$$D \text{ units/h} = \frac{30{,}000 \text{ units}}{500} \times \frac{25}{1 \text{ h}}$$

$$D = 1500 \text{ units/h}$$

STEP C: THINK! . . . IS IT REASONABLE?

Since a dosage strength of 30,000 unit/500 mL provides 60 units/1 mL, and 60 × 25 = 1,500, it is reasonable.

To prevent dosage and administration error, many hospitals use a **heparin protocol.** A heparin protocol is a preprinted order set that guides the administration of IV heparin based on the patient's weight and serum activated partial thromboplastin time (aPTT), a blood clotting value measured in seconds. In the sample weight-based heparin protocol (Table 18-2), used for high-intensity conditions, such as deep vein thrombosis (DVT) or pulmonary embolism (PE), the **loading dose** which is the initial bolus dose given to achieve a therapeutic blood level of heparin, is based on the patient's weight. A maximum dose is provided, so that the patient will not receive a toxic dose of heparin. If the calculated dose of heparin, based on the patient's weight exceeds the maximum dosage, then only the maximum dosage will be administered, followed by the heparin infusion. Notice too, that the infusion rate and all subsequent changes are based on the patient's weight in kg.

TABLE 18-2 Heparin Protocol for DVT, PE, and High intensity Indications GOAL: aPTT 70 – 100

Use premixed heparin sodium 25,000 USP units in 5% dextrose in water 500 mL (50 units/mL) for infusion. Use heparin sodium 1,000 USP units/mL for bolus dose. Obtain baseline CBC and aPTT prior to administering heparin. Obtain aPTT 6 hours after each rate change. If the aPTT is at goal, repeat the aPTT until two consecutive aPTT are at goal, draw aPTT daily while receiving heparin, and aPTT remains between 70 and 100.
Initial bolus dose: 80 units/kg   (maximum 8,000 units)
Initial rate: 18 units/kg/h   (maximum 1,800 units/h = 36 mL/h)

APTT RESULT	IV BOLUS DOSE	# MINUTES TO HOLD INFUSION	AMOUNT TO CHANGE CURRENT INFUSION RATE
Less than 54 Notify AP	80 units/kg (max. 8,000 units)	Do not hold	Increase by 4 units/kg/h
54–59	40 units/kg (max. 4,000 units)	Do not hold	Increase by 2 units/kg/h

(Continued)

APTT RESULT	IV BOLUS DOSE	# MINUTES TO HOLD INFUSION	AMOUNT TO CHANGE CURRENT INFUSION RATE
60–69	40 units/kg (max. 4,000 units)	Do not hold	Increase by 1 unit/kg/h
70–100 goal	**No bolus dose**	**Do not hold**	**Do not change current infusion rate**
101–115	No bolus dose	Do not hold	Decrease by 1 unit/kg/h
116–135	No bolus dose	30	Decrease by 2 units/kg/h
136–150	No bolus dose	60	Decrease by 3 units/kg/h and repeat aPTT 6 hours after infusion resumed
151–200 Notify AP	No bolus dose	90	Decrease by 4 units/kg/h and repeat aPTT 6 hours after infusion resumed

Adapted for calculation purposes only, from (2008) ACCP guidelines; not to be used in clinical practice.

Weight-based Bolus Dose Calculations

To calculate the initial bolus dose of 80 units/kg (maximum dose 8,000 units) follow the ABCs of dosage calculation using the proportion method.

PROPORTION METHOD

EXAMPLE

The patient weighs 154 lb. Using the heparin protocol in Table 18.2, calculate the loading dose.

STEP A: CONVERT

Convert the patients weight in pounds to kilograms:

$$\frac{1 \text{ kg}}{2.2 \text{ lb}} = \frac{x}{154 \text{ lb}}$$

Cross multiply and solve the equation

$1 \text{ kg} \times 154 = 2.2 \times x$

$154 \text{ kg}/2.2 = x$

$70 \text{ kg} = x$

STEP B: CALCULATE

Calculate the bolus dose

$$\frac{80 \text{ units}}{1 \text{ kg}} - \frac{x}{70 \text{ kg}}$$

Cancel kg and multiply

$$\frac{80 \text{ units}}{1 \text{ kg}} \times 70 \text{ kg} = x$$

$5600 \text{ units} = A$

STEP C: THINK! . . . IS IT REASONABLE?

5,600 units is less than the maximum dose of 8,000 units, so it is reasonable.

Next calculate the dose in mL using a supply dose of 1,000 units/mL by following the ABCs of dosage calculation and using any one of the three methods.

PROPORTION METHOD

EXAMPLE

Calculate the dose, 5,600 units, in mL using a supply dose of 1,000 units/mL.

Bolus dose (*D*): 5,600 units

Dosage strength (*H/Q*): 1,000 units/1 mL

Amount to administer (*A*)

STEP A: CONVERT
No conversion necessary

STEP B: CALCULATE
Follow Procedure Checklist 12-1.

1. Fill in the proportion

$$\frac{H}{Q} = \frac{D}{A}$$

$$\frac{1{,}000 \text{ units}}{1 \text{ mL}} = \frac{5{,}600 \text{ units}}{A}$$

2. Cancel Units

$$\frac{1{,}000 \text{ units}}{1 \text{ mL}} = \frac{5{,}600 \text{ units}}{A}$$

3. Cross-multiply and solve

$$1{,}000 \times A = 1 \text{ mL} \times 5{,}600$$

$$1{,}000 (A) = 5{,}600 \text{ mL}$$

$$A = \frac{5{,}600 \text{ mL}}{1{,}000}$$

$$A = 5.6 \text{ mL}$$

STEP C: THINK! . . . IS IT REASONABLE?
Since you want to give 5,600 units, and it is 5.6 times larger than 1,000 units, giving 5.6 mL is reasonable. Administer an IV bolus of 5.6 mL heparin sodium 1,000 USP units/mL from a 10 mL bottle.

DIMENSIONAL ANALYSIS

EXAMPLE

Calculate the dose, 5,600 units, in mL using a supply dose of 1,000 units/mL.

Find the amount to administer.

Ordered: Heparin bolus dose (*D*) 5,600 units.

On hand (*H/Q*): Heparin 1,000 units/1 mL

Amount to administer (*A*)

STEP A: CONVERT
The ordered dose and the supply dose are both measured in units. No conversion factor is necessary.

STEP B: CALCULATE
Follow Procedure Checklist 12-2.

1. The unit of measure for the amount to administer will be in milliliters.

2. No conversion factor necessary.

3. The dosage unit is 1 mL. The dose on hand is 1,000 units. This is the first factor.

$$\frac{1 \text{ mL}}{1,000 \text{ units}}$$

4. The dosage ordered is 5,600 units. Set up the equation.

$$A \text{ mL} = \frac{1 \text{ mL}}{1,000 \text{ units}} \times \frac{5,600 \text{ units}}{1}$$

5. Cancel units.

$$A \text{ mL} = \frac{1 \text{ mL}}{1,000 \text{ units}} \times \frac{5,600 \text{ units}}{1}$$

6. Solve the equation.

$$A = \frac{5,600 \text{ mL}}{1,000}$$

$$A = 5.6 \text{ mL}$$

STEP C: THINK! . . . IS IT REASONABLE?

Since you want to give 5,600 units, and it is 5.6 times larger than 1,000 units, giving 5.6 mL is reasonable. Administer an IV bolus of 5.6 mL heparin sodium 1,000 USP units/mL from a 10 mL bottle.

FORMULA METHOD

EXAMPLE

Find the amount (A) of subcut heparin to administer.

Find the amount to administer.

Ordered: Heparin bolus dose (D) 5,600 units

On hand (H/Q): Heparin 1,000 units/1 mL

Amount to administer (A)

STEP A: CONVERT

The ordered dose and the supply dose are both measured in units; no conversion necessary.

STEP B: CALCULATE
Follow Procedure Checklist 12-3
D = 5,600 units, H = 1,000 units, Q = 1 mL

1. Fill in the formula.

$$\frac{5,600 \text{ units}}{1,000 \text{ units}} \times 1 \text{ mL} = A$$

2. Cancel units.

$$\frac{5,600 \text{ units}}{1,000 \text{ units}} \times 1 \text{ mL} = A$$

3. Solve for the unknown.

$$5.6 \text{ mL} = A$$

STEP C: THINK! . . . IS IT REASONABLE?

Since you want to give 5,600 units, and it is 5.6 times larger than 1,000 units, giving 5.6 mL is reasonable. Administer an IV bolus of 5.6 mL heparin sodium 1,000 USP units/mL from a 10 mL bottle.

Weight-based Intravenous Rates

After calculating the initial bolus dosage and bolus volume, you will now use the weight-based heparin protocol to determine the initial intravenous infusion rate.

RULE 18-8

To find the flow rate based upon weight:

1. Convert pounds to kilograms, if necessary.

2. Determine the desired dose:

   Ordered Dose × weight in kg = Desired Dose

   unit of measurement/kg/h × kg = unit of measurement/h

   For example: units/kg/h × kg = D

3. Utilizing the proportion method, calculate the flow rate in mL/h using the dosage strength H/Q (IV solution) 25,000 units/500 mL or 50 units/mL per protocol.

PROPORTION METHOD

EXAMPLE

Establish the initial infusion rate for a patient that weighs 70 kg.

1. Since weight is in kg, no conversion is necessary.

2. Determine desired dose (units/h) from protocol: 18 units/kg/h

   18 units/kg/h × 70 kg = 1,260 units/h

3. Calculate the flow rate in mL/h.

STEP A: CONVERT

The desired dose, 1,260 units/h, is in units and the dose on hand, 50 units/mL IV solution, is in units. No conversion necessary.

STEP B: CALCULATE

Follow Procedure Checklist 12-1

1. Fill in the formula

   $$\frac{H}{Q} = \frac{D}{A}$$

   $$\frac{50 \text{ units}}{1 \text{ mL}} = \frac{1,260 \text{ units/h}}{A}$$

2. Cancel units

   $$\frac{50 \text{ units}}{1 \text{ mL}} = \frac{1,260 \text{ units/h}}{A}$$

3. Cross-multiply and solve for unknown

   $$50 \times A = 1,260 \text{ mL/h}$$

   $$A = 25.2 \text{ mL/h}$$

Most infusion pumps infuse to the tenth mL, so 25.2 mL/h can be programmed into the pump. For infusion pumps that only infuse full mL/h, round down to 25 mL/h.

For a patient that weighs 70 kg the loading dose would be 5,600 units administered as a 5.6 mL IV bolus, using a heparin concentration 1,000 units/mL. The initial infusion would be started at 1,260 units/h, which is 25.2 mL/h using a heparin concentration 25,000 units in 500 mL (50 units/mL).

Verify the rate by finding mL/h of 1 unit/kg/h and multiplying it by 18 (the desired rate).
Find the rate in mL/h for 1 unit/kg/h.
Dosage strength is 50 units/1 mL

Patient's weight is 70 kg

$$1 \text{ unit/kg/h} \times 70 \text{ kg} = 70 \text{ units/h}$$

Convert units to mL

$$\frac{50 \text{ units}}{1 \text{ mL}} = \frac{70 \text{ units/h}}{A}$$

$$50 \times A = 1 \text{ mL} \times 70/\text{h}$$

$$A = \frac{70 \text{ mL/h}}{50}$$

$$A = 1.4 \text{ mL/h}$$

The infusion rate of 1 unit/kg/h for a 70 kg is 1.4 mL/h.

1.4 mL/h × 18 = 25.2 mL/h, so the infusion rate is reasonable.

Weight-based Intravenous Rate Adjustment

Refer to the heparin protocol (Table 18-2) to determine the rate change. If the infusion is running at 25.2 mL/h, and the aPTT result is 120 seconds, according to the protocol, the IV rate must be decreased by 2 units/kg/h. Use the following method to determine the new rate.

To find the new rate, subtract the rate adjustment from the initial or current IV rate, which for this example is 18 units/kg/h:

18 units/kg/h − 2 units/kg/h = 16 units/kg/h

Find the rate for 16 units/kg/h as previously demonstrated for 18 units/kg/h:

16 units/kg/h × 70 kg = 1120 units/h

$$\frac{50 \text{ units}}{1 \text{ mL}} = \frac{1120 \text{ units/h}}{A}$$

A = 22.4 mL/h

GO TO . . . Open the CD-ROM that accompanies your textbook, and select Chapter 18, Bolus Dose Calculation (LO 18.4). Review the animation and example problems, then complete the practice problems. Continue to the next section of the book once you have mastered the information presented.

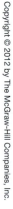

18.4 Intravenous Heparin Dosages

For Exercises 1–5, find the flow rate in mL/h via infusion pump.

1. Ordered: Heparin 1,000 units/h
   On hand: 20,000 units in 1500 mL of 5% DW

2. Ordered: Heparin 1,000 units/h
   On hand: 20,000 units in 500 mL of D5W

3. Ordered: Heparin 850 units/h
   On hand: 40,000 units in 1500 mL of 5% DW

4. Ordered: Heparin 1500 units/h
   On hand: 30,000 units 500 mL of 5% D 0.45% NS

5. Ordered: Heparin 750 units/h
   On hand: 30,000 units in 1000 mL of 5% DW

For Exercises 6–10, find the hourly dosage for the heparin orders.

6. An IV with 60,000 units in 1500 mL of 5% DW infusing at 25 mL/h

7. An IV setup delivering 45 mL/h from 25,000 units in 2500 mL of D5NS

8. 40,000 units in 1800 mL of 5% DW delivered at 25 mL/h

9. 30,000 units in 1500 mL of 5% D 0.45% NS delivered at 20 mL/h

10. 50,000 units in 500 mL NS infusing at 25 mL/h

For Exercises 11–15 calculate the requested bolus doses and IV rate using the heparin protocol in Table 18-2 for a patient who weighs 50 kg.

11. Calculate the loading dose.

12. Calculate the initial rate.

13. Calculate the bolus dose if the patient's aPTT was 57.

14. Calculate the rate change if the patient's aPTT was 57.

15. The IV is infusing at 24 mL/h; calculate the rate change if the patient's aPTT was 110.

For Exercises 16–20 use the heparin protocol in Table 18-2. The patient weighs 120 kg.

16. Calculate the loading dose.

17. Calculate the initial rate.

18. Calculate the bolus dose if the patient's aPTT was 60.

19. Calculate the rate change if the patient's aPTT was 60.

20. The IV is infusing at 36 mL/h; calculate the rate change if the patient's aPTT was 120.

To check your answers, see the Answer section at the end of the book, which starts on page A-1.

CHAPTER 18 SUMMARY

LEARNING OUTCOME	KEY POINTS
18.1a Identify important information on the insulin label. Pages 520–521	The label identifies insulin type (regular, NPH . . .), the manufacturer, brand name, storage information and the expiration date. Insulin labels also contain the concentration written as units/mL (100 units/mL-also called U-100, or 500 units/mL - also called U-500.).
18.1b Read calibration on insulin syringes. Pages 521–524	Standard U-100, 1-mL syringe is calibrated for every 2 units. U-100, 0.5-mL and 0.3-mL syringes are calibrated for every 1 unit; the calibrations and numbers are larger, making them easier for accuracy with smaller doses.
18.1c Explain the procedure for combining insulin. Pages 524–532	Calculate the total dose of insulin (mealtime + basal = total dose) Wash hands; roll the cloudy insulin vial between palms—mix until uniformly cloudy; draw up air equal to intermediate dose and inject in basal (cloudy) insulin—do not draw up dose, withdraw syringe and draw up air equal to the mealtime dose, inject it into the mealtime insulin and withdraw mealtime dose. Now, without injecting any of the mealtime insulin, insert the needle into the basal (cloudy) insulin, and withdraw the cloudy insulin until the leading ring reaches the calibration for the total dose of insulin. *Remember, draw up the clear (mealtime) before the cloudy (basal).*
18.2 Identify information on heparin labels. Pages 532–534	Heparin is manufactured and labeled in different strengths (10 units/mL, 100 units/mL, 1,000 units/mL, 5,000 units/mL, 10,000 units/mL) and different volumes (1 mL, 10 mL, 30 mL). Harmful and deadly errors have occurred when heparin of the wrong strength has been administered. It is imperative that careful attention is paid to the concentration, and not just the volume of heparin in the bottle.

LEARNING OUTCOME	KEY POINTS
18.3 Calculate subcutaneous dosages of heparin. Pages 535–537	Use any of the three methods of dosage calculation, and follow the ABCs of dosage calculation when preparing subcutaneous dosages of heparin. Pay special attention to the concentration of heparin, so that the total volume of the dose is less than or equal to 1 mL (max. subcut volume of injection). *Remember: Desired dose (**D**), Dosage strength (**H/Q**), and Amount to administer (**A**)* **Proportion Method:** $$\frac{H}{Q} = \frac{D}{A}$$ **Dimensional Analysis:** $$A = \text{Conversion factor} \times \frac{Q}{H} \times D$$ **Formula Method:** $$\frac{D}{H} \times Q = A$$
18.4 Calculate intravenous dosages of heparin. Pages 537–545	To calculate weight-based heparin bolus doses: 1. Convert the patient's weight to kg $$\frac{1 \text{ kg}}{2.2 \text{ lb}} = \frac{x}{\text{patient's weight in pounds}}$$ 2. Calculate the desired dose: $$\frac{\text{Ordered dose}}{1 \text{ kg}} = \frac{\text{desired dose}}{\text{patient's weight}}$$ 3. Calculate the amount to administer in mL using one of the three methods: **Proportion Method:** $$\frac{H \text{ (units on hand)}}{1 \text{ mL}} = \frac{D \text{ (desired dose in units)}}{A}$$ **Dimensional Analysis:** No conversion factor needed $$A = \frac{1 \text{ mL}}{H \text{ (units on hand)}} \times \frac{D \text{ (desired dose in units)}}{1}$$ **Formula Method:** $$\frac{D \text{ (desired dose in units)}}{H \text{ (units on hand)}} \times Q \text{ (quantity in mL)} = A$$ To calculate heparin dosage in units/h follow rule 18-6 to infuse heparin with an infusion pump that administers

LEARNING OUTCOME	KEY POINTS
	in mL/h, use proportion method, dimensional analysis, or formula method where:

D = rate of desired dose (units/h)

Q = dosage unit (mL)

H = dose on hand (units)

A = amount to administer (mL/h)

To calculate weight-based heparin rate,

follow Rule 18-8 to find the IV flow rate based upon weight.

1. Convert pounds to kilograms, if necessary.

2. Determine the desired dose:

   Ordered Dose × weight in kg = Desired Dose

   unit of measurement/kg/h × kg = unit of measurement/h e.g. units/kg/h × kg = D

3. Calculate the flow rate.

For example: The patient weighs 220 lb and the rate to infuse is 16 units/kg/h, and the concentration is heparin 25,000 units/500 mL D5W (50 units/mL).

1. Convert:

$$220 \text{ lb} \times \frac{1 \text{ kg}}{2.2 \text{ lb}} = 100 \text{ kg}$$

2. Determine desired dose:

   16 units/kg/h × 100 kg = 1600 units/h

3. Calculate the flow rate:

$$\frac{50 \text{ units}}{1 \text{ mL}} = \frac{1,600 \text{ units/h}}{A}$$

$A = 32$ mL/h

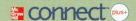
Answer the following questions.

1. Explain what U-100 and U-500 mean when referring to insulin. (LO 18.1a)

2. List the steps in preparing a combined insulin dose. (LO 18.1c)

3. Calculate the total units of insulin if the order is for 16 units Novolin® R and 30 units of Humulin® N. What type and size of syringe would you select. (LO 18.1c)

For Exercises 4-10, refer to labels A to D.

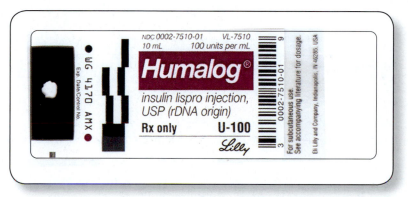

Label A

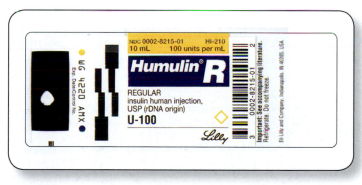

Label B

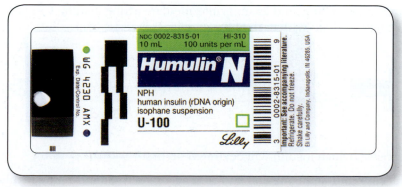

Label C

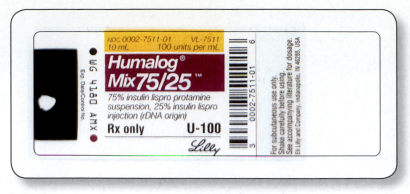

Label D

4. Administer 20 units of NPH insulin. Use label _____. Demonstrate where the syringe will be filled. (LO 18.1a, b)

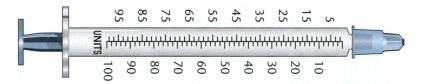

5. Administer 5 units of regular insulin. Use label _____. Demonstrate where the syringe will be filled. (LO 18.1a, b)

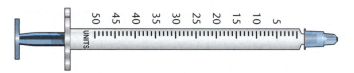

6. Administer 3 units of Humulog insulin. Use label _____. Demonstrate where the syringe will be filled. (LO18.1a, b)

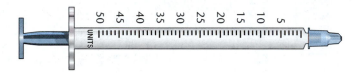

7. Administer 20 units of Humalog 75/25. Use label _____. In this dose how many units of lispro protamine suspension, and how many units of lispro injection will be administered? Insulin lispro protamine suspension_____, insulin lispro injection _____. (LO 18.1a)

8. Administer 10 units short-acting, and 25 units intermediate-acting insulin. Use labels _____. Demonstrate where the syringe will be filled with each of the insulin. (LO 18.1a, b, c)

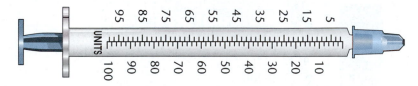

9. Referring to Exercise 8, which insulin will be drawn up first? _____. (LO 18.1c)

10. Administer 5 units of rapid-acting insulin and 30 units of intermediate-acting insulin. Use labels _____. Which insulin will be drawn up first? _____ (LO 18.1a, c)

Use the identified drug labels and package inserts to answer the following questions: (LO 18.2 and 18.3)

11. Refer to Label E. If the order is for 1,500 units heparin subcut, which concentration should you choose, and what amount would you administer?

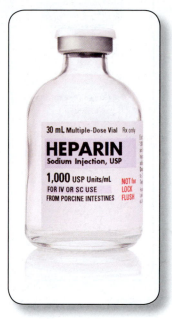

30 mL Multiple-Dose Vial   Rx only

HEPARIN
Sodium Injection, USP

1,000 USP Units/mL   NOT for
FOR IV OR SC USE   LOCK
FROM PORCINE INTESTINES   FLUSH

Label E

For Exercises 12–13 find the flow rate using an infusion pump.

12. Ordered: Heparin 1,500 units/h
    On hand: Heparin 50,000 units in 1000 mL D5W (LO 18.4)

13. Ordered: Heparin 1,500 units/h
    On hand: Heparin 100,000 units in 1000 mL NS (LO 18.4)

For Exercises 14–15 find the hourly dosage for the heparin orders. Determine whether the dosage is within the safe daily range for adults.

14. Heparin 20,000 units in 1000 mL D5W infusing at 30 mL/h. (LO 18.4)

15. Heparin 30,000 units in 1000 mL NS infusing at 10 mL/h. (LO 18.4)

16. Refer to label F. If the bolus dose was heparin 40 units/kg and the patient weighed 80 kg, how many units would you administer and how many mL would you administer? (LO18.2 and 18.4)

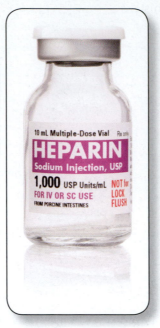

Label F

17. Per weight-based heparin protocol, the 90 kg patient has heparin 25,000 units in 500 mL D5W (50 units/mL) infusing at 24 units/kg/h. The aPTT is 130 and the protocol is to decrease the rate by 2 units/kg/h. What is the new infusion rate in mL/h? (LO 18.4)

For Exercises 18–20, refer to the weight-based heparin protocol; the 60 kg patient has heparin 25,000 units in 500 mL D5W (50 units/mL) infusing at 18 units/kg/h. The aPTT is 65 seconds, and the protocol is to bolus with heparin 40 units/kg (max. 4,000 units) and to increase the infusion by 1 unit/kg/h.

18. How many units is the bolus dose? (LO 18.4)

19. Using heparin from label B, how many mL of heparin would be administered? (LO 18.2)

20. What is the new infusion rate in mL/h? (LO 18.4)

CHECK UP

For Exercises 1–6, refer to labels A–F. Select the label corresponding to each exercise. Then mark the desired amount of insulin on the syringe. (LO 18.1a, b)

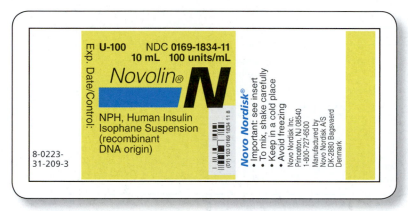

A

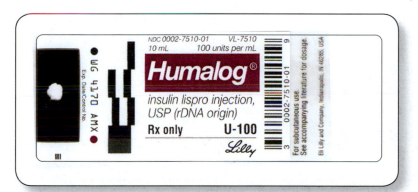

B

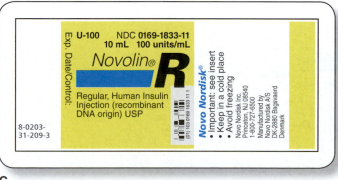

C

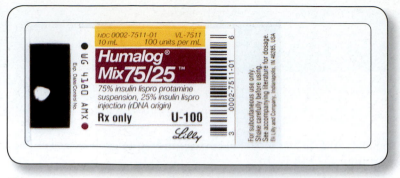

D

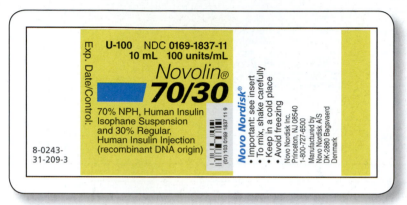

E

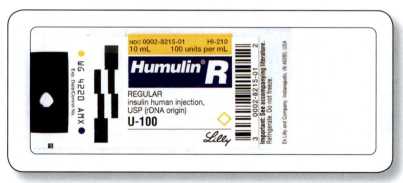

F

1. Ordered: Humulin® R 11 units subcut before breakfast

Select vial: _____

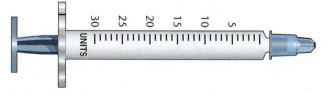

2. Ordered: Humalog 75/25 48 units subcut before dinner

Select vial: _____

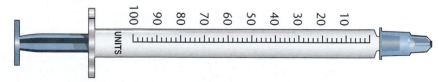

3. Ordered: Novolin® 70/30 57 units subcut before breakfast

Select vial: _____

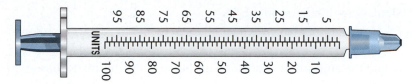

4. Ordered: Humalog® 24 units subcut daily

Select vial: _____

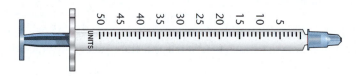

5. Ordered: Novolin® N 65 units subcut before dinner

Select vial: _____

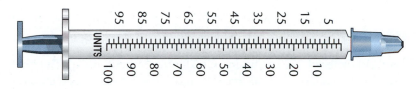

6. Ordered: Novolin® R insulin 21 units subcut before dinner

Select vial: _____

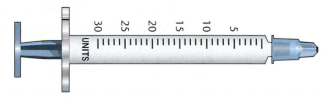

For Exercises 7 and 8, first mark on the syringe the dose of shorter-acting insulin ordered. Then mark where the leading ring will be after you draw up the intermediate-acting insulin into the same syringe. (LO 18.1b)

7. Humulin® N 27 units and Humulin® R 8 units subcut qam

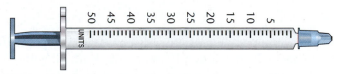

8. Novolin® R 13 units and Novolin® N 57 units subcut qam

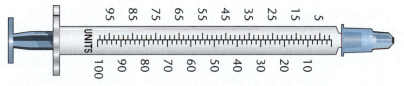

For Exercises 9 and 10 find the flow rate using an infusion pump. (LO 18.4)

9. Ordered: Heparin 1,200 units/h IV

On hand: 40,000 units in 500 mL D5W

10. Ordered: Heparin 800 units/h IV

On hand: 20,000 units in 1000 mL NS

For Exercises 11 and 12, find the hourly dosage for the heparin orders. Determine whether the dosage is within the safe daily range for adults. (LO 18.4)

11. 40,000 units in 1000 mL NS infusing at 40 mL/h.

12. 50,000 units in 500 mL D5W infusing at 10 mL/h.

For Exercises 13–14, calculate the amount of subcutaneous heparin to administer, based on the corresponding label. (LO 18.2 and 18.3)

13. Administer heparin 8,000 units subcut. _____

14. Administer heparin 4,000 units subcut. _____

For Exercises 15–16, use the following to calculate the answer in units and mL: The patient weighs 165 lb, the concentration of heparin for bolus dose is 1,000 units/mL, and the concentration of the heparin infusion is 25,000 units/500 mL (50 units/mL). (LO 18.4)

15. Administer a bolus dose of heparin 80 units/kg (max. 8,000 units). _____

16. Administer a heparin infusion at 18 units/kg/h (max. 1,800 units/h). _____

CRITICAL THINKING APPLICATION

The authorized prescriber (AP) ordered "Humulin insulin 20 units subcut, now." The healthcare practitioner, unaware that Humulin insulin is available in both regular and NPH forms, administered Humulin R, regular insulin at, 5 p.m. At 8 p.m. the patient experienced symptoms of hypoglycemia with a blood glucose level of 42. The blood sugar was treated with orange juice and food and rechecked until it was normal (which occurred within one hour).

The next morning, the fasting blood sugar was elevated, so the AP increased the dose. Again the patient experienced a low blood sugar at bedtime and a high blood sugar in the morning (LO 18.1).

1. What error did the AP make?

2. What error did the healthcare practitioner make?

3. How could have the healthcare practitioner prevented this error?

4. Why was the patient's blood sugar low at bedtime?

5. Why was the patient's blood sugar high in the morning?

CASE STUDY

The pharmacy technician stocks the automated medication dispenser with heparin 10,000 units/mL, 1 mL fill bottle in the slot designated for heparin flush solution 10 units/mL, 1 mL fill bottle. The day-shift nurse retrieves the heparin but does not check the label for concentration, looking only at the concentration on the computer screen. The nurse flushes both of the patient's heparin locks with 1 mL each of the heparin 10,000 units/mL solution. The patient also receives her q12h dose of heparin 5000 units subcut. The patient received an IV antibiotic at 1000 and a different IV antibiotic at 1400. Each time after the antibiotic had infused, the nurse flushed the heparin lock with 1 mL of heparin 10,000 units/mL. By the end of the nurse's shift the patient had blood in her urine and was bleeding from her gums. The patient, frightened by this, bumped her head on the door in her haste to call the nurse. Later, on the evening shift, the patient's level of consciousness decreased, due to a subdural hemorrhage. After the patient died, a root cause analysis revealed the errors of the pharmacy technician and the nurse. It was determined that the patient had received 45,000 units of heparin during the nurse's 8-hour shift (LO 18.2).

1. What is the highest safe dosage of heparin for a patient to receive in 24 hours?

2. What could the pharmacy technician have done to prevent the error?

3. What could the nurse have done to prevent the error?

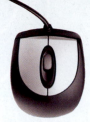

Search the Internet for "insulin and hypoglycemia" to answer the following:

1. What are the signs and symptoms of a hypoglycemic reaction?
2. How could hypoglycemia be treated?

To check your answers, see the Answer section at the end of the book, which starts on page A-1.

GO TO . . . Open the CD-ROM that accompanies your textbook, and complete a final review of the learning outcomes, practice problems, games, slideshow, and other activities presented for this chapter. For a final evaluation, take the chapter test and email or print your results for your instructor. A score of 95 percent or above indicates mastery of the chapter concepts.

Critical Care IV Calculations

Great works are performed not by strength but by perseverance.

—SAMUEL JOHNSON

Learning Outcomes

Upon completion of Chapter 19, you will be able to:

19.1 Calculate the hourly flow rate for IV infusions ordered in dosage per time (Examples: mcg/min, mg/h).

19.2 Calculate IV flow rates for medications ordered based on body weight over a specified period of time (Examples: mg/kg/min or mcg/kg/min).

19.3 Calculate IV flow rates for titrated medications.

KEY TERMS

Antiarrhythmic medications

Dry weight

Hemodynamics

Titrate

Vasoactive medications

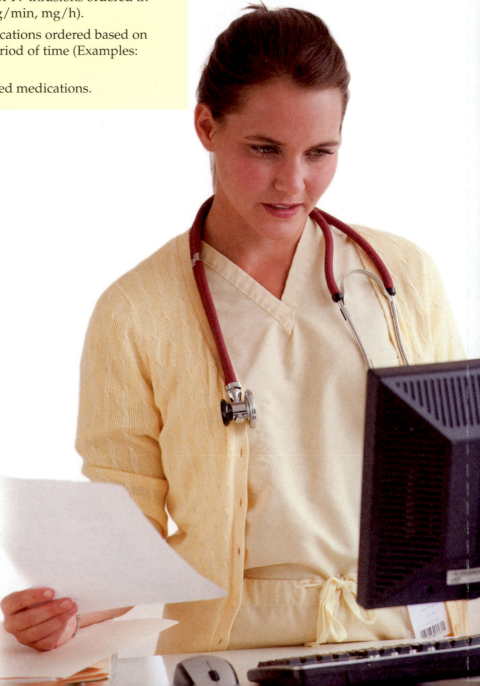

INTRODUCTION

Controlling vital functions of critically ill patients is difficult and requires constant nursing intervention. Often **vasoactive medications** (medications that cause the blood vessels to dilate or constrict) are administered IV to keep the patient's blood pressure within the normal range. These medications may have a side effect on the patient's heart rate. While these medications are administered, the nurse continuously monitors the patient's blood pressure and heart rhythm and rate to **titrate** (adjust) the dosage of medication in response the patient's vital signs. In addition to vasoactive medications, **antiarrhythmic medications** may be given to regulate the patient's heart rate and/or rhythm, and analgesics to relieve pain, sedatives to relieve anxiety, and paralytics to decrease oxygen consumption, may also be infused. These medications may be administered at a constant rate, or the rate may be titrated to patient response. Other IV medications, such as antibiotics or electrolyte replacements, must be administered no faster than a specified rate to prevent serious or life-threatening side effects. For example, too rapid infusion of potassium chloride, a high-alert medication, will result in death. The focus of this chapter is on dosage calculation of medications used in critical care that are administered in small quantities, by patient weight, and/or over time (minute or hour). These medications are administered by an electronic infusion pump. See Figure 19-1.

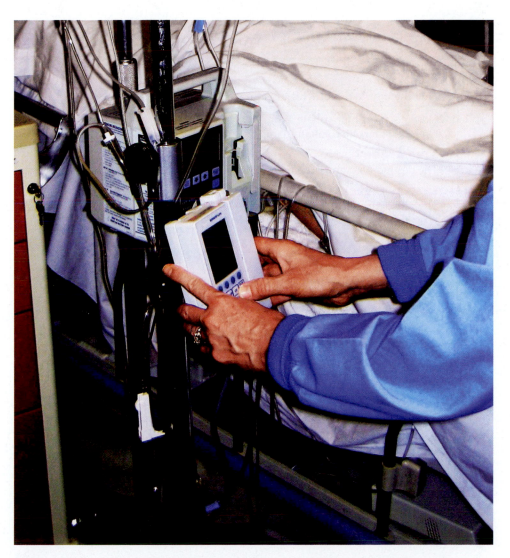

Figure 19-1 Using an electronic infusion pump, a critical care nurse may need to titrate (adjust the dose of a medication) in response to the patient's vital signs.

19.1 Hourly Flow Rates for Dosage per Time Infusions

Dosage per Hour

You have learned to calculate heparin units/h in Chapter 18. The same method can be applied to critical care IV medications.

RULE 19-1

Converting Dosage/h to mL/h.
Determine the following:

> D = rate of desired dose (mcg/h, mg/h, g/h, units/h)
>
> Q = dosage unit (mL)
>
> H = dose on hand (total number of mcg or mg. . .)
>
> A = amount to administer (mL/h)

Use the proportion method, dimensional analysis, or formula method to find the hourly flow rate.

PROPORTION METHOD

EXAMPLE

Find the hourly rate at which to administer IV morphine sulfate.

Ordered: morphine sulfate 4 mg/h
On hand: morphine sulfate 10 mg/100 mL D5W

STEP A: CONVERT
The desired dose and dose on hand are both in mg, so no conversion is necessary.

STEP B: CALCULATE
The rate of the desired dose D is 4 mg/1 h. The dosage unit Q is 100 mL. The dose on hand H is 10 mg. A is the amount (volume) to administer/h.
Follow Procedure Checklist 12-1.

1. Fill in the proportion.

$$\frac{H}{Q} = \frac{D}{A}$$

$$\frac{10 \text{ mg}}{100 \text{ mL}} = \frac{4 \text{ mg/h}}{A}$$

    Fill in the ratio

$$H{:}Q = D{:}A$$

$$10 \text{ mg} : 100 \text{ mL} = 4 \text{ mg/h} : A$$

3. Cancel the units, leaving mL/h

$$\frac{10 \; \cancel{\text{mg}}}{100 \text{ mL}} = \frac{4 \; \cancel{\text{mg}}/h}{A}$$

$$10 : 100 \text{ mL} = 4/h : A$$

4. Cross-multiply and solve for the unknown.

$$10 \times A = 100 \text{ mL} \times 4/h$$

$$A = \frac{400 \text{ mL/h}}{10}$$

$$A = 40 \text{ mL/h}$$

    Multiply the means and the extremes and solve for the unknown.

$$10 \times A = 100 \text{ mL} \times 4 / h$$

$$A = \frac{400 \text{ mL/h}}{10}$$

$$A = 40 \text{ mL/h}$$

STEP C: THINK! . . . IS IT REASONABLE?
Since the dosage strength is 1 mg to 10 mL, and 4 × 10 is 40, it is reasonable that a 4 mg/h dose would equal 40 mL/h.

DIMENSIONAL ANALYSIS

EXAMPLE

Find the hourly rate at which to administer IV morphine sulfate.

Ordered: morphine sulfate 4 mg/h
On hand: morphine sulfate 10 mg/100 mL D5W

STEP A: CONVERT
The desired dose and dose on hand are both in mg, so no conversion factor is needed.

STEP B: CALCULATE
The rate of the desired dose D is 4 mg/h. The dosage unit Q is 100 mL. The dose on hand H is 10 mg. Follow Procedure Checklist 12-2.

$$A = C \times Q/H \times D$$

1. The unit of measure will be in milliliters per hour

    A mL/h

2. No conversion factor is needed.

3. The dosage unit is 100 mL; the dose on hand is 10 mg. This is the first factor.

    $$\frac{100 \text{ mL}}{10 \text{ mg}}$$

4. The desired dose is 4 mg/h. This is the second factor.

    $$A \text{ mL/h} = \frac{100 \text{ mL}}{10 \text{ mg}} \times \frac{4 \text{ mg}}{\text{h}}$$

5. Cancel units. The remaining units on the right side of the equation should be milliliters per hour.

    $$A = \frac{100 \text{ mL}}{10 \ \cancel{\text{mg}}} \times \frac{4 \ \cancel{\text{mg}}}{\text{h}}$$

    $$A = \frac{100 \text{ mL} \times 4}{10 \text{ h}}$$

    $$A = \frac{400 \text{ mL}}{10 \text{ h}}$$

    $$A = 40 \text{ mL/h}$$

STEP C: THINK! . . . IS IT REASONABLE
Since the dosage strength is 1 mg to 10 mL, and 4 × 10 is 40, it is reasonable that a 4 mg/h dose would equal 40 mL/h.

FORMULA METHOD

EXAMPLE

Find the hourly rate at which to administer IV morphine sulfate.

Ordered: morphine sulfate 4 mg/h
On hand: morphine sulfate 10 mg/100 mL D5W

STEP A: CONVERT
The desired dose and dose on hand are both in mg, so no conversion is necessary.

STEP B: CALCULATE
The rate of the desired dose D is 4 mg/h. The dosage unit Q is 100 mL. The dose on hand H is 10 mg.
Follow Procedure Checklist 12-3.
Fill in the formula:

$$\frac{D}{H} \times Q = A$$

$$\frac{4 \text{ mg/h}}{10 \text{ mg}} \times 100 \text{ mL} = A$$

$$\frac{4 \cancel{\text{mg}}/\text{h}}{10 \cancel{\text{mg}}} \times 100 \text{ mL} = A$$

$$\frac{400 \text{ mL/h}}{10} = A$$

$$\frac{40 \text{ mL}}{\text{h}} = A$$

STEP C: THINK! . . . IS IT REASONABLE?

Since the dosage strength is 1 mg to 10 mL, and 4 × 10 is 40, it is reasonable that a 4 mg/h dose would equal 40 mL/h.

GO TO . . . Open the CD-ROM that accompanies your textbook and select Chapter 19, Convert dosage/minute to mL/h (LO 19.1). Review the animation and example problems, then complete the practice problems. Continue to the next section of the book once you have mastered the information presented.

Dosage per Minute

Potent medications may be ordered in amounts per minute. Amounts per minute will need to be converted to milliliters per hour, to program the infusion pump.

RULE 19-2	To convert a per-minute order to an hourly flow rate:
	1. Convert the order to milliliters per minute. Determine the following:
	D = rate of desired dose (mg or mcg/min)
	Q = dosage unit (mL)
	H = dose on hand (total number of mg or mcg)
	A = amount to administer (mL/min)
	Use the proportion method, dimensional analysis, or formula method.
	2. Multiply mg/min × 60 min/h. For Dimensional Analysis, use 60 min/1 h as the conversion factor.

PROPORTION METHOD

EXAMPLE

Find the hourly flow rate.

Ordered: 5000 mg Esmolol in 500 mL of D5W at 8 mg/min via infusion pump

STEP A: CONVERT

Convert mg/min to mg/h

There are 60 minutes in an hour so

$$\text{mg/min} \times 60 \text{ min/h} = \text{mg/h}$$

$$8 \text{ mg/}\cancel{\text{min}} \times 60 \text{ }\cancel{\text{min}}\text{/h} = 480 \text{ mg/h}$$

STEP B: CALCULATE

The rate of the desired dose D is now 480 mg/h. The dosage unit Q is 500 mL. The dose on hand H is 5000 mg

Follow Procedure Checklist 12-1.

1. Fill in the proportion.

$$\frac{H}{Q} = \frac{D}{A}$$

$$\frac{5000 \text{ mg}}{500 \text{ mL}} = \frac{480 \text{ mg/h}}{A}$$

Fill in the ratio

$$H{:}Q = D{:}A$$

$$5000 \text{ mg}{:}500 \text{ mL} = 480 \text{ mg/h}{:}A$$

2. Cancel the units leaving mL/h

$$\frac{5000 \text{ }\cancel{\text{mg}}}{500 \text{ mL}} = \frac{480 \text{ }\cancel{\text{mg}}\text{/h}}{A}$$

$$5000{:}500 \text{ mL} = 480\text{/h}{:}A$$

3. Cross-multiply and solve for the unknown.

$$5000 \times A = 500 \text{ mL} \times 480\text{/h}$$

$$A = \frac{500 \text{ mL} \times 480\text{/h}}{5000}$$

$$A = 48 \text{ mL/h}$$

Multiply the means and the extremes and solve for the unknown.

$$5000 \times A = 500 \text{ mL} \times 480\text{/h}$$

$$A = \frac{500 \text{ mL} \times 480\text{/h}}{5000}$$

$$A = 48 \text{ mL/h}$$

STEP C: THINK! . . . IS IT REASONABLE?

Since the concentration of 5000 mg/500 mL equals 10 mg/mL, and 480 mg/10 = 48, the answer is reasonable.

DIMENSIONAL ANALYSIS

EXAMPLE

Find the hourly flow rate.

Ordered: 5000 mg Esmolol in 500 mL of D5W at 8 mg/min via infusion pump

STEP A: CONVERT

The desired dose D in mg/min should be converted to mg/h, so the conversion factor 60 min/1 h is required.

STEP B: CALCULATE

The rate of the desired dose D is 8 mg/min. The dosage unit Q is 500 mL. The dose on hand H is 5000 mg.

Follow Procedure Checklist 12-2.

1. The unit of measure will be milliliters per hour.

$$A \text{ mL/h} =$$

2. The dosage unit is 500 mL; the dose on hand is 5000 mg. This is the first factor.

$$\frac{500 \text{ mL}}{5000 \text{ mg}}$$

3. The desire dose is 8 mg/min. This is the second factor.

$$A \text{ mL/h} = \frac{500 \text{ mL}}{5000 \text{ mg}} \times \frac{8 \text{ mg}}{1 \text{ min}}$$

4. Use the third factor $\dfrac{60 \text{ min}}{1 \text{ h}}$ to convert the answer from minutes to hours.

$$A \text{ mL/h} = \dfrac{500 \text{ mL}}{5000 \text{ mg}} \times \dfrac{8 \text{ mg}}{1 \text{ min}} \times \dfrac{60 \text{ min}}{1 \text{ h}}$$

5. Cancel units. The remaining units on the right side of the equation should be milliliters per hour.

$$A \text{ mL/h} = \dfrac{500 \text{ mL}}{5000 \text{ mg}} \times \dfrac{8 \text{ mg}}{1 \text{ min}} \times \dfrac{60 \text{ min}}{1 \text{ h}}$$

6. Solve the equation.

$$A \text{ mL/h} = \dfrac{500 \text{ mL}}{5000} \times \dfrac{8}{1} \times \dfrac{60}{1 \text{ h}}$$

$$A = 48 \text{ mL/h}$$

STEP C: THINK! . . . IS IT REASONABLE?

Since the concentration of 5000 mg/500 mL equals 10 mg/mL, and 480 mg/10 = 48, the answer is reasonable.

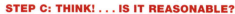 **GO TO . . .** Open the CD-ROM that accompanies your textbook, and select Chapter 19, Per Minute Orders (LO 19.1). Review the animation and example problems, then complete the practice problems. Continue to the next section of the book once you have mastered the information presented.

REVIEW AND PRACTICE

19.1 Hourly Flow Rates for Dosage per Time Infusions

For Examples 1–9 convert the dosage/minute into milliliters/hour.

1. Ordered: xylocaine 2 mg/min IV

    On hand: xylocaine 1 g/500 mL D5W

2. Ordered: nitroglycerin 10 mcg/min IV

    On hand: nitroglycerin 50 mg/250 mL NS

3. Ordered: vasopressin 0.04 units/min IV

    On hand: vasopressin 60 units/50 mL NS

4. Ordered: diltiazem 5 mg/h IV

    On hand: diltiazem 125 mg/125 mL D5W

5. Ordered: epinephrine 2 mcg/min IV

    On hand: epinephrine 1 mg/500 mL NS

6. Ordered: nitroglycerin 10 mcg/min IV

    On hand: nitroglycerin 25 mg in 250 mL D5W

7. Ordered: procainamide 3 mg/min IV

   On hand: procainamide hydrochloride 1 g/250 mL D5W

8. Ordered: morphine 4 mg/h IV

   On hand: morphine 50 mg/100 mL NS

9. Ordered: midazolam 0.5 mg/h

   On hand: midazolam 25 mg/50 mL NS

10. Ordered: nicardipine 7.5 mg/h

    On hand: nicardipine 25 mg/250 mL D5W

To check your answers, see the Answer section at the end of the book, which starts on page A-1.

19.2 IV Flow Rates Based on Body Weight per Time

Many infusions administered to the critically ill patient are ordered by amount/patient's weight/time. In Chapter 18, you learned to calculate heparin units/kg/h. The same procedure can be applied to critical care IV dosage calculation. Round the patient's weight to the nearest tenth.

LEARNING LINK Recall from Chapter 18, Rule 18-8, how to find the IV flow rate based upon weight.

1. Convert pounds to kilograms, if necessary.

2. Determine the desired dose:

   Ordered Dose × weight in kg = Desired Dose (D)

   Unit of measurement/kg/h × kg = unit of measurement/h For example: mg/kg/h × kg = mg/h

3. Calculate the flow rate.

PROPORTION METHOD

EXAMPLE   Find the hourly rate at which to administer dopamine to a 220-lb patient.

Ordered: dopamine 5 mcg/kg/min
On hand: dopamine 400 mg/250 mL NS

STEP A: CONVERT

1. Convert the weight to kilograms.

$$\frac{1 \text{ kg}}{2.2 \text{ lb}} = \frac{x}{220 \text{ lb}}$$

$$\frac{220 \text{ lb} \times 1 \text{ kg}}{2.2 \text{ lb}} = x$$

100 kg = x

The patient weighs 100 kg.

Convert milligrams to micrograms

$$\frac{1000 \text{ mcg}}{1 \text{ mg}} = \frac{x}{400 \text{ mg}}$$

$$\frac{400 \text{ mg} \times 1000 \text{ mcg}}{1 \text{ mg}} = x$$

$$400{,}000 \text{ mcg} = x$$

Therefore 400 mg in 250 mL $= \dfrac{400{,}000 \text{ mcg}}{250 \text{ mL}}$

STEP B: CALCULATE

Determine the desired dose of dopamine.

$$5 \text{ mcg/kg/min} \times 100 \text{ kg} = \dfrac{500 \text{ mcg}}{\text{min}}$$

Use Rule 19-2 to convert mcg/min to mcg/h:

$$\dfrac{500 \text{ mcg}}{\text{min}} \times \dfrac{60 \text{ min}}{\text{h}} = \dfrac{30{,}000 \text{ mcg}}{\text{h}}$$

Calculate the flow rate.
Follow Procedure Checklist 12-1.

$$\dfrac{400{,}000 \text{ mcg}}{250 \text{ mL}} = \dfrac{30{,}000 \text{ mcg/h}}{A}$$

$$400{,}000 \text{ mcg} \times A = 30{,}000 \text{ mcg/h} \times 250 \text{ mL}$$

$$400{,}000 \, A = 7{,}500{,}000 \text{ mL/h}$$

$$A = 18.75 \text{ mL/h}$$

The flow rate is 18.8 mL/h.

STEP C: THINK ! . . . IS IT REASONABLE?

Since the ordered dose, 400,000 mcg, is more than ten times the desired dose, 30,000 mcg/h, and the quantity 250 mL is more than ten times 18.8 mL per hour, the flow rate is reasonable.

DIMENSIONAL ANALYSIS

EXAMPLE

Find the hourly rate at which to administer dopamine to a 220-lb patient.

Ordered: dopamine 5 mcg/kg/min
On hand: dopamine 400 mg/250 mL NS

STEP A: CONVERT

The desired dose is in micrograms and the dose on hand is in milligrams, so a conversion factor, 1 mg/1000 mcg is necessary. To convert minutes to hours, use the conversion factor 60 min/1 h as indicated in Rule 19-2. Convert 220 lb to 100 kg by using the Proportion Method.

STEP B: CALCULATE

Determine the desired dose of dopamine.

$$5 \text{ mcg/kg/min} \times 100 \text{ kg} = 500 \text{ mcg/min}$$

Follow Procedure Checklist 12-2.

$$A \text{ mL/h} = \text{Conversion factors} \times \dfrac{Q}{H} \times D$$

$$A \text{ mL/h} = \dfrac{1 \text{ mg}}{1000 \text{ mcg}} \times \dfrac{60 \text{ min}}{1 \text{ h}} \times \dfrac{250 \text{ mL}}{400 \text{ mg}} \times \dfrac{500 \text{ mcg}}{1 \text{ min}}$$

$$A \text{ mL/h} = 18.75$$

Round to the nearest tenth.

The flow rate is 18.8 mL/h.

STEP C: THINK! . . . IS IT REASONABLE?

Since the ordered dose, 400,000 mcg, is more than ten times the desired dose, 30,000 mcg/h, and the quantity 250 mL is more than ten times 18.8 mL per hour, the flow rate is reasonable.

FORMULA METHOD

EXAMPLE

Find the hourly rate at which to administer dopamine to a 220-lb patient.

Ordered: dopamine 5 mcg/kg/min
On hand: dopamine 400 mg/250 mL NS

STEP A: CONVERT
Convert the 220 lb to 100 kg using the Proportion Method.
Convert 400 mg to 400,000 mcg using the Proportion Method.

STEP B: CALCULATE
Determine the desired dose of dopamine.

5mcg/kg/min × 100 kg = 500 mcg/min

Use Rule 19-2 to convert mcg/min to mcg/h.

500 mcg/min × 60 min/h = 30,000 mcg/h

Calculate the flow rate.
Follow Procedure Checklist 12-3.

$$\frac{D}{H} \times Q = A$$

$$\frac{30,000 \text{ mcg/h}}{400,000 \text{ mcg}} \times 250 \text{ mL} = 18.75 \text{ mL/h}$$

Round to the nearest tenth.

The flow rate is 18.8 mL/h.

STEP C: THINK! . . . IS IT REASONABLE?
Since the ordered dose, 400,000 mcg, is more than ten times the desired dose, 30,000 mcg/h, and the quantity 250 mL is more than ten times 18.8 mL per hour, the flow rate is reasonable.

RULE 19-3	Sometimes it is necessary to convert the rate from mL/h to mL/min to verify a safe dosage. To calculate the rate in mL/minute, divide the rate in mL/h by 60 min/h or multiply the rate in mL/h by the conversion factor 1 h/60 min.
Example	If the rate = 18.8 mL/h, the rate in mL/min is calculated: 18.8 mL/h ÷ 60 min/h = 0.31 mL/min OR 18.8 mL/h × 1h/60 min = 0.31 mL/min

RULE 19-4	If you know the total amount of medication in the total volume of solution (supply dose) as well as the volume of solution that the patient has received, then you can use a proportion to calculate the amount of medication the patient has received (the dose). $$\frac{\text{Total amount of medication}}{\text{Total volume of solution}} = \frac{\text{amount of medication received}}{\text{volume of solution received}}$$
Example 1	A pregnant patient has been given increasing rates of Pitocin® to induce labor. Since her arrival at the hospital, she has received 50 mL of a solution of Pitocin® that contains 20 units in 1000 mL LR. How much Pitocin® has she received? The total amount of medication is 20 units, the total volume of solution is 1000 mL, and the volume of solution received is 50 mL.

$$\frac{20 \text{ units}}{1000 \text{ mL}} = \frac{x \text{ units}}{50 \text{ mL}}$$

20 units × 50 = 1000 × x

1000 units = 1000 × x

1 unit = x

The patient has received 1 unit of Pitocin®.

Example 2	Your patient is receiving dopamine titrated to maintain his blood pressure. His infusion started with dopamine 800 mg/D5W 250 mL at a rate of 5 mL/h. Over the last 3 hours you have titrated the dopamine up to 12 mL/h to maintain the blood pressure. He has received 112 mL of the solution. How much dopamine has the patient received?

The total amount of medication is 800 mg. The total volume of solution is 250 mL. The volume of solution received is 112 mL.

$$\frac{800 \text{ mg}}{250 \text{ mL}} = \frac{x}{112 \text{ mL}}$$

800 mg × 112 = 250 × x

$$\frac{800 \text{ mg} \times 112}{250} = x$$

358.4 mg = x

The patient has received 358.4 mg of dopamine.

GO TO . . . Open the CD-ROM that accompanies your textbook, and select Chapter 19, Calculate the Amount of Medication Received (LO 19.2). Review the animation and example problems, then complete the practice problems. Continue to the next section of the book once you have mastered the information presented.

REVIEW AND PRACTICE

19.2 IV Flow Rates Based on Body Weight per Time

For Exercises 1–4 refer to the following order for a 185-lb patient.

Ordered: vecuronium 1 mcg/kg/min IV
On hand: vecuronium 10 mg/100 mL NS

1. What is the patient's weight in kg?

2. What is the desired dose?

3. What is the flow rate?

4. What is the rate in mL/min?

For Exercises 5–9 refer to the following order for a 140 lb patient.

Ordered: nitroprusside 0.5 mcg/kg/min IV
On hand: nitroprusside 50 mg/250 mL D5W

    5. What is the patient's weight in kg?

    6. What is the desired dose?

    7. What is the flow rate?

    8. What is the rate in mL/min?

For Exercises 10–14 refer to the following order for a 113-lb patient.

Ordered: nesiritide 0.02 mcg/kg/min IV
On hand: nesiritide 1.5 mg/250 mL D5W

    9. What is the patient's weight in kg?

    10. What is the desired dose?

    11. What is the flow rate?

    12. What is the rate in mL/min?

For Exercises 13–17 refer to the following order for a 150-lb patient.

Ordered: dobutamine 1 mcg/kg/min IV
On hand: dobutamine HCl 250 mg/500 mL D5W

    13. What is the patient's weight in kg?

    14. What is the desired dose?

    15. What is the flow rate?

    16. What is the rate in mL/min?

For Exercises 17–18, find the amount of medication that has already been administered to the patient.

    17. Ordered: Lidocaine® 2 g in 1000 mL of D5W.

        The patient has received 400 mL.

    18. Ordered: Remicade® 300 mg in 250 mL of NaCl.

        The patient has received 150 mL.

To check your answers, see the Answer section at the end of the book, which starts on page A-1.

19.3 IV Flow Rates for Titrated Medications

The goal is to administer the least amount of medication to achieve the desired effect. The amount of many critical care IV medications needed to achieve the desired effect varies. For this reason, many critical care IV medication dosages are titrated (adjusted) to the effect on the patient's **hemodynamics** (forces of blood flow), and/or heart rhythm. This requires constant observation of the patient's response, and frequent adjustment (**titration**) of the rate. To make dosage changes quickly and accurately, many nurses create a titration table with medication dosages at different rates within the ordered dosage range (see Table 19-1).

When the dosage of a medication is to be titrated, the AP orders the drug, dosage range (the maximal dose and the minimal dose), the starting dose (which is often the minimal dose), and the desired effect. There also may be limitations that would stop an increased dose, even though the desired effect has not been achieved. For example, Dopamine 400 mg in 500 mL NS, to infuse at 5–20 mcg/kg/min IV to keep systolic blood pressure greater than 90 mm Hg. Keep HR less than 100. Start at 5 mcg/kg/min and titrate to effect.

TABLE 19-1 Titration Table with Dopamine Dosages for a Patient Who Weighs 100 kg	
DOPAMINE DOSAGE (mcg/100 kg)	**IV RATE (mL/h) 1600 mcg/1 mL**
5 mcg/kg/min	18.8 mL/h
10 mcg/kg/min	37.5 mL/h
15 mcg/kg/min	56.3 mL/h
20 mcg/kg/min	75 mL/h

ERROR ALERT!

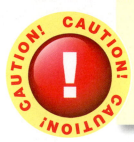

Dry Weight for Weight-based Calculations

The patient's weight may fluctuate frequently due to changes in volume status. Base calculations on the patient's "**dry weight**" (weight when properly hydrated) when titrating IV rates. Sometimes this can be determined by noting the patient's weight when discharged from the last hospital stay.

RULE 19-5

For safe titration:

1. Calculate the starting rate.

2. Calculate the minimum allowable rate.

3. Calculate the maximum allowable rate.

4. Begin infusion at the starting rate.

5. Titrate (adjust) dosage, based on patient response.

6. Do not exceed maximum rate (call AP for new order if the patient does not have the desired response at the maximum rate).

7. If the patient's response exceeds the prescribed parameters at the minimal dose, discontinue the infusion and notify the AP.

Example

Using the titration Table 19-1, find the minimum rate, the maximum rate, and the starting rate to set the IV infusion pump for a 100 kg patient.

Ordered: Dopamine 400 mg in 500 mL NS (1600 mcg/mL), to infuse at 5–20 mcg/kg/min IV to keep systolic blood pressure greater than 90. Keep heart rate less than 100. Start at 5 mcg/kg/min and titrate according to blood pressure (BP) and heart rate (HR). According to Table 19-1, the rates should be:

Minimum rate: 18.8 mL/ h

Maximal rate: 75 mL/h

Starting rate: 18.8 mL/ h

Example	**Titrating a dopamine IV infusion**
	Ordered: Dopamine 400 mg in 500 mL NS (1600 mcg/mL), to infuse at 5–20 mcg/kg/min IV to keep systolic blood pressure greater than 90. Keep heart rate less than 100. Start at 5 mcg/kg/min and titrate according to blood pressure (BP) and heart rate (HR).
	Calculate the minimum rate (follow Rule 18-8, using the proportion method, dimensional analysis, or formula method).

PROPORTION METHOD

EXAMPLE

Ordered: Dopamine 400 mg in 500 mL NS (1600 mcg/mL), to infuse at 5–20 mcg/kg/min IV to keep systolic blood pressure greater than 90. Keep heart rate less than 100. Start at 5 mcg/kg/min and titrate according to blood pressure (BP) and heart rate (HR).

STEP A: CONVERT
Convert milligrams to micrograms

$$\frac{1000\ \text{mcg}}{1\ \text{mg}} = \frac{x\ \text{mcg}}{400\ \text{mg}}$$

$$400\ \text{mg} \times 1,000\ \text{mcg} = 1\ \text{mg} \times x$$

$$400,000\ \text{mcg} = x$$

The concentration is 400,000 mcg/250 mL which can be reduced to 1600 mcg/1 mL. This is the dose on hand (*H*) over the dosage unit (*Q*)

STEP B: CALCULATE
Determine the starting rate (desired dose) of dopamine.

$$5\text{mcg/kg/min} \times 100\ \text{kg} = D$$

$$500\ \text{mcg/min} = D$$

The desired dose *D* = 500 mcg/min.

Use Rule 19-1 to convert mcg/min to mcg/h:

$$\frac{500\ \text{mcg}}{\text{min}} \times \frac{60\ \text{min}}{\text{h}} = 30,000\ \text{mcg/h}$$

Calculate the flow rate:
Follow Procedure Checklist 12-1.

$$\frac{H}{Q} = \frac{D}{A} \qquad\qquad H{:}Q = D{:}A$$

$$\frac{1600\ \text{mcg}}{1\ \text{mL}} = \frac{30,000\ \text{mcg/h}}{A} \qquad\qquad 1600\ \text{mcg}{:}1\ \text{mL} = 30,000\ \text{mcg/h}{:}A$$

$$\frac{1600\ \text{mcg}}{1\ \text{mL}} = \frac{30,000\ \text{mcg/h}}{A} \qquad\qquad \frac{1600\ \text{mcg}}{1\ \text{mL}} = \frac{30,000\ \text{mcg/h}}{A\ \text{mL}}$$

$$1600 \times A = 30,000\ \text{mL/h} \qquad\qquad 1600 \times A\ \text{mL} = 30,000\ \text{mL/h}$$

$$A = 18.75\ \text{mL/h} \qquad\qquad A = 18.75\ \text{mL/h}$$

The minimal flow rate is 18.8 mL/h.   The minimal flow rate is 18.8 mL/h.

STEP C: THINK! . . . IS IT REASONABLE?
Since the ordered dose, 400,000 mcg, is more than ten times the desired dose, 30,000 mcg/h, and the quantity 250 mL is more than ten times 18.8 mL per hour, the flow rate is reasonable.

Calculate the maximum rate (follow Rule 18-8 using the proportion method, dimensional analysis, or formula method).

FORMULA METHOD

Ordered: Dopamine 400 mg in 500 mL NS (1600 mcg/mL), to infuse at 5–20 mcg/kg/min IV to keep systolic blood pressure greater than 90. Keep heart rate less than 100. Start at 5 mcg/kg/min and titrate according to blood pressure (BP) and heart rate (HR).

STEP A: CONVERT
Convert milligrams to micrograms

$$\frac{1000\ \text{mcg}}{1\ \text{mg}} = \frac{x}{400\ \text{mg}}$$

$$\frac{400\ \cancel{\text{mg}} \times 1000\ \text{mcg}}{1\ \cancel{\text{mg}}} = x$$

$$400,000\ \text{mcg} = x$$

STEP B: CALCULATE
Determine the maximum rate (desired dose) of dopamine.

$$20\ \text{mcg}/\cancel{\text{kg}}/\text{min} \times 100\ \cancel{\text{kg}} = 2000\ \text{mcg}/\text{min}$$

The desired dose $D = 2000$ mcg/min.

Use Rule 19-2 to convert mcg/min to mcg/h:

$$\frac{2000\ \text{mcg}}{\cancel{\text{min}}} \times \frac{60\ \cancel{\text{min}}}{\text{h}} = 120,000\ \text{mcg}/\text{h}$$

Calculate the flow rate:
Follow Procedure Checklist 12-3.

$$\frac{D}{H} \times Q = A$$

$$\frac{120,000\ \cancel{\text{mcg}}/\text{h}}{1600\ \cancel{\text{mcg}}} \times 1\ \text{mL} = A$$

$$75\ \text{mL}/\text{h} = A$$

The maximum flow rate is 75 mL/h.

STEP C: THINK! . . . IS IT REASONABLE?
Since the maximum dose is four times the size of the minimum dose and 75 is four times larger than 18.74, the answer is reasonable.

Calculate the starting rate
The starting rate is the same as the minimum rate, so no calculation is necessary.

Based on the patient's blood pressure and heart rate, the rate of dopamine may be titrated up to 75 mL/h and be within the prescribed guidelines.

GO TO . . . Open the CD-ROM that accompanies your textbook, and select Chapter 19, Safe Titration (LO 19.3). Review the animation and example problems, then complete the practice problems. Continue to the next section of the book once you have mastered the information presented.

19.3 IV Flow Rates for Titrated Medications

For Exercises 1–3 refer to the following order, and calculate the requested rates.

Ordered: xylocaine 1 g in 250 mL D5W; start IV infusion at 2 mg/min and titrate to absence of ventricular dysrhythmia; dosage range 1 mg/min–4 mg/min.

1. Calculate the minimum dose.

2. Calculate the maximum dose.

3. Calculate the starting dose.

For Exercises 4–5, the following applies:

Ordered: dopamine: Begin infusion of 2 mcg/kg/min for bradycardia and systolic BP less than 90. Increase infusion up to 10 mcg/kg/min as needed.

You have a premixed bag of dopamine with 200 mg in 500 mL of D5W. The patient weighs 165 lb.

4. At what flow rate in milliliters per hour should you start the IV?

5. The BP remains low, and you increase the flow rate to 35 mL/h. What is the dosage that the patient is receiving at this time?

For Exercises 6–10 calculate the IV flow rate in mL/h based on the following order:

Ordered: nicardipine 25 mg/250 mL normal saline IV; start at 5 mg/h and infuse for 30 minutes. Titrate to systolic BP greater than or equal to 90 by increasing rate 3 mg/h every 5 to 15 minutes. Maximum infusion rate 15 mg/h.

Maintenance rate: After 30 minutes, while systolic BP is greater than or equal to 90 mm Hg, decrease rate to 3 mg/h; may increase rate by 2.5 mg every 5 to 15 minutes until systolic BP is greater than or equal to 90. Maximum infusion rate 15 mg/h.

6. Calculate the minimum dose.

7. Calculate the maximum dose.

8. Calculate the starting dose.

9. The nicardipine was started 15 minutes ago and is infusing at 80 mL/h. The patient's systolic BP is 74. Should the infusion be titrated? If so, what is the new rate?

10. The patient's systolic BP is 94, and the nicardipine infusion has been infusing for 30 minutes. How many mL/h should be infused now?

To check your answers, see the Answer section at the end of the book, which starts on page A-1.

LEARNING OUTCOMES	KEY POINTS
19.1 Calculate the hourly flow rates for IV infusions ordered in dose per time (e.g., mg/min, mcg/min). Page 562–566	▶ Refer to Rule 19-1. D = rate of desired dose (e.g. mcg/h) H = dose on hand A = amount to administer (mL/h) Follow procedure 12-1, 12-2, or 12-3 to calculate the flow rate. Refer to Rule 19-2. To convert a minute flow rate to an hourly flow rate: Multiply per minute order by 60 min/h. For Dimensional Analysis, use the conversion factor 60 min/1 h.
19.2 Calculate IV flow rates for medications ordered based on body weight over a specified period of time (e.g., mg/kg/min or mcg/kg/min). Page 567–571	▶ Refer to Rule 18-8 to find a flow rate based upon weight. 1. Convert pounds to kilograms, if necessary. 2. Determine the desired dose: Ordered dose × weight in kg = Desired Dose, e.g. mg/kg/min × kg = D 3. Calculate the flow rate (mL/h). Refer to Rule 19-3. To convert mL/h to mL/min: mL/h ÷ 60 min/h or multiply mL/h by the conversion factor of 1 h/60 min. Refer to Rule 19-4. To calculate the amount of medication the patient has received over a given time when the flow rate and supply dose are known: H/Q = Dose received (D)/Volume administered (A)
19.3 Calculate IV flow rates for titrated medications. Page 571–582	▶ Refer to Rule 19-5. For safe titration: 1. Calculate the starting rate. 2. Calculate the maximum allowable rate. 3. Calculate the minimum allowable rate. 4. Begin infusion at the starting rate. 5. Titrate (adjust) dosage, based on patient response. 6. Do not exceed maximal rate (call AP for new order if the patient does not have the desired response at the maximal rate). 7. If the patient's response exceeds the prescribed parameters at the minimal dose, discontinue the infusion and notify the AP.

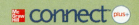
For Exercises 1–3, find the flow rates for an infusion pump. (LO 19.1)

    1. Vasopressin 60 units/50 mL NS infusing at 0.3 units/min.

    2. Ordered: 250 mg dobutamine HCl in 50 mL LR infusing at 1.5 mg/min.

    3. Ordered: 2000 mg lidocaine in 500 mL NS infusing at 2 mg/min.

For Exercises 4–5, find the appropriate flow rate using an infusion pump. (LO 19.2)

    4. Nitroglycerin 50 mg/250 mL D5W infusing at 27 mcg/min.

    5. Levophed® 8 mg/250 mL D5W infusing at 10 mcg/min

    6. Find the amount of medication that has already been administered to the patient. (LO 19-2)

    Ordered: Dobutrex® 250 mg in 1000 mL of D5W.

    The patient has received 120 mL.

    7. Based on the following, what is the dosage the patient is receiving at this time? (LO 19.3)

    Ordered: Dopamine: Begin infusion of 2 mcg/kg/min for bradycardia and systolic BP < 90 mmHg. Increase infusion up to 10 mcg/kg/min as needed.

    You have a premixed bag of dopamine with 200 mg in 500 mL of D5W. The patient weighs 195 lb. The blood pressure remains low and you increase the rate to 65 mL/h.

For Exercises 8–9, calculate the flow rate in mL/h.

    8. Ordered: procainamide 2 mg/min IV. On hand: procainamide 2 g/500 mL D5W. (LO 19.1)

    9. Ordered: nesritide 1.8 mcg/kg/h. On hand: nesritide 1.5 mg/250 mL D5W; the patient weighs 70 kg. (LO 19.2)

    10. Calculate the hourly flow rate in mL/h for the following titrated dose:

    Dobutamine 250 mg/500 mL D5W , 2.5 mcg/kg/min–20 mcg/kg/min IV to keep cardiac index greater than 1.8. Start at 2.5 mcg/kg/min.

    The dobutamine is currently infusing at 2.5 mcg/kg/min in a 50 kg patient. The new cardiac index is 1.4 and the infusion needs to be titrated to 4 mcg/kg/min. What is the new hourly rate? (LO 19.3)

CHAPTER 19 REVIEW

CHECK UP

For Exercises 1–3, find the flow rates for an infusion pump. (LO 19.1)

1. Ordered: 3000 mg lidocaine in 750 mL D5W to infuse at 3 mg/min.

2. Ordered: 500 mg dobutamine HCl in 100 mL of D5W to infuse at 2.4 mg/min.

3. Ordered: epinephrine 1 mg/500 mL to infuse at 3 mcg/min.

For Exercises 4–6, find the appropriate flow rate using an infusion pump. (LO 19.2)

4. Ordered: Neosynephrine® 0.5 mcg/kg/min. On hand: Neosynephrine® 40 mg/250 mL 0.9% NaCl. The patient weighs 214 lb.

5. Ordered: Inocor® 8 mcg/kg/min. On hand: Inocor® 300 mg/120 mL 0.9% NaCl. The patient weighs 152 lb.

6. Primacor® 0.375 mcg/kg/min. On hand: Primacor® 20 mg/100 mL D5W. The patient weighs 165 lb.

7. Find the amount of medication that has already been administered to the patient. (LO 19.2)

   Ordered: procainamide 1 g/250 mL D5W

   The patient has received 105 mL.

For Exercises 8–9 the following applies (LO 19.3):

Ordered: dopamine: Begin infusion of 2 mcg/kg/min for bradycardia and systolic BP < 90 mmHg. Increase infusion up to 10 mcg/kg/min as needed.

You have a premixed bag of dopamine with 200 mg in 500 mL of D5W. The patient weighs 185 lb.

8. At the end of your shift the patient has received 425 mL of the premixed bag of 200 mg in 500 mL of D5W. What is the total amount of dopamine the patient has received on your shift?

9. What is the maximum flow rate at which the IV should run?

For Exercises 10-15, calculate the flow rate in mL/h (LO 19.1, 19.2)

10. Ordered: nitroglycerin 15 mcg/min IV. On hand: nitroglycerin 25 mg in 500 mL D5W.

11. Ordered: xylocaine 3 mg/min IV. On hand: xylocaine 2 g/500 mL D5W.

12. Ordered: epinephrine 4 mcg/min. On hand: epinephrine 1 mg in 500 mL of NS.

13. Ordered: nesritide 0.6 mcg/kg/h (the patient weighs 80 kg). On hand: nesritide 1.5 mg/250 mL D5W.

14. Ordered: dobutamine 4 mcg/kg/min (the patient weighs 95 kg). On hand: dobutamine 1000 mg/250 mL D5W.

15. Ordered: amiodarone 0.5 mg/min. On hand: amiodarone 450 mg/250 mL D5W.

For Exercises 16–20 calculate the hourly flow rate in mL/h; refer to the following order to titrate the dosage: (LO 19.3)

While receiving mechanical ventilation: to achieve Richmond Agitation Sedation Scale (RASS) Level 0, administer lorazepam loading dose 1 mg IVP. Begin lorazepam 50 mg/250 mL D5W IV to infuse at 0.5 mg–2 mg/h. Titrate q 1–2 h, as needed, in 0.5 mg/h increments, to achieve RASS level 0. Rebolus with lorazepam 1 mg IVP prior to making each rate increase.

16. Calculate the minimum dose.

17. Calculate the maximum dose.

18. The patient's RASS is 2, so the patient needs increased sedation. The current infusion rate is 5 mL/h. What is the new rate? _____ Should the patient receive a bolus dose?

19. Two hours have passed since the rate change in question 18, and the patient's RASS is 1, so the patient needs increased sedation. Should the patient receive more lorazepam? If so, how much?

20. Two hours have passed since the rate change in question 19, and the patient's RASS is −1, so the patient needs less sedation. What is the new rate? Should the patient receive a bolus dose prior to this rate adjustment?

CRITICAL THINKING APPLICATION

A patient with malignant hypertension is being treated in the critical care unit. The physician writes the following order: nitroprusside 50 mg in 250 mL D5W to start at 1 mcg/kg/min, and titrate to maintain the systolic BP under 180. (When you measure a patient's blood pressure, the first number represents the systolic blood pressure.) The patient weighs 176 lb. According to the product insert, the maximum safe dose of nitroprusside is 8 mcg/kg/min (for no longer than 10 minutes) and the average dose is 3 mcg/kg/min. Nitroprusside's effect on BP can be seen in 1–2 minutes.(LO 19.3)

1. At what rate should you initially set the infusion?

2. What is the maximum safe rate for the infusion?

3. At 1600, the patient's BP is 220/110. The nitroprusside infusion is running at 165 mL/h. What should you do?

4. At 1610, the patient's BP is 198/96. The nitroprusside infusion is running at 192 mL/h. What should you do?

CASE STUDY

A patient has a PCA pump with fentanyl 1500 mcg in 30 mL in D5W. Hospital policy requires you to document the dose of fentanyl administered every 4 hours. When you came on duty, the pump showed that 13 mL had infused. After 4 hours, the pump shows that 21 mL has infused. How much fentanyl did the patient receive during your shift? (LO 19.2)

INTERNET ACTIVITY

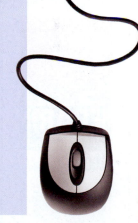

You are working in an intensive care unit that uses many IV critical care drugs. Checking the safe ranges of these drugs during emergency situations is both inconvenient and time-consuming. You and your coworkers decide to search the Internet for guides to dosages of commonly used drugs. Try to find answers to the following questions online.

1. What is the usual adult loading dose of amiodarone IV?
2. You are administering nitroglycerin IV and titrating the dose.
   a. By how many micrograms can you increase the dose at a time?
   b. How often can you increase the dose?
3. What treatment must be in place before tubocurarine is given?

To check your answers, see the Answer section at the end of the book, which starts on page A-1.

GO TO . . . Open the CD-ROM that accompanies your textbook, and complete a final review of the learning outcomes, practice problems, games, slideshow, and other activities presented for this chapter. For a final evaluation, take the chapter test and email or print your results for your instructor. A score of 95 percent or above indicates mastery of the chapter concepts.

For Questions 1–2 refer to labels A–E.

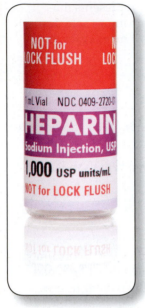

Label A Heparin Sodium 1,000 USP units/mL, 1 mL bottle

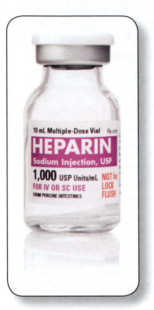

Label B Heparin Sodium 1,000 USP units/mL, 10 mL bottle

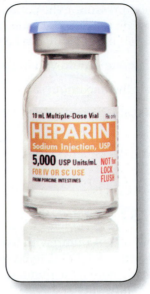

Label C Heparin Sodium 5,000 USP units/mL, 10 mL bottle

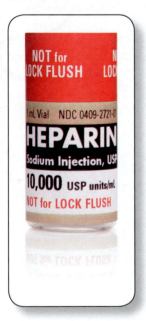

Label D Heparin Sodium 10,000 USP units/mL, 1 mL bottle

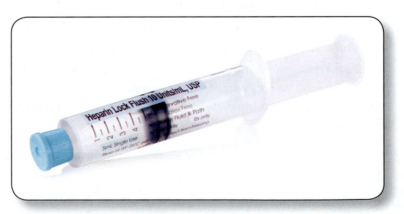

Label E Heparin Lock Flush 10 units/ mL, USP

For Questions 1 and 2 refer to the following: Ordered: Heparin 8,000 units subcut.

1. Which concentration of heparin should you choose? Label _____

2. How much heparin will you administer? _____ mL

For Questions 3–6, refer to the heparin protocol in the table below. The patient's aPTT is 50, weight is 70 kg, and currently heparin is infusing at 1,200 units/h.

3. Which label represents the heparin to be used for the bolus? _____

4. What is the bolus dose of heparin? _____ units

5. What is the current rate? _____ mL/h

6. What is the new rate? _____ mL/h

Heparin Protocol for DVT, PE, and High-Intensity Indications
GOAL: aPTT 70–100

Use premixed heparin sodium 25,000 USP units in 5% dextrose in water 500 mL (50 units/ mL) for infusion. Use heparin sodium 1,000 USP units/mL for bolus dose. Obtain baseline CBC and aPTT prior to administering heparin. Obtain aPTT 6 hours after each rate change. If the aPTT is at goal, repeat the aPTT until two consecutive aPTT are at goal, draw aPTT daily while receiving heparin, and aPTT remains between 70 and 100.
Initial bolus dose: 80 units/kg (maximum 8,000 units)
Initial rate: 18 units/kg/h (maximum 1,800 units/h = 36 mL/h)

aPTT result	IV bolus dose	Number of minutes to hold infusion	Amount to change current infusion rate
Less than 54 Notify AP	80 units/kg (max. 8,000 units)	Do not hold	Increase by 4 units/kg/h
54–59	40 units/kg (max. 4,000 units)	Do not hold	Increase by 2 units/kg/h
60–69	40 units/kg (max. 4,000 units)	Do not hold	Increase by 1 unit/kg/h
70–100 goal	**No bolus dose**	**Do not hold**	**Do not change current infusion rate**
101–115	No bolus dose	Do not hold	Decrease by 1 unit/kg/h
116–135	No bolus dose	30	Decrease by 2 units/kg/h
136–150	No bolus dose	60	Decrease by 3 units/kg/h and repeat aPTT 6 hours after infusion resumed
151–200 Notify AP	No bolus dose	90	Decrease by 4 units/kg/h and repeat aPTT 6 hours after infusion resumed

Adapted for calculation purposes only, from (2008) ACCP guidelines; not to be used in clinical practice.

For Questions 7–9 refer to labels through F to I.

Order: Humalog® 7 units subcut and Humulin® N 30 units subcut

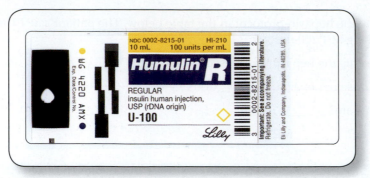

Label F   Humulin® R

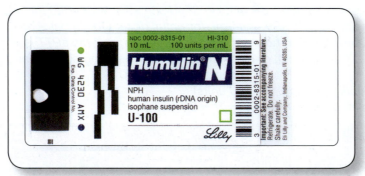

Label G   Humulin® N

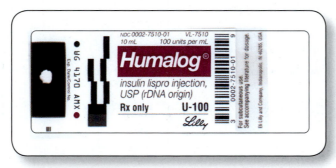

Label H   Humalog®

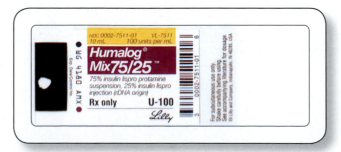

Label I   Humalog® Mix 75/25™

7. Which insulin would you draw up first?   Label _____

8. Which insulin would you inject air into first? Label _____

9. Mark on the syringe how many units of each insulin you administer.

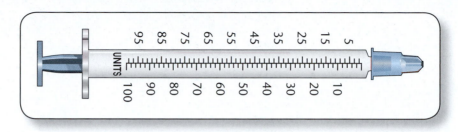

10. Using the heparin protocol in the table on p. 581, how many units of heparin will a patient who weighs 120 kg receive? _____ units

11. Write a recipe for 100 mL of 2% lidocaine solution.

12. Calculate the amount of solute and solvent needed to prepare a one-day supply of ¾ strength Sustacal® 60 mL to be administered q4h.

13. Using saline as a solvent, calculate the total amount of solute and solvent needed to prepare a wound irrigation solution with 4 oz of 1/4 strength hydrogen peroxide t.i.d. × 3 days.

14. Identify the pharmacokinetic process described below:
    a. The process by which a medication leaves the body
    b. The process that moves a medication from the site where it is given into the bloodstream
    c. The process that chemically changes the medication in the body
    d. The process that moves a medication into other body tissues and fluids

15. Ordered: tobramycin 3 mg/kg/day given in three divided doses to a 15 kg child.
    Administer: _____ mg/day or _____ mg/dose

16. Ordered: cephalexin 150 mg PO q6h for a child who weighs 44 lb.
    Recommended dose range: 25–50 mg/kg/day in four divided doses
    Is the dose ordered safe? _____

17. Ordered: enalapril 2.5 mg PO daily for a 76 year old, 5 ft 3 in tall, 195 lb, CL_{CR} of 55 mL/min, diagnosed with hypertension and renal impairment whose ideal weight is 152 lb.

    On hand: enalapril 5 mg (scored) tablets

    According to the package insert, the usual dose for patients with normal renal function (over 80 mL/min creatinine clearance) is 5 mg/day; for mild impairment (30 to 80 mL/min)—2.5 mg/day; for moderate to severe impairment (< 30 mL/min)—2.5 mg/day

    Is the dose ordered safe? _____ If the dose is safe, administer _____ tablet(s)

18. What is the safe dose of interferon for a child with a BSA of 0.28 m^2 if the recommended dose is 2 million units/m^2? _____ units

19. Calculate the daily maintenance fluid needs (DMFN) for a child who weighs 24 kg. _____ mL

20. An 11 lb, 8 oz infant is taking 3 oz formula every 4 hours. Is he meeting his DMFN? _____

The Alligation Method

It is sometimes necessary to combine two solutions in order to produce a solution with a concentration that falls between the solutions available. For example, you may have a 3% and a 10% solution of a medication on hand, but need a 4% solution. The alligation method will allow you to determine the quantities of the available solutions that need to be mixed in order to produce the desired concentration.

1. Write out a tic-tac-toe grid, and fill in the following values.

The concentration of the **more** concentrated solution		Parts of the **more** concentrated solution needed ←	The difference between the concentration needed and the concentration of the LESS concentrated solution. (The **diagonal** difference)
	The concentration needed		
The concentration of the **less** concentrated solution.*		Parts of the **less** concentrated solution needed ←	The difference between the concentration needed and the concentration of the MORE concentrated solution. (The **diagonal** difference)

When you are diluting with water, the less concentrated solution has a concentration of zero.

2. Find the total number of parts in the solution by adding the two values in the right column.
3. Find the volume of one part by dividing the total number of parts into the volume needed.
4. Multiply the volume of one part (answer from step 3) by the number in the top right of the grid. The result is the amount of the more concentrated solution needed.
5. Add a sufficient quantity of the less concentrated solution to bring the final volume up to the desired volume.

Example 1   How would you prepare 500 mL of 50% ethanol from 90% ethanol? (You will use water as a diluent.)

Before you do the calculation, break down the problem to find the information that is needed.

- The volume needed is 500 mL.
- The concentration needed is 50%.
- The concentrations available are 90% and 0%.

1. Write the concentration of the more concentrated solution in the upper left, the concentration of the less concentrated solution in lower left, and the concentration needed in the center of a tic-tac-toe grid, and then take the differences diagonally.

90		50
	50	
0		40

2. Add the numbers in the right column to find the total number of parts.

   50 + 40 = 90 parts total

3. Determine the volume of 1 part by dividing the volume needed by the total number of parts.

   $$\frac{500 \text{ mL}}{90 \text{ parts}} = 5.56 \text{ mL/part}$$

4. Determine how much of the more concentrated solution is needed.

   5.56 mL/part × 50 parts of concentrate = 278 mL

   So 278 mL of the 90% solution is needed to prepare 500 mL of a 50% solution.

5. Since the desired volume is 500 mL, you would dilute the 90% solution by adding water up to a final volume of 500 mL.

Example 2 How would you prepare 100 mL of 5% iodine from 10% and 2% iodine solutions?

1. Write the concentration of the more concentrated solution in the upper left, the concentration of the less concentrated solution in the lower left, and the concentration needed in the center of a tic-tac-toe grid, and then take the differences diagonally.

10		3
	5	
2		5

2. Add the numbers in the right column to find the total number of parts.

   3 + 5 = 8 parts total

3. Determine the volume of 1 part by dividing the volume needed by the total number of parts.

   $$\frac{100 \text{ mL}}{8 \text{ parts}} = 12.5 \text{ mL/part}$$

4. Determine how much of the more concentrated solution is needed.

   12.5 mL/part × 3 parts of 10% solution = 37.5 mL

   So 37.5 mL of the 10% solution is needed to prepare 100 mL of a 10% solution.

5. Since the desired volume is 100 mL, you would dilute the 10% solution by adding 2% iodine up to a final volume of 100 mL.

COMPREHENSIVE EVALUATION

The following test will help you check your mastery of the major learning outcomes for this text. Applying this information will help prevent dosage calculation and medication administration errors.

For Exercises 1–6, refer to MAR 1. (LO 9.1, 9.3, 11.1)

1. What dose of Neurontin® should be administered?

2. By what route should Desyrel® be administered?

3. When should Reglan® be administered?

4. Indicate the time of day, in traditional time, that each medication should be given. Why are no times listed for Ativan? (LO 7.2)

5. Are any of the orders incomplete? If so, what information is missing? (LO 9.2, 11.3)

6. Which order contains an error-prone abbreviation? Correct this abbreviation. (LO 11.4)

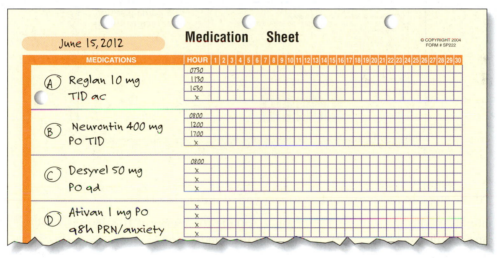

MAR 1

7. Identify the rights of medication administration. (LO 11.6)

8. Describe the three checks of medication administration. (LO 11.5)

For Exercises 9–12, refer to label A. (LO 10.1)

9. What is the generic name of the drug?

10. At what temperature should the drug be stored?

11. What is the dosage strength?

12. If an adult took twice the usual adult dose, how long would the container last?

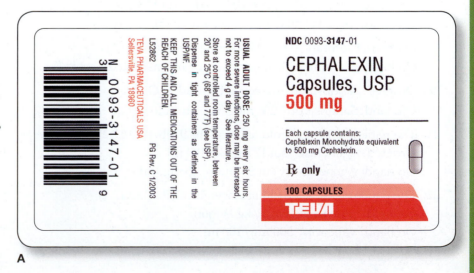

A

For Exercises 13 and 14, refer to label B. (LO 10.1, 10.2)

13. How much fluid is used to reconstitute the entire container of suspension?

14. If the dosage prescribed for a child is 250 mg, how many doses are in the container?

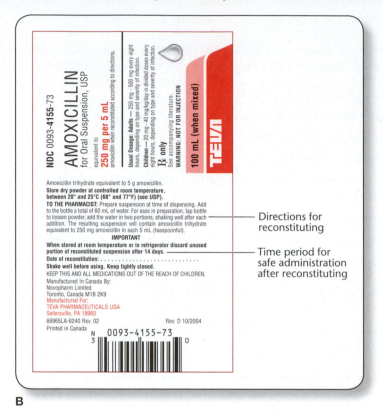

B

15. Name the three steps in receiving and writing a verbal order. (LO 11.2)

16. The patient was medicated with acetaminophen 650 mg for a fever of 102 degrees F. What follow-up observations should be made after administering this medication?

For Exercises 17–28, calculate the amount to administer.

17. Ordered: Zoloft® 75 mg PO daily
    On hand: Zoloft® 50-mg scored tablets

18. Ordered: Zovirax® 0.2 g PO q4h 5x/day (LO 13.2)
    On hand: Zovirax® suspension 200 mg/5 mL

19. Ordered: Claforan® 0.6 g IM 30 min pre-op (LO 14.1)
    On hand: Claforan® 300 mg/mL when reconstituted

20. Ordered: Sandostatin® 0.3 mg subcut tid. (LO 14.1)
    On hand: Sandostatin® 200 mcg/mL multidose vial

21. The patient is 14 years old and weighs 97 lb. (LO 17.2)
    Ordered: Agenerase® sol 17 mg/kg PO tid
    On hand: Agenerase® Oral Solution, 15 mg/mL

22. The patient is 10 years old and weighs 62 lb. (LO 17.2)
    Ordered: Vancocin® 10 mg/kg IV q6h
    On hand: Vancocin® 500 mg/100 mL

23. Ordered: ampicillin 375 mg IV q6h.

On hand: 500 mg vial of ampicillin reconstituted with 1.8 mL sterile water to yield a supply dose of 250 mg/mL. (LO 14.3)

24. The patient is 7 years old and weighs 49 lb. (LO 17.2)

Ordered: Zinacef® 20 mg/kg IM q6h

On hand: Zinacef® 220 mg/mL when reconstituted

25. Ordered: phenytoin extended 300 mg PO daily (LO 13.1)

On hand: Refer to label C.

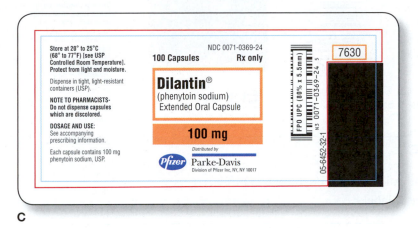

C

26. The patient is 7 years old and weighs 55 lb.

Ordered: Trileptal® 10 mg/kg PO bid. (LO 17.2)

On hand: Refer to label D.

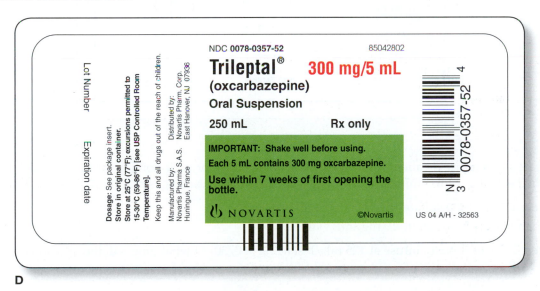

D

27. Ordered: Biaxin® XL 1 g PO q12h. (LO 13.1)

On hand: Refer to label E.

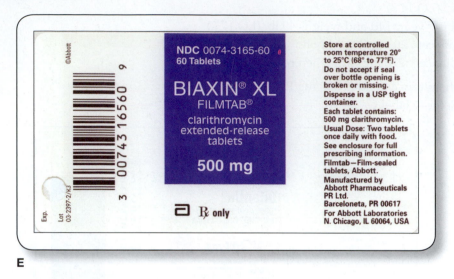

E

28. Ordered: Levothroid® 0.1 mg PO daily. (LO 13.1)

On hand: Refer to label F.

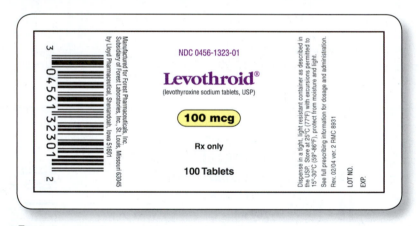

F

29. You are discharging a patient from the walk-in clinic with a prescription for ear drops, which requires a medicine dropper for administration. What specific patient teaching is required? (LO 8.1, 11.8)

30. Ordered: Morphine sulfate 15 mg subcut q4h prn/pain

On hand: Morphine sulfate 10 mg/mL vial

31. Ordered: 1 L $D_5 \frac{1}{2}$ NS to infuse at 125 mL/h starting at 0730. At what time will the infusion be complete? (LO 15.4)

32. Which of the following insulins is shorter-acting? (LO 18.1)
   Refer to labels G and H.

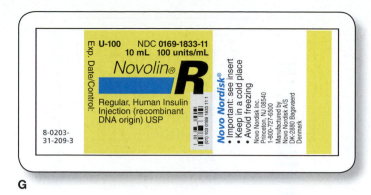

G

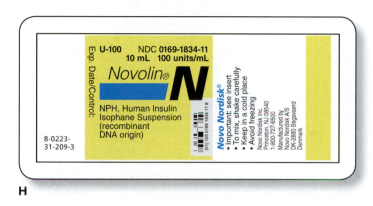

H

33. In what order will you draw the insulin into the syringe for the following order? (LO 18.1)
   Ordered: Humulin® N 46 units and Humulin® R 8 units subcut ac breakfast

In Exercises 34–41, find the flow rate.

34. Ordered: 1000 mL RL over 8 hours, using an infusion pump. (LO 15.3)

35. Ordered: 600 mL 5%D NS over 4 h, 15 gtt/mL tubing. (LO 15.3)

36. Ordered: norepinephrine 4 mg/1000 mL D5/NS 0.5–30 mcg/min IV. Start infusion at 1 mcg/min and titrate in 1 mcg/min increments to keep systolic BP greater than 90 mmHg.
   The patient's systolic BP is 86 mm Hg, and the above IV is infusing at 30 mL/h. What should be the new infusion rate? (LO 19.3)

37. Find the flow rate in mL/h for a child who weighs 68 lb. (LO 17.2)
   Ordered: Zofran® 0.1 mg/kg IV over 4 min
   On hand: Zofran®, premixed with 32 mg in 5% dextrose, 50 mL, and 10 gtt/mL tubing

38. Ordered: nitroglycerin 18 mcg/min IV
   On hand: nitroglycerin 200 mg/500 mL D5W
   What is the flow rate in mL/h? (LO 19.1)

39. Ordered: Rocephin® 750 mg in 100 mL NS IVPB over 30 min q8h via infusion pump. (LO 15.5)
On hand: Refer to label I.

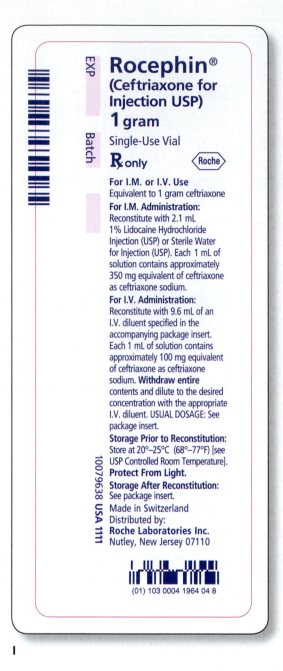

I

40. Ordered: Heparin 23 units/kg/h IV.
On hand: heparin sodium 25,000 units/500 mL D5W
Patient's weight: 212 lb. (LO 18.4)

41. Refer to labels O, P, and Q:

Ordered heparin 7500 units subcut q12h. (LO 18.2, 18.8)

label O, heparin sodium 1,000 USP units/mL 10 mL fill bottle

label P heparin sodium 5,000 USP units/mL, 10 mL fill bottle

label Q heparin sodium 10,000 USP units/mL, 1 mL fill bottle

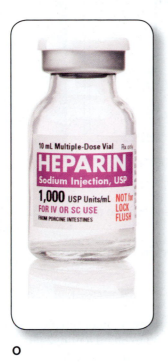

O

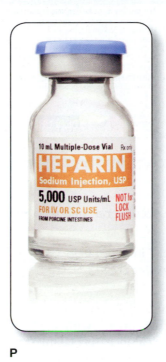

P

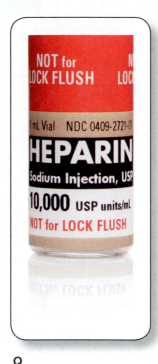

Q

42. Find the amount of medication that has already been administered to the patient. (LO 19.1)

Ordered: nitroprusside 40 mg in 500 mL D5W

The patient has received 175 mL.

43. Calculate the original flow rate for the following order. Then determine if an adjustment is necessary and calculate the adjusted flow rate. (LO 15.3)

Ordered: 650 mL NS over 8 h (15 gtt/mL tubing)

With 5 h remaining, 490 mL of NS remains in the IV bag.

44. Ordered: D_5LR at 80 mL/h started at 1130. At 2245, what volume will be infused? (LO 15.4)

45. Write a recipe for 1000 mL $\frac{1}{2}$ NS (0.45% NS). (LO 16.1)

46. The adult patient's height is 150 cm and weight is 61 kg. (LO 17.4)

Ordered: BiCNU 200 mg/m² IV over 2 h

How many milligrams of BiCNU should be administered?

47. The adult patient's height is 60 in. and weight is 103 lb. What is the flow rate in mL/h? (LO 17.4)

Ordered: leucovorin calcium 200 mg/m^2 IV over 6 min

On hand: Refer to label J.

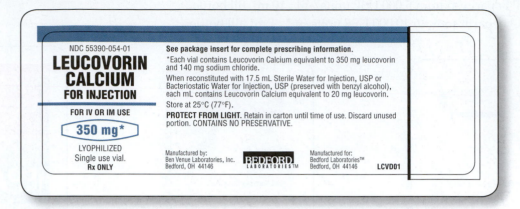

J

48. Find the daily maintenance fluid needs for a child who weighs 18 kg. Then find the microdrip tubing flow rate for DMFN. (LO 17.5)

49. The patient: 78-year-old male, 5 ft 7 in. tall, 148 lb, CL$_{CR}$ of 48 mL/min. Determine if the order is safe. If it is, then find the amount to administer. (LO 17.1)

Ordered: Timentin® 1.7 g IV q4h

On hand: Timentin® reconstituted to 20 mg/mL

According to the package insert, for patients with renal impairment, the following maintenance dosages are recommended: for creatinine clearance over 60 mL/min, 3.1 g q4h; for 30 to 60 mL/min, 2 g q4h; for 10 to 30 mL/min, 2 g q8h; for less than 10 mL/min, 2 g q12h. For patients with more advanced impairments, lower dosages are recommended.

50. Ordered: epinephrine 0.1 mg subcut stat.

On hand: epinephrine 1: 1000 solution.

What volume in mL will you administer?

Score 2 points for each exercise you have answered correctly. To check your answers, see the Answer section at the end of the book, which starts on page A-1.

ANSWERS

PRETEST ANSWERS

1. $4\frac{2}{3}$
2. $\frac{31}{8}$
3. $1\frac{3}{5}$
4. $\frac{11}{4}$
5. 6
6. 18
7. $\frac{2}{5}$
8. $\frac{3}{8}$
9. $4\frac{4}{5}$
10. $3\frac{1}{3}$
11. $1\frac{7}{40}$
12. $2\frac{1}{21}$
13. $\frac{9}{20}$
14. $5\frac{11}{12}$
15. $\frac{1}{15}$
16. 14
17. $\frac{5}{6}$
18. 2
19. $\frac{7}{12}$
20. $1\frac{5}{8}$

21. $5\frac{5}{8}$
22. $1\frac{2}{3}$
23. 1.009
24. 14
25. 6.1
26. 19.20
27. 3.8
28. $\frac{9}{200}$
29. 1.015
30. 7.125
31. 3
32. $3\frac{3}{5}$
33. 15.3
34. 5.112
35. 14.7
36. 99.43
37. 0.224
38. 20
39. 4.975
40. 2.1

41. 0.525
42. 0.008
43. 99 percent
44. $2\frac{3}{5}$
45. 112.5 percent
46. $7 : 12 = \frac{7}{12}$
47. $1 : 5$
48. 0.08
49. $2 : 5$
50. 37.5 percent rounded to 38 percent
51. $1 : 200$
52. $2\frac{2}{3}$
53. 3:20
54. 105%
55. $\frac{3}{200}$
56. $x = 4$
57. $x = 15$
58. $x = 6$
59. $x = 8$

60. $x = 1$
61. The healthcare professional gives 6 teaspoons each day.
62. The desired supply is short by $2\frac{1}{2}$ bottles. The healthcare professional will order 3 bottles.
63. 58.7 milliliters (mL) remains in the bottle.
64. The patient receives 1.875 milligrams (mg) over 5 days.
65. 200 mL/h
66. 3 mg
67. 8.32 mcg
68. 5 mg : 500 mL = 1 mg : 100 mL
69. 25 mg : 1 tablet
70. 125 mg : 3 mL
71. 12 days
72. 2 mg : 1 mL

CHAPTER 1 ANSWERS

Review and Practice

1.1 Fractions and Mixed Numbers

1. 17
2. 8
3. 100
4. 1

5a. $\frac{4}{12}$

$$\frac{part}{whole}$$
$$= \frac{patients\ with\ type\ A\ blood}{all\ patients}$$
$$= \frac{4}{12}$$

5b. $\frac{8}{12}$

6a. $\frac{6}{20}$
6b. $\frac{14}{20}$
7. $\frac{16}{3}$

  $16 \div 3$ is "sixteen divided by three", or $\frac{16}{3}$

8. $\frac{4}{15}$

9. $\frac{3}{4}$
10a. =
10b. <

  Because $24 < 32$, $\frac{24}{32} < 1$

10c. >
11a. >
11b. <
11c. =

12. $7\frac{1}{6}$

$\frac{43}{6} = 43 \div 6 = 7\ R\ 1$

$\frac{remainder}{denominator} = \frac{1}{6}$

$\frac{43}{6} = 7 + \frac{1}{6} = 7\frac{1}{6}$

13. $5\frac{2}{3}$

14. 5

15. 1

16. $1\frac{3}{5}$

17. $6\frac{17}{25}$

18. $1\frac{4}{12} = 1\frac{1}{3}$

19. $\frac{50}{17}$

$17 \times 2 = 34$

$34 + 16 = 50$

$2\frac{16}{17} = \frac{50}{17}$

20. $\frac{80}{9}$

21. $\frac{11}{10}$

22. $\frac{33}{8}$

23. $\frac{311}{3}$

24. $\frac{55}{8}$

25. $\frac{41}{5}$

Review and Practice

1.2 Equivalent Fractions

For Exercises 1–8, answers may vary.

1. $\frac{8}{10}, \frac{16}{20}, \frac{20}{25}$

$4 \times \frac{2}{5} \times 2 = \frac{8}{10}$

$4 \times \frac{4}{5} \times 4 = \frac{16}{20}$

$4 \times \frac{5}{5} \times 5 = \frac{20}{25}$

2. $\frac{2}{20}, \frac{3}{30}, \frac{10}{100}$

3. $\frac{2}{1}, \frac{8}{4}, \frac{16}{8}$

4. $\frac{5}{3}, \frac{30}{18}, \frac{45}{27}$

5. $\frac{18}{2}, \frac{27}{3}, \frac{81}{9}$

6. $\frac{48}{2}, \frac{72}{3}, \frac{96}{4}$

7. $\frac{14}{6}, \frac{21}{9}, \frac{28}{12}$

8. $\frac{11}{3}, \frac{66}{18}, \frac{99}{27}$

9. $\frac{14}{24}, \frac{21}{36}, \frac{28}{48}, \frac{42}{72}, \frac{70}{120}$

10. $\frac{34}{8}, \frac{51}{12}, \frac{68}{16}, \frac{85}{20}, \frac{119}{28}$

11. 6

$16 \div 8 = 2$

$\frac{3}{8} = 3 \times \frac{2}{8} \times 2 = \frac{6}{16}$

missing numerator = 6

12. 9

13. 4

14. 6

15. 12

16. 60

17. 210

18. 17

19. 16

20. 8

Review and Practice

1.3 Reducing Fractions

1. $\frac{5}{6}$

$10 \div \frac{2}{12} \div 2 = \frac{5}{6}$

2. $\frac{1}{2}$

3. $\frac{1}{3}$

4. $\frac{1}{2}$

5. $\frac{1}{10}$

6. $\frac{11}{20}$

7. $\frac{4}{5}$

8. $\frac{6}{17}$

9. $\frac{7}{9}$

10. $\frac{7}{10}$

11. $\frac{8}{15}$

12. $\frac{7}{12}$

13. $\frac{5}{14}$

14. $\frac{5}{8}$

15. $\frac{1}{3}$

16. $\frac{5}{7}$

17. $\frac{3}{8}$

18. $\frac{7}{11}$

19. $\frac{1}{4}$

20. $\frac{6}{11}$

Review and Practice

1.4 Common Denominators

1. LCD: 21

$\frac{7}{21}$ and $\frac{3}{21}$

multiples of 3: 3, 6, 9, 12, 15, 18, 21, 24

multiples of 7: 7, 14, 21, 28

2. LCD: 40

$\frac{8}{40}$ and $\frac{5}{40}$

3. LCD: 200

$\frac{8}{200}$ and $\frac{5}{200}$

4. LCD: 72

$\frac{3}{72}$ and $\frac{2}{72}$

5. LCD: 12

$\frac{6}{12}$ and $\frac{1}{12}$

6. LCD: 18

$\frac{3}{18}$ and $\frac{1}{18}$

7. LCD: 42

$\frac{35}{42}$ and $\frac{24}{42}$

8. LCD: 8

$\frac{6}{8}$ and $\frac{5}{8}$

9. LCD: 36

$\frac{4}{36}$ and $\frac{1}{36}$

10. LCD: 96

$\frac{20}{96}$ and $\frac{9}{96}$

11. LCD: 55

$\frac{44}{55}$ and $\frac{45}{55}$

12. LCD: 12

$\frac{10}{12}$ and $\frac{7}{12}$

13. LCD: 240

$\frac{88}{240}$ and $\frac{63}{240}$

14. LCD: 144

$\frac{15}{144}$ and $\frac{14}{144}$

15. LCD: 12

$\frac{6}{12}, \frac{4}{12},$ and $\frac{3}{12}$

16. LCD: 72

$\frac{12}{72}, \frac{32}{72},$ and $\frac{39}{72}$

18. LCD: 48

$\frac{12}{48}, \frac{40}{48},$ and $\frac{21}{48}$

19. LCD: 20

$\frac{4}{20}, \frac{6}{20},$ and $\frac{7}{20}$

20. LCD: 120

$\frac{20}{120}, \frac{25}{120},$ and $\frac{27}{120}$

17. LCD: 45

$\frac{30}{45}, \frac{20}{45},$ and $\frac{21}{45}$

Review and Practice

1.5 Comparing Fractions

1. $<$

$1 < 3$ therefore $\frac{1}{5} < \frac{3}{5}$

2. $>$

3. $=$

4. $>$

$\frac{7}{10} = 7 \times \frac{2}{10} \times 2 = \frac{14}{20}$

$\frac{14}{20} > \frac{7}{20},$ therefore $\frac{7}{10} > \frac{7}{20}$

5. $=$

6. $>$

7. $>$

8. $>$

9. $<$

10. $<$

11. $>$

12. $<$

13. $<$

14. $>$

15. $=$

16. $\frac{5}{6}, \frac{3}{4}, \frac{4}{7}, \frac{2}{5}$

The LCD of 4, 5, 6, and 7 is 420.

$\frac{3}{4} = 3 \times \frac{105}{4} \times 105 = \frac{315}{420}$

$\frac{2}{5} = 2 \times \frac{84}{5} \times 84 = \frac{168}{420}$

$\frac{5}{6} = 5 \times \frac{70}{6} \times 70 = \frac{350}{420}$

$\frac{4}{7} = 4 \times \frac{60}{7} \times 60 = \frac{240}{420}$

$\frac{5}{6} > \frac{3}{4} > \frac{4}{7} > \frac{2}{5}$

17. $\frac{4}{7}, \frac{5}{9}, \frac{1}{2}, \frac{1}{3}$

18. $\frac{5}{2}, 2\frac{1}{10}, 1\frac{3}{16}, \frac{9}{8}$

19. $2\frac{1}{2}, 1\frac{5}{6}, \frac{5}{3}, \frac{12}{9}$

20. $\frac{6}{7}, \frac{5}{8}, \frac{3}{5}, \frac{1}{2}$

21. Too little

22. Yes, $\frac{25}{125} = \frac{1}{5}$

23. North wing

24. Martha

25. You have more time since $1\frac{3}{4}$ equals $1\frac{9}{12}$ hours.

Review and Practice

1.6 Adding Fractions

1. $\frac{1}{2}$

$\frac{1}{8} + \frac{3}{8} = 1 + \frac{3}{8} = \frac{4}{8} = \frac{1}{2}$

2. $\frac{4}{7}$

3. $\frac{2}{7}$

4. $\frac{2}{3}$

5. $\frac{13}{24}$

6. $\frac{12}{25}$

7. $1\frac{5}{24}$

8. $1\frac{11}{18}$

9. $2\frac{4}{5}$

10. $3\frac{8}{11}$

11. $1\frac{5}{6}$

12. $2\frac{23}{40}$

13. $1\frac{19}{36}$

14. $5\frac{29}{35}$

15. $3\frac{5}{8}$

16. $\frac{33}{40}$

17. $\frac{47}{60}$

18. $1\frac{17}{24}$

19. $1\frac{23}{30}$

20. $\frac{19}{20}$

21. $160\frac{1}{4}$ pounds

22. $11\frac{1}{4}$ ounces

23. $2\frac{2}{3}$ cups

24. 2 tablespoons

25. 12 hours

Review and Practice

1.7 Subtracting Fractions

1. $3\frac{1}{5}$

Subtract the whole numbers:

$7 - 4 = 3$

Subtract the fractional part:

$\frac{7}{15} - \frac{4}{15}$

$= 7 - \frac{4}{15}$

$5\frac{3}{15} = \frac{1}{5}$

$7\frac{7}{15} - 4\frac{4}{15} = 3\frac{1}{5}$

2. $\frac{1}{5}$

3. $3\frac{1}{3}$

4. $\frac{3}{7}$

5. $\frac{7}{18}$

6. $\frac{7}{12}$

7. $1\frac{5}{8}$

8. $2\frac{1}{8}$

9. $5\frac{1}{2}$

10. $3\frac{3}{4}$

11. $11\frac{17}{30}$

12. $4\frac{9}{35}$

13. $20\frac{15}{16}$

14. $4\frac{19}{20}$

15. $5\frac{1}{3}$

16. $6\frac{4}{7}$

17. $4\frac{2}{5}$

18. $\frac{1}{6}$

19. $9\frac{11}{15}$

20. $7\frac{1}{12}$

21. $\frac{3}{8}$ cup

22. $\frac{5}{8}$ cup

23. $2\frac{3}{4}$ bottles

24. $143\frac{3}{4}$ pounds

25. $2\frac{3}{4}$ degrees

Review and Practice

1.8 Multiplying Fractions

1. $\frac{1}{48}$

   $\frac{1}{6} \times \frac{1}{8} = 1 \times \frac{1}{6} \times 8 = \frac{1}{48}$

2. $\frac{6}{35}$

3. $\frac{3}{8}$

4. $\frac{1}{9}$

5. $\frac{1}{6}$

6. $\frac{1}{6}$

7. 1

8. $1\frac{1}{2}$

9. $4\frac{1}{2}$

10. $2\frac{1}{2}$

11. $1\frac{1}{2}$

12. 2

13. $19\frac{7}{12}$

14. $14\frac{3}{10}$

15. $\frac{7}{24}$

16. $\frac{9}{56}$

17. $\frac{3}{4}$

18. $\frac{1}{2}$

19. $\frac{2}{5}$

20. 1

21. 234 doses

22. $1\frac{1}{8}$ grains

23. a. $1\frac{1}{3}$ teaspoons

    b. $\frac{3}{4}$ teaspoon

    c. $\frac{7}{12}$ teaspoon

24. 30 ounces

25. 1750 milligrams

Review and Practice

1.9 Dividing Fractions

1. $\frac{28}{45}$

   $\frac{4}{9} \div \frac{5}{7} = \frac{4}{9} \times \frac{7}{5} = \frac{28}{45}$

2. $\frac{15}{44}$

3. $\frac{3}{4}$

4. $\frac{2}{9}$

5. $2\frac{2}{5}$

6. $1\frac{7}{15}$

7. $1\frac{1}{2}$

8. 1

9. $2\frac{5}{8}$

10. $\frac{1}{2}$

11. $1\frac{7}{9}$

12. $2\frac{4}{5}$

13. $\frac{5}{24}$

14. $9\frac{3}{5}$

15. $1\frac{1}{8}$

16. $1\frac{7}{9}$

17. $1\frac{1}{7}$

18. $1\frac{1}{6}$

19. $6\frac{1}{4}$

20. $2\frac{2}{15}$

21. 160 doses

22. 60 doses

23. 16 times

24. 48 vials

25. $12\frac{3}{4}$

Chapter 1 Review

Check up

1. $\frac{19}{8}$

   $8 \times 2 = 16$

   $16 + 3 = 19$

   $2\frac{3}{8} = \frac{19}{8}$

2. $\frac{9}{7}$

3. $\frac{99}{10}$

4. $\frac{155}{12}$

5. $\frac{1}{3}$

   $\frac{12}{36} = 12 \div \frac{12}{36} \div 12 = \frac{1}{3}$

6. $\frac{13}{16}$

7. 5

8. $7\frac{1}{4}$

9. LCD: 10

   $\frac{3}{10}$ and $\frac{8}{10}$

$\frac{3}{10}$ *already has the LCD*

$\frac{4}{5} = 4 \times \frac{2}{5} \times 2$

$= \frac{8}{10}$

10. LCD: 18

    $\frac{15}{18}$ and $\frac{8}{18}$

11. LCD: 24

    $\frac{9}{24}, \frac{18}{24},$ and $\frac{4}{24}$

12. LCD: 60

    $\frac{42}{60}, \frac{15}{60},$ and $\frac{40}{60}$

13. $>$

    $\frac{3}{10} = 3 \times \frac{8}{10} \times 8 = \frac{24}{80}$

    $\frac{3}{16} = 3 \times \frac{5}{16} \times 5 = \frac{15}{80}$

    $\frac{24}{80} > \frac{15}{80}$ *therefore* $\frac{3}{10} > \frac{3}{16}$

14. $<$

15. =

16. <

17. $2\frac{11}{12}$

$$\frac{9}{4} = 9 \times \frac{3}{4} \times 3 = \frac{27}{12}$$
$$\frac{2}{3} = 2 \times \frac{4}{3} \times 4 = \frac{8}{12}$$
$$\frac{27}{12} + \frac{8}{12} = 27 + \frac{8}{12}$$
$$= \frac{35}{12} = 2\frac{11}{12}$$

18. 2

19. $\frac{29}{100}$

20. $7\frac{3}{8}$

21. $\frac{8}{9}$

$\frac{11}{9}$ *already has the*
LCD
$$\frac{1}{3} = 1 \times \frac{3}{3} \times 3 = \frac{3}{9}$$
$$\frac{11}{9} - \frac{3}{9} = 11 - \frac{3}{9} = \frac{8}{9}$$

22. $\frac{1}{20}$

23. $1\frac{3}{8}$

24. $2\frac{5}{7}$

25. $\frac{5}{9}$

$$\frac{5}{6} \times \frac{2}{3} = 5 \times \frac{2}{6} \times 3$$
$$= \frac{10}{18} = \frac{5}{9}$$

26. $\frac{1}{6}$

27. 8

28. $4\frac{1}{8}$

29. $\frac{4}{21}$

$$\frac{1}{7} \div \frac{3}{4} = \frac{1}{7} \times \frac{4}{3}$$
$$= 1 \times \frac{4}{7} \times 3 = \frac{4}{21}$$

30. 16

31. $15\frac{3}{4}$

32. $\frac{4}{15}$

33. Type O— $\frac{4}{9}$

Type A— $\frac{5}{18}$

Type AB— $\frac{1}{9}$

Type B— $\frac{1}{6}$

34. Receives $\frac{2}{3}$ cup; amount is $\frac{5}{6}$ cup less than the patient should receive.

35. $8\frac{3}{4}$ cups

36. a. 64 doses

Critical Thinking Applications

$$\frac{1}{16}, \frac{1}{8}, \frac{3}{16}, \frac{1}{4}, \frac{5}{16}, \frac{7}{16}, \frac{1}{2}$$

$\frac{3}{8}$-diameter instrument is missing.

Case Study

Day 2, 8:00 a.m.	$+1\frac{1}{2}$ pounds
Day 3, 8:00 a.m.	$+1\frac{3}{4}$ pounds
Day 3, 2:00 p.m.	-1 pound
Day 4, 8:00 a.m.	-2 pounds
Day 4, 4:00 p.m.	$-2\frac{1}{4}$ pounds

CHAPTER 2 ANSWERS

Review and Practice

2.1 Writing and Comparing Decimals

1. 0.2
   two-tenths is 0.2

2. 0.17

3. 6.5

4. 7.19

5. 0.003

6. 0.023

7. 5.067

8. 7.151

9. >
   The whole number 4 is the same. In the tenths place, 2 > 0 so that 4.27 > 4.02

10. >

11. <

12. >

13. <

14. >

15. >

16. <

17. <

18. >

19. >

20. <

Critical Thinking on the Job

Rounding Errors with 9

Because the healthcare professional forgets to carry a unit from the tenths place into the ones place, an error results. The patient does not receive a full dose of medication. With correct rounding, the patient should receive 5.0 mL, not 4.0 mL.

Review and Practice

2.2 Rounding Decimals

1. 14.3

   The digit to the right of the tenths place is 4. Do not change the digit in the tenths place

2. 3.5

3. 0.9

4. 0.2

5. 1

6. 0.2

   The digit to the right of the tenths place is 0. Do not change the digit in the tenths place

7. 152.7

8. 9.29

9. 55.17

10. 4.01

11. 2.21

12. 5.52

13. 12.00

   Remember that, according to Rule 2.2, trailing zeros after the decimal point should be dropped, and this number would be rewritten as 12.

14. 767.46

15. 11

16. 20

17. 2

18. 51

19. 3.8 milliliters

20. 0.38 milliliters

Review and Practice

2.3 Converting Fractions into Decimals

1. 0.4

   $\frac{2}{5} = 2 \div 5 = 0.4$

2. 0.35

3. 0.75

4. 0.5

5. 0.333

6. 0.444

7. 0.556

8. 0.583

9. 1.5

10. 2.2

11. 2.333

12. 1.125

13. $\frac{1}{8}$

   $1\frac{4}{5} = 1 + \frac{4}{5}$

   $= 1 + (4 \; 4 \; 5)$

   $= 1 + 0.8 = 1.8$

14. 2.1

15. 6.75

16. 3.5

17. 0.875

18. 0.2

19. 2.857

20. 7.667

Review and Practice

2.4 Converting Decimals into Fractions

1. $1\frac{1}{5}$

   The number 1 to the left of the decimal point is the whole number. The number 2 to the right of the decimal point is the numerator. 2 is in the tenths place so that 10 is the denominator.

   $1.2 = 1\frac{2}{10} = 1\frac{1}{5}$

2. $98\frac{3}{5}$

3. $\frac{3}{10}$

4. $\frac{221}{500}$

5. $5\frac{3}{100}$

6. $\frac{301}{1000}$

7. $100\frac{1}{25}$

8. $206\frac{7}{100}$

9. $10\frac{17}{25}$

10. $7\frac{11}{25}$

Review and Practice

2.5 Adding and Subtracting Decimals

1. 10.82

   $\begin{array}{r} 7.58 \\ + \; 3.24 \\ \hline 10.82 \end{array}$

2. 165.12

3. 13.66

4. 26.512

5. 2.51

6. 2.305

7. 0.805

8. 4.025

9. 14.25

10. 14.625

11. 5.57

12. 13.8

13. 0.82

14. 11.228

15. 7.924

16. 11.98

17. 9.6

18. 177.79

19. 65.99

20. 518.69

21. 1.9 degrees

22. $7.45

23. 2.25 grams

24. 37.4 mL

25. 74.62 kg

Review and Practice

2.6 Multiplying Decimals

1. 60.68

    $$\begin{array}{r} 70.4 \\ \times\ 8.2 \\ \hline 148 \\ 592 \\ \hline 6068 \end{array}$$

    The factors have 2 decimal places.

2. 9.031

3. 1.26

4. 0.1216

5. 0.275

6. 0.0108

7. 0.00006

8. 0.1875

9. 14.42

10. 1.08

11. 0.062

12. 0.16004

13. 16.12

14. 37.5 milliliters

15. 4.48 milliliters

16. 1.125 milligrams

17. 0.2 milligrams

18. 191.4 ounces

Critical Thinking on the Job

Placing Decimals Correctly

The healthcare professional got confused when placing the decimal in the answer. She followed the rule for addition rather than that for multiplication of decimals. The result, had the error not been caught, could have been a disastrous overdose. The baby should have received 1.5625 g of medication, which rounds to 1.56 g.

Review and Practice

2.7 Dividing Decimals

1. 2

    $3.2 \div 1.6 = \frac{3.2}{1.6} = \frac{32}{16} = 2$

2. 27

3. 122.5

4. 2

5. 2.5

6. 0.4

7. 0.0125 rounded to 0.013

8. 3.15

9. 50

10. 0.1

11. 0.2905 rounded to 0.291

12. 0.00348 rounded to 0.003

13. 1322.2

14. 6060

15. 0.8887 rounded to 0.889

16. 1.231016 rounded to 1.231

17. 80 doses

18. 80 doses

19. 0.25 grams per dose

20. 3.75 pounds per month

Chapter 2 Review

Check Up

1. >

    The whole number 5 is the same. In the tenths place, 7 > 0 so that 5.7 > 5.09

2. >

3. =

4. <

5. 0.23

    The digit to the right of the hundredths place is 9. Round the digit in the hundredths place up one unit: 0.23

6. 7.09

7. 46

8. 9.89

9. 4.3

10. 3.7

11. 7.0

    Remember that, according to Rule 2.2, trailing zeros after the decimal point should be dropped, and this number would be rewritten as 12.

12. 0.1

13. 9

14. 21

15. 1

16. 12

17. 0.5

    $\frac{7}{14} = 7 \div 14$

    $= 0.5$

18. 0.625

19. 2.6

20. 8

21. $\frac{41}{50}$

22. $\frac{13}{20}$

23. $\frac{41}{50}$

    0.82 has no whole number. 82 is the numerator. 2 is in the hundredths place: 0.82

    $= \frac{82}{100} = \frac{41}{50}$

24. $1\frac{1}{1000}$

25. 19.61

    $$\begin{array}{r} 7.23 \\ +\ 12.38 \\ \hline 19.61 \end{array}$$

26. 4.79

27. 1.021

28. 13.704

29. 7.11

30. 0.89

31. 0.242

32. 13.222

33. 11.27

    $$\begin{array}{r} 2.3 \\ \times 4.9 \\ \hline 207 \\ 92 \\ \hline 1127 \end{array}$$

    The factors have 2 decimal places.

34. 0.00066

35. 4.995

36. 12.07005

37. 18.5

38. 1.5

39. 20

40. 20

41. The bottle contains 40 doses of 1.2 mL.

Critical Thinking Applications

0.125, 0.25, 0.375, 0.625, 0.75, 0.875, 1.0

0.5-diameter instrument is missing.

Case Study

Day 3, 8:00 a.m.	+1.75 pounds
Day 3, 2:00 p.m.	−1 pound
Day 4, 8:00 a.m.	−2 pounds
Day 4, 4:00 p.m.	−2.25 pounds

CHAPTER 3 ANSWERS

Review and Practice

3.1 Percents

1. 0.14
   *Add a decimal, move it
   two places to the left and
   drop the percent sign.
   14% = 14.% = .14
   = 0.14*

2. 0.3

3. 0.02

4. 0.09

5. 1.03

6. 3

7. 0.0021

8. 0.004

9. 0.425

10. 0.038

11. 0.045

12. 2.508

13. 0.237

14. 0.018

15. 0.145

16. 404%
   *Multiply by 100 and add
   the percent symbol.
   4.04 × 100% = 404%*

17. 230%

18. 70%

19. 33%

20. 6%

21. 1.3%

22. 1500%

23. 3200%

24. 12,100%

25. $\frac{11}{50}$
   *Write the value of the
   percent as the numerator
   and 100 as the denominator.*
   $22\% = \frac{22}{100}$
   *Reduce the fraction to its
   lowest terms.*
   $\frac{22}{100} = \frac{11}{50}$

26. $\frac{1}{25}$

27. $1\frac{29}{50}$

28. 3

29. $\frac{1}{1000}$

30. $\frac{1}{125}$

31. $\frac{9}{1000}$

32. $\frac{7}{500}$

33. $\frac{3}{1000}$

34. 75%
   *Convert the fraction to a
   decimal.*
   $\frac{6}{8} = 0.75$
   *Convert the decimal to a
   percent.*
   $0.75 \times 100\% = 75\%$

35. 80%

36. 17%

37. 56%

38. 110%

39. 225%

40. 175%

41. 40%

42. 567%

Review and Practice

3.2 Ratios

1. $\frac{3}{4}$
   *Write the first value in the
   ratio as the numerator and
   the second value as the
   denominator.*
   $3 : 4 = \frac{3}{4}$

2. $\frac{4}{9}$

3. $1\frac{2}{3}$

4. $\frac{10}{1}$

5. $\frac{1}{20}$

6. $\frac{1}{250}$

7. $\frac{1}{3}$

8. 2 : 3
   *Write the numerator as
   the first value and the
   denominator as the second.
   Separate the values with
   a colon.*
   $\frac{2}{3} = 2 : 3$

9. 6 : 7

10. 5 : 4

11. 7 : 3

12. 15 : 8

13. 10 : 3

14. 3 : 5

15. 2 : 3

16. 1 : 50

17. 1 : 75

18. 29 : 5

19. 0.25

Write the ratio as
a fraction.

$1 : 4 = \frac{1}{4}$

Convert the fraction
to a decimal.

$\frac{1}{4} = 1 \div 4 = 0.25$

20. 0.13

21. 0.75

22. 0.4

23. 50

24. 12.5

25. 2.67

26. 0.83

27. 0.07

28. 9 : 10

Write the decimal
as a fraction.

$0.9 = \frac{9}{10}$

Reduce the fraction
to lowest terms.

$\frac{9}{10}$ is already reduced
to lowest terms.

Restate the fraction
as a ratio.

$\frac{9}{10} = 9 : 10$

29. 3 : 10

30. 1 : 100

31. 9 : 20

32. 6 : 1

33. 12 : 5

34. 8 : 1

35. 49 : 5

36. 25%

Convert the ratio to a
decimal.

$1 : 4 = \frac{1}{4} = 0.25$

Multiply by 100 and add
the percent symbol.

$0.25 \times 100\% = 25\%$

37. 4%

38. 22%

39. 41%

40. 2000%

41. 750%

42. 37.5%

43. 7 : 50

Write the percent as
a fraction.

$14\% = \frac{14}{100}$

Reduce the fraction
to lowest terms.

$\frac{14}{100} = \frac{7}{50}$

44. 13 : 20

45. 4 : 1

46. 7 : 4

47. 3 : 500

48. 9 : 5000

49. 21 : 25

50. 57 : 10,000

Review and Practice

3.3 Proportions

1. $\frac{4}{5} = \frac{8}{10}$

   Convert both ratios to
   fractions.

   $4 : 5 = 8 : 10 \rightarrow \frac{4}{5} = \frac{8}{10}$

2. $\frac{5}{12} = \frac{10}{24}$

3. $\frac{1}{10} = \frac{100}{1000}$

4. $\frac{2}{3} = \frac{20}{30}$

5. $\frac{50}{25} = \frac{10}{5}$

6. $\frac{6}{4} = \frac{18}{12}$

7. $\frac{5}{24} = \frac{10}{48}$

8. $\frac{75}{100} = \frac{150}{200}$

9. $\frac{4}{16} = \frac{16}{64}$

10. $\frac{125}{100} = \frac{375}{300}$

11. $3 : 4 = 75 : 10$

    Convert both fractions
    to ratios.

    $\frac{3}{4} = \frac{75}{100} \rightarrow$

    $3 : 4 = 75 : 100$

12. $1 : 5 = 3 : 15$

13. $8 : 4 = 2 : 1$

14. $8 : 7 = 24 : 21$

15. $18 : 16 = 9 : 8$

16. $10 : 1 = 40 : 4$

17. $5 : 7 = 15 : 21$

18. $45 : 5 = 9 : 1$

19. $1 : 100 = 100 : 10,000$

20. $36 : 12 = 72 : 24$

Critical Thinking on the Job

Setting Up the Correct Proportion

The healthcare professional realizes while solving the equation that he will not be able to cancel any units, and that his answer will contain both milligrams and milliliters. After looking at the proportion once again, he discovers that he has set up the proportion incorrectly, and that the first fraction is written upside down. He rewrites the proportion as 125 mg/mL = 250 mg/x. After canceling the milligrams in the numerator, he solves the equation and correctly determines that the dose is 10 mL. Critical thinking is especially important when you use a calculator. Had the healthcare professional ignored the units and simply punched in the numbers, he would have come up with the wrong dose. Always include the units when you perform drug calculations.

Review and Practice

3.4 Using Proportions to Solve for an Unknown Quantity

1. True
   Multiply means and extremes. Compare the products.
   $12 \times 12 = 6 \times 24$
   $144 = 144$

2. Not true

3. Not true

4. True

5. True

6. Not true
   Cross multiply, then compare the products.
   $7 \times 48 = 16 \times 28$
   $336 = 448$

7. True

8. True

9. Not true

10. Not true

11. 16
    Multiply means and extremes and then solve the equation.
    $5 \times x = 10 \times 8$
    $5x = 80$
    $x = 16$

12. 8

13. 100

14. 20

15. 35

16. 4

17. 9

18. 65

19. 4

20. 4

21. 1
    Cross multiply and then solve the equation.
    $15 \times x = 3 \times 5$
    $15x = 15$
    $x = 1$

22. 25

23. 24

24. 150

25. 200

26. 1

27. 1

28. 9

29. 6

30. 30

31. 42 tablets

32. 300 mg

33. 24 h

34. 250 mg

35. 1250 mL

Critical Thinking on the Job

Confusing Multiplying Fractions with Cross-Multiplying

The healthcare professional realizes that mixing 10,000 g for a solution with 500 mL is not reasonable. Looking at her work, she realizes she has treated the problem as if she were multiplying fractions rather than solving a proportion problem. She has mistakenly multiplied the two numerators and set their product equal to the product of the two denominators.

To calculate correctly, the healthcare professional should cross-multiply $100 \times x$ and 5×500.

$$100 \times x = 2500$$
$$x = 25$$

She will need 25 g, *not* 10,000 g, of dextrose. The healthcare professional did not double-check her answer by making sure that the answer gave a true proportion. If she had, she would have found that $\frac{5\,g}{100\,mL}$ is not equal to $\frac{10,000\,g}{500\,mL}$. Fortunately, the answer that she calculated was not reasonable, and she was able to detect the error. Sometimes, however, even a wrong answer can be reasonable. *Always double-check your answer when performing dosage calculations.*

Chapter 3 Review

Check Up

Exercise	Fraction	Decimal	Ratio	Percent
1.	$\frac{2}{3}$	0.67	2 : 3	67%
2.	$\frac{5}{4}$	1.25	5 : 4	125%
3.	$\frac{28}{100}$	0.28	28 : 100	28%
4.	$\frac{3}{100}$	0.03	3 : 100	3%

Exercise	Fraction	Decimal	Ratio	Percent
5.	$\frac{40}{8}$	5	40 : 8	500%
6.	$\frac{4}{12}$	0.33	4 : 12	33%
7.	$\frac{9}{27}$	0.33	9 : 27	33%
8.	$1\frac{4}{10}$	1.4	14 : 10	140%
9.	$\frac{1}{200}$	0.005	1 : 200	0.5%
10.	$\frac{3}{50}$	0.06	3 : 50	6%
11.	$\frac{1}{4}$	0.25	1 : 4	25%
12.	$\frac{6}{1}$	6	6 : 1	600%
13.	$\frac{1}{9}$	0.11	1 : 9	11%
14.	$\frac{150}{100}$	1.5	3 : 2 or 150 : 100	150%
15.	$\frac{6}{97}$	0.06	6 : 97	6%
16.	$\frac{128}{10}$	12.8	64 : 5 or 128 : 10	1280%

17. 40
Use means and extremes to solve.
$1 \times x = 10 \times 4$
$1x = 40$
$x = 40$

18. 1

19. 4

20. 25

21. 48

22. 1

23. 2

24. 5

25. 75 mg
Set the problem up as a proportion, where the unknown is the number of milligrams in 3 tablets.
$\frac{1\ tablet}{25\ mg} = \frac{3\ tablets}{x}$
Cancel units.
$\frac{1\ tablet}{25\ mg} = \frac{3\ tablets}{x}$
Cross multiply to solve the equation.
$25\ mg \times 3 = 1 \times x$
$75\ mg = x$

26. 300 mL

27. 25 g

28. 150 mL

29. 2 mL

30. 105 g

Critical Thinking Applications

5 g

Case Study

1. 250 mg

2. 10 mL

Internet Activity

Answers may vary.
Solutions: (1) Auralgan otic solution, (2) Eye irrigating solution, (3) SSKI solution
Lotions: (1) Cordran® lotion, (2) Hytone® lotion, (3) Klaron lotion
Creams: (1) Bactroban® cream, (2) Benzashave cream, (3) Silvadene® 1% cream
Suspensions: (1) Carafate® suspension, (2) Betaxon opthalmic suspension, (3) Codeine suspension
Ointments: (1) Cetamide ointment, (2) Cortosporin® ointment, (3) Neosporin® opthalmic ointment

UNIT ONE ASSESSMENT ANSWERS

1a. <	5. 3	11. 42	16. 17.5
1b. <	6. $\frac{37}{5}$	12. 3	17. $4\frac{1}{2}$
1c. =	7. 600 mg	13. $\frac{3}{4}$	18. 5.75
2. 57%	8. 4:10 (or 2 : 5)	14. $8\frac{3}{8}$	19. 200 mg
3. 8	9. 6%	15. 30	20. 1.425
4. 12	10. 0.035		

CHAPTER 4 ANSWERS

Review and Practice

4.1 Metric Notation

1. d
   Choice "a" is incorrect because the K is capitalized.
   Choice "b" is incorrect because the value is wrong.
   Choice "c" is incorrect because the fraction should be converted to a decimal.

2. d	7. d	12. 0.62 g	17. 157 km
3. c	8. b	13. 0.75 mL	18. 7.75 cm
4. d	9. c	14. 0.7 m	19. 93 mcg
5. b	10. a	15. 12 L	20. 0.08 mg
6. c	11. 4.5 mL	16. 0.75 kg	

Critical Thinking on the Job

Placing the Decimal Point Correctly

When you convert quantities from one unit of measure to another, pay close attention to the decimal point. In going from milligrams (mg) to micrograms (mcg), the quantity should be multiplied by 1000; the decimal should move three places to the right. The problem should have been calculated as follows:

$$0.05 \text{ mg} \times 1000 = 50 \text{ mcg}$$

$$0.050 \text{ mg} = 50 \text{ mcg}$$

Be even more careful when the patient is a child. Dosages that are perfectly safe for adults may be life-threatening for children. As you will learn in Chapter 10, you must carefully read the labels on all drugs. In the case of Lanoxin®, both the elixir and the injection have labels marked in both micrograms (mcg) and milligrams (mg). A careful look at the labels would help prevent this error.

Review and Practice

4.2 Converting Within the Metric System

1. 7000 mg	3. 0.023 kg	9. 0.5 km	15. 60,000 mcg
You are converting from a larger unit to a smaller unit, so you need to multiply.	4. 8000 g	10. 3250 m	16. 500,000 mcg
	5. 8010 mL	11. 250 mcg	17. 0.008 g
	6. 0.1 L	12. 462,000 mcg	18. 0.02 g
$7 \text{ g} \times 1000 = 7000 \text{ mg}$	7. 3600 mm	13. 0.25 mg	19. 56.2 cm
2. 1.2 g	8. 5.233 m	14. 0.075 mg	20. 0.0432 m

Chapter 4 Review

Check Up

1. 25.5 kg
2. 0.45 cm
3. 40 mcg
4. 0.75 L
5. 0.9 mg
6. 1.5 mm
7. 0.375 g
8. 12 mL

9. 60 mg

   You are converting from a larger unit to a smaller, so you need to multiply.

   0.06 g × 1000 = 60 mg

10. 0.125 mg

    You are converting from a smaller unit to a larger, so you need to divide.

    125 mcg ÷ 1000 = 0.125 mg

11. 4 m
12. 7.5 mm
13. 0.965 L
14. 8 mL
15. 320 g
16. 50 mcg
17. 0.988 km
18. 0.01725 km

19. 0.368 g
20. 0.247 kg

Critical Thinking Applications

The patient would take 2 of the 250 mg tablets.

Case Study

1. The patient will take 45 mL of medication each day.

2. If the patient is taking 45 mL a day for 10 days, they will need 450 mL to complete the order. Therefore, 0.5 L bottle will contain enough medication to complete 10 days of treatment.

Internet Activity

1. × 1,000,000
2. × 1/1,000,000,000,000
3. × 1,000,000,000,000,000,000,000,000

4. × 1/1,000,000,000
5. × 100

CHAPTER 5 ANSWERS

Review and Practice

5.1 Apothecary System

1. 7 grains or gr vii

   Using Rule 5-1, seven grains can be written out or the abbreviation "gr" can be used. When using the abbreviation and Roman numerals, the value should be written after the unit.

2. 8 ounces or 8 oz
3. 5 drams
4. 14 grains or gr xiv
5. $\frac{1}{2}$ grain or $\frac{1}{2}$ gr
6. $5\frac{1}{2}$ ounces or $5\frac{1}{2}$ oz

7. 480 grains

   1 oz = 480 gr (from Table 5-1)

8. 1 drams
9. 1 fluid ounce
10. 16 ounces

Review and Practice

5.2 Household System

1. 2 tsp or 2 t

   Refer to Table 5-3 for the appropriate abbreviations.

2. $3\frac{1}{2}$ tbsp, $3\frac{1}{2}$ tbs, or $3\frac{1}{2}$ T
3. 75 lb
4. 4 fluid oz
5. 2 gtt

6. 1 gal
7. 960

   1 pt 5 480 mL (from Table 5-4)

   Solve the problem as a proportion.

   $\frac{x}{2} pt = \frac{480 mL}{1 pt}$

   $x = 960 mL$

   Refer to Chapter 3 if you need help solving proportions.

8. 2
9. 6
10. 2

Review and Practice

5.3 Equivalent Measurements

1. 6.6

   1 kg = 2.2 lb (From Table 5-4)

   Solve the problem as a proportion.

   $\frac{x}{3}\,kg = \frac{2.2\,lb}{1\,kg}$

   $x = 6.6\,lb$

   Refer to Chapter 3 if you need help solving proportions.

2. 2

3. 2

4. 3

5. 1440

6. 10

7. 4

8. 45

9. 454

10. 60

Chapter 5 Review

Check Up

1. $14\frac{1}{4}$ oz
2. 2 T or 2 tbsp or 2 tbs
3. 15 gr or xv gr
4. 3.5 gal or $3\frac{1}{2}$ gal
5. 2 drops or 2 gtt
6. 75 lb
7. $1\frac{1}{2}$ t, 1.5 t, $1\frac{1}{2}$ tsp, or 1.5 tsp
8. 2 pt
9. 480
10. 15
11. 30
12. 2
13. 480
14. 60
15. 8
16. 2.2
17. 16
18. 3
19. 16
20. 5

Critical Thinking Applications

1. 8 teaspoons
2. 2 bottles
3. 1 bottle

Case Study

3 mL

Internet Activity

Try *refdesk.com*. Click on "Convert anything" on bottom of left column

1. Answer varies based upon weight.
2. 1 oz

CHAPTER 6 ANSWERS

Review and Practice

6.1 Writing Conversion Factors from Equivalent Measurements

1. 60 mg/1 gr, 60 mg:1 gr
2. 454 g/1 lb, 454 g:1 lb
3. 1 tsp/5 mL, 1 tsp:5 mL
4. 1000 mg/1 g, 1000 mg:1 g
5. 2 tbsp/1 oz, 2 tbsp:1 oz
6. 2.2 lb/1 kg, 2.2 lb:1 kg
7. 1 L/1000 mL, 1 L:1000 mL
8. 240 mL/1 cup, 240 mL:1 cup
9. 1000 mcg/1 mg, 1000 mcg:1 mg
10. 15 mL/1 tbsp, 15 mL:1 tbsp

6.2 Converting Units using the Proportion Method

1. 2 tbsp

   Using ratios:

   Write the conversion factor 1 tbsp : 15 mL

   Set up the proportion x : 30 mL = 1 tbsp : 15 mL

   Cancel units x : 30 m̶L̶ = 1 tbsp : 15 m̶L̶

   Solve for the unknown x = 2 tbsp

   Using fractions:

   Write the conversion factor 1 tbsp/15 mL

   Set up the proportion x/30 mL = 1 tbsp/15 mL

   Cancel units x/30 m̶L̶ = 1 tbsp/15 m̶L̶

   Solve for the unknown x = 2 tbsp

2. 25
3. 24
4. 0.24
5. 0.25
6. 900
7. 0.01
8. 37.5
9. 92.4
10. 20
11. 180
12. 1.5 pints
13. 10 mL
14. 143 lb
15. 85 kg
16. 4 tbsp
17. 960 mL
18. 180 mg
19. 0.5 grains
20. 22.5 mL

Critical Thinking on the Job
Selecting the Correct Conversion Factor

Even though Greg set up the proportion correctly, he used the wrong conversion factor. Certain equivalent measures, such as 1 tsp = 5 mL, are so commonly used that you should memorize them. When you are using a conversion chart, always double-check that you select the correct unit of measure and be sure that you read across the same line. Had Greg used the correct conversion, 1 tsp/5 mL, he would have calculated as follows:

$$x/30 \text{ mL} = 1 \text{ tsp}/5 \text{ mL}$$
$$x/30 \text{ m̶L̶} = 1 \text{ tsp}/5 \text{ m̶L̶}$$
$$x \times 5 = 1 \text{ tsp} \times 30$$
$$x = 6 \text{ tsp}$$

The patient would be told to take 6 tsp of medication, not 2 tsp.

Review and Practice
6.3 Converting Units using Dimensional Analysis

1. 2 tbsp

   x tbsp = 1 tbsp/15 mL $\times$ 30 mL/1

   x = 2 tbsp

2. 25
3. 24
4. 0.24
5. $\frac{1}{4}$
6. 900
7. 0.01
8. $37\frac{1}{2}$
9. 92.4
10. 20
11. 180
12. 1.5 pints
13. 10 mL
14. 143 lb
15. 85 kg
16. 4 tbsp
17. 960 mL
18. 180 mg
19. 0.5 grains
20. 22.5 mL

Chapter 6 Review
Check Up

1. 1 kg/2.2 lb, 2.2 lb/1 kg, 1 kg:2.2 lb, and 2.2 lb:1 kg

2. 1 oz/30 mL, 30 mL/1 oz, 1 oz:30 mL, and 30 mL:1 oz

3. 1000 mcg/1 mg, 1 mg/1000 mcg, 1000 mcg:1 mg, and 1 mg:1000 mcg

4. 1 gr/60 mg, 60 mg/1 gr, 1 gr:60 mg, and 60 mg:1 gr

5. 1 tsp/5 mL, 5 mL/1 tsp, 1 tsp:5 mL, and 5 mL:1 tsp

6. 1000 mL/1 L, 1 L/1000 mL, 1000 mL:1 L, and 1 L:1000 mL

7. 2 tbsp/1 oz, 1 oz/2 tbsp, 2 tbsp:1 oz, and 1 oz:2 tbsp

8. 1 tbsp/15 mL, 15 mL/1 tbsp, 1 tbsp:15 mL, and 15 mL:1 tbsp

9. 120

Using ratios:	*Using fractions:*
Write the conversion factor 15 gr : 1 g	Write the conversion factor 15 gr/1 g
Set up the proportion $x : 8\ g = 15\ gr : 1\ g$	Set up the proportion $x/8\ g = 15\ gr/1\ g$
Cancel units $x : 8\ \not{g} = 15\ gr : 1\ \not{g}$	Cancel units $x/8\ \not{g} = 15\ gr/1\ \not{g}$
Solve for the unknown $x = 120\ gr$	Solve for the unknown $x = 120\ gr$
	Using dimensional analysis:
	$x\ gr = 15\ gr/1\ g \times 8\ g/1$
	$x = 120\ gr$

10. 150	14. 40	18. 103.4	22. 45 mL
11. 6	15. 9	19. 325 mg	23. $2\frac{1}{2}$ qt per day
12. 25	16. 45	20. 20 kg	24. 90 kg
13. 240	17. 81	21. 15 mL	

Critical Thinking Applications

1. $1\frac{1}{2}$ tsp

2. The patient will need a total of 450 mL in order to complete 10 days of treatment, which means that 3 bottles will be needed.

Case Study

1. 1310 mL

2. You need to order 2 pint bottles.

Internet Activity

1. approximately 2.11 quarts

2. approximately 8.45 ounces

3. approximately 71 mL

CHAPTER 7 ANSWERS

Review and Practice

7.1 Converting Temperature

1. 93.2°F
   $5F - 160 = 9 \times 34$
   $5F - 160 = 306$
   $\quad\quad 5F = 306 + 160$
   $\quad\quad 5F = 466$
   $\quad\quad\ F = 93.2$

2. 105.8°F

3. 35°C
   $(5 \times 95) - 160 = 9C$
   $475 - 160 = 9C$
   $315 = 9C$
   $35 = C$

4. 38.9°C

5. 7.4°C

6. 100°C

7. 77°F

8. 212°F

9. 15°C

10. 152.6°F

Review and Practice

7.2 Converting Time

1. 0235
   Remove the colon and the abbreviation a.m. Write the hour 2 with two digits, starting with zero.
   2:35 a.m. = 0235

2. 0757

3. 0008

4. 0055

5. 1349

6. 1514

7. 2354

8. 2219

9. 1859

10. 0426

11. 12:11 a.m.

12. 12:36 a.m.

13. 3:25 a.m.

14. 8:49 a.m.

15. 1:13 p.m.
   Insert a colon to separate the hour from the minutes. Subtract 12 from the hour, and add the abbreviation p.m.
   1313 = 1:13 p.m.

16. 3:27 p.m.

17. 9:45 p.m.

18. 11:59 p.m.

19. 8:37 p.m.

20. 6:18 p.m.

Chapter 7 Review
Check Up

1. 36.4°C
   $(5 \times 97.6) - 160 = 9C$
   $488 - 160 = 9C$
   $328 = 9C$
   $36.4 = C$

2. 22.2°C

3. 14.1°C

4. 28.2°C

5. 75.2°F
   $5F - 160 = 9 \times 24$
   $5F - 160 = 216$
   $5F = 216 + 160$
   $5F = 376$
   $F = 75.2$

6. 110.8°F

7. 60.1°F

8. 47.8°F

9. 0321
   Remove the colon and the abbreviation a.m. Write the hour 3 with two digits, starting with zero.
   3:21 a.m. = 0321

10. 1642

11. 2247

12. 1120

13. 12:29 a.m.

14. 2:17 p.m.
   Insert a colon to separate the hour from the minutes. Subtract 12 from the hour, and add the abbreviation p.m.
   1417 = 2:17 p.m.

15. 8:53 p.m.

16. 9:12 a.m.

Critical Thinking Applications

1. 3:30 p.m. and 11:30 p.m.

2. 1530 and 2330

Case Study

Between 2.2°C and 5°C

UNIT TWO ASSESSMENT ANSWERS

1. 0.15 mg
2. 10 kg
3. 59°F
4. 120 mL
5. 12.5 mL
6. 2.4 L
7. 520 mg
8. 3:30 pm
9. 340 cm
10. 4 tbsp
11. 8000 g
12. 20 oz
13. 12.8°C
14. 1415
15. 480 mL
16. Yes, his weight changed. Bill lost 3.5 pounds (or 1.6 kg).
17. 4 days
18. 975 mg
19. No – only $3\frac{1}{2}$ fl oz remain in the bottle.
20a. 428°F
20b. 1915

CHAPTER 8 ANSWERS

Critical Thinking on the Job

Use the Correct Dropper

This error could easily be avoided. During the initial visit, the father should have been instructed to use *only* the dropper that accompanies the medication. When he calls two days later, he should be asked if the *correct equipment* was used.

Review and Practice

8.1 Enteral Medication Administration Devices

1. False. Syringes with needles should not be used for oral medication administration.

2. False. Medicine cups should be used for doses over 5 mL.

3. False. Oral syringes are labels for oral use, have a off-center, or flexible tip.

4. True

5. False. Drop sizes can vary between droppers; never substitute a dropper provided by the manufacturer.

6. False. Calibrated spoons are best, however measuring spoons for baking can be used.

7. True

8. True

9. False. One mL equals 1 cubic centimeter.

10. False. You must convert the prescribed dose to the same unit of measure as the calibrated device used to deliver the dose.

11. False. Measure the quantity of liquid at the meniscus.

12. False. Calibrated droppers may be used to delivery medications to the eyes, ears, and nose.

13. True

14. False. Gelcaps and extended-release medications cannot be crushed to be delivered through the nasogastric tube.

15. d
16. c
17. d
18. b
19. c
20. d

Critical Thinking on the Job

Finishing What You Start

This overdose could be avoided. The first healthcare professional should check the prescribed dose and immediately discard the extra medication from the syringe. He should personally deliver the dose or in some cases identify its contents prior to leaving the room. The second healthcare professional also should take extra precautions. She should confirm directly with the first healthcare professional the amount to deliver and check the patient's chart before administering medication. She should not have administered from a syringe unless she was certain that its contents matched the amount ordered.

Review and Practice

8.2 Parenteral Medication Administration Devices

1. Tenths of a mL (0.1 mL)
2. Units (1 unit or 0.01 mL)
3. Hundredths of a mL (0.01 mL)
4. Two-tenths of a mL (0.2 mL)
5. True
6. True
7. False
8. True
9. False
10. False
11. False
12. False
13. True

14. Type: standard, volume: 1 mL
15. Type: insulin, volume: 49 units
16. Type: tuberculin, volume: 0.05 mL
17. Type: large-capacity, volume: 4.2 mL
18. Type: standard, volume: 2.2 mL
19. Type: insulin, volume: 22 units
20. Type: tuberculin, volume: 0.8 mL
21. Type: standard, volume: 3 mL
22. Type: large-capacity, volume: 9.5 mL or 9.4 mL (closest calibration mark)
23. Type: tuberculin, volume: 0.2 mL
24. Type: large-capacity, volume: 2.8 mL
25. Type: insulin, volume: 1 unit

Chapter 8 Review

Check Up

1. a and c
2. c
3. d
4. c and d
5. d
6. a
7. c
8. b
9. a
10. d
11. True
12. False
13. False
14. True
15. True
16. False
17. True
18. False
19. False
20. False

21.

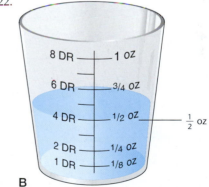

22.

23.

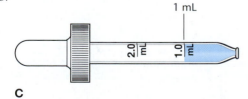

24.

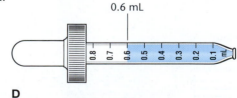

25.

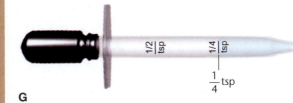

E

26.

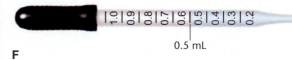

0.5 mL

F

27.

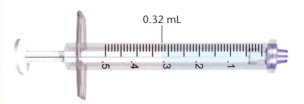

G

28.

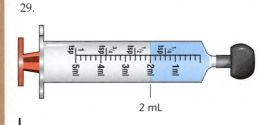

0.32 mL

H

29.

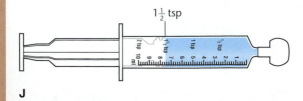

2 mL

I

30.

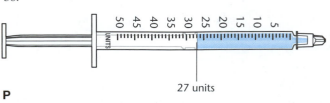

$1\frac{1}{2}$ tsp

J

31.

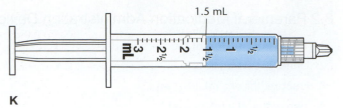

1.5 mL

K

32.

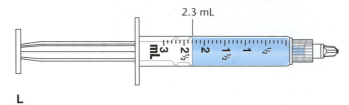

2.3 mL

L

33.

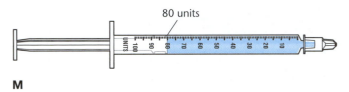

80 units

M

34.

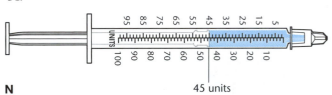

45 units

N

35.

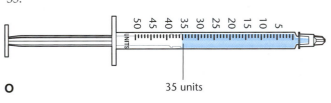

35 units

O

36.

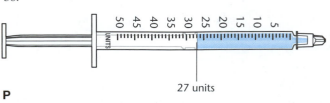

27 units

P

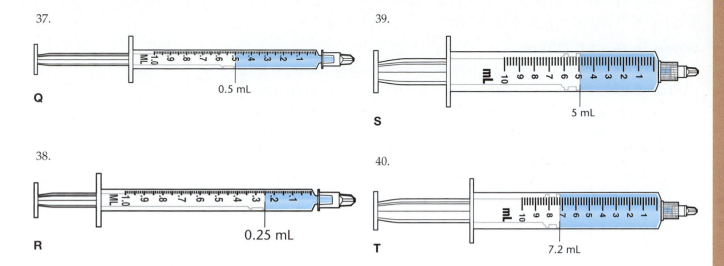

37.

Q

0.5 mL

38.

R

0.25 mL

39.

S

5 mL

40.

T

7.2 mL

Critical Thinking Applications

1. Standard, safety, or needleless syringe
2. 50-unit (0.5 mL) Insulin syringe
3. Tuberculin syringe
4. Oral syringe
5. Medicine cup, calibrated spoon, or oral syringe
6. Standard, safety, or needleless syringe
7. Medicine cup, calibrated spoon, or oral syringe
8. Large-capacity syringe
9. Transdermal patch
10. Dropper or oral syringe
11. Teaspoon dropper, calibrated spoon, or oral syringe

Case Study

The dose to be administered is 0.75 tsp. It could be measured in a calibrated spoon. Another acceptable form of administration would be 3.75 mL in an oral syringe.

Internet Activity

Your report should indicate knowledge of at least two needleless systems or types of safety syringes. Try *www.safetysyringes.com, www.bd.com.*

CHAPTER 9 ANSWERS

Review and Practice

9.1 Medical Abbreviations

1. One Bactrim® (400 mg sulfamethoxazole and 80 mg trimethoprim) tablet by mouth every 12 hours for 10 days.
2. One 0.1 mg tablet Catapres® (clinidine hydrochloride) by mouth twice a day, once in the morning and once at bedtime.
3. One 1 mg tablet of Lunesta® (eszopiclone) by mouth every evening at bedtime, as needed for insomnia.
4. One $\frac{1}{150}$ grain tablet of Nitrostat® (nitroglycerin) sublingual as needed for relief of chest pain; may repeat dose in 5 minutes if chest pain continues, not to exceed a maximum of 3 tablets per episode of chest pain.
5. Two 20 mg tablets of Mevacor® (loavastatin) by mouth once a day.

Critical Thinking on the Job

Understanding the Order of Roman Numerals

The numeral with the smaller value comes immediately before the one with the larger value. Instead of adding i and x, the healthcare professional should subtract i from x to calculate the correct dose of 9 gr.

Critical Thinking on the Job

When in Doubt, Check

1. The patient's date of birth and the AP's signature are missing from the order in Figure 9.2.

2. The healthcare practitioner is questioning the dose of 600 mg of the order in Figure 9.2.

3. By using her critical thinking skills, the healthcare professional has prevented a serious error.

The Lasix® order appears to be 600 mg. However, she realizes that the second zero of 600 is actually the loop of the *q* from the digoxin order. The intended dose of Lasix® is 60 mg. If she had not checked the medication orders, she might have given 10 times more than the prescriber intended. When in doubt, always verify the order written on the chart. In this case if "daily" had been used instead of "qd", the error would not have occurred.

Review and Practice

9.2 Components of a Medication Order

1. e
2. f
3. c
4. b
5. g
6. h
7. d
8. a

Review and Practice

9.3 Medication Administration Records

1. Check if the patient's systolic blood pressure is below 110.

2. 5 mg.

3. 0630 (6:30 a.m.).

4. Subcut or subcutaneous injection.

5. The Maalox® is administered 2 h after meals and at bedtime.

6. 30 mL.

7. 45 units.

Chapter 9 Review

Check Up

1. One 25 mg tablet of Aldoactone® (spironolactone) by mouth once a day.

2. 400 mg of Neurontin® (gabapentin) oral solution, 250 mg/5 mL strength, by mouth three times a day.

3. One 150 mg tablet Boniva® (ibandronate sodium) by mouth, before breakfast, every month.

4. 20 mg of a 10 mg/5 mL suspension of Paxil® (paroxetine hydrochloride) by mouth once a day in the morning.

5. Chew one 5 mg tablet of Singulair® (montelukast sodium) by mouth once a day.

6. Two 5 grain tablets of aspirin by mouth every 4 hours as needed for headache.

7. One 40 mg tablet of Protonix® (pantoprazole sodium) by mouth once a day.

8. One inch of Nitrong® (nitroglycerin) to skin every 8 hours—remove at bedtime for eight hours.

9. One 250 mg tablet of Naprosyn® (naproxen) by mouth every eight hours.

10. One 50 mg tablet of Cozaar® (losartan potassium) by mouth once a day.

11. October 30, 2012.

12. lisinopril.

13. Every morning.

14. Oral.

15. Robert Byron.

16. 5 mg.

17. Betsy Robertson.

18. January 1, 1952.

19. Stat—immediately.

20. Both eyes.

21. IVPB or via intravenous piggyback.

22. Dilantin®, Ancef®, Viroptic®.

23. Adalat® 3 doses, Dilantin® 3 doses, Ancef® 3 doses, Viroptic® 6 doses, furosemide 1 dose.

24. Six.

25. furosemide and Ancef®.

Critical Thinking Application

1. Tablet, one, by mouth, immediately.

2. Patient name, DOB, time order was written, complete dosage, signature of AP.

3. The eight components of a medication order must be present to ensure that the right patient receives the right drug in the right amount via the right route at the right time/frequency. The signature identifies the name and credentials of the AP. Date and time are necessary to provide a reference point for medication administration.

Case Study

Eight components of a medication order: patient's name, date, DOB, name of medication, dose, route, frequency, AP signature.

Patient: Katherine Drexel

DOB (today's date minus 20 years)

Date & time : (today's date and time)

Medication, dose, route, & frequency: Motrin® (ibuprofen) 800 mg po q8h prn pain.

AP's signature: L. Pingree, RN, APN, CNM

Internet Activity

Go to http://www.quia.com/mc/405408.html and practice matching the medical terminology with the correct abbreviations.

CHAPTER 10 ANSWERS

Critical Thinking on the Job

Read Labels Carefully

When a patient questions a medication, the healthcare professional should not administer the medication until verification is obtained. In this example, the healthcare professional made an initial mistake. He did not carefully compare the drug order with the drug label. Looking at Figures 10-19 and 10-20, you may think that the healthcare professional's error was reasonable given the similarity between the labels. Still, this error should have been avoided. The healthcare professional should have read the label carefully before trying to administer the drug. This rule is especially important when you administer a drug that is available in different dosage strengths or is designed for different routes of administration.

Fortunately, the patient gave the healthcare professional an opportunity to catch the error. When she questioned the color, the healthcare professional listened to the patient and rechecked his work.

However, if he had not listened, or if the patient had not alerted him, he may have administered 3 times the amount of the drug that was ordered.

Review and Practice

10.1 Information on Drug Labels and Package Inserts

1. There is no trade name.
2. Erythromycin
3. Multiple doses, 100 capsules
4. Abbott
5. 250 mg/capsule
6. 0074-6301-13
7. clorazepate dipotassium
8. Tranxene
9. 15 mg/tablet
10. T-tabs
11. 3 67386 30301 0
12. Protected from moisture, stored below 77°F (25°C), bottle kept tightly closed, dispense in USP tight, light-resistant container
13. There is no trade name; the generic name is methadone hydrochloride.
14. Vial
15. 10 mg/1 mL
16. Injection
17. 20 mL
18. In the package insert
19. Azithromycin
20. Orally
21. Label does not state; refer to the package insert.
22. 200 mg/5 mL
23. 1 tsp
24. 3 days (2 bottles = 30 mL; 10 mL/ day × 3 days = 30 mL)
25. Furosemide
26. There is no trade name.
27. Intramuscular (IM) or intravenous (IV) injection
28. Protect from light, do not use if discolored, use only if solution is clear and seal is intact, and store at controlled room temperature 20 to 25°C (68 to 77°F).
29. 40 mg
30. One (single dose vial)
31. 75 mL
32. Cefprozil
33. Oral suspension
34. 125 mg/5 mL
35. Teva
36. 15 doses
37. Because there is no registered trademark, this is a generic drug and, therefore, has no trade name.
38. Metformin hydrochloride is the generic name of the drug.
39. 500 mg/tablet
40. At 15 to 30°C or 59 to 86°F in a light-resistant container
41. Orally. The label states that the medication is a tablet.
42. 90 tablets in the bottle divided by 30 tablets in each prescription equals three prescriptions per bottle.
43. Caraco is the manufacturer.
44. B, G
45. A, B, D, F, G
46. A
47. D, F
48. C, E
49. D, F
50. A, C, E, F, G

Review and Practice

10.2 Label Information Related to Medication Routes

1. 57664-474-99
2. 1000 mg/tablet
3. Yes
4. 90
5. Levoxyl®
6. King Pharmaceuticals
7. 50 mcg/tablet
8. 100

9. Famotidine

10. Intravenously

11. 20 mg/2 mL

12. One (single dose vial)

13. 60 mL

14. 250 mg/5 mL

15. 100 mL

16. 14 days

17. Rimantadine hydrochloride

18. 100 mg/tablet

19. Flumadine®

20. Controlled room temperature 15°–30°C (59°–86°F)

21. B, E

22. C, D (NOTE: tablets can only be broken if they are scored)

23. A, B, D, E

24. A, B, D, E

25. C

26. 5 mg/mL

27. IM or IV administration

28. Colorless to light yellow

29. 10 mL

30. 0.3 mg/tablet

31. Wyeth

32. Conjugated estrogens

33. No, check the package insert for usual dose, timing of medication administration, etc.

34. Store at or below 25 °C

35. 25 mg/capsule

36. Orally

37. 30 doses (each dose is 2 capsules)

38. rDNA origin

39. 100 units/mL

40. Insulin lispro injection

41. 3 mL

42. 100 mg/mL

43. Trimethobenzamide HCl

44. Each dose is 1 mL, 20-mL multidose vial would hold 20 doses.

45. Storage should be at 25°C (77°F).

46. Neomycin and polymyxin B sulfates and hydrocortisone

47. In the ears (otic suspension)

48. Shake well before using

49. Store at 15–25°C (59–77°F)

50. Topically

51. Store refrigerated 2 to 8°C (36 to 46°F)

52. 0.01%

53. Becaplermin

54. In the eyes (ophthalmic solution)

55. Sulfacetamide solution and prednisolone sodium phosphate

56. 10 mL

57. Falcon Pharmaceuticals

58. Transdermally

59. 100 mcg/h for 72 h

60. Opioid-tolerant

61. 5

62. Calcitonin-salmon

63. 200 units/spray

64. Intranasal use only

65. 30

Chapter 10 Review

Check Up

1. The generic name is the one official name recognized by the USP and the NF. Brand or trade names can be registered with the U.S. Patent and Trademark Office. A drug may have several different trade names, but only one generic name.

2. Trade name

3. IM means intramuscular, or into the muscle. IV means intravenously, or into the vein.

4. Unscored tablets, gelcaps, caplets, enteric-coated tablets, and controlled-, sustained-, or extended-release capsules; breaking them would change the action or absorption of the drug

5. Use a package insert, when the label does not have enough information to administer the drug correctly.

6. A lot number provides a code that enables a company to know when and where the drug was manufactured. A company can use the lot number to recall a product in case of contamination.

7. 36 mg/tablet

8. 100 tablets

9. McNeil Pediatrics

10. Orally

11. Flunisolide

12. By oral inhalation

13. 250 mcg per activation

14. 50 metered inhalations

15. Orally

16. 2 mcg/capsule

17. Zemplar (paricalcitol)

18. 30 capsules

19. rDNA origin

20. R (regular), which means shorter acting

21. By injection

22. 100 units/mL

Critical Thinking Application

The tablets would probably be preferable for an adult homeless patient. The oral suspension needs refrigeration, a condition that would not be available to someone living on the streets or in a shelter. In addition, a homeless person might not have adequate facilities to wash the medicine cup. Finally, the tablets can be stored in a much smaller container than the liquid and are, therefore, more portable.

Case Study

1. Read the package insert, check any warnings on the package insert, and note any warnings on the label. Note that this medication is for pediatric patients and must be diluted for IV use.

2. The drug will need to be administered intravenously. It will need to be diluted before it is administered. You will need to check the label and the package insert for specific directions.

3. This is a single-dose vial. Dispose of the container, following the guidelines at your facility. Destroy leftover medication.

Internet Activity

Pages on the Internet may change. By doing a search using words such as *coumadin* and *interactions,* you will find a variety of sites. Sample sites include

http://www.druginfonet.com/faq/faqcouma.htm
http://www.drugs.com/pdr/coumadin.html
http://www.coumadin.com

CHAPTER 11 ANSWERS

Review and Practice

11.1 Prescription/Medication Order

1. The prescription is complete.

2. 90

3. Three times a day

4. 50 mg

5. 180 days or approximately 6 months; *Note:* The current prescription lasts 30 days and five refills will last an additional 150 days.

6. The dosage strength

7. 100 mL, but dosage strength must be included

8. One tsp

9. It cannot be refilled.

10. Every 8 hours

11. Patient name–Jane Doe, patient date of birth–3/15/55, drug name–Letters A to D, dose, route, time/frequency– Letters A to D, date/time order is written 1/3/10 8 AM, signature of authorized prescriber–Mak Sanger MD

12. A. dose, B. route, C. time/frequency, D. drug

Review and Practice

11.2 Verbal Orders

Step 1: The receiver writes: cefixime 200 mg   q12h for 10 days

   The receiver asks: "By what route?"

Step 2: "OK, that is: cefixime 200 mg po q12h for 10 days"

Step 3: "Is that correct?"

Review and Practice

11.3 Safe Medication Order Transcription

- Write on MAR "Probanthine 15 mg po tid"; insert times in the "HOUR" column – 6 a.m., 2 p.m., 10 p.m.
- Write on MAR "heparin 10,000 units subcut daily"; insert time – 10 a.m.
- Write on MAR "diphenhydramine 50 mg po at bedtime"; insert time – 10 p.m.

Review and Practice

11.4 Error-Prone Abbreviations and Symbols

1. OS, QD, HS
2. Give Coumadin® 5 mg p.o. daily
3. Morphine sulfate 4 mg subcut q4h prn pain
4. Vitamin D 1,000 international units every other day
5. Digoxin 0.125 mg (125 micrograms) p.o. daily

Review and Practice

11.5 The Three Checks of Medication Administration

1. 3rd check
2. 2nd check
3. 1st check
4. 3rd check
5. 1st check

Critical Thinking on the Job

The Importance of the Right Drug

The healthcare practitioner should have read the label three times to be certain that he had the correct drug. If he had also shown the label to the physician, the error could have been avoided.

Critical Thinking on the Job

The Importance of the Right Dose

The pediatrician made the initial error by not specifying the dose. This error does not relieve the healthcare practitioner of her responsibilities. All should have recognized that one of the rights of medication – the right dose – was missed in this order. The pediatrician should have been contacted to clarify the desired dose.

Review and Practice

11.6 The Rights of Medication Administration

1. d
2. g
3. a
4. f
5. h
6. c
7. e
8. b
9. d/j

Critical Thinking on the Job

The Importance of the Right Drug and Right Reason

- The nurse failed to double-check a medication label that did not match the MAR.
- The nurse made an inappropriate assumption and rationalization about a medication order discrepancy instead of thinking critically about this incident.
- The nurse violated the *right reason* of medication administration by not recognizing that this patient did not need quinidine, but did need quinine.
- The nurse violated the *right to know* of medication administration. Patient teaching would have likely have led to an inquiry regarding the rationale for quinidine administration and may have averted a serious medication error.

Review and Practice

11.7 Observation

1. Observe the IV access to ensure it is able to receive the intravenous medication.
2. Check and observe that each eye drop went into the space between the lower lid and the eye.
3. Observe for untoward reactions and desired effect.
4. Observe that the patient can swallow.
5. Observe that the tube is functioning properly.

Review and Practice

11.8 Patient Teaching

1. e
2. a, b, c
3. d
4. c
5. b

Chapter 11 Review

Check Up

1. Using the three checks of medication administration, administer one 2 mg tablet of Dilaudid® orally every four hours when necessary for pain.
2. Using the three checks of medication administration, administer one 30 mg tablet of codeine orally 4 times a day.
3. Instill two drops in the right eye 4 times a day.
4. Twice
5. Instilled into the right eye
6. "For ophthalmic use"
7. Every eight hours
8. By inhalation, using a metered dose inhaler
9. 10:00 a.m.
10. 8 tablets
11. 200 mg
12. Twice a day
13. Intravenous
14. 10 mg
15. Trental® and Rocephin®
16. Three times a day
17. 8:00 a.m.
18. Order C (route), order D (frequency)
19. qd; Rocephin® 1 g daily (include route)
20. Subcutaneous
21. 1.25 mg
22. 8 a.m., 2 p.m., 8 p.m.
23. Heparin and Proventil®
24. 0600
25. Every eight hours
26. New times would be marked 8 a.m., 2 p.m., 8 p.m. (8 a.m., 4 p.m., 12 a.m. is also acceptable)
27. Bleph-10® does not include the dose and Premarin® does not include the route.

28. OD should be written right eye

29. Determine if the patients ate at lunchtime. Determine if any medications must be taken on an empty stomach. Double-check any calculations. Use appropriate measuring device to administer medications. Ensure that medications can be administered after a meal.

30. Ask patients their names; verify their names with their identification bracelets. Do not administer drugs prescribed for the elderly to children or vice versa.

31. Step 1: The receiver writes: Tylenol 650 mg pr

   The receiver asks: "What frequency?"

   Step 2: "OK, that is: Tylenol 650 mg pr q4h prn headache"

   Step 3: "Is that correct?"

32. 3rd check

33. 1st check

34. Observe the site for suitability, presence of adipose tissue, and lack of fatty necrosis.

35. Observe for proper effect and untoward reaction.

36. Teach patient to report any occurrence of yellow vision to AP, because dose may need to be changed.

37. Enter on MAR: "Lasix 40 mg po daily"; insert time—8 a.m.

38. Enter on MAR: "nifedipine 10 mg po tid": insert times—0600, 1400, 2200

39. Enter on MAR "ampicillin 1 g IV q6h": insert times—2400 (or 0000), 0600, 1200, 1800

Critical Thinking Applications

Contact the order writer to find the strength that should be given. Administer the tablet immediately. Be sure that the revised order is signed. Also note that there is not a patient's name on the order sheet.

Case Study

1. Tell Mr. Burke to take one Xanax® tablet with breakfast, lunch, and dinner.

2. Give 120 tablets at one time. You may refill the prescription once.

Internet Activity

According to the article on cephalexin, the usual adult dose of cephalexin is 1 to 4 g daily, in divided doses. If the patient receives 500 mg q6h, the patient will receive 500 mg every 6 hours or four times a day. Four doses of 500 mg is a total of 2000 mg, or 2 g, per day. This amount is within the acceptable range. You may want to check for more information by using *cephalexin* as your search word.

UNIT THREE ASSESSMENT ANSWERS

1. Montelukast one 10 mg tablet by mouth every evening.

2. Morphine Sulfate 10 mg suppository per rectum every 4 hours as needed for pain

3. Frequency (daily)

4. Dose

5. Rosuvastatin and cefuroxime sodium

6. 5 mL

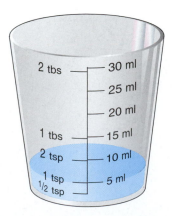

7. 0.5 mL

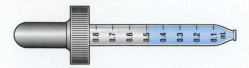

8. U-100, 1-mL syringe; 20 units

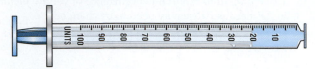

9. U-100, 0.5-mL syringe; 10 units

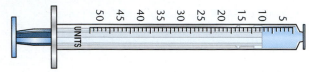

10. 1.5 mL

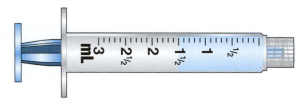

11. a. Brand name: Aranesp®; generic name: darbepoetin alfa.

b. 40 mcg/1 mL

c. Both the lot number and expiration date are imprinted on the far right side of the label.

d. One, this is "single-use vial"

e. Store at 2 to 8°C.

12. a. By mouth; orally

b. Intramuscular injection route

c. Intravenous injection route

d. Subcutaneous injection route

e. Sublingually; under the tongue

13. a. Indications—identifies conditions for which the medication would be prescribed.

b. Contraindications—conditions under which the medication should not be given.

c. Warnings—information about serious, possibly fatal, side effects.

d. Precautions—drug interactions and conditions that may cause unwanted side effects.

e. Adverse reactions—less serious, anticipated, side effects.

14. a. Patient name (RIGHT PATIENT).

b. Date of birth.

c. Medication name (RIGHT DRUG).

d. Dosage of medication (RIGHT DOSE).

e. Route by which the drug is to be given (RIGHT ROUTE).

f. Frequency or time the medication is to be given (RIGHT TIME).

g. Date and time the order was written.

h. Signature of the authorized prescriber.

15. RIGHT PATIENT: The healthcare professional will check the patient's name and date of birth on the name band; have the patient state his/her name.
RIGHT MEDICATION: The healthcare professional will check the medication label three times: when pulling the medication from the storage container; when measuring it/matching it to the MAR; just prior to administering the medication to the patient.

16. "This medication should be taken three times per day with food." (Also include dose, side effects, precautions, etc.)

17. The nurse will check the patient's pain level before and (30 minutes to 1 hour) after medication administration. The nurse will also observe the patient for side effects of this medication such as nausea or diarrhea.

18. a. OD—mistaken as AD—use right eye.

   b. qhs—mistaken as qhr—use nightly.

   c. QD—mistaken as QID—use daily.

   d. SC—mistaken as SL—use subcut.

   e. U—mistaken as the number 0—use unit

19. If the decimal point is not written clearly, the transcriber may write 50 mg or the reader may interpret 50 mg. The authorized prescriber should be reminded that trailing zeros should be dropped. The order should be written as "Coumadin 5 mg PO daily."

20. a. Write the order.

   b. Read the order.

   c. Confirm the order.

CHAPTER 12 ANSWERS

Review and Practice

12.1 Information Needed to Perform Dosage Calculations

	Dose on hand	Dosage unit	Conversion factor	Desired dose
1.	125 mg	capsule	1000 mg/1 g	250 mg
2.	500 mg	tablet	1000 mg/1 g	500 mg
3.	15 mg	tablet	no conversion	30 mg
4.	500 mg	tablet	1000 mg/1 g	250 mg
5.	300 mcg	tablet	1000 mcg/1 mg	150 mg
6.	150 mg	15 mL	5 mL/1 teaspoon	2 teaspoon
7.	mL	mL	5 mL/1 teaspoon	10 mL
8.	500 mg	tablet	1000 mg/1g	1000 mg
9.	15 mg	tablet	no conversion	30 mg
10.	50 mcg	tablet	1000 mcg/1 mg	50 mcg
11.	88 mcg	tablet	1000 mcg/1 mg	88 mcg
12.	125 mg	tablet	1000 mg/1 g	500 mg
13.	125 mcg	tablet	no conversion	250 mcg
14.	200 mg	5 mL	5 mL/1 tsp	7.5 mL
15.	125 mg	5 mL	1 teaspoon/5 mL	1.5 teaspoon
16.	137 mcg	tablet	1000 mcg/1 mg	137 mcg
17.	112 mcg	tablet	1000 mcg/mg	112 mcg

	Dose on hand	Dosage unit	Conversion factor	Desired dose
18.	0.5 mg	tablet	1 mg/1000 mg	250 mcg
19.	0.5 mg	tablet	1 mg/1000 mcg	750 mcg
20.	500 mg	tablet	1000 mg/1 g	1000 mg

Critical Thinking on the Job

When in Doubt, Check

As he looked at his answer of 4 tsp, Jorge's initial thought was that 4 tsp was a lot of medication to give the patient. First, Jorge rechecked his calculations, which were correct. Still not sure that 4 tsp was an appropriate amount to give the patient, Jorge went to the physician in charge and confirmed the order. In this case, Jorge heard the order correctly. The usual first dose of aminocaproic acid is large: 5 g, which amounts to either 4 tsp of Amicar syrup 25% or 10 of the 500-mg Amicar capsules.

Because of the unusually large volume of liquid or number of tablets, Jorge was correct to reconfirm the order. Since the order was given orally in an emergency situation, it was important that he check directly with the ordering physician before administering the drug. If Jorge's question had arisen in another circumstance, when a physician was not readily available, Jorge could consult the pharmacist or refer to the PDR (*Physicians' Desk Reference*) or another reliable reference to check the usual dose.

Review and Practice

12.2 Dosage Calculations

1. Amount to administer: 2 tablets

   Proportion Method:

   Step A: Convert. Ordered dosage and desired dose are both in mg, so conversion is not necessary.

   Step B: Calculate.

   $10 \text{ mg}/1 \text{ tab} = 20 \text{ mg}/x$ $\qquad$ $10 \text{ mg} : 1 \text{ tab} = 20 \text{ mg} : x$

   $10 \times x = 1 \text{ tab} \times 20$ $\qquad\qquad$ $1 \text{ tab} \times 20 = 10 \times x$

   $x = 20 \text{ tab}/10 \text{ or } 2 \text{ tab}$ $\qquad$ $20 \text{ tab}/10 = x \text{ or } 2 \text{ tab}$

   Step C: Think! . . . Is It Reasonable? Since the dosage ordered is twice as large as the dose on hand, and two tablets are twice as much as one tablet, it is reasonable.

   Dimensional Analysis:

   Step A: Convert. Ordered dosage and desired dose are both in mg, so conversion is not necessary.

   Step B: Calculate.

   $x = 1 \text{ tab}/10 \text{ mg} \times 20 \text{ mg}$

   $x = 2 \text{ tab}$

   Step C: Think! . . . Is It Reasonable? Since the dosage ordered is twice as large as the dose on hand, and two tablets are twice as much as one tablet, it is reasonable.

   Formula Method:

   Step A: Convert. Ordered dosage and desired dose are both in mg, so conversion is not necessary.

   Step B: Calculate.

   $20 \text{ mg}/10 \text{ mg} \times 1 \text{ tab} = x$

   $2 \text{ tab} = x$

2. Amount to administer: 10 mL

3. Amount to administer: 10 mL

4. Amount to administer: 2 tablets

5. Amount to administer: 5 mL

6. Amount to administer: 2 tablets

7. Amount to administer: 2 capsules

8. Amount to administer: 2 capsules

9. Amount to administer: 2 tablets

10. Amount to administer: 1 capsule

11. Amount to administer: 10 mL

12. Amount to administer: $1\frac{1}{2}$ or 1.5 mL

13. Amount to administer: $\frac{1}{2}$ tablet

14. Amount to administer: 0.5 mL

15. Amount to administer: 3.75 mL

16. Amount to administer: 2 tablets

17. Amount to administer: 3 mL

18. Amount to administer: $\frac{28}{100}$ mL = 0.28 mL or 28 units

19. Amount to administer: 3 tablets

20. Amount to administer: 1 capsule

Chapter 12 Review

Check Up

1. Desired dose: 5 mg

   Amount to administer: $2\frac{1}{2}$ tablets

2. Desired dose: 16 mg

   Amount to administer: 2 tablets

3. Desired dose: 400 mg

   Amount to administer: 2 tablets

4. Desired dose: 800 mg

   Amount to administer: 2 tablets

5. Desired dose D: 2 mg

   Amount to administer: 2 tablets

6. Desired dose D: 7.5 mg

   Amount to administer: 2 tablets

7. Desired dose D: 0.1 mg

   Amount to administer: 2 tablets

8. Desired dose D: 250 mg

   Amount to administer: $2\frac{1}{2}$ tablets

9. Desired dose D: 7.5 mg

   Amount to administer: 3 tablets

10. Desired dose D: 500 mg

    Amount to administer: 2 tablets

11. Desired dose D: 20 mg

    Amount to administer: 2 tablets

12. Desired dose D: 500 mg

    Amount to administer: 2 capsules

13. Desired dose D: 250 mg

    Amount to administer: 1 capsule

14. Desired dose: 60 mg

    Amount to administer: 2 capsules

15. Desired dose: 40 mg

    Amount to administer: 2 tablets

16. D: 125 mg, A: 2.5 mL or $\frac{1}{2}$ tsp

17. D: 1000 mg, A: 12.5 mL or $2\frac{1}{2}$ tsp

18. D: 5 mg, A: 1 tablet

19. D: 200 mg, A: 8 mL

20. D: 500 mg, A: 71.4 mL

21. D: 4 mg, A: 20 mL or 4 tsp

22. D: 100 mg, A: 10 mL (This is a large amount to give IM. You should check with pharmacist or physician to verify this order.)

23. D: 20 mg, A: 2 tablets

Critical Thinking Applications

1. Amount to administer: 1 tablet

2. Amount to administer: 2 tablets

3. Amount to administer: 1 tablet

4. #1 6 tablets

   #2 40 tablets

   #3 120 tablets

Case Study

1. Amount to administer: 1 of the 5 mg tablets and 1 of the 2 mg tablets.

2. The patient should take 2 tablets 3 times a day orally for 7 days. This would be total of 42 tablets. The patient will need 21 of the 2 mg tablets and 21 of the 5 mg tablets.

3. The order now calls for 15 mg, rather than 7 so the patient would need one 5 mg and one 10 mg tablet per dose. Each dose is given three times a day for seven days for a total of 21 of each of the 5 mg and 10 mg tablets.

Internet Activity

Answers will vary. Some examples of medications with different dosage strengths are:

Avandia®	Valium®	Metformin	Nitroglycerin
Augmentin®	Aerobid®	Biaxin®	Levothroid®
Amoxil®	Dilaudid®	Univasc®	Coumadin®

CHAPTER 13 ANSWERS

Review and Practice

13.1 Solid Oral Medications

1. 2 tablets

   Proportion Method:

   Step A: Convert. Since the medication is ordered in mg, and the dosage unit is mg, no conversion is necessary.

   Step B: Calculate. The desired dose (D) is 400 mg. The dosage unit (Q) is 1 tablet. The dose on hand H is 200 mg.

   1. *Fill in the proportion.*   *Fill in the ratio.*

   $$\frac{H}{Q} = \frac{D}{A}$$ $$H:Q = D:A$$

   $$\frac{200 \ mg}{1 \ tab} = \frac{400 \ mg}{A}$$ $200 \ mg: 1 \ tab = 400 \ mg/: A$

   2. *Cancel the units*

   $$\frac{200 \ \cancel{mg}}{1 \ tab} = \frac{400 \ \cancel{mg}}{A}$$ $200 \ \cancel{mg}: 1 \ tab = 400 \ \cancel{mg}/: A$

   3. *Cross-multiply and solve*   *Multiply the means and the extremes*
      for the unknown.   *and solve for the unknown.*

   $$200 \ A = \frac{400}{1 \ tab}$$ $400 \ tab = 200 \ A \ \cancel{tab}$

   $$A = \frac{400}{200} \ tab$$ $\frac{400}{200} \ tab = A \ \cancel{tab}$

   $$A = 2 \ tab$$ $2 \ tab = A \ \cancel{tab}$

   Step C: Think! . . . Is It Reasonable? Since the amount ordered is twice as much as the dose on hand, it is reasonable that the amount to administer is twice as much as the dosage unit.

   Dimensional Analysis:

   Step A: Convert. Since the medication is ordered in mg, and the dosage unit is mg, no conversion is necessary.

   $$A = \frac{Q}{H} \times \frac{D}{1}$$

   $$A = \frac{1 \ tab}{200 \ \cancel{mg}} \times \frac{400 \ \cancel{mg}}{1}$$

   $$A = \frac{400 \ tab}{200}$$

   $$A = 2 \ tab$$

   Step C: Think! . . . Is It Reasonable? Since the amount ordered is twice as much as the dose on hand, it is reasonable that the amount to administer is twice as much as the dosage unit.

   Formula Method:

   Step A: Convert. Since the medication is ordered in mg, and the dosage unit is mg, no conversion is necessary.

   Step B: Calculate.

   $$\frac{D}{H} \times Q = A$$

   $$\frac{400 \ mg}{200 \ mg} \times 1 \ tab = A$$

   $$2 \ tab = A$$

Step C: Think! . . . Is It Reasonable? Since the amount ordered is twice as much as the dose on hand, it is reasonable that the amount to administer is twice as much as the dosage unit.

2. 3 tablets   8. $1\frac{1}{2}$ tablets   14. 2 tablets   19. 2 tablets

3. $1\frac{1}{2}$ tablets   9. $1\frac{1}{2}$ tablets   15. use 2 tablets, 0.5 mg dosage strength   20. $\frac{1}{2}$ tablet

4. $1\frac{1}{2}$ tablets   10. 2 tablets   21. b

5. $1\frac{1}{2}$ tablets   11. $\frac{1}{4}$ tablet   16. 2 tablets   22. d

6. 2 tablets   12. 1 tablet   17. 3 tablets   23. a

7. $2\frac{1}{2}$ tablets   13. 2 tablets   18. $\frac{1}{2}$ tablet   24. c

25. **Splitting** pills is done when it is necessary to divide a tablet or caplet to give a smaller dose as ordered. Pills may be split only if they are scored as scored tablets have the medication distributed evenly throughout. **Crushing** pills is done when it is necessary for patients that have difficulty swallowing medication. With appropriate authorization, a crushed pill can be mixed with soft food or liquid. Pills can also be crushed and dissolved to administer via a nasogastric tube. It is important to note that some medications cannot be crushed and, therefore, a drug reference or pharmacist should be consulted prior to crushing any medication.

Critical Thinking on the Job

Reconstituting Powders

The healthcare professional correctly determined that 150 mL of medication was needed for 5 days, and therefore, should have selected the Amoxicillin in Figure 13–13. Mixing a medication requires that the individual read the reconstitution instructions on the medication label or package insert (see Rule 13–5). When checking the label on Figure 13–13, the healthcare professional should have realized that 90 mL , not 150 mL of diluent (water), was required. Furthermore, only $\frac{1}{2}$ of the water, or 45 mL, should have been added at first to wet the powder, followed by the remaining 45 mL. One cannot assume that the amount needed for administration is equal to the amount needed for reconstitution. Powder most often will expand the volume once the liquid is added, therefore, it is imperative that the manufacturer's instructions are followed. In this example, the patient's medication was over diluted, decreasing the dosage strength. In addition, when the medication overflowed, the exact dosage would be incalculable and, therefore, the medication would need to be discarded.

Review and Practice

13.2 Liquid Oral Medications

1. 4 mL

     Proportion Method:

     Step A: Convert. Since the medication is ordered in mg, and the dosage unit is mg, no conversion is necessary.

     Step B: Calculate. The desired dose (D) is 400 mg. The dosage unit (Q) is 5 mL. The dose on hand H is 500 mg.

     1. Fill in the proportion.   *Fill in the ratio.*

$$\frac{H}{Q} = \frac{D}{A} \qquad\qquad\qquad H{:}Q = D{:}A$$

     2. Cancel the units

$$\frac{500 \ \cancel{mg}}{5 \ mL} = \frac{400 \ \cancel{mg}}{A} \qquad\qquad 500 \ \cancel{mg} : 5 \ mL = 400 \ \cancel{mg}{:} \ A$$

     3. Cross-multiply and solve   *Multiply the means and the extremes*
        for the unknown.   *and solve for the unknown.*

$$500 \ A = 400 \times 5 \ mL \qquad\qquad 5 \ mL \times 400 = 500 \ A$$

$$A = \frac{2000 \ mL}{500} \qquad\qquad\qquad \frac{2000 \ mL}{500} = A$$

$$A = 4 \ mL \qquad\qquad\qquad\qquad 4 \ mL = A$$

Step C: Think! . . . Is It Reasonable? Since the concentration of mg/5 mL equals 100 mg/mL, and 100 mg 3 4 5 400 mg, it is reasonable that 4 mL equals 400 mg.

Dimensional Analysis:

Step A: Convert. Since the medication is ordered in mg, and the dosage unit is mg, no conversion is necessary.

Step B: Calculate. The desired dose (D) is 400 mg. The dosage unit (Q) is 5 mL. The dose on hand H is 500 mg.

$$A = \frac{5 \ mL}{500 \ \cancel{mg}} \times \frac{400 \ \cancel{mg}}{1}$$

$$A = \frac{2000 \ mL}{500}$$

$$A = 4 \ mL$$

Step C: Think! . . . Is It Reasonable? Since the concentration of 500 mg/5 mL equals 100 mg/mL, and 100 mg 3 4 5 400 mg, it is reasonable that 4 mL equals 400 mg.

Formula Method:

Step A: Convert. Since the medication is ordered in mg, and the dosage unit is mg, no conversion is necessary.

Step B: Calculate. The desired dose (D) is 400 mg. The dosage unit (Q) is 5 mL. The dose on hand H is 500 mg.

$$\frac{400 \ \cancel{mg}}{500 \ \cancel{mg}} \times 5 \ mL = A$$

$$\frac{2000 \ mL}{5} = A$$

$$4 \ mL = A$$

Step C: Think! . . . Is It Reasonable? Since the concentration of 500 mg/5 mL equals 100 mg/mL, and 100 mg 3 4 5 400 mg, it is reasonable that 4 mL equals 400 mg.

2. 7.5 mL
3. 5 mL
4. 0.75 mL
5. 10 mL

6. 30 mL
7. 6.3 mL
8. 5.4 mL
9. 12.5 mL

10. 2.5 mL
11. 5 mL
12. 2.5 mL
13. 6.3 mL

14. 20 mL or 4 tsp
15. 10 mL or 2 tsp
16. 12.5 mL or $2\frac{1}{2}$ tsp
17. 20 mL or 4 tsp

18. 10 mL or 2 tsp
19. 1.3 mL
20. 15 mL or 3 tsp

Chapter 13 Review

Check Up

1. $\frac{1}{2}$ tablet; 16 mg/day
2. 2 tablets; 2.5 mg/day
3. $\frac{3}{4}$ tablet; 1350 mg/day
4. 6 mL; 600 mg/day
5. 7.5 mL; 3 mg/day
6. 2 tablets; 10 mg/day
7. 2.5 mL; 125 mg/day
8. $1\frac{1}{2}$ tablets; 270 mg/day
9. 10 mL; 1000 mg (1 g)/day
10. $1\frac{1}{2}$ tablets; 450 mcg (0.45 mg)/day
11. 2 tablets; 2250 mcg (2.25 mg)/day
12. $\frac{1}{2}$ tablet; 1000 mg (1 g)/day
13. 3 tablets; 1500 mg (1.5 g)/day
14. 3.3 mL; 1200 mg (1.2 g)/day
15. 1 tablet; 175 mcg (0.175 mg)/day

16. $\frac{1}{2}$ tablet; 500 mg (0.5 g)/day
17. 1 teaspoon or 5 mL; 375 mg/day
18. Two 2-mg tablets and one 1-mg tablet
19. 2000 mg or 2 g
20. Add 140 mL in 2 portions. Amount to administer: 3 teaspoons or 15 mL
21. Use: H Administer: 7.5 mL
22. Use: E, Administer: $\frac{1}{2}$ tablet
23. Use: G, Administer: 2 tablets
24. Use: F, Administer: 4 mL
25. Use: O, Administer: 2 capsules
26. Use: J, Administer: 2 tablets
27. Use: M, Administer: 3 tablets
28. Use: L, Administer: 12.5 mL
29. Use: K, Administer 1 tablet

Critical Thinking Applications

1. a. Depakote® ER: 1 tablet, b. Valium®: 2 tablets, c. Vistaril®: 10 mL, d. cephalexin: 1 capsule

2. Depakote® ER

3. Valium® would be crushed and dissolved in water. The cephalexin capsules would be opened and the powder dissolved in water. These two medications would then be administered through the tube. The vistaril could be administered directly into the tube since it is in liquid form.

4. Consult either the pharmacist or a drug reference. Depakote® is now available in multiple forms. Consult the physician about how to handle the Depakote® order.

Case Study

1. First add one-half of 55 mL of water to the powdered drug, and shake. Then add the other half of the water, and shake again.

2. 7.5 mL

3. An oral syringe, calibrated spoon, or medicine cup marked in tenths of a milliliter

4. 187.5 mg/dose × 4 doses (qid) = 750 mg/day

Internet Activity

Pages on the Internet may change. Try these sites:

http://www.northeastessexpct.nhs.uk/guidelines/May%202009%20NEEMMC%20GUIDELINES%20FOR%20TABLET%20CRUSHING1.pdf

http://www.mndgp.org.au/programs/documents_links/Aged%20Care/to%20crush%20or%20not%20to%20crush.pdf

CHAPTER 14 ANSWERS

Critical Thinking on the Job

Confirming the Physician's Order

The healthcare professional realizes that the physician has ordered a quantity of solution rather than a quantity of drug. She checks with the physician, who clarifies that the intended dose is 50 mg. If the healthcare professional administers the injection without thinking, the patient receives 100 mg, twice the intended dose. The healthcare professional calculates that 1 mL of 50 mg/mL solution contains the 50-mg dose. She discards 1 mL of the original dose and administers the remaining 1 mL.

Review and Practice

14.1 Calculating Parenteral Dosages in Solution

1. Administer: 1 mL Syringe: standard 3-mL syringe

2. Administer: 0.7 mL Syringe: 1-mL or standard 3-mL tuberculin syringe

3. Administer: 2 mL Syringe: standard 3-mL syringe

4. Administer: 0.4 mL Syringe: 1-mL or 0.5-mL tuberculin syringe

5. Administer: 0.3 mL Syringe: 1-mL or 0.5-mL tuberculin syringe

6. Administer: 0.8 mL Syringe: 1-mL or standard 3-mL tuberculin syringe

7. Administer: 0.88 mL Syringe: 1-mL tuberculin syringe

8. Administer: 0.6 mL Syringe: 1-mL or standard 3-mL tuberculin syringe

9. Administer: 0.6 mL Syringe: 1-mL or standard 3-mL tuberculin syringe

10. Administer: 1 mL Syringe: standard 3 mL syringe

11. Administer: 4 mL Syringe: two standard 3-mL syringes, dose divided evenly between syringes, 2 mL each, given in two injections

12. Administer: 0.35 mL Syringe: 1 mL or 0.5-mL tuberculin syringe

13. Administer: 1.5 mL Syringe: standard 3-mL syringe

14. Administer: 2 mL Syringe: standard 3-mL syringe

15. Administer: 0.63 mL Syringe: 1-mL tuberculin syringe

16. Administer: 2 mL Syringe: standard 3-mL syringe

Critical Thinking on the Job

Confusing the Amount of Solution with the Dosage Unit

The actual solution strength is 5 mg/1 mL, not 5 mg/5 mL. When 5 mL is administered, the patient receives 25 mg of Compazine®, 5 times the desired dose. This error would have been avoided if the healthcare professional had read the label three times. The healthcare professional must take extra care not to confuse the total volume in the vial (5 mL) with the dosage unit (1 mL), as indicated by the dosage strength (5 mg/mL).

Review and Practice

14.2 Calculate Medication Doses Expressed in Percent or Ratio Format

1. Administer 3.8 mL in 2 syringes.

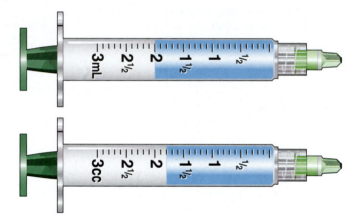

Proportion Method:

Step A: Convert. Convert the supply dose of a 20% solution to 20 g (H) per 100 mL (Q).

Convert the dosage ordered, 750 mg, to the same unit of measure as the dose on hand, grams. $\dfrac{1\ g}{1000\ mg} = \dfrac{D}{750\ mg}$

$\dfrac{750\ g}{1000} = D$

$0.75\ g = D$

Step B: Calculate.

$\dfrac{20\ g}{100\ mL} = \dfrac{0.75\ g}{A}$ 　　　　 or 　　　　 $20\ g{:}100\ mL = 0.75\ g{:}A$

$20A = 75\ mL$ 　　　　　　　　　　　　　　 $75\ mL = 20A$

$A = 3.75\ mL$, round to 3.8 mL 　　　　　　 $3.75\ mL = A$, round to 3.8 mL

Step C: Think! . . . Is It Reasonable? 200,000 mg in 100 mL is a 2000mg/mL solution. Since 750 mg is less than half of 2000 mg but more than a quarter of 2000 mg, and 3.8 is less than 5 mL but more than 2.5 mL, the answer is reasonable.

Dimensional Analysis:

Step A: Convert. Convert the supply dose of a 20% solution to 20 g (H) per 100 mL (Q).

Use the conversion factor: $\dfrac{1g}{1000\ mg}$

Step B: Calculate.

$$A\ mL = \frac{1\ \cancel{g}}{1000\ \cancel{mg}} \times \frac{100\ mL}{20\ \cancel{g}} \times \frac{750\ \cancel{mg}}{1}$$

$$A\ mL = \frac{75,000\ mL}{20,000}$$

$$A\ mL = 3.8\ mL$$

Step C: Think! . . . Is It Reasonable? 200,000 mg in 100 mL is a 2000mg/mL solution. Since 750 mg is less than half of 2000 mg but more than a quarter of 2000 mg, and 3.8 is less than 5 mL but more than 2.5 mL, the answer is reasonable.

Formula Method:

Step A: Convert. Convert the supply dose of a 20% solution to 20 g (H) per 100 mL (Q).

Convert the dosage ordered to grams

$$\frac{1\ g}{1000\ \cancel{mg}} = \frac{D}{750\ \cancel{mg}}$$

$$750\ g = 1000\ D$$

$$0.75\ g = D$$

Step B: Calculate.

$$\frac{0.75\ \cancel{g}}{20\ \cancel{g}} \times 100\ mL = A$$

$$0.0375 \times 100\ mL = A$$

$$3.75\ mL = A.\ round\ to\ 3.8\ mL$$

Step C: Think! . . . Is It Reasonable? 200,000 mg in 100 mL is a 2000mg/mL solution. Since 750 mg is less than half of 2000 mg but more than a quarter of 2000 mg, and 3.75 is less than 5 mL but more than 2.5 mL, the answer is reasonable.

2. Administer 2 mL.

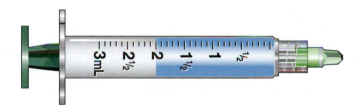

3. Administer 0.3 mL.

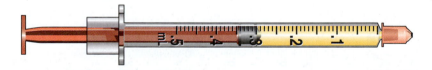

Proportion Method:

Step A: Convert. Convert ratio to grams per milliliter.

$$\frac{1\ g}{1000\ mL}$$

Convert supply dose and dose ordered to like units of measurement. Remember 1 g = 1000 mg, so $\frac{1\ g}{1000\ mL}$ can be converted to $\frac{1000\ mg}{1000\ mL}$ (which reduces to $\frac{1\ mg}{1\ mL}$).

Step B: Calculate.

$$\frac{1\ \cancel{mg}}{1\ mL} = \frac{0.3\ \cancel{mg}}{A} \qquad or \qquad 1\cancel{mg}: 1mL = 0.3\ \cancel{mg}: A$$

$$A = 0.3\ mL \qquad\qquad\qquad 0.3\ mL = A$$

Step C: Think! . . . Is It Reasonable? Since the supply dose of 1: 1000 (1g: 1000 mL) is a one-to-one ratio of mg to mL, it is reasonable that 0.3 mg would be in 0.3 mL.

Following rule 14-1, a 0.5 mL tuberculin syringe should be used.

Dimensional Analysis:

Step A: Convert. Convert ratio to grams per milliliter.

$$\frac{1\ g}{1000\ mL}$$

Convert supply dose and dosage ordered to like units of measurement, using the conversion factor $\frac{1\ g}{1000\ mg}$.

Step B: Calculate.

$$A\ mL = \frac{1\ \cancel{g}}{1000\ \cancel{mg}} \times \frac{1000\ mL}{1\ \cancel{g}} \times \frac{0.3\ \cancel{mg}}{1}$$

$$A = 0.3\ mL$$

Step C: Think! . . . Is It Reasonable? Since the supply dose of 1: 1000 (1g: 1000 mL) is a one-to-one ratio of mg to mL, it is reasonable that 0.3 mg would be in 0.3 mL.

Following rule 14-1, a 0.5 mL tuberculin syringe should be used.

Formula Method:

Step A: Convert. Convert ratio to grams per milliliter.

$$\frac{1\ g}{1000\ mL}$$

Convert supply dose and dose ordered to likes units of measurement. Remember 1 g = 1000 mg, so $\frac{1\ g}{1000\ mL}$ *can be converted to* $\frac{1000\ mg}{1000\ mL}$ *(which reduces to* $\frac{1\ mg}{1\ mL}$*).*

$$\frac{1\ g}{1000\ mL}$$

Step B: Calculate.

$$\frac{0.3\ \cancel{mg}}{1000\ \cancel{mg}} \times 1000\ mL = A$$

$$0.3\ mL = A$$

Step C: Think! . . . Is It Reasonable? Since the supply dose of 1: 1000 (1g: 1000 mL) is a one-to-one ratio of mg to mL, it is reasonable that 0.3 mg would be in 0.3 mL.

Following rule 14-1, a 0.5 mL tuberculin syringe should be used.

4. Administer 0.5 mL.

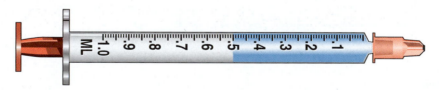

5. Administer 0.8 mL.

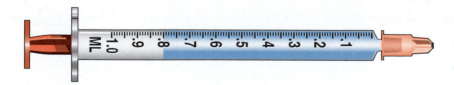

6. Administer 1 mL.

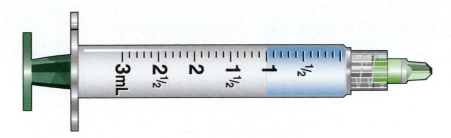

7. Administer 1.6 mL.

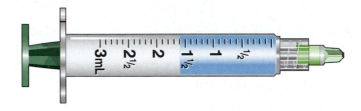

8. Administer 0.5 mL.

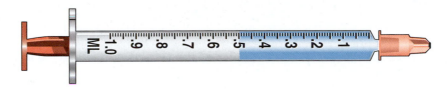

9. Administer 0.5 mL.

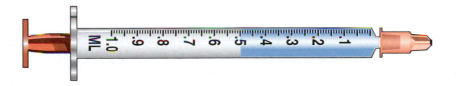

Critical Thinking on the Job

Recording Accurate Information

While the healthcare professional has followed instructions carefully, she has mislabeled the vial. She used 5 mL of sterile diluent, not 1 mL. Her label should indicate 5 mg/5 mL so that her calculation should be:

$$\frac{2 \text{ mg}}{5 \text{ mL}} \times 5 \text{ mL} = A$$

$$2 \text{ mL} = A$$

She would administer this amount using a 3 mL syringe. Because of her labeling error, the patient received only $\frac{1}{5}$ of the amount of medication ordered.

Review and Practice

14.3 Reconstituting Parenteral Medications

1. 17.5 mL of sterile diluent

2. 20 mg/1 mL

3. Sterile water or bacteriostatic water for injection

4. 0.75 mL

   Ordered: 15 mg IM; find the amount to administer using a supply dose of 20 mg/1 mL.

   Proportion Method

   Step A: Convert. No conversion needed

   Step B: Calculate.

   $$\frac{15 \text{ mg}}{A} = \frac{20 \text{ mg}}{1 \text{ mL}} \qquad \text{or} \qquad 15 \text{ mg}:A = 20 \text{ mg}:1 \text{ mL}$$

   $$15 \text{ mL} = 20\,A \qquad\qquad\qquad 20\,A = 15 \text{ mL}$$

   $$0.75 \text{ mL} = A \qquad\qquad\qquad A = 0.75 \text{ mL}$$

   Step C: Think! . . . Is It Reasonable? Since the dose ordered is $\frac{3}{4}$ of the dose on hand it is reasonable that the amount to administer is $\frac{3}{4}$ of the dosage unit or 0.75 mL.

   Dimensional Analysis:

   Step A: Convert. No conversion needed

   Step B: Calculate.

   $$A \text{ mL} = \frac{1 \text{ mL}}{20 \text{ mg}} \times \frac{15 \text{ mg}}{1}$$

   $$A = 0.75 \text{ mL}$$

   Step C: Think! . . . Is It Reasonable? Since the dose ordered is $\frac{3}{4}$ of the dose on hand it is reasonable that the amount to administer is $\frac{3}{4}$ of the dosage unit or 0.75 mL.

   Formula Method:

   Step A: Convert. No conversion needed

   Step B: Calculate.

   $$\frac{15 \text{ mg}}{20 \text{ mg}} \times 1 \text{ mL} = A$$

   $$0.75 \text{ mL} = A$$

   Step C: Think! . . . Is It Reasonable? Since the dose ordered is $\frac{3}{4}$ of the dose on hand it is reasonable that the amount to administer is $\frac{3}{4}$ of the dosage unit or 0.75 mL.

5. Sterile water for injection

6. 1 mL

7. 100 mg/mL

8. Exp. 1/3/13, 1600 plus initials; usually dose is given immediately—only stable 6 h

9. 0.75 mL

10. 0.9% sodium chloride injection

11. 5 mL

12. 38 mg/mL

13. 2400 on 6/6/2012

14. At a controlled room temperature. Do not refrigerate.

15. 2.6 mL

16. 8.2 mL

17. 750,000 units/mL

18. Exp.11/27/13, 1200

19. 2 mL

20. 1% lidocaine hydrochloride or sterile water injection

21. 2.1 mL

22. 350 mg/mL

23. Discard at 1600 on October 7, 2013

24. 2.1 mL

Review and Practice

14.4 Other Medication Forms and Equipment

1. F
2. A
3. E
4. B
5. G

6. B
7. C
8. D
9. A, F, B, G
10. C

11. 5 mL

   Proportion Method:

   Step A: Convert. Convert the supply dose of a 20% solution to 20 g (H) per 100 mL (Q).

   The dosage ordered is in the same unit of measure as the dose on hand, grams, so no conversion is needed.

   Step B: Calculate.

   $$\frac{20\,g}{100\ mL} = \frac{1\,g}{A} \qquad \text{or} \qquad 20\,g : 100\ mL = 1\,g : A$$

   $$20\,A = 100\ mL \qquad\qquad 100\ mL = 20\,A$$

   $$A\,5 = mL \qquad\qquad\qquad 5\ mL = A$$

   Step C: Think! . . . Is It Reasonable? Since only 1 g is needed of a 20 g per 100 mL solution, one twentieth of the solution is needed. One twentieth of 100 is 5, so 5 mL is reasonable.

   Dimensional Analysis:

   Step A: Convert. Convert the supply dose of a 20% solution to 20 g (H) per 100 mL (Q).

   The dosage ordered is in the same unit of measure as the dose on hand, grams, so no conversion factor is needed.

   Step B: Calculate.

   $$A\ mL = \frac{100\ mL}{20\,g} \times \frac{1\,g}{1}$$

   $$A\ mL = \frac{100\ mL}{20}$$

   $$A\ mL = 5\ mL$$

   Step C: Think! . . . Is It Reasonable? Since only 1 g is needed of a 20 g per 100 mL solution, one twentieth of the solution is needed. One twentieth of 100 is 5, so 5 mL is reasonable.

   Formula Method:

   Step A: Convert. Convert the supply dose of a 20% solution to 20 g (H) per 100 mL (Q).

   The dosage ordered is in the same unit of measure as the dose on hand, grams, so no conversion is needed.

   Step B: Calculate.

   $$\frac{1\,g}{20\,g} \times 100\ mL = A$$

   $$5\ mL = A$$

   Step C: Think! . . . Is It Reasonable? Since only 1 g is needed of a 20 g per 100 mL solution, one twentieth of the solution is needed. One twentieth of 100 is 5, so 5 mL is reasonable.

12. 0.5 mL
13. 1.25 mL
14. 2 suppositories
15. One 10 mg and one 5 mg suppository
16. $\frac{1}{2}$ suppository. Check manufacturer's directions to verify that suppository can be divided before administration.

17. 2 patches
18. One TTS-3 patch and one TTS-2 patch
19. One 0.1 mg/day patch with one 0.05 mg/day patch, or two 0.75 mg/day patches
20. One 0.2 mg/h patch with one 0.1 mg/h patch

Chapter 14 Review

Check Up

1. Administer 2 mL.

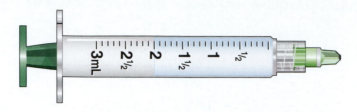

2. Administer 1.2 mL.

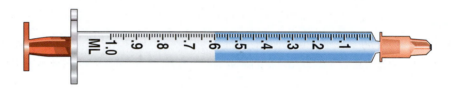

3. Administer 0.6 mL.

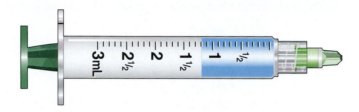

4. Administer 0.7 mL.

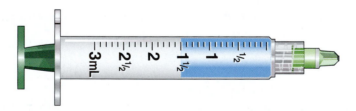

5. Administer 1.5 mL.

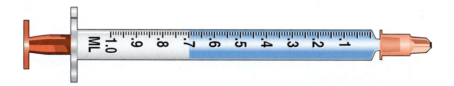

6. Administer 2.5 mL.

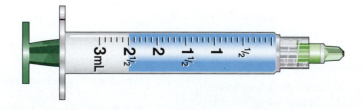

7. Administer 0.8 mL.

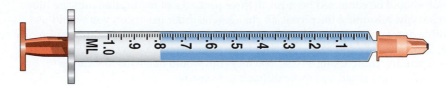

8. Administer 0.75 mL.

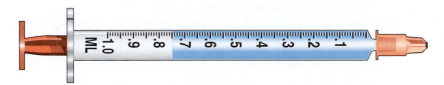

9. Administer 0.75 mL.

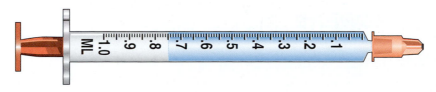

10. Administer 0.1 mL.

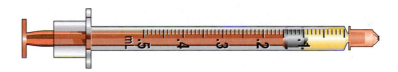

11. Administer: 0.4 mL Syringe: 1-mL or 0.5-mL tuberculin syringe

12. Administer: 0.24 mL Syringe: 1-mL or 0.5-mL tuberculin syringe

13. Administer: 0.38 mL Syringe: 1-mL or 0.5-mL tuberculin syringe

14. Administer: 0.3 mL Syringe: 1-mL or 0.5-mL tuberculin syringe

15. Administer: 2 mL Syringe: standard 3-mL syringe

16. Administer: 0.4 mL Syringe: 1-mL or 0.5-mL tuberculin syringe

17. Administer: 1.5 mL Syringe: standard 3-mL syringe

18. Administer: 2 mL Syringe: standard 3-mL syringe

19. Administer: 0.63 mL Syringe: 1-mL syringe

20. Administer: 2 mL Syringe: standard 3-mL syringe

21. Administer: 0.5 mL Syringe: 1-mL tuberculin syringe

22. One vial of label H (40 mg/4 mL) or two vials of label I (20 mg/2 mL). For either medication you would administer 4 mL of medication.

23. Sterile water

24. 2.1 mL

25. 1 mL

26. 1 hour

27. 8 mL

28. 0.25 mL

29. Two 25-mg suppositories

30. 2 suppositories

31. 2 patches

32. One 0.2 mg/h patch with one 0.1 mg/h patch

Critical Thinking Applications

1. Using the diluent that is provided with the vial—sterile water

2. Supplied 1.25 mL, used 0.7 mL

3. Discard

4. Subcutaneously

5. Stored at a temperature of 2 to 8°C (36 to 46°F) for up to 24 h

Case Study

First of all, the physician should be contacted because all three packages of medication indicate they are for subcutaneous use only. Assuming the physician changes the order to subcut, you would use the package 14-15a with a dosage strength of 100 mcg/mL and administer 0.75 mL in a tuberculin syringe. Using 14-15b, 50 mcg/mL would cause the amount to administer to be over 1 mL, which is not acceptable for a subcut injection. Using 14-15c, 500 mcg/mL would make the amount to administer only 0.15, which is very small and more difficult to measure.

Internet Activity

Answer found at manufacturer's web site GlaxoKlineSmith at *www.gks.com.*
Intramuscular use (concentration of approximately 385 mg/mL): For initial reconstitution use sterile water for injection, USP, sodium chloride injection, USP, or 1% lidocaine hydrochloride solution (without epinephrine).
Each gram of ticarcillin should be reconstituted with 2 mL of sterile water for injection, USP, sodium chloride injection, USP, or 1% lidocaine hydrochloride solution (without epinephrine) and used promptly. Each 2.6 mL of the resulting solution will then contain 1 g of ticarcillin. Amount to administer: 0.5 mL.

CHAPTER 15 ANSWERS

Review and Practice

15.1 IV Solutions

1. 100 g

   1000 mL D10W _____ *g Dextrose*

   D10W = 10% dextrose in water; 10% = 10 g/100 mL

   $$\frac{10\ g}{100\ mL} = \frac{x}{1000\ mL}$$

   $$100x = 10{,}000\ g$$

   $$x = 100\ g\ Dextrose$$

2. 25 g dextrose; 2.25 g sodium chloride

   500 mL D5 $\frac{1}{2}$ NS _____ *g Dextrose* _____ *g NaCl*

   D5 $\frac{1}{2}$ NS = 5% dextrose in 0.45% sodium chloride (NaCl); 5% = 5 g/100 mL; 0.45% = 0.45 g/100 mL

   $$\frac{5\ g}{100\ mL} = \frac{x}{500\ mL} \qquad\qquad \frac{0.45\ g}{100\ mL} = \frac{x}{500\ mL}$$

   $$100x = 2{,}500\ g \qquad\qquad\qquad 100x = 225\ g$$

   $$x = 25\ g\ Dextrose \qquad\qquad\quad x = 2.25\ g\ NaCl$$

3. 12.5 g dextrose; 2.25 g sodium chloride

4. 50 g

5. 25 g dextrose; 1.125 g sodium chloride

Critical Thinking on the Job

Checking Compatibility

The healthcare professional suspects that the additive is not compatible with the IV solution. She stops the administration, then uses a compatibility chart to verify her suspicions. After that, she calls the physician to obtain a new order. In this case, the healthcare professional was fortunate that a change in the fluid's appearance alerted her to the problem. However, in many cases, failing to verify compatibility **before** introducing an additive can have severe consequences for the patient, including death.

Review and Practice

15.2 IV Equipment

1. Injection port
2. Roller or screw clamp
3. Slide clamp
4. Infusion pump
5. Microdrip tubing
6. PCA pump
7. Syringe pump
8. Burette
9. If a patient needed a large amount of fluids, a rapid infusion of medication, an infusion of highly concentrated solutions, or long-term IV therapy

10. Flow rate, whether an ordered medication has been infused properly, times at which an IV bag needs to be changed, and signs of infiltration or phlebitis
11. Swelling, coolness, or discomfort at the IV site
12. Irritation of the vein by additives, movement of the needle or catheter, and long-term IV therapy
13. 36 inches above the heart
14. Rate controller, infusion pump, syringe pump, patient-controlled analgesia device
15. To add medications or additives to an IV

Critical Thinking on the Job

Adjusting the Flow Rate

Pat's error could have serious consequences for the patient by providing far too much solution in a limited time period. The new flow rate of 28 gtt/min is a 75 percent increase over the original flow rate of 16 gtt/min. Instead of making up the entire schedule in 1 h, Pat should have adjusted the remainder of the entire schedule. The IV bag still had 450 mL of fluid with 4 h of infusion time remaining. The calculation should be:

$$10 \text{ gtt/mL} \times 450 \text{ mL/4 h} \times 1 \text{ h/60 min} = 18.75 \text{ gtt/min} = 19 \text{ gtt/min}$$

Review and Practice

15.3 Calculating Flow Rates

1. 167 mL/h

    Formula Method:

    $$F = V/T$$

    $$F = \frac{1000 \text{ mL}}{6 \text{ h}} = 167 \text{ mL/h}$$

2. 150 mL/h

3. 125 mL/h

4. 133 mL/h

    To use Formula Method, first convert 45 min to 0.75 h, by using the Proportion Method:

    $$1 \text{ h/60 min} = x/45 \text{ min}$$

    $$60 x = 45 \text{ h}$$

    $$x = 0.75 \text{ h}$$

    Formula Method:

    $$F = \frac{V}{T}$$

    $$F = \frac{100 \text{ mL}}{0.75 \text{ h}}$$

    $$F = 133 \text{ mL/h}$$

    Dimensional Analysis:

    $$F \text{ mL/h} = \frac{100 \text{ mL}}{45 \text{ min}} \times \frac{60 \text{ min}}{1 \text{ h}}$$

    $$F \text{ mL/h} = 100 \times \frac{60}{45}$$

    $$F \text{ mL/h} = \frac{6000}{45} = 133$$

Copyright © 2012 by The McGraw-Hill Companies, Inc.

5. 125 mL/h

6. 83 mL/h

7. 94 mL/h

8. 100 mL/h

9. 75 mL/h

10. 83 mL/h

11. 14 gtt/min

Formula Method:

$$F = \frac{V}{T}$$

$$F = \frac{1000\ mL}{24\ h} = 42\ mL/h$$

$$f = \frac{F \times C}{60}$$

$$f = \frac{42\ mL/h \times 20\ gtt/mL}{60\ min}$$

$$f = \frac{840}{60} = 14\ gtt/min$$

Dimensional Analysis:

$$f\ gtt/min = \frac{1000\ mL}{24\ h} \times \frac{1\ h}{60\ min} \times \frac{20\ gtt}{mL}$$

$$f\ gtt/min = \frac{20{,}000}{1440}$$

$$f\ gtt/min = 14\ gtt/min$$

12. 8 gtt/min

13. 31 gtt/min

14. 14 gtt/min

15. 50 gtt/min

16. 16 gtt/min

17. 21 gtt/min

18. 50 gtt/min

19. 50 gtt/min

20. 50 gtt/min

21. 28 gtt/min

22. 23 gtt/min

23. Original flow rate: 21 gtt/min; Adjusted flow rate: 17 gtt/min

Original Flow Rate Using Formula Method:

$$F = \frac{V}{T}$$

$$F = \frac{375\ mL}{3\ h} = 125\ mL/h$$

$$f = \frac{F \times C}{60\ min/h}$$

$$f = \frac{125\ mL/h \times 10\ gtt/mL}{60\ min/h}$$

$$f = \frac{1250}{60} = 21\ gtt/min$$

Original Flow Rate Using Dimensional Analysis:

$$f\ gtt/min = \frac{375\ mL}{3\ h} \times \frac{1\ h}{60\ min} \times \frac{10\ gtt}{mL}$$

$$f\ gtt/min = \frac{3750}{180}$$

$$f\ gtt/min = 21\ gtt/min$$

To calculated the adjusted IV rate, determine the volume remaining and the time remaining:

$$375\ mL - 175\ mL = 200\ mL$$

$$3\ h - 1\ h = 2\ h$$

To use the formula method, convert 2 h to 120 minutes by using the Proportion Method:

$$\frac{1\ h}{60\ min} = \frac{2\ h}{x}$$

$$x = 120\ min$$

Adjusted Flow Rate Using Formula Method:

$$f = \frac{C \times V}{T}$$

$$f = \frac{10\ gtt/mL \times 200\ mL}{120\ min}$$

$$f = \frac{2000}{120} = 17\ gtt/min$$

Adjusted Flow Rate Using Dimensional Analysis:

$$f\ gtt/min = \frac{200\ mL}{2\ h} + \frac{1\ h}{60\ min} \times \frac{10\ gtt}{mL}$$

$$f\ gtt/min = \frac{2000}{120}$$

$$f\ gtt/min = 17\ gtt/min$$

Flow rate must be decreased from 21 gtt/min to 17 gtt/min

24. Original flow rate: 42 gtt/min; Adjusted flow rate: 37 gtt/min

25. Original flow rate: 31 gtt/min; Adjusted flow rate: 38 gtt/min

26. 33 gtt/min

Formula Method:

$$f = \frac{F \times C}{60}$$

$$f = \frac{200 \text{ mL/h} \times 10 \text{ gtt/mL}}{60 \text{ min}}$$

$$f = \frac{2000}{60} = 33 \text{ gtt/min}$$

or

$$f = \frac{C \times V}{T}$$

$$f = \frac{10 \text{ gtt/mL} \times 200 \text{ mL}}{60 \text{ min}}$$

$$f = \frac{2000}{60} = 33 \text{ gtt/min}$$

Dimensional Analysis:

$$f \text{ gtt/min} = \frac{200 \text{ mL}}{h} \times \frac{1 h}{60 \text{ min}} \times \frac{10 \text{ gtt}}{mL}$$

$$f \text{ gtt/min} = \frac{2000}{60}$$

$$f \text{ gtt/min} = 33 \text{ gtt/min}$$

27. 31 gtt/min

28. 38 gtt/min

29. 75 gtt/min

30. 17 gtt/min

Review and Practice

15.4 Infusion Time and Volume

1. 12 h, 3 min

Formula Method:

$$T = \frac{V}{F}$$

$$T = \frac{1000 \text{ mL}}{83 \text{ mL/h}}$$

$$T = 12.05 \text{ h}; \ 0.05 \text{ h} \times 60 \text{ min/h} = 3 \text{ min}$$

$$T = 12 \text{ h } 3 \text{ min}$$

Dimensional Analysis:

$$T \text{ h} = 1000 \text{ mL} \times \frac{1 h}{83 \text{ mL}}$$

$$T \text{ h} = \frac{1000}{83} = 12.05 \text{ h}; \ 0.05 \text{ h} \times 60 \text{ min/h} = 3 \text{ min}$$

$$T = 12 \text{ h } 3 \text{ min}$$

2. 4 h

3. 24 h, 12 min

4. 5 h

5. $2\frac{1}{2}$ h

6. The infusion will be finished at 0800 the next day.

Formula Method:

$$T = \frac{V}{F}$$

$$T = \frac{1500 \text{ mL}}{75 \text{ mL/h}}$$

$$T = 20 \text{ h}$$

12 Noon + 20 h, 00 min = 1200 + 2000 = 3200; 3200 − 2400 = 0800 or 8 a.m. the next day

Dimensional Analysis:

$$T \text{ h} = 1500 \text{ mL} \times \frac{1 h}{75 \text{ mL}}$$

$$T \text{ h} = \frac{1500}{75} = 20 \text{ h}$$

7. The infusion will finished the next day at 11:30 a.m.

8. The infusion will be finished at 0100 the next day.

9. The infusion will be finished at 4 a.m. the next day.

10. The infusion will be finished at 2255 or 10:55 p.m.

11. 187.5 mL

    Formula Method:

    Convert T to hours: 30 ~~min~~ ÷ 60 ~~min~~/h = 0.5 h

    $V = T \times F$

    $V = 2.5\,\cancel{h} \times 75\ mL/\cancel{h} = 187.5\ mL$

    Dimensional Analysis:

    $V\ mL/h = 2.5\,\cancel{h}/1 \times 75\ mL/\cancel{h} = 187.5\ mL$

12. 800 mL

13. 1500 mL

14. 150 mL

Review and Practice

15.5 Intermittent IV Infusions

1. Neither is appropriate for a heparin flush.

2. A

3. 3 mL

4. 5 mL

    Proportion Method:

    $\dfrac{H}{Q} = \dfrac{D}{A}$

    $\dfrac{1{,}000\ \text{units}}{1\ mL} = \dfrac{5{,}000\ \text{units}}{A}$

    $1{,}000\,A = 5{,}000$

    $A = 5\ mL$

    Dimensional Analysis:

    $x = \dfrac{1\ mL}{1{,}000\ \text{units}} \times \dfrac{5{,}000\ \text{units}}{1}$

    $x = \dfrac{5{,}000}{1{,}000} = 5\ mL$

    Formula Method:

    $\dfrac{D}{H} \times Q = A$

    $\dfrac{5{,}000\ \text{units}}{1{,}000\ \text{units}} \times 1\ mL = A$

    $\dfrac{5{,}000}{1{,}000} = A$

    $5\ mL = A$

5. 3.9 mL added to 500 mL NS

    (NOTE: Gemzar is reconstituted to 38 mg/mL, per Label D.)

    Proportion Method:

    $\dfrac{H}{Q} = \dfrac{D}{A}$

    $\dfrac{38\ mg}{1\ mL} = \dfrac{150\ mg}{A}$

    $38\,A = 150$

    $A = 3.9$

    $x = 3.9\ mL$ to be added to the 500 mL NS

    Dimensional Analysis:

    $x = \dfrac{1\ mL}{38\ mg} \times \dfrac{150\ mg}{1} = 3.9\ mL$

    Formula Method:

    $\dfrac{D}{H} \times Q = A$

    $\dfrac{150\ mg}{38\ mg} \times 1\ mL = 3.9\ mL$

    NOTE: For accuracy, remove 3.9 mL of NS before adding 3.9 mL of medication.

6. 250 mL/h

    Flow rate (F) in mL per hour:

    $F = \dfrac{V}{T}$

    $F = \dfrac{500\ mL}{2\ h}$

    $F = 250\ mL/h$

7. 63 gtt/min

    Flow rate (f) in gtt/min:

    (NOTE: Tubing calibration is 15 gtt/mL per Label C).

    $f\ gtt/min = \dfrac{250\ \cancel{mL}}{\cancel{h}} \times \dfrac{1\,\cancel{h}}{60\ min} \times \dfrac{15\ gtt}{\cancel{mL}} = 63\ gtt/min$

8. 7.5 mL

9. 107.5 rounded to 108 mL/h (or 100 mL/h if 7.5 mL of IV solution is withdrawn prior to adding 7.5 mL of medication)

10. 17 gtt/min

Chapter 15 Review

Check Up

1. g

2. d

3. a

4. e

5. c

6. f

7. b

8. Flow rate = 125 mL/h

9. Flow rate = 63 mL/h

10. Flow rate = 100 mL/h

11. Flow rate = 63 mL/h

12. Flow rate = 67 mL/h

13. Flow rate = 100 mL/h

14. 23 gtt/min

15. 6 gtt/min

16. 42 gtt/min

17. 50 gtt/min

18. 31 gtt/min

19. 50 gtt/min

20. Original flow rate: 31 gtt/min; Adjusted flow rate: 36 gtt/min

21. Original flow rate: 17 gtt/min; Adjusted flow rate: 18 gtt/min

22. Original flow rate: 63 gtt/min; Adjusted flow rate: 75 gtt/min

23. 8 h

24. 16 h

25. 24 h

26. 17 h, 8 min or 17 h, 9 min

27. The infusion will be finished at 1713.

28. The infusion will be finished at 9 PM.

29. The infusion will be finished the next day at 0121 or 0122.

30. The infusion will be finished the next day at 1:25 to 1:26 PM

31. 688 mL

32. 300 mL

33. 938 mL

34. 667 mL

Critical Thinking Applications

1. You use 2 mL of medication from one vial (300 mg) and 1.3 mL (200 mg) from a second vial of clindamycin for a total of 3.3 mL. Add this to 100 mL of diluent.

2. $x = 3.3$ mL

3. No. For pneumonia, the package insert suggests the patient should receive 2400 to 2700 mg per day. The order is for 500 mg three times a day (1500 mg), which is less than the lowest recommended dose.

4. Any product that contains benzyl alcohol.

5. According to the package insert, the medication can be used for up to 24 h with no refrigeration. You should label the IV bag with the date and time of expiration, the solution strength, and your initials.

6. To run a 500 mg dose, you would select the 100 mL diluent to run over 20 minutes.

$$\frac{100 \text{ mL}}{20 \text{ min}} \times \frac{60 \text{ min}}{h} = 300 \text{ mL/h}$$

Case Study

The patient received 4.5 mg of morphine sulfate during the shift.

Internet Activity

Internet sites include various IV fluids and equipment. Try the following site as part of your research:

www.tpub.com/content/medical/14274/css/14274_204.htm

UNIT FOUR ASSESSMENT ANSWERS

1. 30
2. d. oral syringe
3. The bottom
4. 10
5. Calibrated spoon
6. A 1-mL or 0.5 mL tuberculin syringe
7. A standard 3-mL syringe
8. A 10-mL or 12-mL syringe
9. A 1-mL, U-100 insulin syringe
10. A 1-mL tuberculin syringe
11. $\frac{1}{2}$ tablet
12. 2 tablets

13. 4 tsp
14. 1.5 oz
15. 12.5 mL
16. a. Dextrose 5%; sodium chloride 0.9%
    b. Dextrose 10%
    c. Dextrose 5%; sodium chloride 0.45%
    d. Dextrose 5%; sodium chloride 0.225%
17. a. iii   b. iv   c. v   d. ii   e. i
18. a. 125   b. 67   c. 25   d. 300   e. 14
19. a. 2300   b. 250 mL   c. 0745   d. 300 mL
20. a. 150   b. 150   c. 100   d. 300

CHAPTER 16 ANSWERS

Review and Practice

16.1 Preparation of Solutions

1.

0.9% Sodium chloride	
NaCl	4.5g
Water	qsad 500 mL

0.9% Sodium chloride	
NaCl	4.5g
Water	qsad 500 mL

Proportion Method:

$$\frac{0.9\ g}{100\ mL} = \frac{x\ g}{500\ mL}$$

$$100\ x = 450$$

$$x = 4.5\ g$$

Dimensional Analysis:

$$x = \frac{0.9\ g}{100\ mL} \times \frac{500\ mL}{1}$$

$$x = 0.9 \times \frac{500}{100} = \frac{450}{100} = 4.5\ g$$

2.

2% Lidocaine	
Lidocaine	1 g
Water	qsad 50 mL

3.

3% Hydrocortisone ointment	
Hydrocortisone	3 g
Petroleum jelly	97 g

4.

0.45% Sodium chloride	
NaCl	1.125 g
Water	qsad 250 mL

5.

20% Zinc oxide ointment	
Zinc oxide	15 g
Petroleum jelly	60 g

Proportion Method:

$$\frac{20\ g}{100\ g} = \frac{x\ g}{75\ g}$$

$$100\ x = 1500$$

$$x = 15\ g$$

Dimensional Analysis:

$$x = \frac{20\ \cancel{g}}{100\ \cancel{g}} \times \frac{75\ g}{1} = \frac{1500}{100} = 15\ g$$

75 g of 20% zinc oxide contains 15 g of zinc oxide and 60 g of petroleum jelly.

Critical Thinking on the Job

Order: Give 90 mL $\frac{1}{2}$ Strength Sustacal® Now

The nurse misinterpreted $\frac{1}{2}$ strength formula as 1 part formula to 2 parts water instead of interpreting the concentration (fraction) as 1 of 2 equal parts. Therefore, the patient received a more dilute solution ($\frac{1}{3}$ strength instead of $\frac{1}{2}$ strength) leading to a decreased caloric intake. Also, a mistaken assessment of patient tolerance of $\frac{1}{2}$ strength formula (which was actually $\frac{1}{3}$ strength formula), may lead to premature advancement to full-strength formula which may result in digestion problems.

$$V = 90;\ C = \tfrac{1}{2};\ St = 45;\ Sv = 45$$

The nurse should have prepared the order with 45 mL of Sustacal® + 45 mL water.

Review and Practice

16.2 Preparing a Dilution from a Concentrate

1. $V = 960$ mL; $C = \frac{1}{2}$; $St = 480$ mL; $Sv = 480$ mL

   Recipe: 480 mL acetic acid + 480 mL NS = 960 mL total solution

   Calculate total volume: $\dfrac{4\ ounces}{\cancel{dose}} \times \dfrac{4\ \cancel{doses}}{\cancel{day}\ (q6h)} \times 2\ \cancel{days} = 32\ ounces$

   Convert 32 ounces to mL: $\dfrac{1\ oz}{30\ mL} = \dfrac{32\ oz}{x}$; $x = 960$ mL

   $C \times V = St$

   $\frac{1}{2} \times 960$ mL $= 480$ mL solute (St)

   $V - St = Sv$

   960 mL $- 480$ mL $= 480$ mL solvent (Sv)

2. $V = 1080$ mL; $C = \frac{1}{3}$; $St = 360$; $Sv = 720$

   Recipe: 360 mL H_2O_2 + 720 mL NS = 1080 mL total solution

3. $V = 1680$ mL; $C = \frac{1}{4}$; $St = 420$; $Sv = 1260$ mL

   Recipe: 420 mL sodium hypochlorite + 1260 mL NS = 1680 mL total solution

4. $V = 1260$ mL; $C = \frac{3}{4}$; $St = 945$ mL; $Sv = 315$ mL

   Recipe: 945 mL H_2O_2 + 315 mL NS = 1260 mL total solution

5. $V = 720$ mL; $St = 480$ mL; $Sv = 240$ mL

   Recipe: 480 mL povidine-iodine solution + 240 mL NS = 720 mL total solution

6. $V = 1620$ mL; $C = \frac{1}{4}$; $St = 405$ mL; 1215 mL

   Recipe: 405 mL Enfamil + 1215 mL water = 1620 mL total nutritional formula

7. $V = 1920$ mL; $C = \frac{3}{4}$; $St = 1440$ mL; $Sv = 480$ mL

   Recipe: 1440 mL Boost + 480 mL water = 1920 mL total nutritional formula

8. $V = 1680$ mL; $C = \frac{1}{3}$; $St = 560$ mL; $Sv = 1120$ mL

   Recipe: 560 mL Ensure + 1120 mL water = 1680 mL total nutritional formula

9. $V = 720$ mL; $C = \frac{2}{3}$; $St = 480$ mL; $Sv = 240$

   Recipe: 480 mL Sustacal + 240 mL water = 720 mL total nutritional formula

10. $V = 1440$ mL; $C = \frac{1}{2}$; $St = 720$; $Sv = 720$

   Recipe: 720 mL Similac + 720 mL water = 1440 mL total nutritional formula

Chapter 16 Review

Check Up

1. c

2. e

3. d

4. a

5. b

6. Dextrose (*St*), water (*Sv*)

7. NaCl (*St*), water (*Sv*)

8. Zinc powder (*St*), petroleum jelly (*Sv*)

9. Lidocaine (*St*), water (*Sv*)

10. Ensure (*St*), water (*Sv*)

11. Dextrose—50 g, Water—qsad 500 mL

12. NaCl—0.45 g, Water—qsad 100 mL

13. Zinc oxide powder—40 g, petroleum jelly—160 g

14. Lidocaine—0.5 g, Water—qsad 50 mL

15. Hydrocortisone powder—2 g, petroleum jelly—98 g

16. 600 mL H_2O_2 (*St*); 600 mL NS (*Sv*)

17. 360 mL Enfamil (*St*); 1080 mL water (*Sv*)

18. 2250 mL Pulmocare (*St*); 750 mL water (*Sv*)

19. 70 mL povidine-iodine (*St*); 140 mL NS (*Sv*)

20. 240 mL Sustacal (*St*); 120 mL water (*Sv*)

Critical Thinking Applications

1. 64 oz = 1920 mL; need 1440 mL formula; 1440 mL divided by 240 mL/can = 6 cans

2. 480 mL water = 2 cups

Case Study

1. Day 1—50 mL/h × 24 h = 1200 mL; 600 mL of Ensure.

   Day 2—75 mL/h × 24 h = 1800 mL; 900 mL of Ensure.

   Day 3—75 mL/h × 24 h = 1800 mL; 900 mL of Ensure.

   Day 4—75 mL/h × 24 h = 1800 mL; 1800 mL of Ensure.

   Day 5—75 mL/h × 24 h = 1800 mL; 1800 mL of Ensure.

   Day 6—100 mL/h × 24 h =2400 mL; 2400 mL of Ensure.

   Day 7—100 mL/h × 24 h =2400 mL; <u>2400 mL</u> of Ensure.

   TOTAL: 10,800 mL of Ensure = 10,800 calories

2. 10,800 calories/week divided by 7 days = 1543 calories per day

3. No

   • 130 lb divided by 2.2 lb/kg = 59.1 kg

   • 40 cal/kg/day × 59.1 kg = 2364 calories

   • The actual average daily caloric intake of 1543 calories did not meet the need of 2364 calories

4. Yes, the patient will receive 2400 mL Ensure per day, or 2400 calories per day, which will provide a bit more than the required 2364 calories per day.

Internet Activity

1. Pulmocare® (for patients with COPD)
2. Jevity® (for patients requiring a high protein, high fiber diet)
3. Glucerna® (for patients with diabetes)
4. Sustacal® (for patient with increased calorie requirements)

CHAPTER 17 ANSWERS

Review and Practice

17.1 Factors that Impact Dosing and Medication Administration

1. e	6. i	11. G
2. a	7. h	12. G
3. d	8. j	13. P
4. c	9. g	14. P
5. b	10. f	15. P, G

Review and Practice

17.2 Dosages Based on Body Weight

1. 30 kg

   66 lb × 1 kg/2.2 lb = 30 kg

2. 35 kg

3. 24.5 kg

4. 16.8 kg

5. 69.1 kg

6. 91.8 kg

10. 6.5 kg

7. 7.4 kg

   First convert 4 oz to 0.25 lb:
   16 oz/1 lb = 4 oz/x
   16 x = 4
   x = 0.25 lb
   Then convert 16.25 lb to kg:
   16.25 lb × 1 kg/2.2 lb = 7.38 or 7.4 kg

8. 5.3 kg

9. 4.5 kg

11. Two doses of 5 mg, or 10 mg/day, are within a safe range. Amount to administer: 0.5 mL

   Step A: *Convert 6 lb 5 oz to 6.3 lb (5/16 oz = 0.3 lb)*
      Convert 6.3 lb to kg: 6.3 lb ÷ 2.2 lb/kg 5 2.9 kg
   Step B: *Calculate the desired dose (safe amount) to administer:*
      4 mg/kg/day × 2.9 kg = 11.6 mg/day
   Step C: *Think! . . . Is It Reasonable? 11.6 mg/day is safe; 10 mg/day (5 mg q12h) is ordered. The order is safe.*

   Calculate the ordered amount to administer:

   Proportion Method: **Dimensional Analysis:**
   H/Q = D/A   *A mL = 2 mL/20 mg × 5 mg/1 = 10/20 = 0.5 mL*
   20 mg/2 mL = 5 mg/A
   20 x = 10
   x = 0.5 mL

12. The order is above the appropriate starting dosage for a patient of this weight. Consult the authorized prescriber.

13. The order of 750 mg per dose is above the safe dose for children with a severe infection. According to the dosage regimen, the child should receive between 290 mg to 580 mg of medication. Consult the authorized prescriber.

14. The ordered dose of 30 mg is within a safe range. Amount to administer: 1.2 mL

15. The ordered dose is safe to administer to this child. Amount to administer: 4 mL

16. The safe range is 300 to 600 mg/day or 75 to 150 mg/dose qid. This order is within the safe range. Amount to administer: $\frac{1}{2}$ tablet

17. Based on the patient's weight of 20 kg, the safe range is 1 to 8 mg. This order is within the safe range. Amount to administer: 1.5 mL

18. The order of 1 mg IM is safe. Administer 1 mL IM to the patient.

19. Dose is safe. Amount to administer: 1.6 mL

20. Dose is unsafe, call the authorized prescriber. 160 mg × 3 doses/day = 480 mg/day. Safe dose range is 246–410 mg/day for an 18 lb (8.2 kg) child.

21. 0.64 mL/dose

22. 5.4 mL/dose

Critical Thinking on the Job

Consulting the Authorized Prescriber

Karen should have immediately contacted the authorized prescriber to discuss the order. As it turns out, the prescriber did not consider the chronic renal failure when prescribing the medication for the pneumonia. A new order is written: Tazidime 500 mg q24h.

If Karen had administered the original amount of Tazidime, Mrs. Bekins would probably have developed an accumulation of the drug, producing symptoms of toxicity such as seizures. By using her critical thinking skills, Karen helped the patient to receive the correct dosage.

Review and Practice

17.3 Dosages Based on Ideal Weight

1. Safe

   According to the package insert, patients with normal renal function may be administered 7.5 mg/kg q12h or 5 mg/kg q8h. This patient has normal renal function.

   Step A: *Convert 130 lb to kg: 130 lb × 1 kg/2.2 lb = 59.1 kg*

   Step B: *Calculate the desired (safe) amount to administer: 7.5 mg/kg × 59.1 kg = 443.25 mg q12h is safe*

   Step C: *Think! . . . Is It Reasonable? Since the ordered dose 375 mg is less than the desired (safe) amount to administer, 443 mg, the dosage ordered is (low, but) safe.*

2. Safe

3. Safe

   According to the package insert, the daily dosage for patients with normal renal function is 2 g divided into doses q6h or q12h. The daily dosage for patients with impaired renal function is 1545 mg/24 h for creatinine clearance of 100 mL/min; 1390 mg/24 h for 90 mL/min; 1235 mg/24 h for 80 mL/min; 1080 mg/24 h for 70 mL/min; 925 mg/24 h for 60 mL/min; 770 mg/24 h for 50 mL/min; 620 mg/24 h for 40 mL/min; 425 mg/24 h for 30 mL/min; 310 mg/24 h for 20 mL/min; and 155 mg/24 h for 10 mL/min.

   Step A: *No conversion is necessary as the desired (safe) amount to administer is based on CL_{CR}*

   Step B: *Calculate the ordered daily dose: 150 mg/dose × 4 doses/day = 600 mg/day*

   Step C: *Think! . . . Is It Reasonable? 600 mg/day is ordered and 925 mg/24 h is safe for patients with impaired renal function and a CL_{CR} of 60 mL/min; The dose ordered is (low, but) safe.*

4. Safe

5. Safe; Amount to administer: $\frac{1}{2}$ tablet

6. Safe; Amount to administer: 10 mL q4h

Review and Practice

17.4 Dosages Based on Body Surface Area (BSA)

1. 0.57 m²

88 cm and 13.2 kg

$$BSA \ in \ m^2 = \sqrt{\frac{(ht \ (cm) \times wt \ (kg))}{3600}}$$

$$m^2 = \sqrt{\frac{(88 \times 13.2)}{3600}}$$

$$m^2 = \sqrt{\frac{1161.6}{3600}}$$

$$m^2 = \sqrt{0.32}$$

$$m^2 = 0.568 = 0.57$$

2. $0.57 \ m^2$

3. $0.25 \ m^2$

4. $0.37 \ m^2$

5. $1 \ m^2$

   52 in and 64 lb

$$BSA \ in \ m^2 = \sqrt{\frac{(ht \ (in) \times wt \ (lb))}{3131}}$$

$$m^2 = \sqrt{\frac{(52 \times 64)}{3131}}$$

$$m^2 = \sqrt{\frac{3328}{3131}}$$

$$m^2 = \sqrt{1.06}$$

$$m^2 = 1$$

6. $0.69 \ m^2$

7. $0.36 \ m^2$

8. $0.42 \ m^2$

9. 143.5 mcg

   The child's BSA is 0.82 m^2. The recommended dosage is 175 mcg/m^2.

   175 mcg/m^2 3 0.82 m^2 = 143.5 mcg

10. 0.26 mg

11. 14.5 mcg

12. 0.18 mg

13. 14.7 mL

$$BSA \ in \ m^2 = \sqrt{\frac{(ht \ (in) \times wt \ (lb))}{3131}}$$

$$m^2 = \sqrt{\frac{(42 \times 71)}{3131}}$$

$$m^2 = \sqrt{\frac{2982}{3131}}$$

$$m^2 = \sqrt{0.952}$$

$$m^2 = 0.98$$

Calculate the ordered dose:

6 mg/m^2/day q12h

6 mg/m^2 × 0.98 m^2 = 5.88 mg or 5,880 mcg per day ÷ 2 doses/day (q12h) = 2940 mcg/dose

Calculate the amount to administer:

Proportion Method:

$H/Q = D/A$

$200 \text{ meg}/1 \text{ mL} = 2{,}940 \text{ meg}/A$

$\quad\quad 200\, x = 2{,}940$

$\quad\quad\quad\quad x = 14.7 \text{ mL}$

Dimensional Analysis:

$A \text{ mL} = 1 \text{ mL}/200 \text{ meg} \times 2{,}940 \text{ meg}/1 = 14.7 \text{ mL}$

14. 1.7 mL/dose

15. 1.1 mL/dose

16. 2.6 mL/dose

17. The ordered dose of 800 mg is within this range, but may be too low—contact the authorized prescriber; if authorized, administer 21 mL. (Note: you will need 4 vials.)

    BSA: 1.3 m²; D: 1250 mg;

18. The ordered dose of 125 mg is within this range and safe.

    Amount to administer: 125 mL

    Lower range: 1.6 m² × 75 mg/m² = 120 mg; Upper range: 1.6 m² × 100 mg/m² = 160 mg

Review and Practice

17.5 Daily Maintenance Fluid Needs

1. 800 mL

   8 kg

   100 mL/kg × 8 kg = 800 mL

2. 1760 mL

   33 kg

   1500 mL + (20 mL/kg × 13 kg) = 1500 mL + 260 mL = 1760 mL

3. 1341 mL

   37 lb × 1 kg/2.2 lb/kg = 16.8 kg

   1000 mL + (50 mL/kg × 6.8 kg) = 1000 mL + 340 mL = 1340 mL

4. 1627 mL

5. 2200 mL

6. 63 gtt/min

   21 kg

   1500 mL + (20 mL/kg × 1 kg) = 1500 mL + 20 mL = 1520 mL daily

   F (mL/h) = V/T

   F = 1520 mL/24 h (daily = 24 h)

   F = 63 mL/h

   Microdrip tubing has a calibration of 60 gtt/mL

   f gtt/min = 63 mL/h × 1 h/60 min × 60 gtt/mL = 63 gtt/min

7. 52 gtt/min

8. 32 gtt/min

9. 60 gtt/min

10. 108 gtt/min

11. 72 mL/h

    180 lb × 1 kg/2.2 lb = 81.8 kg

    1500 mL + (20 mL/kg × 61.8 kg) = 1500 mL + 1236 mL + 2736 mL

    2736 mL − 1000 mL (oral intake) = 1736 mL/24 h to maintain daily fluids

    1736 mL/day × 1 day/24 h= 72 mL/h

12. 63 mL/h

Chapter 17 Review

Check Up

1. 22.3 kg

2. 27.7 kg

3. 3 kg

4. 5.8 kg

5. 0.74 m^2

6. 0.5 m^2

7. 0.66 m^2

8. 0.47 m^2

9. The safe dose is 204 mg/day (15 mg/kg/day × 13.6 kg). The ordered dose of 100 mg q12h (200 mg/day) is safe. Amount to administer: 2 mL

10. The safe dose is 1.6 mg (0.1 mg/kg/day × 16 kg) tid. The ordered dose of 1.6 mg tid is safe. Amount to administer: 4 mL

11. The safe dose is 1320 International Units (82.5 International Units/kg × 16 kg). The ordered dose of 1300 International Units is safe. Amount to administer: 1.7 mL

12. The safe dose is 465 mg/day. The ordered dose of 225 mg q12h (450 mg/day) is safe. Amount to administer: 4.5 mL

13. The safe dose range is 240 mg to 300 mg per day (8–10 mg/kg/day × 30 kg) The ordered dose of 150 mg BID (300 mg/day) is safe. Amount to administer: 2.5 mL

14. The safe dose is 792 mg to 1320 mg/day (30–50 mg/kg/day × 26.4 kg) is doubled for severe infections: 1584 mg to 2640 mg/day. The ordered dose of 650 mg tid (1950 mg/day) is safe. Amount to administer 8.125 mL, rounded to 8.1 mL

15. The safe dose is 125 mcg/day (5 mcg/kg/day × 25 kg). The ordered dose of 125 mcg is safe. Amount to administer: 0.21 mL

16. DMFN: 1580 mL, flow rate: 66 mL/h

17. DMFN: 1386 mL, flow rate: 58 mL/h

18. DMFN: 2100 mL − 800 mL taken orally = 1300 mL, flow rate: 54 mL/h

19. The rate at which the kidneys remove waste from the body. The faster the rate, the faster the elimination of medication from the body.

20. Safe; amount to administer: 1 tablet

21. Safe; amount to administer: 2 mL

22. Safe; amount to administer: 9 mL

23. Safe; amount to administer: 100 mL

24. Not safe: consult the authorized prescriber

25. Safe; amount to administer: 100 mL

Critical Thinking Applications

1. The dose for patient A is not safe. He has a creatinine clearance of 37 mL/min and nosocomial pneumonia. He should receive 3.375 g q6h. The dose for patient B is safe.

2. For patient B, you would select the 3.375 g vial and mix it with 15 mL of any of the compatible reconstitution solutions. Always double-check the package instructions with any medication you are going to reconstitute.

3. For patient A, you would contact and inform the authorized prescriber that the patient's creatinine clearance is 37 mL/min.

4. For patient B, you end up with a volume of 165 mL (15 mL in the syringe and 150 mL of diluent) to infuse over $\frac{1}{2}$ hour. The flow rate would be 330 mL per hour.

Case Study

1. Upper range: 1365 mg/day (75 mg/kg/day × 18.2 kg)

   Lower range: 910 mg/day (50 mg/kg/day × 18.2 kg)

2. The hourly flow rate is 30 mL/h

3. The ordered dose of 1200 mg (600 mg twice a day) is within the accepted range of 910 to 1365 mg and is safe to administer.

Internet Activity

Some height-to-weight ratio charts can be found at:

http://www.healthchecksystems.com/heightweightchart.htm

http://www.halls.md/ideal-weight/met.htm

http://www.changingshape.com/resources/references/idealbodyweight.asp

CHAPTER 18 ANSWERS

Critical Thinking on the Job

Timing is Essential

1. Both NPH and regular insulin

2. 19 units

3. U-100 50 unit-syringe or 30 unit-syringe.

4. The regular insulin will start to peak and the NPH insulin will start to take effect before the patient gets breakfast. This may result in the blood sugar dropping too low. To prevent the blood sugar from dropping too low, you could administer some milk (which contains both sugar and protein) or other food at 0800, then remove the equivalent food from the patient's breakfast tray when it arrives. Notify AP and recheck blood sugar as ordered, administer dextrose 50% water (D50W) if ordered.

Review and Practice

18.1 Insulin Administration

1. Vial D

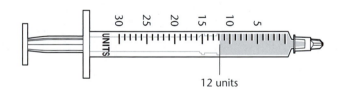

12 units

2. Vial A

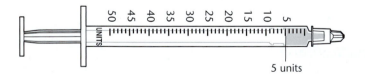

5 units

3. Vial C

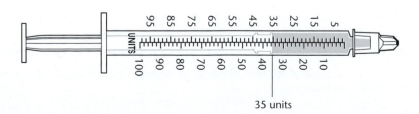

35 units

4. Vial B

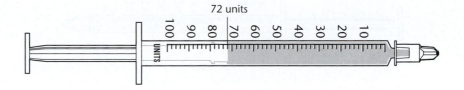

72 units

5. Vial G

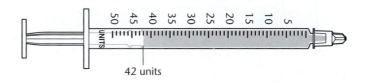

42 units

6. Vial E

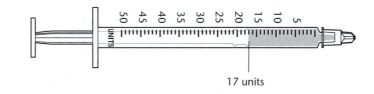

17 units

7. Vial F

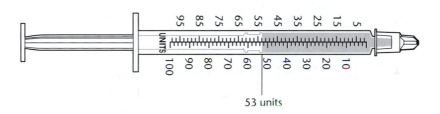

53 units

8. Vial F

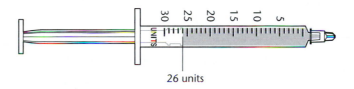

26 units

9. Vial B

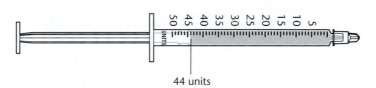

44 units

10. Vial A

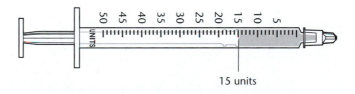

15 units

11. Vial C

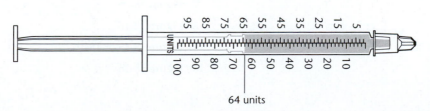

64 units

12. Vial G

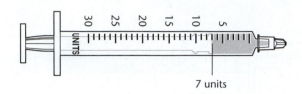

36 units

13. Vial E

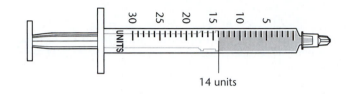

7 units

14. Vial D

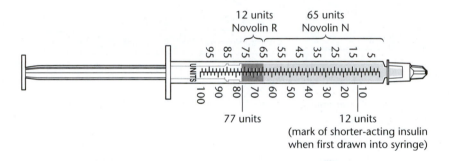

14 units

15.

12 units   65 units
Novolin R   Novolin N

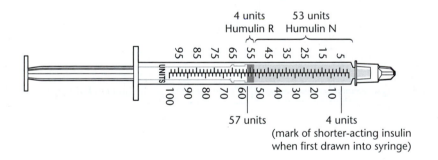

77 units   12 units
                        (mark of shorter-acting insulin
                        when first drawn into syringe)

16.

4 units   53 units
Humulin R   Humulin N

57 units   4 units
                        (mark of shorter-acting insulin
                        when first drawn into syringe)

Review and Practice

18.2 Heparin Labels

1. Figure 18-1 or 18-18

2. Figure 18-20

3. Figure 18-14

4. Figure 18-16 or 18-20

5. Figure 18-18

6. Figure 18-15, 18-16; 18-17

7. Figure 18-20

8. Figure 18-16

9. Figure 18-15 or 18-16

10. Figure 18-16

18.3. Calculating Subcutaneous Heparin Dosages

1. 1 mL

2. 0.75 mL

   Proportion Method:

   Step A: Convert. Desired dose and the supply dose are both in units, so no conversion is needed.

   Step B: Calculate.

   $$\frac{10{,}000 \text{ units}}{1 \text{ mL}} = \frac{7{,}500 \text{ units}}{A} \qquad or \qquad 10{,}000 \text{ units} : 1 \text{ mL} = 7{,}500 \text{ units} : x \text{ mL}$$

   $$10{,}000\, A = 7{,}500 \qquad\qquad\qquad 7{,}500 = 10{,}000A$$

   $$A = \frac{7{,}500}{10{,}000} \qquad\qquad\qquad \frac{7{,}500}{10{,}000} = A$$

   $$A = 0.75 \qquad\qquad\qquad\qquad 0.75 = A$$

   Administer 0.75 mL

   Step C: Think! . . . Is It Reasonable? Since the desired dose is $\frac{3}{4}$ as much as the dose on hand, it is reasonable that the amount to administer is $\frac{3}{4}$ of the dosage unit or 0.75 mL.

   Dimensional Analysis:

   Step A: Convert. Desired dose and the supply dose are both in units, so no conversion factor is needed.

   Step B: Calculate.

   $$A = \frac{1 \text{ mL}}{10{,}000 \text{ units}} \times \frac{7{,}500 \text{ units}}{1}$$

   $$A = 0.75 \text{ mL}$$

   Step C: Think! . . . Is It Reasonable? Since the desired dose is $\frac{1}{4}$ as much as the dose on hand, it is reasonable that the amount to administer is $\frac{3}{4}$ of the dosage unit or 0.75 mL.

   Formula Method:

   Step A: Convert. Desired dose and the supply dose are both in units, so no conversion is needed.

   Step B: Calculate.

   $$\frac{7{,}500 \text{ units}}{10{,}000 \text{ units}} \times 1 \text{ mL} = A$$

   $$0.75 \text{ mL} = A$$

   Step C: Think! . . . Is It Reasonable? Since the desired dose is $\frac{3}{4}$ as much as the dose on hand, it is reasonable that the amount to administer is $\frac{3}{4}$ of the dosage unit or 0.75 mL

3. 0.5 mL

4. 0.4 mL

5. 0.5 mL

Review and Practice

18.4 Intravenous Heparin Dosages

1. 75 mL/h

2. 25 mL/h

3. 32 mL/h

4. 25 mL/h

5. 25 mL/h

6. The hourly dose is 1,000 units/h.

7. The hourly dose is 450 units/h.

8. The hourly dose is 556 units/h.

9. The hourly dose is 400 units/h.

10. The hourly dose is 2,500 units/h.

11. 4,000 units, which is 4 mL of 1,000 unit/mL solution

Proportion Method:

Step A: Convert. Since the patient's weight is in kg and the ordered dose is per kg, no conversion is necessary.

Since the ordered dose is in units and the dose on hand is in units no conversion is necessary.

Step B: Calculate.

$80 \text{ units}/1 \text{ kg} = x/50 \text{ kg}$ $\qquad\qquad$ $80 \text{ units}: 1 \text{ kg} = x:50 \text{ kg}$

$80 \text{ units} \times 50 = x \times 1$ $\qquad\qquad$ $1 \times x = 80 \text{ units} \times 50$

$\qquad 4,000 \text{ units} = x$ $\qquad\qquad\qquad$ $x = 4,000 \text{ units}$

Since 4,000 units is less than the maximum dose of 8,000 units, proceed to calculate the amount to administer from Heparin 1,000 USP units/mL:

$1,000 \text{ units}/1 \text{ mL} = 4,000 \text{ units}/A$ $\qquad\qquad$ $1,000 \text{ units}:1 \text{ mL} = 4,000 \text{ units}:A$

$\qquad 1,000 A = 1 \text{ mL} \times 4,000$ $\qquad\qquad$ $1 \text{ mL} \times 4,000 = 1,000 A$

$\qquad\qquad A = 4,000 \text{ mL}/1,000$ $\qquad\qquad$ $4,000 \text{ mL}/1,000 = A$

$\qquad\qquad\qquad A = 4 \text{ mL}$ $\qquad\qquad\qquad\qquad$ $4 \text{ mL} = A$

Step C: Think!. . .Is It Reasonable? 4 mL of a 1,000 units/mL solution is 4,000 units, which is less than the maximum dose of 8,000 units, so it is reasonable.

Dimensional Analysis:

Step A: Convert. Since the patient's weight is in kg and the ordered dose is per kg, no conversion factor is necessary.

Since the ordered dose is in units and the dose on hand is in units no conversion factor is necessary

Step B: Calculate.

$A = 1 \text{ mL}/1,000 \text{ units} \times 80 \text{ unit/kg} \times 50 \text{ kg}$

$A = 4,000 \text{ mL}/1,000$

$A = 4 \text{ mL}$

Step C: Think! . . . Is It Reasonable? 4 mL of a 1,000 units/mL solution is 4,000 units, which is less than the maximum dose of 8,000 units, so it is reasonable.

Formula Method:

Step A: Convert. Since the patient's weight is in kg and the ordered dose is per kg, no conversion is necessary.

Since the ordered dose is in units and the dose on hand is in units no conversion is necessary.

Step B: Calculate. The desired dose is 80 unit/kg

$$\frac{80 \text{ units}}{1 \text{ kg}} = \frac{x}{50 \text{ kg}} \qquad\qquad 80 \text{ unit}: 1 \text{ kg} = x:50 \text{ kg}$$

$\qquad 80 \text{ units} \times 50 = x$ $\qquad\qquad$ $x = 80 \text{ units} \times 50$

$\qquad\qquad 4,000 \text{ units} = x$ $\qquad\qquad$ $x = 4,000 \text{ units}$

$\dfrac{4,000 \text{ units}}{1,000 \text{ units}} \times 1 \text{ mL} = A$

$\qquad\qquad 4 \text{ mL} = A$

Step C: Think! . . . Is It Reasonable? 4 mL of a 1,000 USP units/mL solution is 4,000 units, which is less than the maximum dose of 8,000 units, so it is reasonable.

12. 900 units/h, which is 18 mL/h of a 50 unit/mL solution

Proportion Method:

Step A: Convert. Since the patient's weight is in kg and the ordered dose is per kg, no conversion is necessary.

Since the ordered dose is in units and the dose on hand is in units no conversion is necessary.

Calculate. Calculate. Calculate the desired dose

18 units/1 k̶g̶/h × 50 k̶g̶ = D

18 units/h × 50 = 900 units/h

The amount to administer is 900 units/h.

Calculate the flow rate (using the IV concentration in the protocol: 50 units/mL).

$$\frac{50 \text{ units}}{1 \text{ mL}} = \frac{900 \text{ units}/h}{A}$$ $$50 \text{ units} : 1 \text{ mL} = 900 \text{ units}/h : A$$

$$50 A = 900 \text{ mL}/h$$ $$900 \text{ mL}/h = 50 A$$

$$A = \frac{900 \text{ mL}/h}{50}$$ $$\frac{900 \text{ mL}/h}{50} = A$$

$$x = 18 \text{ mL}/h$$ $$18 \text{ mL}/h = A$$

Step C: Think! . . . Is It Reasonable? 900 units/hour is less than the maximum dose of 1800 units/h , so it is reasonable.

Dimensional Analysis:

Step A: Convert. Since the patient's weight is in kg and the ordered dose is per kg, no conversion is necessary.

Since the ordered dose is in units and the dose on hand is in units no conversion is necessary.

Step B: Calculate. Calculate the desired dose

18 units/1 k̶g̶/h × 50 k̶g̶ = D

18 units/h × 50 = 900 units/h

Calculate the amount to administer

$$A = \frac{500 \text{ mL}}{25,000 \text{ units}} \times \frac{900 \text{ units}/h}{1}$$

$$A = \frac{450,000 \text{ mL}/h}{25,000}$$

$$A = 18 \text{ mL}/h$$

Step C: Think! . . . Is It Reasonable? 900 units/hour is less than the maximum dose of 1800 units/h, so it is reasonable.

Formula Method:

Step A: Convert. Since the patient's weight is in kg and the ordered dose is per kg, no conversion is necessary.

Since the ordered dose is in units and the dose on hand is in units no conversion is necessary.

Step B: Calculate. Calculate the desired dose

18 units/1 k̶g̶/h × 50 k̶g̶ = D

18 units/h × 50 = 900 units/h

Calculate the amount to administer

$$\frac{900 \text{ units}/h}{25,000 \text{ units}/h} \times 500 \text{ mL} = A$$

$$450,000 \text{ mL}/25,000 = A$$

$$18 \text{ mL} = A$$

Step C: Think! . . . Is It Reasonable? 900 units/hour is less than the maximum dose of 1800 units/h, so it is reasonable.

13. 2,000 units, which is 2 mL

14. 1,000 units/kg/h; 20 mL/h

Calculate the desired dose

18 units/kg/h + 2 units/kg/h = 20 units/kg/h

  20 units/kg/h × 50 kg = 1,000 units/h

Calculate the amount to administer

1,000 units/h/25,000 units × 500 mL = A

A = 20 mL/h

15. 1,150 units/h; 23 mL/h

16. 9,600 units (max. 8,000 units); give 8,000 units (8 mL of heparin sodium 1,000 units/mL)

17. 2,160 units/h (max. 1800 units/h); infuse 1800 units/h at 36 mL/h

18. 4,800 units exceeds the maximum dose of 4,000 units; administer 4 mL of heparin sodium, 1,000 units/mL.

19. 1,920 units/h; 38.4 mL/h

20. 1,560 units/h; 31.2 mL/h

Chapter 18 Review

Check Up

1. Vial F

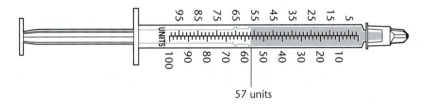

11 units

2. Vial D

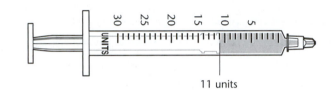

48 units

3. Vial E

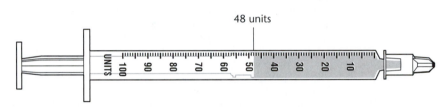

57 units

4. Vial B

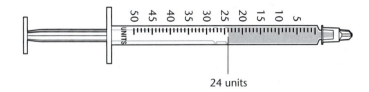

24 units

5. Vial A

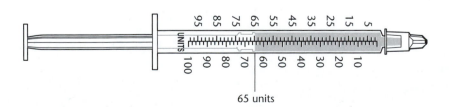

65 units

6. Vial C

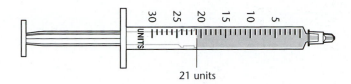

21 units

7.

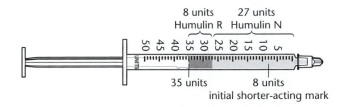

8 units   27 units
Humulin R Humulin N

35 units   8 units
          initial shorter-acting mark

8.

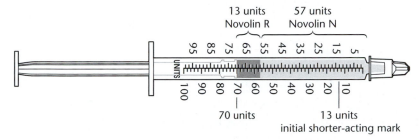

13 units   57 units
Novolin R   Novolin N

70 units   13 units
          initial shorter-acting mark

9. 15 mL/h

10. 40 gtt/min

11. 1600 units/h is 38,400 units/24h.

12. 1000 units/h

13. 0.8 mL of label G

14. 0.8 mL of label H

15. 6,000 units; 6 mL

16. 1,350 units/h; 27 mL/h

Critical Thinking Applications

1. The AP failed to write the full name of the insulin ordered.

2. The healthcare practitioner failed to question either the order or the insulin when the insulin label did not match the order exactly (Humulin insulin v. Humulin R regular insulin).

3. The healthcare practitioner should have sought clarification from the AP when a discrepancy between the order and the insulin label was noticed.

4. Regular insulin peaks 1–3 hours after administration.

5. Regular insulin has a shorter duration than NPH insulin. Since Humulin R was administered instead of Humulin N, the effects of the insulin had worn off before the morning blood sugar was measured. The patient needed an evening dose of basal insulin for adequate blood sugar regulation.

Case Study

1. 20,000–40,000 units

2. The pharmacy technician should have read the label including the concentration as he pulled the heparin from his stock, compared this to the computer's bin label.

3. The nurse should have checked the label including the concentration, when she pulled the medication from the drawer, she also should have checked the label before she withdrew the dose from the vial, and again as she put the vial down.

Internet Activity

1. The common symptoms of hypoglycemia include:

   • Shakiness

   • Dizziness

- Weak feeling
- Sweating
- Nervousness
- Fast heart rate
- Pale skin color
- Hunger
- Difficulty paying attention or confusion
- Headache
  - —Sudden moodiness or behavior changes
  - —Tingling sensations around the mouth

2. Treat low blood sugar with 3 glucose tablets, one-half cup of fruit juice, or 5 to 6 pieces of hard candy. If none of these are available, drink one-half can of regular soda, one-half cup of low-fat milk, or eat some other form of carbohydrate. Contact AP and administer glucagon and D50W IV if ordered, and follow blood sugar as ordered.

CHAPTER 19 ANSWERS

Review and Practice

19.1 Hourly Flow Rates for Dosage per Time Infusions

For Exercises 1–9 convert the dosage/minute into milliliters/hour.

1. 60 mL/h

   Proportion Method:

   Step A: Convert. Convert g to mg (1g = 1000 mg)

   $$\frac{1g}{500\ mL} = \frac{1000\ mg}{500\ mL}$$

   Convert mg/min to mg/h

   $$\frac{60\ \cancel{min}}{h} \times \frac{2\ mg}{\cancel{min}} = 120\ mg/h$$

   Step B: Calculate. The rate of the desired dose (D) is now 120 mg/1 h. The dosage unit (Q) is 500 mL. The dose on hand H is 1,000 mg.

1. Fill in the proportion.	*Fill in the ratio.*

   $$\frac{H}{Q} = \frac{D}{A}$$

   $$H:Q = D:A$$

   $$\frac{1,000\ mg}{500\ mL} = \frac{120\ mg/h}{A}$$

   $$1,000\ mg:500\ mL = 120\ mg/h:A$$

   2. Cancel the units leaving mL/h

   $$\frac{1,000\ \cancel{mg}}{500\ mL} = \frac{120\ \cancel{mg}/h}{A}$$

   $$1,000\ \cancel{mg}:500mL = 120\ \cancel{mg}/h:A$$

   3. Cross-multiply and solve.

   Multiply the means and the extremes for the unknown.

   $$1,000 \times A = 500 \times 120\ mL/h$$

   $$1,000 \times A = 500\ mL \times 120/h$$

   $$A = \frac{500\ mL \times 120/h}{1,000}$$

   $$A = \frac{500\ mL \times 120/h}{1,000}$$

   $$A = \frac{60,000\ mL/h}{1,000}$$

   $$A = \frac{60,000\ mL/h}{1,000}$$

   $$A = 60\ mL/h$$

   $$A = 60\ mL/h$$

   Step C: Think! . . . Is It Reasonable? Since the concentration of 1,000 mg/500 mL equals 2 mg/mL, then 1 mL/min would equal 2 mg/min, and because there are 60 minutes in 1 hour, then 60 mL/h would equal 1 mL/min, so the answer is reasonable.

Dimensional Analysis:

Step A: Convert. The conversion factor 1 g/1000 mg is needed to convert g to mg.

The conversion factor 60 min/1 h is needed to convert minutes to hours.

Step B: Calculate.

$$A\ mL/h = \frac{1\ g}{1000\ \cancel{mg}} \times \frac{500\ mL}{1\ \cancel{g}} \times \frac{2\ \cancel{mg}}{1\ \cancel{min}} \times \frac{60\ \cancel{min}}{1\ h}$$

$$A\ mL = \frac{60,000\ mL}{1,000\ h} = 60\ mL/h$$

Step C: Think! . . . Is It Reasonable? Since the concentration of 1,000 mg/500 mL equals 2 mg/mL, then 1 mL/min would equal 2 mg/min, and because there are 60 minutes in 1 hour, then 60 mL/h would equal 1 mL/min, so the answer is reasonable.

Formula Method:

Step A: Convert. Convert g to mg (1g = 1000 mg)

$$\frac{1\ g}{500\ mL} = \frac{1000\ mg}{500\ mL}$$

Convert mg/min to mg/h (60 minutes = 1 hour)

$$\frac{60\ min}{h} \times \frac{mg}{min} = \frac{mg}{h}$$

$$\frac{60\ \cancel{min}}{h} \times \frac{2\ mg}{1\ \cancel{min}} = \frac{120\ mg}{1h}$$

Step B: Calculate.

$$\frac{D}{H} \times Q = A$$

$$\frac{120\ \cancel{mg}/h}{1000\ \cancel{mg}} \times 500\ mL = A$$

$$\frac{60,000\ mL/h}{1000} = A$$

$$60\ mL/h = A$$

Step C: Think! . . . Is It Reasonable? Since the concentration of 1,000 mg/500 mL equals 2 mg/mL, then 1 mL/min would equal 2 mg/min, and because there are 60 minutes in 1 hour, then 60 mL/h would equal 1 mL/min, so the answer is reasonable.

2. 3 mL/h
3. 2 mL/h
4. 5 mL/h
5. 60 mL/h
6. 6 mL/h
7. 45 mL/h
8. 8 mL/h
9. 1 mL/h
10. 75 mL/h

Review and Practice

19.2 IV Flow Rates Based on Body Weight per Time

1. 84.1 kg

$$\frac{1\ kg}{2.2\ \cancel{lb}} = \frac{x}{185\ \cancel{lb}}$$

$$\frac{185\ kg}{2.2} = x$$

84.09 or 84.1 kg = x round to the nearest tenth

84.1 kg

2. 84.1 mcg/min

Convert milligrams to micrograms

$$\frac{1,000\ mcg}{1mg} = \frac{x}{10\ mg}$$

$$\frac{10\ mg \times 1{,}000\ mcg}{1\ mg} = x$$

$10{,}000\ mcg = x$

The concentration is 10,000 mcg/100 mL or 100 mcg/1 mL

Determine the desired dose of vecuronium

1 mcg/kg/min × 84.1 kg = x

1 mcg/kg/min × 84.1 kg = x

$$\frac{84.1\ mcg}{min} \times \frac{60\ min}{h} = 5046\ mcg/h$$

The desired dose D = 84.1 mcg/min or 5046 mcg/h

3. 50.5 mL/h (50.46 mL/h rounded to the nearest tenth)

4. 0.841 mL/min

   50.5 mL/h ÷ 60 min/h = 0.84 mL/min

Proportion Method:

Step A: Convert. See question 1 for lb to kg conversion. Convert milligrams to micrograms

$$\frac{1{,}000\ mcg}{1mg} = \frac{x\ mcg}{10\ mg}$$

$$\frac{10\ mg \times 1{,}000\ mcg}{1\ mg} = x\ mcg$$

$10{,}000\ mcg = x\ mcg$

The concentration is 10,000 mcg/100 mL or 100 mcg/1 mL

Step B: Calculate.

$$\frac{H}{Q} = \frac{D}{A}$$

$$\frac{10{,}000\ mcg}{100\ mL} = \frac{5046\ mcg/h}{A}$$

10,000 mcg × A 5 5046 mcg/h × 100 mL

10,000 A = 504,600 mL/h

A = 50.46 mL/h or 50.5 mL/h

Step C: Think! . . . Is It Reasonable? Since 50.46 mL = 5046 mcg, and 5046 mcg divided by 60 min equals 84.1 mcg/min, and the patient weighs 84.1 kg, it is reasonable that a flow rate of 50.5 mL/h [rounded] delivers approximately 1 mcg/kg/min.

Dimensional Analysis:

Step A: Convert. The desired dose is in micrograms and the dose on hand is in milligrams, the conversion factor 1 mg/1000 mcg, is necessary.

Convert 185 lb to 84.1 kg using the Proportion Method.

Use Rule 18-8 to determine the Desired Dose, D

1 mcg/kg/min × 84.1 kg − 84.1 mcg/min

Use Rule 19-2 to convert mcg/min to mcg/h:

$$\frac{84.1\ mcg}{min} \times \frac{60\ min}{h} = 5046\ mcg/h$$

Step B: Calculate. Determine the values for Q, H, and D.

Q = 100 mL

H = 10 mg

D = 1 mcg/kg/min

Determine the amount to administer (A) as flow rate in mL/h.

$$A = Conversion\ factor \times \frac{Q}{H} \times D$$

$$A = \frac{1\ \cancel{mg}}{1000\ \cancel{mcg}} \times \frac{100\ mL}{10\ \cancel{mg}} \times \frac{5046\ \cancel{mcg}}{h}$$

$$A = \frac{504{,}600\ mL}{10{,}000\ h}$$

$A = 50.46\ mL/h$

Rounded to the nearest tenth: A = 50.5 mL/h

Step C: Think! . . . Is It Reasonable? Since 50.45 mL = 5045 mcg, and 5045 mcg divided by 60 min equals 84.08 mcg/min which rounds to 84.1 mcg, and the patient weighs 84.1 kg, it is reasonable that a flow rate of 50.5 mL/h [rounded] delivers approximately 1 mg/kg/min

5. 63.6 kg

6. 31.8 mcg/min

7. 0.159 mL/min

8. 9.5 mL/h (9.54 mL/h rounded to nearest tenth)

9. 51.4 kg (51.36)

10. 1.028 mcg/min

11. 0.1713 mL/min

12. 10.3 mL/h (10.27)

13. 68.2 kg

14. 68.2 mcg/min

15. 0.1364 mL/min

16. 8.2 mL/h (8.184)

17. 0.8 g

18. 180 mg

Review and Practice

19.3 IV Flow Rates for Titrated Medications

1. 15 mL/h

   Proportion Method:

   Step A: Convert. Convert grams to milligrams

   1 g = 1000 mg, so the concentration can be rewritten as 1000 mg/250 mL.

   Convert the desired dose from mg/min to mg/h

   60 min/h × 4 mg/min = 240 mg/h

   Step B: Calculate. Calculate the flow rate by converting 240 mg into mL then placing it over 1 hour e.g. A/h

   $$\frac{H}{Q} = \frac{D}{A}$$ $H:Q = D:A$

   $$\frac{1{,}000\ \cancel{mg}}{250\ mL} = \frac{240\ \cancel{mg}/h}{A}$$ $1{,}000\ \cancel{mg}:250\ mL = 240\ \cancel{mg}/h:A$

   $1{,}000 \times A = 250\ mL \times 240/h$ $250\ mL \times 240/h = 1{,}000 \times A$

   $$A = \frac{60{,}000\ mL/h}{1{,}000}$$ $$\frac{60{,}000\ mL/h}{1{,}000} = A$$

   $A = 60\ mL/h$ $60\ mL/h = A$

   The flow rate is 60 mL/h

   Step C: Think!...Is It Reasonable? Since the concentration of 1000 mg/250 mL equals 4 mg/mL and the maximum dose is 4mg/min, then 1 mL/min equals 4 mg/min. And since there are 60 minutes in 1 hour, it is reasonable that the rate per hour would be 60 times the minute rate or 60 mL/h, so it is reasonable.

   Dimensional Analysis:

   Step A: Convert. Since the desired dose is in milligrams and the dose on hand is in grams, use the conversion factor 1g/1000 mg.

   Since the desired dose is in minutes and the pump infuses per hour, convert desired dose D from mg/min to mg/h, use the conversion factor 60 min/1 h

   $$\frac{4\ mg}{\cancel{min}} \times \frac{60\ \cancel{min}}{h} = 240\ mg/h$$

$$A = \frac{1\,g}{1000\,mg} \times \frac{250\,mL}{1\,g} \times 240\,mg/h$$

$$A = \frac{60{,}000\,mL}{1000\,h}$$

$$A = 60\,mL/h$$

Formula Method:

Step A: Convert. Convert grams to milligrams

1 g = 1000 mg, so the concentration can be rewritten as 1000mg/250 mL.

Convert the desired dose from mg/min to mg/h

$$\frac{4\,mg}{min} \times \frac{60\,min}{h} = 240\,mg/h$$

Step B: Calculate.

$$\frac{D}{H} \times Q = A$$

$$\frac{240\,mg/h}{1000\,mg} \times 250\,mL = A$$

$$\frac{60{,}000\,mL}{1000\,h} = A$$

$$60\,mL/h = A$$

Step C: Think! . . . Is It Reasonable? Since the concentration of 1000 mg/250 mL equals 4 mg/mL and the maximum dose is 4mg/min, then 1 mL/min equals 4 mg/min. And since there are 60 minutes in 1 hour, it is reasonable that the rate per hour would be 60 times the minute rate or 60 mL/h, so it is reasonable.

2. 60 mL/h

3. 30 mL/h

4. 22.5 mL/h

5. 3.1 mcg/kg/min

6. 30 mL/h

7. 150 mL/h

8. 50 mL/h

9. Yes, increase the rate to 105 mL/h (10.5 mg/h)

10. 30 mL/h

Chapter 19 Review

Check Up

1. 45 mL/h

2. 28.8 mL/h

3. 90 mL/h

4. 18.2 mL/h

5. 13.3 mL/h (13.2672 rounded to the nearest tenth)

6. 8.4 mL/h

7. 420 mg

8. 170 mg or 170,000 mcg

9. 126.2 mL/h

10. 18 mL/h

11. 45 mL/h

12. 120 mL/h

13. 8 mL/h

14. 5.7 mL/h

15. 16.7 mL/h (16.66)

16. 2.5mL/h

17. 10 mL/h

18. 5 mL/h; yes

19. Yes, rebolus with 1 mg, and increase the infusion to 7.5 mL/h

20. 5 mL/h. No, the bolus should only be given if the rate is increased.

Critical Thinking Application

1. 24 mL/h

2. 194 mL/h for less than or equal to 10 minutes.

3. Increase the rate, since the nitroprusside is infusing at 6.88 mcg/kg/min, which is less than the maximum rate.

4. Notify the AP, since the nitroprusside has been administered at the maximal rate, and the patient's BP is still too high. Since the response should be quick, and it is not safe to infuse at the maximum rate for more than 10 minutes, place the call as the infusion is trending up, beyond the average dose of 3 mcg/kg/min. Additionally, verify the blood pressure, and troubleshoot for problems with the infusion:

- Ask another nurse to check the calculated rate.

- Check the IV site, tubing, and infusion pump to ensure the medication is infusing into the patient.

- Consider administering a fresh bag of nitroprusside.

Case Study

400 mcg

Internet Activity

You are working in an intensive care unit that uses many IV critical care drugs. Checking the safe ranges of these drugs during emergency situations is both inconvenient and time-consuming. You and your coworkers decide to search the Internet for guides to dosages of commonly used drugs. Try to find answers to the following questions online.

1. 150 min over 10 minutes followed by 360 mg over the next 6 hours

2. a. 5 to 10 mcg

   b. Every 5 to 10 minutes.

3. Mechanical ventilator support should be in place.

UNIT FIVE ASSESSMENT ANSWERS

1. Figure D
2. 0.8
3. Figure B
4. 5600
5. 24
6. 29.6
7. H
8. G
9.

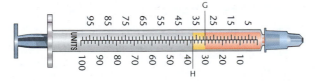

10. 8000
11. 2 g lidocaine + qsad water 100 mL
12. 270 mL Sustacal®/solute; 90 mL water/solvent
13. 270 mL peroxide/solute; 810 mL saline/solvent
14. a. Elimination
    b. Absorption
    c. Biotransformation (Metabolism)
    d. Distribution
15. 45 mg/day; 15 mg/dose
16. Yes
17. Yes, $\frac{1}{2}$ tablet
18. 560,000
19. 1580
20. Yes

COMPREHENSIVE EVALUATION ANSWERS

1. 400 mg

2. Orally (po)

3. 0730, 1130, and 1630

4. Reglan® 7:30 a.m., 11:30 a.m., 4:30 p.m.; Neurontin® 8:00 a.m., 12:00 p.m., 5:00 p.m.; Desyrel® 8:00 a.m.; Ativan® has no scheduled times because it is order prn (as needed).

5. The order for Reglan is incomplete. It does not list the route.

6. The Desyrel® frequency was transcribed as "qd," but should have been transcribed as "daily" or "once a day."

7. 1. Right patient, 2. Right drug, 3. Right dose, 4. Right route, 5. Right time, 6. Right documentation, 7. Right reason, 8. Right to know, 9. Right to refuse, 10. Right technique.

8. 1st check: when you take it from the storage container and match it to the MAR

   2nd check: when you prepare it

   3rd check: just before you administer the medication to the patient when you are taking it out of the package, or just before you put it back on the shelf or drawer when you take it from a multidose vial in the medication room.

9. Cephalexin

10. The drug should be stored at controlled room temperature 20 to 25°C (68° to 77°F).

11. 500 mg/capsule

12. The usual adult dose is 250 mg every 6 hours, which is 2 capsules per day since each capsule is 500 mg. Twice the usual dose would be 4 capsules per day. The container would last 100 ÷ 4 or 25 days.

13. 60 mL

14. The total volume is 100 mL. The dosage strength is $\frac{250 \text{ mg}}{5 \text{ mL}}$. Dividing 100 mL total by 5 mL per dose equals 20 doses.

15. Write the order as it is received.

    Read the order back to the authorized prescriber.

    Confirm the order with the authorized prescriber.

16. Observe for untoward effects, and that the desired effect (fever reduction) has occurred. A follow-up temperature reading is indicated.

17. $\frac{50 \text{ mg}}{1 \text{ tab}} = \frac{75 \text{ mg}}{A}$

    $50 \times A = 1 \text{ tablet} \times 75$

    $A = 1\frac{1}{2} \text{ tablets}$

18. 200 mg : 5 mL = 200 mg : A

    $200 \times A = 5 \text{ mL} \times 200$

    $A = 5 \text{ mL}$

19. $\frac{300 \text{ mg}}{1 \text{ mL}} = \frac{600 \text{ mg}}{A}$

    $300 \times A = 1 \text{ mL} \times 600$

    $A = 2 \text{ mL}$

20. 200 mcg : 1 mL = 300 mcg : A

    $200 \times A = 1 \text{ mL} \times 300$

    $A = 1.5 \text{ mL}$

21. $97 \text{ lb} \times \frac{1 \text{ kg}}{2.2 \text{ lb}} = 44 \text{ kg}$

    $44 \text{ kg} \times \frac{17 \text{ mg}}{\text{kg}} = 748 \text{ mg}$

    $A \text{ mL} = \frac{1 \text{ mL}}{15 \text{ mg}} \times \frac{748 \text{ mg}}{1}$

    $A = 49.9 \text{ mL rounded to } 50 \text{ mL}$

22. $62 \text{ lb} \times \frac{1 \text{ kg}}{2.2 \text{ lb}} = 28.2 \text{ kg}$

    $28.2 \text{ kg} \times \frac{10 \text{ mg}}{\text{kg}} = 282 \text{ mg}$

    $A = \frac{282 \text{ mg}}{500 \text{ mg}} \times 100 \text{ mL}$

    $A = 56.4 \text{ mL} = 56 \text{ mL}$

23. 1.5 mL

24. $49 \text{ lb} \times \frac{1 \text{ kg}}{2.2 \text{ lb}} = 22.3 \text{ kg}$

    $22.3 \text{ kg} \times \frac{20 \text{ mg}}{\text{kg}} = 446 \text{ mg}$

    1 mL : 220 mg = A : 446 mg

    220 mg : 1 mL = 445 mg : A

    $220 \times A = 1 \text{ mL} \times 446$

    $A = 2 \text{ mL}$

25. $A = \frac{1 \text{ capsule}}{100 \text{ mg}} \times \frac{300 \text{ mg}}{1}$

    $A = 3 \text{ capsules}$

26. $55 \text{ lb} \times \frac{1 \text{ kg}}{2.2 \text{ lb}} = 25 \text{ kg}$

    $25 \text{ kg} \times \frac{10 \text{ mg}}{\text{kg}} = 250 \text{ mg}$

    $\frac{300 \text{ mg}}{5 \text{ mL}} = \frac{250 \text{ mg}}{A}$

$300 \times A = 5 \text{ mL} \times 250$

$A = 4.2 \text{ mL}$

27. $500 \text{ mg} : 1 \text{ tablet} = 1000 \text{ mg} : A$

$500 \times A = 1 \text{ tablet} \times 1000$

$A = 2 \text{ tablets}$

28. $\dfrac{1 \text{ mg}}{1000 \text{ mcg}} = \dfrac{0.1 \text{ mg}}{x}$

Desired dose $(x) = 100$ mcg or 1 tablet

29. • Name of medication, including generic and brand name

   • Purpose of the medication

   • Dose and use of calibrated equipment (ear dropper). The patient must be instructed to only use the ear dropper provided with the medication, since not all droppers are calibrated the same, and the patient might receive the wrong dose.

   • Route and self-administration guidelines, as needed

   • Medication schedule, related to food intake

   • Drug-drug interactions

   • Side effects and other reportable concerns.

   • Where to procure the medication

30. $\dfrac{10 \text{ mg}}{15 \text{ mg}} \times 1 \text{ mL} = 1.5 \text{ mL}$

31. $T = \dfrac{V}{F}$

   $T = 1000 \text{ mL} / 125 \text{ mL per h}$

   $T = 8 \text{ h}$

   $0730 + 8 \text{ h} = 1530$

32. GK. Novolin R is a shorter-acting insulin.

33. Draw the shorter-acting insulin (G) into the syringe first, then the intermediate-acting insulin (H).

34. $\dfrac{1000 \text{ mL}}{8 \text{ h}} = \dfrac{125 \text{ mL}}{1 \text{ h}}$

   Administer: 125 mL/h

35. $\dfrac{15 \text{ gtt}}{1 \text{ mL}} \times \dfrac{600 \text{ mL}}{4 \text{ h}} \times \dfrac{1 \text{ h}}{60 \text{ min}}$

   $\dfrac{\overset{1}{\cancel{15}} \text{ gtt}}{1 \text{ mL}} \times \dfrac{\overset{150}{\cancel{600}} \text{ mL}}{\underset{1}{\cancel{4}} \text{ h}} \times \dfrac{1 \cancel{\text{ h}}}{\underset{4}{\cancel{60}} \text{ min}}$

   $= 1 \text{ gtt} \times 150 \times \dfrac{1}{4} \text{ min}$

   $= \dfrac{150 \text{ gtt}}{4 \text{ min}} = 37.5 \text{ gtt/min}$

   Flow rate: 38 gtt/min

36. Increase the rate by 1 mcg/min:

   $A \text{ mL/h} = \dfrac{1 \text{ mg}}{1000 \text{ mcg}} \times \dfrac{1000 \text{ mL}}{4 \text{ mg}} \times \dfrac{1 \text{ mcg}}{1 \text{ min}} \times \dfrac{60 \text{ min}}{1 \text{ min}}$

   $A \text{ mL/h} = \dfrac{60,000 \text{ mL}}{4,000 \text{ h}} = 15 \text{ mL/h}$

   30 mL/h (existing rate) + 15 mL/h
   $= 45 \text{ mL/h}$ (new rate)

37. $68 \text{ lb} \times \dfrac{1 \text{ kg}}{2.2 \text{ lb}} = 31 \text{ kg}$

   $31 \text{ kg} \times \dfrac{0.1 \text{ mg}}{\text{kg}} = 3.1 \text{ mg}$

   $A \text{ mL/h} = \dfrac{50 \text{ mL}}{32 \text{ mg}} \times \dfrac{3.1 \text{ mg}}{4 \text{ min}} \times \dfrac{60 \text{ min}}{1 \text{ h}}$

   $A \text{ mL/h} = \dfrac{9300 \text{ mL}}{128 \text{ h}} = 73 \text{ mL/h}$

38. $A \text{ mL/h} = \dfrac{1 \text{ mg}}{1000 \text{ mcg}} \times \dfrac{500 \text{ mL}}{200 \text{ mg}} \times \dfrac{18 \text{ mcg}}{1 \text{ min}} \times \dfrac{60 \text{ min}}{1 \text{ h}}$

   $A \text{ mL/h} = \dfrac{540,000 \text{ mL/h}}{200,000} = 2.7 \text{ mL/h}$

39. You want to administer 750 mg Rocephin in 100 mL of NS over 30 minutes. According to the drug label you must add 9.6 mL of diluent; then each 1 mL contains 100 mg. Adding 7.5 mL to 100 mL of NS, you will have 107.5 mL to infuse over 30 minutes. Your flow rate will be 215 mL/h.

40. a. Convert the weight to kilograms, if needed.　96.4 kg (96.36)

   b. Determine the desired dose.　23 units/kg/h

   c. Calculate the amount to administer.　2217.2 units/h

   d. Calculate the flow rate.　44.3 mL/h

41. Label Q 0.75 mL

42. $\dfrac{40 \text{ mg}}{500 \text{ mL}} = \dfrac{x}{175 \text{ mL}}$

   $40 \text{ mg} \times 175 = 500 \times x$

   $14 = x$

   The patient has received 14 mg of nitroprusside.

43. $\dfrac{15 \text{ gtt}}{1 \text{ mL}} \times \dfrac{650 \text{ mL}}{8 \text{ h}} \times \dfrac{1 \text{ h}}{60 \text{ min}} = F$

   $\dfrac{\overset{1}{\cancel{15}} \text{ gtt}}{1 \text{ mL}} \times \dfrac{\overset{325}{\cancel{650}} \text{ mL}}{\cancel{8} \text{ h}} \times \dfrac{1 \cancel{\text{ h}}}{\underset{4}{\cancel{60}} \text{ min}} = \dfrac{20.31 \text{ gtt}}{\text{min}}$

   The original flow rate is 20 gtt/min.

   The amount of solution remaining is 490 mL. Recalculate the flow rate for 490 mL over 5 h.

   $\dfrac{15 \text{ gtt}}{\text{mL}} \times \dfrac{490 \text{ mL}}{5 \text{ h}} \times \dfrac{1 \text{ h}}{60 \text{ min}} = F$

   $\dfrac{\overset{1}{\cancel{15}} \text{ gtt}}{1 \text{ mL}} \times \dfrac{\overset{98}{\cancel{490}} \text{ mL}}{\underset{1}{\cancel{5}} \text{ h}} \times \dfrac{1 \cancel{\text{ h}}}{\underset{4}{\cancel{60}} \text{ min}} = \dfrac{24.5 \text{ gtt}}{\text{min}}$

The adjusted flow rate should be 25 gtt/min. Checking if it is within 25% of the original flow rate,

$$25\% \times 20 = 5$$

Because 25 gtt/min is 5 gtt/min more than the original flow rate, 25 gtt/min is within the acceptable range.

44. $V = T \times F$

$T = 2245 - 1130 = 11$ hr, 15 min or 11.25 h

$V = 11.25$ h $\times 80$ mL/h

$V = 900$ mL

45. $\dfrac{0.45 \text{ g}}{100 \text{ mL}} = \dfrac{x}{1000 \text{ mL}}$

$100\,x = 450$

$x = 4.5$ g sodium chloride (NaCl)

NaCl	4.5 g
Water	qsad 1000 mL

46. BSA $= \sqrt{\dfrac{150 \times 61}{3600}}$ m² $= \sqrt{\dfrac{9150}{3600}}$ m² $= 1.594$ m²

rounded to 1.6 m²

1.594 m² $\times \dfrac{200 \text{ mg}}{\text{m}^2} = 318.8$ mg

47. BSA $= \sqrt{\dfrac{60 \times 103}{3131}}$ m² $= \sqrt{\dfrac{6180}{3131}}$ m² $= 1.4$ m²

1.4 m² $\times \dfrac{200 \text{ mg}}{\text{m}^2} = 280$ mg

You want to administer 280 mg of leucovorin calcium. According to the label, the reconstituted leucovorin will have a dosage strength of 20 mg/mL.

$A = \dfrac{280 \text{ mg}}{20 \text{ mg}} \times 1$ mL

$A = 14$ mL

48. $1000 \text{ mL} + \left[\dfrac{50 \text{ mL}}{1 \text{ kg}} \times (18 - 10) \right]$

$= 1000 \text{ mL} + \left[\dfrac{50 \text{ mL}}{1 \text{ kg}} \times 8 \right]$

$= 1000 \text{ mL} + 400 \text{ mL} = 1400 \text{ mL}$

DMFN = 1400 mL; for microdrip tubing,

$\dfrac{1400 \text{ mL}}{1 \text{ day}} \times \dfrac{1 \text{ day}}{24 \text{ h}} = \dfrac{1400 \text{ mL}}{24 \text{ h}} = 58$ mL/h

$\dfrac{58 \text{ mL}}{60 \text{ min}} \times 60$ gtt/mL $= 58$ gtt/min

49. The patient's CL_{CR} is 48 mL/min. The recommended maintenance dosage is 2 g q4h. This amount is more than the order, which is safe to administer.

$1.7 \text{ g} \times \dfrac{1000 \text{ mg}}{1 \text{ g}} \times \dfrac{1 \text{ mL}}{20 \text{ g}} = 85$ mL

50. $1 : 1000 = \dfrac{1 \text{ g}}{1000 \text{ mL}}$ or $\dfrac{1000 \text{ mg}}{1000 \text{ mL}}$

$\dfrac{1000 \text{ mg}}{1000 \text{ mL}} = \dfrac{1 \text{ mg}}{\text{mL}}$

$\dfrac{0.1 \text{ mg}}{x \text{ mL}} = \dfrac{1 \text{ mg}}{1 \text{ mL}}$

$0.1 \text{ mL} = x$

Administer 0.1 mL subcut

24-hour time A system in which time is indicated with four digits; the first two digits indicate hours since midnight, and the last two digits indicate minutes.

A

Absorption Movement of a drug from the site where it is given into the bloodstream.

Absorption rate Movement of a drug from the site where it is given into the bloodstream.

Alligation One method for calculating dilutions.

Amount to administer The volume of liquid or number of solid dosage units that contains the desired dose.

Ampule Sealed container that usually holds 1 dose of liquid medication.

Antiarrhythmic medications Medications given to regulate a patient's heart rate and/or rhythm.

Anticoagulant A class of medication that reduces the blood's ability to clot.

Apothecary system An older system of measurement based upon a grain of wheat; other common units are the ounce, minim, and dram.

Authorized prescriber (AP) Licensed health care professional who has the authority to write medication orders, or prescriptions.

B

Bar code Code on a medication label that is used to identify the drug electronically; helps ensure that an individual receives the correct medication.

Biotransformation Chemical changes of a drug in the body; metabolism.

Body surface area (BSA) Surface area of a patient's body, factoring in both height and weight, stated in square meters, or m^2.

Bolus A volume administered rapidly via IV push to attain a therapeutic blood level of a drug.

C

Calibrated spoons Specially marked spoons used to administer oral medications with accuracy.

Calibrations Markings on medication equipment at various intervals.

Caplet Oval-shaped pill similar to a tablet but having a coating for easy swallowing.

Capsule Oval-shaped gelatin shell, usually in two pieces, that contains powder or granules.

Cartridge Prefilled container shaped like a syringe barrel, generally used with a reusable syringe.

Celsius A temperature scale on which water freezes at 0 degrees and boils at 100 degrees.

Centi (c) Metric prefix that indicates $\frac{1}{100}$ of the basic unit.

Centigrade A temperature scale similar to the Celsius scale. Values on this scale are within 0.1 degree of the values on the Celsius scale. For general purposes, the two scales are used interchangeably; however, Celsius is preferred.

Central line An IV line that administers large amounts of medications to major veins.

Complex fraction A fraction in which the numerator and the denominator are themselves fractions.

Conventional time A 12-hour system that uses a.m. and p.m. to indicate "before noon" or "after noon."

Conversion factor A fraction or ratio made of two quantities that are equal to each other but expressed in different units; for example, 7 days/1 week.

Critical care Area of a medical facility in which patients are more seriously ill and fast-acting, potent medications are given.

Cross-multiplying Multiplying the numerator of each fraction by the denominator of the other; for example, $\frac{A}{B} = \frac{C}{D}$ or $A \times D = B \times C$.

Cubic centimeter Measure of volume that is the same as a milliliter (mL).

D

D5W solution Intravenous solution of 5% dextrose in water.

Daily maintenance fluid needs (DMFN) Amount of fluids a patient needs over 24 h, including maintenance fluids (both oral and parenteral), medications, diluent for medications, and fluids used to flush the injection port.

Denominator The bottom number of a fraction; represents the whole.

Desired dose Amount of drug to be given at one time; the ordered dose.

Diluent A substance used to dilute; a liquid used to dissolve other chemicals when making a solution; also known as a solvent.

Dilution A solution created from an already prepared concentrated solution.

Dimensional analysis A method of dosage calculations that utilizes a series of conversion factors to calculate dosages.

Distribution Movement of a drug from the bloodstream into other body tissues and fluids.

Dividend In a division problem, the number you divide into.

Divisor The number you divide by in a division problem.

Dosage ordered The amount of drug to be given and how often it is to be given. The desired dose converted to the same unit of measurement as the dose on hand (supply dose).

Dosage strength Dose on hand per dosage unit; the amount of drug over the form of the drug; for example, 500 mg/tablet or 250 mg/5 mL; ratio strength.

Dosage unit The quantity of solid or liquid in which the dose is supplied.

Dose on hand Amount of drug contained in each dosage unit.

Dram Common unit of volume in the apothecary system; 1 dram = 60 minims

Drip chamber An area on the IV equipment where the drop of fluid is visualized during an infusion.

Dry weight Patient's weight when properly hydrated.

Duration The length of time the effect of a medication, such as insulin, lasts.

E

Eccentric Off-center.

Electronic medication administration record (eMAR) Medication administration record that can be viewed and completed on an electronic device.

Elimination Process in which the drug leaves the body.

Embolism A traveling blood clot.

Enema Means of delivering medication or fluids into the rectum.

Enteral Absorbed through the gastrointestinal tract.

Enteric-coated Medications that only dissolve in an alkaline environment, such as the small intestine.

Equivalent fractions Two fractions that have the same value even though they are written differently: $\frac{3}{6} = \frac{5}{10}$

F

Fahrenheit A temperature scale on which water freezes at 32 degrees and boils at 212 degrees.

Formula A method of dosage calculation that utilizes a set equation (formula) to calculate the amount to administer; $\frac{D}{H} \times Q = A$

Fraction proportion Mathematical statement that indicates two fractions are equal.

Frequency The time(s) of day and how often a medication is to be given.

G

Gelcap Medication, usually liquid, in a gelatin shell that is not designed to be opened.

Generic name A drug's official name.

Geriatric Describes patients who are age 65 and over.

Grain Basic unit for measurement of weight in the apothecary system.

Gram Basic unit for measurement of weight in the metric system.

H

Hemodynamics The study of the circulation of blood in the body.

Heparin An anticoagulant medication that reduces the blood's ability to clot.

Heparin lock An infusion port attached to an already inserted catheter for IV access; flushed with heparin.

Heparin protocol A preprinted order set that guides the administration of IV heparin based on the patient's weight and serum activated partial thromboplastin time (aPTT).

High-alert medication Medication that has a higher risk of devastating harm or death if the dosage is miscalculated.

Household Common system of measurement that utilizes the teaspoon, ounce, cup, pint, quart, and gallon.

Hypertonic Describes fluids that draw fluids from cells and tissues across the cell membrane into the bloodstream, such as 3% saline.

Hypodermic syringe Syringe used to administer injections.

Hypotonic Describes fluids that move across the cell membrane into surrounding cells and tissues, such as 0.45% NS and 0.33% NS.

I

Infiltration Delivery of fluid from an IV infusion outside of a blood vessel into the surrounding tissue.

Infusion pumps Devices that apply pressure to maintain the rate of an IV infusion, using a sensor to monitor both the rate and when the bag is empty.

Inhalant Medication that is inhaled; administered directly to the lungs, usually through a metered-dose inhaler or nebulizer.

Instillations Drops; used to deliver medications to the nose, eyes, and ears.

Institute for Safe Medication Practice (ISMP) A healthcare organization whose mission includes the promotion of patient safety; devoted to supporting the safe use of medications and preventing medication errors.

Insulin A pancreatic hormone that stimulates glucose metabolism.

International unit (IU) Amount of medication needed to produce a certain effect; standardized by an international agreement.

Intradermal (ID) Describes medication administered between layers of the skin.

Intramuscular (IM) Describes medication administered into a muscle by injection.

Intravenous (IV) Describes medication delivered directly to the bloodstream through a vein.

Isotonic Describes fluids that do not affect the fluid balance of the surrounding cells or tissues, such as D5W, NS, and lactated Ringer's.

J

Jejunostomy tube Tube that delivers medication and nutrients directly into the small intestine.

K

Kilo (k) Metric prefix that indicates the basic unit times 1000.

KVO or TKO fluids "Keep veins open" or "to keep open"; fluids that provide access to the vascular system for emergency situations.

L

Leading ring The wide ring on the tip of the plunger of a syringe that is closest to the needle; the medication is measured here.

Least common denominator The smallest number that is a common multiple of all the denominators in a group of fractions.

Liter (L) The basic unit for measurement of volume in the metric system.

Loading dose An initial bolus dose given to achieve a therapeutic blood level of a drug.

M

Macrodrip tubing Type of IV tubing that delivers 10, 15, or 20 drops of fluid per milliliter.

Maintenance fluids Fluids that help patients maintain fluid and electrolyte balance.

Means and extremes For the equation $A : B = C : D$, A and D are the extremes (ends) and B and C are the means (middle).

Medication Administration Record (MAR) A legal document that contains all the information on a medication order, specifies the actual times to administer the medication, and provides a place to document that each medication has been given.

Medication order form Written or computerized form for medication orders used in an inpatient facility; can list multiple medications.

Medicine cup A calibrated cup used to measure and deliver medications that usually holds 30 mL or 1 oz.

Meniscus A slight curve in the surface of a liquid.

Meter (m) Basic unit for measurement of length in the metric system.

Metered-dose inhaler (MDI) Device to deliver medication into the lungs.

Metric A widely used system of measurements based upon the meter for length, gram for weight, and liter for volume.

Micro (mc) Metric prefix that indicates $\frac{1}{1,000,000}$ of the basic unit.

Microdrip tubing Type of IV tubing that delivers 60 drops of fluid per milliliter.

Milli (m) Metric prefix that indicates $\frac{1}{1000}$ of the basic unit.

Milliequivalents (mEq) A unit of measure based upon the chemical combining power of the substance; defined as $\frac{1}{1000}$ of an equivalent of a chemical.

Minim ℳ Common unit of volume in the apothecary system.

Mixed number A fraction with a value greater than 1 that combines a whole number with a fraction.

N

Nasogastric Type of tube that carries medication through the nose to the stomach.

Nomogram A special chart used to determine a patient's body surface area (BSA).

Numerator The top number of a fraction; represents parts of the whole.

O

Onset Moment when a medication begins its effect, such as when insulin begins to lower the glucose (blood sugar) level.

Ounce Generally implies a fluid ounce volume when discussing medications; 1 fluid ounce = 8 drams.

P

Package insert Paper insert that provides complete and authoritative information about a medication.

Parenteral Route of administration other than oral; medications that are delivered outside of the digestive tract; most often refers to injections.

Patient-controlled analgesia (PCA) Technique that allows the patient to control the amount of pain medication delivered through an IV within limits set by the authorized prescriber.

Peak The time when a medication has its strongest effect, such as insulin's effect on the glucose level.

Pediatric Describes patients under the age of 18 years.

PEG tube Percutaneous endoscopic gastrostomy tube; delivers medication directly into the stomach.

Percent Per 100 or divided by 100.

Percent strength Represents the number of grams or milliliters of medication contained in 100 mL of a mixture.

Peripherally inserted central catheter (PICC) IV line that is inserted in an arm vein and threaded into a central vein, often by a specially trained nurse.

Pharmacokinetics The study of what happens to a drug after it is administered to a patient.

Phlebitis Inflammation of a vein, which can be caused by an irritated IV site.

Physician order form Written or computerized form for medication orders used in an inpatient facility; can list multiple medications.

***Physicians' Desk Reference* (PDR)** A compilation of information from package inserts of medications; contains information about most currently available prescription drugs.

Polypharmacy The practice of taking many medications at one time.

Port-A-Cath A device placed surgically under the skin in the chest in order to deliver drugs into a large, central vein.

Prefilled syringes Syringes that come from the manufacturer with the medication already inside; usually marked in milliliters (mL) and milligrams (mg).

Prescription Written or computerized form for medication orders.

Primary line The main tubing that delivers an IV infusion, usually consisting of a drip chamber, clamp, and injection port(s).

Prime number Number other than 1 that can be evenly divided by only itself and 1, such as 2, 3, 5, 7, 11, 13, 17, 19, 23, and 29.

Proportion A mathematical statement that two ratios are equal.

Q

Qsad   Abbreviation of a Latin phrase meaning "a sufficient quantity to adjust the dimensions to . . ."; used when preparing solutions.

Quotient   The answer to a division problem.

R

Rate controller   Device that controls the rate of an IV infusion by using a pincher and sensor; the infusion relies on gravity.

Ratio   Expression of the relationship of a part to the whole.

Ratio proportion   Mathematical statement that indicates two ratios are equal.

Ratio strength   The amount of drug in a solution or the amount of drug in a solid dosage such as a tablet or capsule; dosage strength.

Reconstitute   Add liquid to a powder medication; must be done shortly before administering.

Reconstitution   The process of adding liquid to a powder medication.

Rectal   Describes medication administered through the rectum, usually a suppository.

Replacement fluids   Fluids that replace electrolytes or fluids lost from dehydration, hemorrhage, vomiting, or diarrhea.

Roman numerals   A numeral system in which letters indicate numbers; I = 1, V = 5, and X = 10

Route   Path by which a drug is brought into the body.

S

Saline lock   An infusion port attached to an already inserted catheter for IV access; flushed with saline.

Scored   Describes medications having indented lines indicating where they may be broken to divide the medication evenly.

Secondary line   Line used to add medications or other additives to an existing IV or infusion port; also known as piggyback (IVPB).

Sig   Indicates the instructions for the container; found on a prescription.

Solute   Chemicals dissolved in a solvent, making a solution; drug or substance being dissolved in a solution.

Solution   A liquid mixture containing two or more different chemicals.

Solution strength   The amount of dry drug in grams per 100 mL of solution.

Solvent   Liquid used to dissolve other chemicals, making a solution; also called a diluent.

Spansule   Special capsule that contains granules with different coatings that delay the release of some of the medication.

Subcutaneous (subcut)   Describes medication administered under the skin by an injection.

Sustained release   Describes medication that is released slowly into the bloodstream over several hours.

Syringe   Device used to deliver parenteral medications that includes a barrel, plunger, hub, leading ring, and needle.

Syringe pumps   Pumps that provide precise control of IV infusions via a syringe inside of a pump.

T

Tablet   A solid disk or cylinder that contains a drug plus inactive ingredients.

The Joint Commission (TJC)   A healthcare organization whose mission includes the promotion of patient safety. TJC's goal is to continuously improve health care by setting standards and by evaluating and accrediting healthcare organizations.

Therapeutic fluids   IV fluids that deliver medication to patients.

Titrate   Adjust the dosage of medication in response to the patient's vital signs.

Titrated medications   Medications that are adjusted or regulated based upon their effect.

Topical medication   Medication applied to the skin.

Trade name   Name of a drug owned by a specific company; also called *brand name*.

Trailing ring   The ring on the plunger of the syringe farthest from the needle. Do *not* measure medication from this ring.

Transcription   The process of taking the information from the prescribing practitioner's order (prescription) and transferring it to the prescription label (in outpatient settings) or to the medication administration record (in inpatient settings).

Transdermal   Describes medication administered through the skin.

Tuberculin syringe   A small syringe used for delivering 1 mL of medication or less parenterally.

U

U-100   Common concentration of insulin in which 100 units of insulin are contained in 1 mL of solution.

U-500   Concentration of insulin in which 500 units of insulin are contained in 1 mL of solution.

Unit   Also known as USP unit; amount of a medication required to produce an effect.

United States Pharmacopeia   A medication guide or reference for health care professionals.

Universal solvent   Water.

V

Vaporizer   Device that uses boiling water to create a mist from liquid medications; also known as steam inhaler.

Vasoactive medications   Medications that cause the blood vessels to dilate or constrict.

Verbal order   A medication order from an authorized prescriber stated directly, in person or via the telephone, to a nurse or other practitioner whose scope of practice includes the authorization to receive and document such orders.

Vial   Container covered with a rubber stopper, or diaphragm, that holds one or more doses of medication in liquid or powder form.

W

Warnings   Statements found on the medication label that help the health care worker to deliver medications safely.

CREDITS

TEXT, LINE ART, AND DRUG LABELS

Chapter 9

Table 9-1, p. 164–165: © The Joint Commission, 2010. Reprinted with permission.

Chapter 10

Figure 10-1, p. 183 (Provera): Used with permission from Pfizer Inc.

Figure 10-2, p. 184 (EES): Courtesy of Abbott Laboratories and Knoll Labs.

Figure 10-3, p. 184 (Heparin): Hospira Inc., Lake Forest, IL. USA.

Figure 10-4, p. 184 (Amoxicillin): Courtesy of Teva Pharmaceuticals USA.

Figure 10-5, p. 186 (Ritalin): Copyright © Novartis Pharmaceutical Corp. used by permission.

Figure 10-6, p. 186 (Azithromycin): Courtesy of Teva Pharmaceuticals USA.

Figure 10-7, p. 187 (Rocephin): Reprinted with the permission of Roche Laboratories Inc. All rights reserved.

Figure 10-8, p. 188 (Nitrostat): Used with permission from Pfizer Inc.

Figure 10-9, p. 188 (Regranex): Reprinted with permission from Johnson & Johnson Pharmaceutical Research & Development.

Figure 10-10, p. 188 (Tigan): Courtesy of King Pharmaceuticals.

Figure 10-11, p. 189 (Amiodarone): Reprinted with permission of Abraxis BioScience, Inc.

Figure 10-12, p. 189 (Aerobid): Courtesy of Forest Laboratories, Inc.

Figure 10-13, p. 190 (Clozaril): Copyright © Novartis Pharmaceutical Corp. used by permission.

Figure 10-14, p. 190 (Kaletra): Courtesy of Abbott Laboratories and Knoll Labs.

Figure 10-15, p. 191 (Valium): Reprinted with the permission of Roche Laboratories Inc. All rights reserved.

Figure 10-16, p. 192 (Amoxicillin): Courtesy of Teva Pharmaceuticals USA.

Figure 10-17, p. 193 (Vantin): Used with permission from Pfizer Inc.

Figure 10-18, p. 194 (Aricept): Used with permission from Pfizer Inc.

Figure 10-19, p. 196 (Synthroid): Courtesy of Abbott Laboratories and Knoll Labs.

Figure 10-20, p. 196 (Synthroid): Courtesy of Abbott Laboratories and Knoll Labs.

Page 196 (Erythromycin): Courtesy of Abbott Laboratories and Knoll Labs.

Page 197 (Tranxene): Reprinted with permission from Lundbeck Inc. Traxene® is a registered trademark of Lundbeck Inc.

Page 197 (Methadone): Reprinted with permission from Bioniche Pharma USA.

Page 197 (Zithromax): Reprinted with permission of Abraxis BioScience, Inc.

Page 197 (Furosemide): Reprinted with permission of Abraxis BioScience, Inc.

Page 198 (Cefprozil): Courtesy of Teva Pharmaceuticals USA.

Page 198 (Metformin): Courtesy of Caraco Pharmaceutical Laboratories.

Figure 10-21, p. 200 (Depakote): Courtesy of Abbott Laboratories and Knoll Labs.

Figure 10-22, p. 200 (Kytril): Reprinted with the permission of Roche Laboratories Inc. All rights reserved.

Figure 10-23, p. 200 (Vistaril): Used with permission from Pfizer Inc.

Figure 10-24, p. 202: (NuvaRing) Reproduced with permission of N.V. Organon, subsidiary of Merck & Co., Inc. All rights reserved. NuvaRing is a registered trademark of N.V. Organon.

Figure 10-25, p. 202 (Camptosar): Used with permission from Pfizer Inc.

Figure 10-26, p. 202 (Humulin N): © Copyright Eli Lily and Company. All rights reserved. Used with permission. ® Evista, Gemzar, Humalog, Humatrope, Humulin, Prozac, Strattera, and Zyprexa are registered trademarks of Eli Lily and Company.

Figure 10-27, p. 202 (Humulin R): © Copyright Eli Lily and Company. All rights reserved. Used with permission. ® Evista, Gemzar, Humalog, Humatrope, Humulin, Prozac, Strattera, and Zyprexa are registered trademarks of Eli Lily and Company.

Figure 10-28, p. 203 (Sulfactamide): Courtesy of Alcon Research, Ltd.

Figure 10-29, p. 203 (Duragesic): Reprinted with permission from Johnson & Johnson Pharmaceutical Research & Development.

Figure 10-30, p. 204 (Regranex): Reprinted with permission from Johnson & Johnson Pharmaceutical Research & Development.

Page 204 (Metformin): Courtesy of Caraco Pharmaceutical Laboratories.

Page 205 (Levoxyl): Courtesy of King Pharmaceuticals.

Page 205 (Famotidine): Reprinted with permission of Abraxis BioScience, Inc.

Page 288 (Humulin R): © Copyright Eli Lily and Company. All rights reserved. Used with permission. ® Evista, Gemzar, Humalog, Humatrope, Humulin, Prozac, Strattera, and Zyprexa are registered trademarks of Eli Lily and Company.

Page 288 (Ritalin): Copyright © Novartis Pharmaceutical Corp. used by permission.

Page 288 (Targretin): Copyright 2010, Eisai Inc. All rights reserved. Used with permission.

Page 292 (Amoxicillin): Courtesy of Teva Pharmaceuticals USA.

Page 292 (Depakene): Courtesy of Abbott Laboratories and Knoll Labs.

Page 292 (Gleevec): Copyright © Novartis Pharmaceutical Corp. used by permission.

Page 293 (Procardia): Used with permission from Pfizer Inc.

Page 293 (Zemplar): Courtesy of Abbott Laboratories and Knoll Labs.

Page 293 (Zoloft): Used with permission from Pfizer Inc

Page 293 (Risperdal): Reprinted with permission from Johnson & Johnson Pharmaceutical Research & Development.

Page 293 (Cefprozil): Courtesy of Teva Pharmaceuticals USA.

Page 293 (Aranesp): Reprinted with permission from Amgen. Please note that the label(s) in this book may not be current and should not be used for any treatment decisions.

Page 295 (Cipro): "Copyright © 2009 Bayer Inc., 77 Belfield Road, Toronto, Ontario, CANADA, M9W1G6. Used under license from Bayer. All rights reserved".

Page 295 (Lexapro): Courtesy of Forest Laboratories, Inc.

Page 295 (Erythromycin): Courtesy of Abbott Laboratories and Knoll Labs.

Page 296 (Depakene): Courtesy of Abbott Laboratories and Knoll Labs.

Page 296 (Dilantin): Used with permission from Pfizer Inc.

Page 296 (Lisinopril): Courtesy of Teva Pharmaceuticals USA.

Page 297 (Biaxin): Courtesy of Abbott Laboratories and Knoll Labs.

Page 297 (Amoxicillin): Courtesy of Teva Pharmaceuticals USA.

Page 297 (Clarinex): The labels for CLARINEX, INTRON A, PegIntron, REBETOL, DIPROLENE, NASONEX, PROVENTIL, PREGNYL are reproduced with permission of Schering Corporation, subsidiary of Merck, Co., Inc. All rights reserved. CLARINEX, INTRON A, PegItron, REBETOL, DIPROLENE, NASONEX, PROVENTIL, PREGNYL are registered trademarks of Schering Corporation.

Page 298 (Cefprozil): Courtesy of Teva Pharmaceuticals USA.

Page 298 (Acyclovir): Reprinted with permission of Abraxis BioScience, Inc.

Page 298 (Kytril): Reprinted with the permission of Roche Laboratories Inc. All rights reserved.

Page 299 (Furosemide): Reprinted with permission of Abraxis BioScience, Inc.

Page 299 (Lipitor): Used with permission from Pfizer Inc.

Page 299 (Cipro): Copyright © 2009 Bayer Inc., 77 Belfield Road, Toronto, Ontario, CANADA, M9W1G6. Used under license from Bayer. All rights reserved.

Page 300 (Valium): Reprinted with the permission of Roche Laboratories Inc. All rights reserved.

Chapter 13

Figure 13-4, page 307 (Cipro): Copyright © 2009 Bayer Inc., 77 Belfield Road, Toronto, Ontario, CANADA, M9W1G6. Used under license from Bayer. All rights reserved

Page 316 (Clozaril): Copyright © Novartis Pharmaceutical Corp. used by permission.

Page 316 (Xanax): Used with permission from Pfizer Inc.

Page 316 (Valium): Reprinted with the permission of Roche Laboratories Inc. All rights reserved.

Page 316 (Famvir): Copyright © Novartis Pharmaceutical Corp. used by permission.

Page 317 (Aricept): Used with permission from Pfizer Inc.

Page 317 (Prandin): Courtesy of Novo Nordisk Pharmaceuticals, Inc.

Page 318 (Actos): "ACTOS® and RozeremTM are trademarks of Takeda Pharmaceutical Company Limited and are used under license by Takeda Pharmaceuticals North America, Inc. The ACTOS® and RozeremTM labels have been provided courtesy of Takeda Pharmaceuticals North America, Inc."

Page 318 (Lipitor): Used with permission from Pfizer Inc.

Page 318 (Zoloft): Used with permission from Pfizer Inc.

Page 318 (Gleevec): Copyright © Novartis Pharmaceutical Corp. used by permission.

Figure 13-9, page 320 (Kytril): Reprinted with the permission of Roche Laboratories Inc. All rights reserved.

Figure 13-10, page 322 (Erythromycin): Courtesy of Abbott Laboratories and Knoll Labs.

Figure 13-11, page 325 (Amoxicillin): Courtesy of Teva Pharmaceuticals USA.

Figure 13-12, page 328 (Amoxicillin): Courtesy of Teva Pharmaceuticals USA.

Figure 13-13, page 329 (Amoxicillin): Courtesy of Teva Pharmaceuticals USA.

Page 330 (Erythromycin): Courtesy of Abbott Laboratories and Knoll Labs.

Page 330 (Amoxicillin): Courtesy of Teva Pharmaceuticals USA.

Page 330 (Zithromax): Used with permission from Pfizer Inc.

Page 331 (Depakene): Courtesy of Abbott Laboratories and Knoll Labs.

Page 331 (Kytril): Reprinted with the permission of Roche Laboratories Inc. All rights reserved.

Page 331 (CellCept): Reprinted with the permission of Roche Laboratories Inc. All rights reserved.

Page 332 (Erythromycin): Courtesy of Abbott Laboratories and Knoll Labs.

Page 332 (Flumadine Syrup): Courtesy of Forest Laboratories, Inc.

Page 332 (Zithromax): Used with permission from Pfizer Inc.

Page 333 (Depakene): Courtesy of Abbott Laboratories and Knoll Labs.

Page 333 (Trileptal): Copyright © Novartis Pharmaceutical Corp. used by permission.

Page 337 (TopAmax): Reprinted with permission from Johnson & Johnson Pharmaceutical Research & Development.

Page 337 (OxyContin): © Purdue Pharma L.P., used with permission.

Page 338 (Strattera): © Copyright Eli Lily and Company. All rights reserved. Used with permission. ® Evista, Gemzar, Humalog, Humatrope, Humulin, Prozac, Strattera, and Zyprexa are registered trademarks of Eli Lily and Company.

Page 338 (Kytril): Reprinted with the permission of Roche Laboratories Inc. All rights reserved.

Page 338 (Cefprozil): Courtesy of Teva Pharmaceuticals USA.

Page 340 (Synthroid): Courtesy of Abbott Laboratories and Knoll Labs.

Page 340 (Metformin): Courtesy of Caraco Pharmaceutical Laboratories.

Page 340 (Cefprozil): Courtesy of Teva Pharmaceuticals USA.

Page 341 (Cephalexin): Courtesy of Teva Pharmaceuticals USA.

Page 341 (Celexa): Courtesy of Forest Laboratories, Inc.

Page 341 (Cipro): Copyright © 2009 Bayer Inc., 77 Belfield Road, Toronto, Ontario, CANADA, M9W1G6. Used under license from Bayer. All rights reserved.

Page 341 (Depakene): Courtesy of Abbott Laboratories and Knoll Labs.

Page 341 (Norvir): Courtesy of Abbott Laboratories and Knoll Labs.

Page 344 (Prandin): Courtesy of Novo Nordisk Pharmaceuticals, Inc.

Page 344 (Tranxene): Reprinted with permission from Lundbeck Inc. Traxene® is a registered trademark of Lundbeck Inc.

Page 344 (Erythromycin): Courtesy of Abbott Laboratories and Knoll Labs.

Page 344 (Valium): Reprinted with the permission of Roche Laboratories Inc. All rights reserved.

Page 344 (Tricor): Courtesy of Abbott Laboratories and Knoll Labs.

Page 345 (Depakote ER): Courtesy of Abbott Laboratories and Knoll Labs.

Page 345 (Valium): Reprinted with the permission of Roche Laboratories Inc. All rights reserved.

Page 345 (Vistaril): Used with permission from Pfizer Inc.

Page 345 (Cephalexin): Courtesy of Teva Pharmaceuticals USA.

Page 346 (Biaxin): Courtesy of Abbott Laboratories and Knoll Labs.

Chapter 14

Figure 14-5, page 352 (Valium): Reprinted with the permission of Roche Laboratories Inc. All rights reserved.

Figure 14-6, page 352 (Lorazepam): Courtesy of Bedford Laboratories

Page 357 (Thiamine hydrochloride): Reprinted with permission of Abraxis BioScience, Inc.

Page 358 (Heparin): Hospira Inc., Lake Forest, IL. USA.

Page 358 (Tigan): Courtesy of King Pharmaceuticals.

Page 358 (Sandostatin): Copyright © Novartis Pharmaceutical Corp. used by permission.

Page 359 (Neupogen): Reprinted with permission from Amgen. Please note that the label(s) in this book may not be current and should not be used for any treatment decisions.

Page 359 (Epogen): Reprinted with permission from Amgen. Please note that the label(s) in this book may not be current and should not be used for any treatment decisions.

Page 360 (Neulasta): Reprinted with permission from Amgen. Please note that the label(s) in this book may not be current and should not be used for any treatment decisions.

Page 360 (Zemplar): Courtesy of Abbott Laboratories and Knoll Labs.

Page 360 (Oxytocin): Reprinted with permission of Abraxis BioScience, Inc.

Page 361 (Clindamycin): Courtesy of Bedford Laboratories

Page 361 (Synagis): Courtesy of Medimmune, Inc.

Page 361 (Oxytocin): Reprinted with permission of Abraxis BioScience, Inc.

Page 362 (Furosemide): Reprinted with permission of Abraxis BioScience, Inc.

Page 362 (Aranesp): Reprinted with permission from Amgen. Please note that the label(s) in this book may not be current and should not be used for any treatment decisions.

Page 363 (Valium): Reprinted with the permission of Roche Laboratories Inc. All rights reserved.

Figure 14-7, page 376 (Glucagon for injection and diluting solution): © Copyright Eli Lily and Company. All rights reserved. Used with permission. ® Evista, Gemzar, Humalog, Humatrope, Humulin, Prozac, Strattera, and Zyprexa are registered trademarks of Eli Lily and Company.

Figure 14-8, page 376 (Zyprexa): © Copyright Eli Lily and Company. All rights reserved. Used with permission. ® Evista, Gemzar, Humalog, Humatrope, Humulin, Prozac, Strattera, and Zyprexa are registered trademarks of Eli Lily and Company.

Figure 14-9, page 377 (Package insert for Zyprexa): © Copyright Eli Lily and Company. All rights reserved. Used with permission. ® Evista, Gemzar, Humalog, Humatrope, Humulin, Prozac, Strattera, and Zyprexa are registered trademarks of Eli Lily and Company.

Figure 14-10, page 377 (Methylprednisolone—sodium succinate for injection): Courtesy of Bedford Laboratories.

Figure 14-11, page 378 (Package insert for Methylprednisolone): Courtesy of Bedford Laboratories.

Figure 14-12, page 381 (Humatrope): © Copyright Eli Lily and Company. All rights reserved. Used with permission. ® Evista, Gemzar, Humalog, Humatrope, Humulin, Prozac,

Strattera, and Zyprexa are registered trademarks of Eli Lily and Company.

Figure 14-13, page 381 (Sterile diluent for humatrope): © Copyright Eli Lily and Company. All rights reserved. Used with permission. ® Evista, Gemzar, Humalog, Humatrope, Humulin, Prozac, Strattera, and Zyprexa are registered trademarks of Eli Lily and Company.

Page 382 (Leucovorin calcium): Courtesy of Bedford Laboratories

Page 382 (Synagis): Courtesy of Medimmune, Inc.

Page 383 (Gemzar): © Copyright Eli Lily and Company. All rights reserved. Used with permission. ® Evista, Gemzar, Humalog, Humatrope, Humulin, Prozac, Strattera, and Zyprexa are registered trademarks of Eli Lily and Company.

Page 384 (Pfizerpen label and package insert): Used with permission from Pfizer Inc.

Page 385 (Rocephin): Reprinted with the permission of Roche Laboratories Inc. All rights reserved.

Page 395 (Thiamine hydrochloride): Reprinted with permission of Abraxis BioScience, Inc.

Page 396 (Heparin): Hospira Inc., Lake Forest, IL. USA.

Page 396 (Clindamycin): Courtesy of Bedford Laboratories

Page 396 (Rocephin): Reprinted with the permission of Roche Laboratories Inc. All rights reserved.

Page 399 (Thiamine hydrochloride): Reprinted with permission of Abraxis BioScience, Inc.

Page 400 (Heparin): Hospira Inc., Lake Forest, IL. USA.

Page 400 (Furosemide): Reprinted with permission of Abraxis BioScience, Inc.

Page 401 (Oxytocin): Reprinted with permission of Abraxis BioScience, Inc.

Page 401 (Epogen): Reprinted with permission from Amgen. Please note that the label(s) in this book may not be current and should not be used for any treatment decisions.

Page 401 (Clindamycin): Courtesy of Bedford Laboratories

Page 402 (Sandostatin): Copyright © Novartis Pharmaceutical Corp. Used by permission.

Page 402 (Furosemide): Reprinted with permission of Abraxis BioScience, Inc.

Page 403 (Zyprexa label and package insert): © Copyright Eli Lily and Company. All rights reserved. Used with permission. ® Evista, Gemzar, Humalog, Humatrope, Humulin, Prozac, Strattera, and Zyprexa are registered trademarks of Eli Lily and Company.

Page 404 (Pegintron label and package insert): The labels for CLARINEX, INTRON A, PegIntron, REBETOL, DIPROLENE, NASONEX, PROVENTIL, PREGNYL are reproduced with permission of Schering Corporation, subsidiary of Merck, Co., Inc. All rights reserved. CLARINEX, INTRON A, PegItron, REBETOL, DIPROLENE, NASONEX, PROVENTIL, PREGNYL are registered trademarks of Schering Corporation.

Page 405 (Sandostatin): Copyright © Novartis Pharmaceutical Corp. Used by permission.

Chapter 15

Figure 151, p. 409 (Lactated Ringer's): Baxter and Viaflex are registered trademarks of Baxter International Inc.

Figure 15-2, p. 410 (5% dextrose injection): Baxter and Viaflex are registered trademarks of Baxter International Inc.

Figure 15-3, p. 410 (0.9% sodium chloride injection): Baxter and Viaflex are registered trademarks of Baxter International Inc.

Figure 15-4, p. 411 (5% dextrose and 0.45% sodium chloride): Baxter and Viaflex are registered trademarks of Baxter International Inc.

Figure 15-20, p. 437 (5% dextrose injection): Baxter and Viaflex are registered trademarks of Baxter International Inc.

Figure 15-24a, p. 442 (Heparin): Hospira Inc., Lake Forest, IL. USA.

Figure 15-24b, p. 442 (0.9% sodium chloride injection): Baxter and Viaflex are registered trademarks of Baxter International Inc.

Figure 15-25d, p. 443 (Gemzar): © Copyright Eli Lily and Company. All rights reserved. Used with permission. ® Evista, Gemzar, Humalog, Humatrope, Humulin, Prozac, Strattera, and Zyprexa are registered trademarks of Eli Lily and Company.

Figure 15-25e, p. 443: (Gemzar package insert): © Copyright Eli Lily and Company. All rights reserved. Used with permission. ® Evista, Gemzar, Humalog, Humatrope, Humulin, Prozac, Strattera, and Zyprexa are registered trademarks of Eli Lily and Company.

Figure 15-26, p. 444 (Doxycycline): Courtesy of Bedford Laboratories.

Figure 15-26, p. 444 (Doxycycline package insert): Courtesy of Bedford Laboratories.

Figure 15-27, p. 450 (Clindamycin label and package insert): Reprinted with permission of Abraxis BioScience, Inc.

Chapter 17

Figure 17-4a & b, page 484 (Midazolam label and package insert): Courtesy of Bedford Laboratories

Figure 17-5, page 487 (Erythromycin): Courtesy of Abbott Laboratories and Knoll Labs.

Figure 17-6, page 488 (Amoxil): Copyright GlaxoSmithKline. Used with permission.

Page 491 (Amoxicillin): Courtesy of Teva Pharmaceuticals USA.

Page 491 (Ranitodine): Courtesy of Bedford Laboratories.

Page 492 (Cephalexin): Courtesy of Teva Pharmaceuticals USA.

Page 493 (Midazolam): Courtesy of Bedford Laboratories

Page 493 (Erythromycin): Courtesy of Abbott Laboratories and Knoll Labs.

Page 502 (Gemzar): © Copyright Eli Lily and Company. All rights reserved. Used with permission. ® Evista, Gemzar, Humalog, Humatrope, Humulin, Prozac, Strattera, and Zyprexa are registered trademarks of Eli Lily and Company.

Page 503 (CISplatin): This is on log as being granted from APP, but label has that it's owned by Bedford. If it is, then we don't have permission.

Page 509 (Depakene): Courtesy of Abbott Laboratories and Knoll Labs.

Page 510 (Kytril): Reprinted with the permission of Roche Laboratories Inc. All rights reserved.

Page 510 (Clindamycin): Reprinted with permission of Abraxis BioScience, Inc.

Page 510 (Gammagard): Images courtesy of Baxter Healthcare Corporation. All rights reserved.

Page 511 (Camptosar): Used with permission from Pfizer Inc.

Page 512 (Biaxin): Courtesy of Abbott Laboratories and Knoll Labs.

Page 513 (Trileptal): Copyright © Novartis Pharmaceutical Corp. used by permission.

Page 513 (Erythromycin): Courtesy of Abbott Laboratories and Knoll Labs.

Page 514 (Neupogen): Reprinted with permission from Amgen. Please note that the label(s) in this book may not be current and should not be used for any treatment decisions.

Page 515 (Zosyn): Courtesy of Abbott.

Page 517 (Rocephin): Reprinted with the permission of Roche Laboratories Inc. All rights reserved.

Chapter 18

Figure 18-1, page 520: (Humulin R): © Copyright Eli Lily and Company. All rights reserved. Used with permission. ® Evista, Gemzar, Humalog, Humatrope, Humulin, Prozac, Strattera, and Zyprexa are registered trademarks of Eli Lily and Company.

Figure 18-2, page 521: (Intermediate acting Humulin N): © Copyright Eli Lily and Company. All rights reserved. Used with permission. ® Evista, Gemzar, Humalog, Humatrope, Humulin, Prozac, Strattera, and Zyprexa are registered trademarks of Eli Lily and Company.

Figure 18-7, page 523: (Regular Humulin R): © Copyright Eli Lily and Company. All rights reserved. Used with permission. ® Evista, Gemzar, Humalog, Humatrope, Humulin, Prozac, Strattera, and Zyprexa are registered trademarks of Eli Lily and Company.

Figure 18-10, page 525: (Humalog): © Copyright Eli Lily and Company. All rights reserved. Used with permission. ® Evista, Gemzar, Humalog, Humatrope, Humulin, Prozac, Strattera, and Zyprexa are registered trademarks of Eli Lily and Company.

Figure 18-11, page 525: (Novolin): "Courtesy of Novo Nordisk Pharmaceuticals, Inc."

Figure 18-12, page 525: (Humalog Mix): © Copyright Eli Lily and Company. All rights reserved. Used with permission. ® Evista, Gemzar, Humalog, Humatrope, Humulin, Prozac, Strattera, and Zyprexa are registered trademarks of Eli Lily and Company.

Page 527: (Humalog): © Copyright Eli Lily and Company. All rights reserved. Used with permission. ® Evista, Gemzar, Humalog, Humatrope, Humulin, Prozac, Strattera, and Zyprexa are registered trademarks of Eli Lily and Company.

Page 528: (Humulin): © Copyright Eli Lily and Company. All rights reserved. Used with permission. ® Evista, Gemzar, Humalog, Humatrope, Humulin, Prozac, Strattera, and Zyprexa are registered trademarks of Eli Lily and Company.

Page 528: (Novolin N): "Courtesy of Novo Nordisk Pharmaceuticals, Inc."

Page 528: (Novolin R): "Courtesy of Novo Nordisk Pharmaceuticals, Inc."

Page 528: (Humalog Mix): © Copyright Eli Lily and Company. All rights reserved. Used with permission. ® Evista, Gemzar, Humalog, Humatrope, Humulin, Prozac, Strattera, and Zyprexa are registered trademarks of Eli Lily and Company.

Page 529: (Novolin): "Courtesy of Novo Nordisk Pharmaceuticals, Inc."

Page 529: (Humulin R): © Copyright Eli Lily and Company. All rights reserved. Used with permission. ® Evista, Gemzar, Humalog, Humatrope, Humulin, Prozac, Strattera, and Zyprexa are registered trademarks of Eli Lily and Company.

Figure 18-15, page 533: (Heparin): Hospira Inc., Lake Forest, IL. USA

Figure 18-16, page 533: (Heparin): Hospira Inc., Lake Forest, IL. USA

Figure 18-17, page 533: (Heparin): Hospira Inc., Lake Forest, IL. USA

Figure 18-18, page 533: (Heparin): Hospira Inc., Lake Forest, IL. USA

Figure 18-19, page 533: (Heparin): Hospira Inc., Lake Forest, IL. USA

Figure 18-20, page 533: (Heparin): Hospira Inc., Lake Forest, IL. USA.

Label A, page 551: (Humalog): © Copyright Eli Lily and Company. All rights reserved. Used with permission. ® Evista, Gemzar, Humalog, Humatrope, Humulin, Prozac, Strattera, and Zyprexa are registered trademarks of Eli Lily and Company.

Label B, page 551: (Humulin R): © Copyright Eli Lily and Company. All rights reserved. Used with permission. ® Evista, Gemzar, Humalog, Humatrope, Humulin, Prozac, Strattera, and Zyprexa are registered trademarks of Eli Lily and Company.

Label C, page 551: (Humulin N): © Copyright Eli Lily and Company. All rights reserved. Used with permission. ® Evista, Gemzar, Humalog, Humatrope, Humulin, Prozac, Strattera, and Zyprexa are registered trademarks of Eli Lily and Company.

Label D, page 552: (Humalog Mix): © Copyright Eli Lily and Company. All rights reserved. Used with permission. ® Evista, Gemzar, Humalog, Humatrope, Humulin, Prozac, Strattera, and Zyprexa are registered trademarks of Eli Lily and Company.

Label E, page 553: (Heparin): Hospira Inc., Lake Forest, IL. USA.

Label F, page 554: (Heparin): Hospira Inc., Lake Forest, IL. USA.

Page 555: (Novolin N):): "Courtesy of Novo Nordisk Pharmaceuticals, Inc."

Page 555: (Humalog): © Copyright Eli Lily and Company. All rights reserved. Used with permission. ® Evista, Gemzar, Humalog, Humatrope, Humulin, Prozac, Strattera, and Zyprexa are registered trademarks of Eli Lily and Company.

Page 555: (Novolin R): "Courtesy of Novo Nordisk Pharmaceuticals, Inc."

Page 556: (Humalog Mix): © Copyright Eli Lily and Company. All rights reserved. Used with permission. ® Evista, Gemzar, Humalog, Humatrope, Humulin, Prozac, Strattera, and Zyprexa are registered trademarks of Eli Lily and Company.

Page 556: (Novolin): "Courtesy of Novo Nordisk Pharmaceuticals, Inc."

Page 556: (Humulin R): © Copyright Eli Lily and Company. All rights reserved. Used with permission. ® Evista, Gemzar, Humatrope, Humulin, Prozac, Strattera, and Zyprexa are registered trademarks of Eli Lily and Company.

Chapter 19

Label A, page 580: (Heparin): Hospira Inc., Lake Forest, IL. USA

Label B, page 580: (Heparin): Hospira Inc., Lake Forest, IL. USA

Label C, page 580: (Heparin) Hospira Inc., Lake Forest, IL. USA.

Label D, page 580: (Heparin): Hospira Inc., Lake Forest, IL. USA.

Label E, page 580: (Heparin Lock Flush): Reprinted with permission of Abraxis BioScience, Inc.

Label F, page 582: (Humulin R): © Copyright Eli Lily and Company. All rights reserved. Used with permission. ® Evista, Gemzar, Humalog, Humatrope, Humulin, Prozac, Strattera, and Zyprexa are registered trademarks of Eli Lily and Company.

Label G, page 582: (Humulin N): © Copyright Eli Lily and Company. All rights reserved. Used with permission. ® Evista, Gemzar, Humalog, Humatrope, Humulin, Prozac, Strattera, and Zyprexa are registered trademarks of Eli Lily and Company.

Label H, page 582: (Humalog): © Copyright Eli Lily and Company. All rights reserved. Used with permission. ® Evista, Gemzar, Humalog, Humatrope, Humulin, Prozac, Strattera, and Zyprexa are registered trademarks of Eli Lily and Company.

Label I, page 582: (Humalog Mix): © Copyright Eli Lily and Company. All rights reserved. Used with permission. ® Evista, Gemzar, Humalog, Humatrope, Humulin, Prozac, Strattera, and Zyprexa are registered trademarks of Eli Lily and Company.

PHOTOS

Frontmatter

Design Elements(all): © Getty RF.

Chapter **1**
Opener: © Group 3660/Getty Images.

Chapter **2**
Opener: © PhotoDisc/Getty RF.

Chapter **3**
Opener: © Blend Images/Getty RF.

Chapter **4**
Opener: © Jonnie Miles/Getty Images.

Chapter **5**
Opener: © PhotoDisc/Getty RF.

Chapter **6**
Opener: © Digital Vision/Getty RF.

Chapter **7**
Opener: © Stockbyte/Getty RF.

Chapter **8**
Opener: © Vol. 168/Getty RF; 8 4: © Total Care Programming, Inc.; 8.5: Courtesy of Apothecary Products, Inc.; 8.8, 8.9: © Total Care Programming, Inc.; 8.10: Photo provided by the Smiths Medical, ASD, Inc.; 8.11, 8.12, 8.14, 8.15, 8.17: © Total Care Programming, Inc.; 8.18: Courtesy and copyright Becton, Dickinson and Company; 8.19: © Total Care Programming, Inc.

Chapter **9**
Opener: © Custom Medical Stock Photos.

Chapter **10**
Opener: © Stockbyte RF/Getty RF.

Chapter **11**
Opener: © Getty RF.

Chapter **12**
Opener: © Comstock/Getty RF.

Chapter **13**
Opener: © Joos Mind/Getty Images ; 13.1, 13.2, 13.6 (both), 13.7, 13.8: © Total Care Programming, Inc.

Chapter 14

Opener: © image 100/Punchstock RF; 14.14: © Corbis RF; 14.15, 14.16: Photo by Susan Sienkiewicz and Jennifer F. Palmenen; 14.17: © Total Care Programming, Inc.

Chapter 15

Opener: © Blend Images/Getty RF; 15.5: © Corbis RF; 15.6-15.12, 15.15, 15.21: © Total Care Programming, Inc.

Chapter 16

Opener: Getty RF; 16.1: Photo by Susan Sienkiewicz and Jennifer F. Palmenen.

Chapter 17

Opener: © Jose Luis Pelaez/Getty Images; 17.1: © The McGraw-Hill Companies, Inc./Jill Braaten, photographer; 17.2: © Creatis/Punchstock RF; 17.3: © Total Care Programming, Inc.

Chapter 18

Opener: © Joos Mind/Getty Images; 18.14: Reprinted with permission of Abraxis BioScience, Inc.

Chapter 19

Opener: © Getty RF; 19.1: Photo by Susan Sienkiewicz and Jennifer F. Palmenen.

INDEX

Note: 'f' indicates a figure; 't' indicates a table.

0.5-mL tuberculin syringe, 523f
1-mL tuberculin syringe, 144f, 145f, 153
3-mL syringe, 144, 153
24-hour time (24 h), 123
    conversion, 126
    medication administration, 167
30-unit insulin syringe, 522f
50-unit insulin syringe, 522f
100-unit insulin syringe, 141f, 521

A

Abbreviations, 218
    error prone, 140, 165, 228, 229t–232t
    general medical, 164t, 175
    household measures, 102t
    IV solutions, 409t
    medication administration frequency, 165t, 175
    medication administration route, 165t, 175
    medication form, 164t, 175
ABC's of dosage calculation, 261f, 262t, 271–273
    dimensional analysis checklist, 277–280
    formula method checklist, 280–283
    heparin, 535
    proportion procedure checklist, 273–277
    solid oral medications, 305
Absorption, 474, 474t, 505
Absorption rates, 348
Actos (pioglitazone HCl), 318f
Acyclovir, 298f
Addition
    decimals, 45–47, 52
    fractions, 18–21
ADME (absorption, distribution, biotransformation, elimination), 473
Administration needle, 147
a.m. (*ante meridian*), 123
Amount to administer (A)
    dimensional analysis checklist, 277–280
    dosage calculation, 261f, 262t, 271–273
    formula method checklist, 280–283
    heparin, 535, 538, 539
    proportion procedure checklist, 273–277
    solid oral medications, 305
Amicar (aminocaproic acid syrup), 284f
Amoxicillin, 285f, 296f, 292f, 325f, 328f, 329f, 330f
    oral suspension, 75, 491
Amoxil (amoxicillin), oral suspension, 488f
Ampules, 146, 146f, 154
Analgesics, pain, 561

Antiarrhythmic medications, 561
Anticoagulant medication, heparin, 532
Apothecary system of measurement
    converting grains to milligrams, 101f
    description, 99
    equivalent measurements, 103t
    notation, 100, 105
    practice, 101
    units, 99t
Aranesp (darbepoetin alfa), 293f, 362f
Aricept (donepezil HCl), 317f
Atomizers, 387
Authorized prescribers (APs), 164, 167, 171, 281

B

Bar code, medication label, 183f, 184f, 191
Basal insulin, 502t, 526f, 548
Biaxin (clarithromycin), 269f, 270f, 29tf
    oral suspension, 512f
Biotransformation, 474, 474t, 505
Body surface area (BSA), 475, 496, 507
    dosage based on, 496–501
    practice, 501–502
Body weight
    flow rate calculations, 567–571, 576
    dosage based on, 480–490, 506
    dosing practice, 490–493
    potent medication IV infusions, 567–569
Bolus dosage
    calculations, 542–544
    heparin, 533–534, 549
Brand name, 183
Buccal medication, 203

C

Calibrated spoons, 134, 136f, 153
Calibrations, 133
    insulin syringes, 142–143
    medicine cups, 133f
    standard syringes, 140
    tuberculin syringes, 144, 145f
Camptosar (irinotecan HCl), injection, 511f
Caplets, 303, 333
Capsules, 199, 303, 333
    opening, 312
Caregiver, medication information for, 473t
Carpujet, 146
Cartridges, 146, 146f
Ceclor® oral suspension, 83
Cefprozil oral suspension, 293f, 298f
CellCept (mycophenolate mofetil), 331f
Celsius (C) temperature scale, 121–122, 126
Centi- (c), 88t
Central lines, 418, 418f, 445
Cephalexin, oral suspension, 492f

Chewable tablets, 199
Cipro (ciprofloxacin HCl), 295f, 299f, 397f
CISplatin, injection, 502f
Clarinex (desloratadine), 297f
Clindamycin, injection, 361f, 396f, 401f, 450f, 510f
Clozaril (clozapine), 316f
Combination drugs, 184f, 185–186
Combination insulin, 524–525
    error alert, 527
Common denominators, 13–15, 16
Common fractions, 3–4
Comparison
    decimals, 38, 39–40, 51
    fractions, 16–18, 32
Complex fraction, 29
Conventional time (12h), 123
    conversion, 126
Conversion
    decimal to percent, 58–59
    decimal to ratio, 64–65
    dosage ordered (O) to dose on hand (H), 262, 305
    fraction to mixed number, 5
    fraction to percent, 60–61
    grain to milligram, 101f
    hourly to minute potent medications, 569–570
    least common denominator (LCD), 15, 31
    like units of measurement, 262–271
    within metric system, 91–94
    milliequivalents conversions, 105
    percent to decimal, 57–58
    percent to equivalent fraction, 59–60
    ratio from percent, 66–67
    ratio to decimal, 63–64
    ratio to percent, 65–66
    roman numerals to arabic numbers, 166t
Conversion factors
    definition, 109
    dimensional analysis (DA), 113–115
    equivalent measures, 109–110, 261
    proportions, 110–112
Conversion formulas, temperature, 121, 126
CR, controlled release drug, 199
Creatinine clearance (CLCR), 477, 506
Critical care medication administration, 561–566
    time infusion practice, 566–567
Critical thinking applications
    apothecary measures, 107
    conversion factors, 119
    decimals, 54
    dosage calculation, 299
    fractions, 34
    gastrostomy tube medications, 345